To audiology department

El-Khouly

Clinical
Otolaryngology

Clinical Otolaryngology

EDITED BY

A.G.D. MARAN

MD, FRCSE, FACS

Honorary Senior Lecturer, Department of Otolaryngology
University of Edinburgh
Consultant Otolaryngologist
Royal Infirmary, Edinburgh

AND

P.M. STELL

ChM, FRCS

Professor of Otorhinolaryngology
University of Liverpool
Consultant Otolaryngologist
Royal Liverpool Hospital

BLACKWELL
SCIENTIFIC PUBLICATIONS
OXFORD LONDON EDINBURGH
MELBOURNE

© 1979 Blackwell Scientific Publications
Osney Mead, Oxford, OX2 0EL
Editorial offices:
8 John Street, London, WC1N 2ES
9 Forrest Road, Edinburgh, EH1 2QH
214 Berkeley Street, Carlton
Victoria 3053, Australia

First published 1979

British Library Cataloguing in Publication Data
Clinical otolaryngology.
  1. Otolaryngology
  I. Maran, Arnold George D
  II. Stell, Philip Michael
  616.2'1   RF46

  ISBN 0-632-00479-7

Distributed in USA by
Blackwell Mosby Book Distributors
11830 Westline Industrial Drive
St. Louis, Missouri 63141,
in Canada by
Blackwell Mosby Book Distributors
86 Northline Road, Toronto
Ontario M4B 3E5,
and in Australia by
Blackwell Scientific Book Distributors
214 Berkeley Street, Carlton
Victoria 3053

Printed in Great Britain at the Alden Press, Oxford

Contents

PAEDIATRIC OTOLARYNGOLOGY

Contributors

J. ATKINS, MB, ChB, FRCS, FRCSE, *Consultant Otolaryngologist, Eye, Ear & Throat Hospital, Shrewsbury.*

G.D. BEAUMONT, MB, MS, FRCS, FRACS, *Senior Lecturer in Otolaryngology, Flinders University of South Australia, and Chief of Otolaryngology, Flinders Medical Centre, South Australia.*

L. BERNSTEIN, MD, DDS, *Professor and Chairman of Department of Otolaryngology, University of Southern California, Sacramento, USA.*

J.F. BIRRELL, MD, FRCSE, *Formerly Consultant Otolaryngologist, Royal Hospital for Sick Children, Edinburgh.*

D.P. BRYCE, MD, *Otolaryngologist-in-Chief, Toronto General Hospital, Toronto, Canada.*

Y. CACHIN, MD, *Head of the Department of Head and Neck Surgery, Institute Gustave-Roussy, Villejuif, France.*

A.D. CHEESMAN, BSC, MB, BS, FRCS, *Senior Lecturer, Institute of Laryngology and Otology, University of London, Consultant Otolaryngologist, Royal National Throat, Nose and Ear Hospital, London, and Consultant Otolaryngologist and Head and Neck Surgeon, Charing Cross Hospital, London.*

P.P.P. CLIFFORD, MD, MCh, FRCS, *Consultant Head and Neck Surgeon, Royal Marsden Hospital, London, and Consultant Otolaryngologist, King's College Hospital, London.*

The late Rt. Hon. LORD COHEN OF BIRKENHEAD, CH, MD, FRCP, *Formerly Professor of Medicine, University of Liverpool.*

B.H. COLMAN, VRD, BSC, MA, ChM, FRCS, *Clinical Lecturer in Otolaryngology, University of Oxford, and Consultant Otolaryngologist, United Oxford Hospitals.*

P.J. DONALD, MD, FRCSC, *Associate Professor of Otolaryngology, University of Southern California, Sacramento, USA.*

L. FISCH, MD, DLO, *Consultant Audiologist, Hospital for Sick Children, and Consultant Otologist, Royal National Throat and Ear Hospital, London.*

U. FISCH, MD, *Professor of Otolaryngology, University Hospital of Zürich, Zürich, Switzerland.*

A.G. GIBB, MB, ChB, FRCS, *Head of Department of Otolaryngology, University of Dundee, and Consultant Otolaryngologist, Ninewells Hospital, Dundee.*

O. GILAD, MD, *Ear Research Institute, Los Angeles, USA.*

L.P. GRAY, MB, BS, DLO, FRACS, *Consultant Otolaryngologist, Princess Margaret Hospital for Children, Perth, Western Australia.*

R.E. GRISTWOOD, MB, ChB, FRCSE, FRACS, *Clinical Lecturer in Otolaryngology, University of Adelaide and Senior Visiting Otolaryngologist, Royal Adelaide Hospital, Australia.*

L. A. HARKER, MD, *Associate Professor of Otolaryngology and Maxillofacial Surgery, University of Iowa, Iowa City, USA.*

D.F.N. HARRISON, MD, MS, FRCS, *Professor of Laryngology and Otology, Institute of Laryngology and Otology and Consultant Surgeon, Royal National Throat, Nose and Ear Hospital, London.*

J.E. HAWKINS, Jr., MA, PhD, *Professor of Otolaryngology (Physiological Acoustics), University of Michigan, Ann Arbor, USA.*

J. HIBBERT, BChir, MB, FRCS, *Consultant Otolaryngologist, Guy's Hospital, London.*

R. HINCHCLIFFE, MD, FRCPE, DLO, *Professor of Audiological Medicine, Institute of Laryngology and Otology, University of London.*

W.E. HITSELBERGER, MD, *Ear Research Institute, Los Angeles, USA.*

W.F. HOUSE, MD, *Ear Research Institute, Los Angeles, USA.*

T.T.S. INGRAM, MD, FRCP, *Formerly Reader in Paediatric Neurology, Department of Child Life and Health, University of Edinburgh, and Consultant Neurologist, Royal Hospital for Sick Children, Edinburgh.*

I. JACOBSON, MB, BCh, FRCSE, *Honorary Senior Lecturer in Surgical Neurology, University of Dundee, and Consultant Neurosurgeon, Royal Infirmary, Dundee.*

A.G. KERR, MB, Bh, FRCS, *Professor of Otolaryngology, Queen's University of Belfast, and Consultant Otolaryngologist, Royal Victoria Hospital, Belfast, Northern Ireland.*

A.I.G. KERR, MB, ChB, FRCSE, FRCSG, *Honorary Senior Lecturer in Otolaryngology, University of Edinburgh, and Consultant Otolaryngologist, City Hospital, Edinburgh.*

C.J. KRAUSE, MD, *Professor and Chairman, Department of Otolaryngology and Maxillofacial Surgery, University of Michigan, Ann Arbor, USA.*

B.F. MCCABE, MD, *Professor and Head of Department of Otolaryngology and Maxillofacial Surgery, University of Iowa, Iowa City, USA.*

P. MCKELVIE, MD, ChM, FRCS, DLO, *Consultant Otolaryngologist, The London Hospital, London.*

K. MCLAY, MB, ChB, FRCSE, *Honorary Senior Lecturer in Otolaryngology, University of Edinburgh, and Consultant Otolaryngologist, Royal Infirmary, Edinburgh.*

A.G.D. MARAN, MD, FRCSE, FACS, *Honorary Senior Lecturer in Otolaryngology, University of Edinburgh, and Consultant Otolaryngologist, Royal Infirmary, Edinburgh.*

J. MARQUET, MD, *Professor of Otolaryngology, University of Antwerp, Belgium.*

T. PALVA, MD, *Professor of Otolaryngology, University of Helsinki, Finland.*

R. PRACY, MB, BS, FRCS, *Consultant Otolaryngologist, Hospital for Sick Children, London, and Royal National Throat, Nose and Ear Hospital, London.*

H.F. SCHUKNECHT, MD, *Professor of Otology and Laryngology, Harvard Medical School, and Chief of Otolaryngology, Massachusetts Eye and Ear Infirmary, Boston, USA.*

D. E. SCHULLER, MD, *Associate Professor of Otolaryngology, Ohio State University, Columbus, USA.*

G.D.L. SMYTH, DSC, MD, MCh, FRCS, *Honorary Reader in Otolaryngology, Queen's University of Belfast, and Consultant Otolaryngologist, Royal Victoria Hospital, Belfast, Northern Ireland.*

G.B. SNOW, MD, *Professor of Otolaryngology, Free University Hospital, Amsterdam, The Netherlands.*

P.M. SPRINKLE, MD, *Professor and Chairman of the Division of Otolaryngology, West Virginia University, Morgantown, USA.*

P.M. STELL, ChM, FRCS, *Professor of Otolaryngology, University of Liverpool, and Consultant Otolaryngologist, Royal Liverpool Hospital, Liverpool.*

S.F. TAYLOR, MA, DM, MCh, FRCS, *Formerly Dean, Royal Postgraduate Medical School, University of London, and Consultant Surgeon, Hammersmith Hospital, London.*

W. TAYLOR, DSC, MD, FRCPE, *Formerly Professor of Community and Occupational Medicine, University of Dundee, Dundee.*

P. VAN DEN BROEK, MD, *Professor of Otolaryngology, University of Nijmegen, Sint Radboud Hospital, Nijmegen, The Netherlands.*

I. VAN DER WAAL, MD, *Professor of Oral Surgery, Free University Hospital, Amsterdam, The Netherlands.*

R. W. ... MD, *Professor of Microbiology and Otolaryngology, West Virginia University, ...own, USA.*

R. Th. R. WENTGES, MD, *Professor of Otolaryngology, University of Nijmegen, Sint Radboud Hospital, Nijmegen, The Netherlands.*

T... VILMOT, MS, FRCS, *Consultant Otolaryngologist, Tyrone County Hospital, Omagh, Northern Ireland.*

Preface

When we set out to edit this book we tried to picture the needs of a postgraduate student preparing for the final Fellowship examinations in the United Kingdom, Canada and Australia, or the Specialty Board examinations in the United States of America. During the training years the student will have read many excellent monographs in otolaryngology and its related sciences, and several of the atlases of surgery. He will also have acquired a grounding in the basic sciences and will have read basic texts in audiology. We felt, therefore, that towards the end of training there was a need for a comprehensive account in one volume of all aspects of the principles of otolaryngology which correlated previous reading.

A book on the principles *and* practice of otolaryngology must occupy several volumes due to the enormous expansion in the scope of the subject, from audiology and its applied physiological aspects at one end of the spectrum to the treatment of malignancy and reconstructive surgery at the other end. What then have we sacrificed to produce a one-volume text? The primary omission is operative technique. We felt that, due to the requirements of the various examining boards, candidates for final examination will have acquired sufficient knowledge of operative technique. Moreover, this is a skill which is not to be learned from the written word; instruction from teachers and reference to atlases of surgery are thus preferable to reading about it in a book of this type.

Basic sciences have also been pruned down to what might be considered an unacceptable brevity. Again we felt that by the time a candidate is in the final stages of preparation for an examination he should certainly know the relevant surgical anatomy and physiology at a satisfactory level. To have included more surgical anatomy and physiology would have increased the length of the book to unmanageable proportions.

If books that cover the entire principles and practice of otolaryngology are becoming more impossible to produce because of size, the days of one man writing a book on the principles of otolaryngology are certainly over. With the increasing subspecialization in otology, audiology, head and neck surgery and plastic and reconstructive surgery, there must be few general otolaryngologists with a sufficient expertise in all branches to create a book.

We thus had to recruit a team of authors, each of whom was chosen not only for his expertise but also for his international knowledge of the requirements demanded by the various examining boards. We were fortunate in obtaining help from forty-seven of the world's most prominent otolaryngologists. These contributions have inevitably been subject to editing, both to produce a uniformity of style and form and to avoid duplication: the editors are deeply grateful to the contributors for their tolerance of this editing process. Any faults in production of the chapters, therefore, are those of the editors and the authors should be absolved.

The book is subdivided into the four main subspecialties of otolaryngology: otology, rhinology, head and neck surgery, and paediatric otolaryngology. Some duplication was inevitable but we hope that it has been kept to a minimum.

Finally, we wish to record our gratitude to a number of people: to all the contributors; to the staff of Blackwell Scientific Publications, and Mr. Nigel Palmer in particular, for their patience and help; to Dr. John Hibbert for reading the proofs and preparing the index; to numerous registrars for their criticisms at the galley stage; to our secretaries for typing, organizing and portering with good grace; and finally, but by no means least, to our wives.

April 1979   A.G.D. Maran
                                                               P.M. Stell

CHAPTER I

Audiology

AUDITORY SYMPTOMS

The four basic auditory symptoms are *hypoacusis, dysacusis, dysstereoacusis* and *tinnitus*. There are also indirect symptoms, such as *delayed* or *defective speech development, auditory inattention* (or *unresponsiveness*) and *response inconsistency*, which are very important in respect of children. Auditory hallucinations, being psychotic symptoms, are the proper subject of psychiatry.

Hypoacusis

Hypoacusis is an elevation of the threshold of hearing (*anacusis*, if there is no hearing). Hypoacusis indicates either impairment of sound transmission through the external and middle ears to the internal ear or a lesion of the first and/or second cochlear neurone. The term 'deafness' should be reserved, as in its simple everyday use, to a total or severe impairment of hearing [1].

Dysacusis

Dysacusis is best restricted to cover difficulties in hearing other than those due to hypoacusis or dysstereoacusis. Thus, dysacusis comprises *distortion* of sound, *diplacusis binauralis* (difference in pitch of the same tone presented to each ear) *echoing* sensations and abnormal growths of loudness, including *phonophobia* (abnormal sensitivity to suprathreshold sounds). Distortion of sound and diplacusis binauralis indicate lesions of the spiral receptor organ. Phonophobia may occur not only in internal ear disorders but also in conditions where there is no lesion of the auditory system, for example, in paralysis of the nerve to stapedius and in anxiety and other psychological states. The term *paracusis Willisii*

is applied to the symptom of hearing better in noisy environments than in quiet ones. Paracusis Willisii is characteristic not only of otosclerosis but of conductive hearing impairments in general. *Autophony* refers to the perception of one's own voice as though it were originating inside the skull.

Dysstereoacusis

Dysstereoacusis comprises both impaired sound directionalization and impaired distance perception; both of these are rare as presenting symptoms. The symptom may indicate a central lesion which is responsible for failure to integrate sound signals coming to the two ears. Subjects with a sudden incomplete unilateral hearing loss rapidly adapt to the disturbance in sound localization.

Tinnitus

If a patient complains of hearing sounds for which there is no evident external cause, this symptom is referred to as tinnitus. But this term does not include the hearing of organized sounds, which symptom is referred to as an auditory hallucination. On the one hand, tinnitus may be intermittent and the only symptom heralding a tumour of, or pressing on, the vestibulocochlear nerve, and such a tinnitus may be insufficiently annoying for the patient to seek medical help. On the other hand, a sustained tinnitus may be associated with benign aural disease or no evident disease at all and yet, because of its terrifying soul-destroying nature, drive the patient towards suicide.

Objective tinnitus is tinnitus which is also audible to observers other than the patient. It may arise from a foreign body in the external acoustic meatus, or from some physiological disturbance in the head [2]. Mandibular joint dysfunction may present as 'clicking' tinnitus. In Costen's syndrome, a mandibular joint derangement is associated with an internal ear dysfunction, which itself may be characterized by tinnitus. Myogenous tinnitus is experienced with palatal myoclonus (myorhythmia), in tensor tympani disorders, and after facial palsy. Respiratory tinnitus – hearing one's own breathing – occurs in patulous auditory tubal conditions. Vascular tinnitus may be pulsatile or due to a high frequency tone [3].

Subjective tinnitus is far more common than objective tinnitus, and can occur in almost any type of auditory disorder. Conventionally, subjective tinnitus is divided into 'peripheral' and 'central' according to whether or not it can be masked. It is unusual for 'peripheral' subjective tinnitus to be a pure tone, but patients prefer to match the sound that they hear to a pure tone rather than a narrow band of noise.

There are broad similarities between pathological pain states and tinnitus; in particular, both symptoms are very resistant to section of the corresponding sensory nerve, although they are frequently ameliorated by such procedures. Although tinnitus is usually brought to a tolerable level by section of the vestibulocochlear nerve, there has been at least one case where such a procedure accentuated the tinnitus.

AUDIOLOGICAL UNITS

The pitch of a pure tone is a function of its frequency (symbol, f). The frequency of a tone is defined as the number of sound waves passing any point of the sound field each second. Thus, according to the International System of Units, a tone with 2000 waves passing a given point in 1 second is said to have a frequency of 2000 hertz. The symbol for 'hertz' is 'Hz'. Since this unit is the reciprocal of the second, which is an SI base unit, it is said to be a derived unit. Thus a frequency that was formerly referred to as 2000 c.p.s., or 2000 c/s, is now referred to as 2000 Hz.

The intensity (symbol, J) of a sound is expressed in watts per square metre ($W \cdot m^{-2}$) which is also a SI derived unit. The smallest audible intensity is about $10^{-12} W \cdot m^{-2}$. Sound intensities more than one thousand million times greater than this occur in factories where noise hazards exist. A reduced scale is thus required for practical purposes. This is the decibel scale. The decibel (dB) is one-tenth of a bel, which is the logarithm of the ratio of two particular sound intensities. Since the scientist measures sound pressure and not sound intensity, and pressure is proportional to the square root of intensity, the decibel scale is also derived from the ratio of two sound pressures:

i.e. $$L = 10 \log_{10} I_2/I_1 \qquad (1.1)$$

where L = sound level in decibels
    I_1 = reference intensity ($W \cdot m^{-2}$)
and I_2 = intensity of sound in question ($W \cdot m^{-2}$).

$\therefore$ $$L = 10 \log_{10} (p_2/p_1)^2 \qquad (1.2)$$

$\therefore$ $$L = 20 \log_{10} p_2/p_1 \qquad (1.3)$$

where L = sound level in decibels
    p_1 = reference pressure in pascals
and p_2 = pressure of sound in question in pascals.

Equation (1.3) indicates that 1 dB corresponds to a 12% change in sound pressure. Depending on the reference pressure, there are three decibel scales. First, unless stated otherwise, the reference pressure (p_1) is taken to be 20 μPa (micropascals). This latter value was formerly expressed as 0·00002 newtons per square metre (and before that as 0·0002 dynes per square centimetre). The pascal is a derived SI unit. If the reference pressure is 20 μPa, a sound level of, for example, 95 dB should be expressed as 95 dB SPL (sound pressure level). The use of this particular decibel scale is usual when measurements are made of industrial sound levels. In audiometry (see later), the reference pressure depends upon the frequency, since it is the pressure of the faintest sound heard by otologically normal young adults at that frequency. These pressures have now been defined by the International Organization for Standardization. To avoid specifying the reference pressure at each frequency, audiometric sound levels are referred to, for example, as 45 dB *HL* (*hearing level*). A third decibel scale is that which refers sound levels to a particular individual's threshold of hearing at a given frequency, i.e. the scale of *sensation level* (*SL*). Thus, if a patient has an impaired threshold of hearing of 45 dB HL, a tone which is 25 dB above his threshold, i.e. at 70 dB HL, is said to have a level of 25 dB SL.

AUDITORY DIAGNOSTIC TESTS

It is convenient to discuss auditory diagnostic tests under three headings:

(1) Psychoacoustical, i.e. tests of auditory sensation and perception;

(2) Acoustical, i.e. measurement of the acoustical properties of the ear, and changes incurred in these by various stimuli, and

(3) Electrophysiological, i.e. measurement of the electrical changes (evoked potentials) induced by acoustic stimuli.

Psychoacoustical tests are frequently termed *subjective*, since the results depend upon the patient's volunteered responses to acoustic stimuli. *Acoustical* and *electrophysiological* tests are frequently termed *objective*, since they do not require the patient to volunteer a response. Although the second and third groups of tests are objective in respect of the patient, the interpretation of some of these tests requires a decision that is sufficiently subjective that the term 'quasi-objective' would be more appropriate.

Psychoacoustical tests comprise both clinical tests of hearing and tests of hearing using electroacoustic equipment, i.e. conventional audiometry.

Clinical tests

Clinical tests of hearing comprise both speech tests and tuning fork tests.

Clinical speech tests

Clinical speech tests comprise both *forced whisper* and *conversational voice tests*. A forced whisper test uses a whispered voice after a forced expiration by the examiner. When either forced whisper or conversational voice tests are employed, the examiner stands facing the side of the patient. Two precautions to avoid false results must be taken: the patient's eyes must be shielded by the palm of the examiner's hand to prevent lip-reading; the tragus of the ear not being tested should be massaged by the middle finger of the examiner's other hand; this produces a masking noise in the non-tested ear.

When the examiner's hands are so occupied, the maximum distance between the examiner's mouth and the patient's ear is about 50 cm. However, if a patient can hear a forced whisper at this distance under the ambient noise conditions that commonly obtain in clinical examination rooms, the patient is unlikely to have any appreciable impairment of hearing.

Tuning fork tests

The principal tuning fork tests of value to the otological surgeon are three tests (bone-conducted cross-hearing, Teal, and Stenger) to ascertain whether a unilateral hearing loss is non-organic or organic and two tests (Schmalz and Rinne) to determine the nature of organic loss.

The first test for a unilateral suspected non-organic hearing loss is to ascertain whether the patient denies hearing a tuning fork placed on the ipsilateral mastoid process; irrespective of the degree of hearing loss the patient should hear the fork because the interaural attentuation of bone-conducted sound is negligible.

The Teal test. If a patient with a unilateral loss to air conducted sound admits to hearing by bone conduction, the examiner should then retest the patient, who should have his eyes closed, by applying a non-vibrating tuning fork to the ipsilateral mastoid process and simultaneously bringing the prongs of a vibrating fork near to the patient's ear. Usually the patient does not suspect that two tuning forks are being used; he feels the fork applied to the mastoid process and at the same time hears a sound if his hearing is normal; in this case he does not dissociate these two sensations and acknowledges hearing a sound.

The Stenger test. If the two ears of a person with

the same threshold of hearing in each ear are stimulated by a sound of the same frequency but of a different intensity a single sound is heard in the ear that receives the greater sound intensity. Thus, if, in a patient exhibiting a unilateral deafness to air conducted sound, a pair (unknown to the patient) of vibrating tuning forks are so disposed that one is much nearer the deaf ear, the patient will deny hearing anything if the hearing on that side is normal; if the hearing is truly impaired in that ear, the patient will acknowledge hearing a sound but refer it to the opposite ear.

The Schmalz* test ascertains whether a unilateral organic hearing loss is conductive (due to impairment of sound transmission through the external and middle ears), or sensorineural (due to a lesion of the internal ear or the auditory nervous pathway). If, with a unilateral hearing impairment, a vibrating fork is applied to the vertex, a sound will be heard in the impaired ear if the loss is conductive; if the loss is sensorineural, the sound will be heard in the normal ear.

The Rinne test ascertains whether a unilateral or bilateral hearing loss is conductive or sensorineural. An ear is said to exhibit a Rinne positive response if a vibrating tuning fork is heard better by air conduction than by bone conduction (with the footpiece of the fork applied to the mastoid process). This response occurs in normal ears and in those with a sensorineural hearing loss. If the vibrating fork is heard better by bone conduction than by air conduction (Rinne negative response) the test must be repeated with a Bárány noise box applied to the opposite ear; if the same response occurs, then it is said to be a true Rinne negative; if the fork is no longer heard better by bone conduction, then it is said to be a false Rinne negative response. The effect of the noise in the opposite ear is to exclude the possibility of cross-hearing that occurs with severe sensorineural hearing loss. True Rinne negative responses occur with conductive hearing losses.

AUDIOMETRY

An audiometer is an electroacoustic instrument

* Usually, but erroneously, referred to as the Weber test.

specifically designed to measure one or more aspect of auditory sensation or perception for clinical purposes [4]; this definition excludes instruments for measuring the acoustical properties of the ear or for measuring acoustically evoked potentials.

Audiometry [5] may:

(1) be performed by either air-conducted or bone-conducted acoustic stimuli;

(2) if using an air-conduction route, use stimuli delivered by either a loudspeaker or by an earphone;

(3) use tonal or verbal stimuli;

(4) be concerned with threshold or suprathreshold stimuli;

(5) be monaural or binaural;

(6) have the presentation of the stimulus controlled by the tester or by the patient; and

(7) if the presentation of the stimulus is under the control of the patient, use tonal stimuli that may be sustained or interrupted.

By choosing various combinations, a large number of audiometric procedures are possible. In practice, a limited number of tests are in use. Thus, we have:

(1) measurement of the air-conduction threshold of hearing for tones by earphone listening;

(2) the same as (1) but for bone-conducted stimuli;

(3) measurement of auditory adaptation at threshold for fixed frequency tonal stimuli;

(4) measurement of auditory adaptation at threshold for sweep frequency tonal stimuli;

(5) measurement of suprathreshold auditory adaptation for fixed frequency tonal stimuli;

(6) measurement of suprathreshold auditory adaptation for sweep frequency tonal stimuli;

(7) measurement of the recruitment of loudness sensation by

(a) recording the most comfortable loudness level,

(b) recording the threshold of uncomfortable loudness (sometimes referred to as the uncomfortable loudness level or the loudness discomfort level, but, of course, there are many such levels),

(c) alternate binaural loudness matching;

(8) measurement of fused binaural tonal threshold, i.e. audiometric Stenger test [6];

(9) measurement of the ability to hear verbal stimuli as a function of sound intensity (speech audiometry);

(10) measurement of alternate binaural pitch matching.

Measurement of threshold of hearing

The determination of the threshold of hearing by either air conduction or bone conduction is performed by a psychophysical procedure termed the *method of limits*. For a given frequency, this consists of presenting a series of stimuli descending in 10 dB steps from a clearly audible suprathreshold sound. The subject is instructed to respond by raising a finger or pressing a button every time he hears a signal. When the subject no longer hears the sound, a second (ascending) series of stimuli is presented in 5 dB steps [7].

The threshold is not found to be an 'all-or-none' phenomenon associated with a particular sound level, especially for extremely low or high frequencies. The threshold is therefore taken as the mid-point of the 'going up' and the 'coming down' thresholds; a 'two-out-of-four' response is used as the criterion of threshold at a given level.

The results are plotted, using conventional symbols (Table 1.1) on a chart termed an *audiogram*, which may also be used to represent other data relating to auditory or acoustic function. An example is shown in Fig. 1.1.

Erroneous results for the measurement of the threshold of hearing may be obtained when:
  (1) there are instrumental errors;
  (2) there are observer errors;
  (3) the patient does not comprehend instructions;
  (4) the subject chooses either not to respond at all or to respond to a sound that is above threshold;
  (5) 'canal collapse' occurs; or
  (6) cross-hearing occurs.

Instrumental errors arise if there are defects in the audiometer. These can be avoided by proper calibration and constant monitoring of the output [7].

Recommendations for calibrating audiometers have been drawn up by the International

TABLE 1.1. Symbols approved by the British Association of Otolaryngologists and the British Society of Audiologists for denoting the results of various tests on standard audiogram forms

Right	Audiometric symbols (BAO and BSA)	Left
	Unmasked unoccluded bone conduction threshold △	
	Other symbols	
o	Air conduction threshold	×
[	Bone conduction threshold (masked)	]
(	ASRT (reference to stimulated ear)	)
Σ	Most comfortable loudness level	Ɔ
L	Threshold of uncomfortable loudness	⌐

Electrotechnical Commission and the International Organization for Standardization [4].

Observer errors are more likely to arise from the employment of untrained audiometricians; they can be eliminated by automatic, self-recording (Békésy-type) audiometry.

Non-organic hearing loss is the term which encompasses conditions (3) and (4). The possibility of their occurrence should have been indicated by the clinical tests; indeed some types, e.g. unilateral simulated hearing loss, should have been diagnosed with certainty. Again, Békésy-type audiometry can detect the majority of these [8] and, when suitably modified, quantify them [9].

Owing to a variety of anatomical factors, *collapse* of the external acoustic meatus can occur when an earphone is placed on an auricle. This can cause an apparent hearing loss of as much as 30 dB. The pattern is that of a conductive, or of a combined conductive and sensorineural, hearing loss. Again, the prior performance of certain clinical tests of hearing (forced

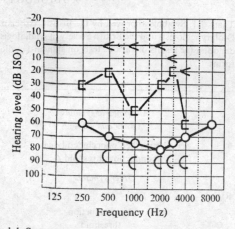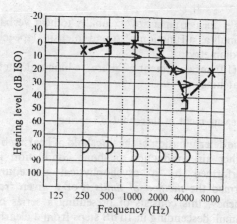

FIG. 1.1. Several measures of auditory and acoustic function plotted on a pure tone audiogram with the format agreed to by the BSA (British Society of Audiology) and the BAO (British Association of Otolaryngologists). Values for the patient's right ear are plotted on the left-hand side and those for the left ear on the right-hand side. This format, like those for the symbols, which are derived from a representation for an earphone, represents the patient's head from the perspective of the clinician, or technician, facing the patient. The symbols used are those shown in Table 1.1, together with a 'greater than' sign (>) or a 'less than' sign (<) to denote thresholds for the slow cortical vertex evoked potential for left and right ears respectively.

The audiogram for the left ear shows normal thresholds up to about 2000 Hz but with a subsequent high tone notch. The bone conduction levels for the left ear are essentially the same as those for the air conduction levels; thus the high tone loss on the left is sensorineural. The volunteered thresholds for air conduction in the left ear have been validated by measurement of the thresholds for the slow cortical evoked potential. The normal acoustic stapedius reflex thresholds (ASRTs) for sounds delivered to the left ear confirms that the site of the lesion at 4000 Hz is in the receptor organ, i.e. the spiral organ.

On first inspection, the audiogram for the right ear might be held to indicate a conductive hearing loss (because of the 'air-bone' gap) together with an associated sensori neural hearing loss (because of the elevated bone conduction threshold). However (1) the air conduction threshold has the form of the 'saucer-shape' curve (this is frequently seen in malingering because of the patient's latching on to an equal loudness contour when deciding to acknowledge that he hears a sound), (2) the bone conduction threshold is erratic, (3) the ASRTs are normal on each side (so there is unlikely to be any conductive component in either ear), (4) there is a very narrow gap between the ASRTs and the air conduction thresholds of hearing (much narrower than one would expect to find in recruiting ears) and, finally, (5) the thresholds for the slow cortical evoked potentials are normal except for a slight high tone loss in that right ear. Thus, the hearing loss in that right ear is predominantly non-organic.

whisper, Rinne and Bing) should have precluded such an artefact passing undetected.

Cross-hearing is the condition in which the response to a particular stimulus is due to stimulation of the opposite ear. Thus it will occur when there is an appreciable (including total) hearing loss on one side and sufficient hearing on the other side to detect the signal after it has been attenuated by its passage across the skull. The detection of a sound by the opposite ear depends only on the bone-conduction hearing level of that ear and not on the air-conduction levels. The mechanism of cross-hearing for either air-conducted or bone-conducted signals is shown in Figs. 1.2 and 1.3 respectively. To prevent cross-

hearing the threshold of hearing must be raised artificially, but temporarily, for the ear not being tested. This can be done by applying another sound signal, termed a *masking noise*, to the non-tested ear.

If cross-hearing is suspected, a *graduated masking procedure* must be followed to ascertain the true value of an air-conduction or bone-conduction threshold of hearing. The measured air-conduction (or bone-conduction) threshold is plotted as a function of masking level (Figs. 1.2 and 1.3) and a plateau is sought in the curve relating these two measures.

Since the interaural attenuation in respect of a bone conduction transducer is minimal (0–10 dB), masking by a graduated masking procedure

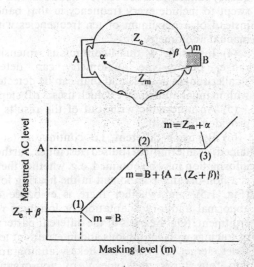

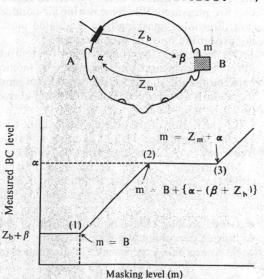

FIG. 1.2. Measurement of air conduction thresholds of hearing by a graduated masking procedure. *Above*: Sketch showing factors operating in cross-hearing and effect of masking the opposite ear. A and B represent air conduction hearing levels, and α and β the corresponding bone conduction levels; Z_e = interaural attenuation for a sound stimulus delivered by an earphone; Z_m = interaural attenuation for the masking noise; m is the level of the masking noise. *Below*: Graph showing measured air conduction threshold of hearing as a function of the masking level (m). The first (horizontal) segment of the graph is that part which covers the increase in the level of masking noise until it becomes audible (1); this is the air conduction hearing level (B) of that non-tested ear. With increasing levels of masking noise, the curve rises at a 45° angle until it reaches point (2); this corresponds to the point where the masking noise has 'freed' the masked ear from cross-hearing. The next segment of the curve is again horizontal; if extended, it cuts the vertical axis at a point corresponding to the true air conduction hearing level (A) of the ear under test. With increasing masking level, a point (3) is eventually reached where the curve again begins to rise at a 45° angle; this is due to the masking noise now reaching the ear under test (overmasking). It will thus be seen that, with this graduated masking procedure, in order to establish the true air-conduction hearing level (A), it is necessary to detect a plateau on the rising curve after the masking noise becomes audible (1). This condition is met if

$$B+\{A-(Z_e+\beta)\} < (Z_m+\alpha)$$

i.e. $\{(A-\alpha)+(B-\beta)\} < (Z_e+Z_m).$

In words, the sum of the two air–bone gaps should be less than the interaural attenuation of the test tone together with the interaural attenuation of the masking noise.

FIG. 1.3. Measurement of bone conduction threshold of hearing by a graduated masking procedure. *Above*: Sketch showing factors operating in cross-hearing and effect of masking the opposite ear. Symbols as in Fig. 1.2; in addition, Z_b is the interaural attenuation for a sound stimulus delivered by a bone conduction transducer (vibrator). *Below*: Graph showing measured bone conduction threshold as a function of masking level (m). The first (horizontal) segment of the graph is that which covers the increase in the level of the masking noise until it becomes audible (1); this is the air-conduction hearing level (B) of that masked ear. With increasing levels of masking noise, the curve rises at a 45° angle until it reaches point (2); this corresponds to the point where the masking noise has 'freed' the masked ear from cross-hearing. The next segment of the curve is again a horizontal line which cuts the vertical axis at a point corresponding to the true bone-conduction hearing level (α) of the ear under test. With increasing masking levels, a point (3) is eventually reached where the curve again begins to rise at a 45° angle; this is due to the masking noise now reaching the ear under test (overmasking). Thus, in order to establish the true bone conduction hearing level (α), it is necessary to detect a plateau subsequent to the point (1) where the masking noise becomes audible. This condition is met if:

$$B+\{\alpha-(\beta+Z_b)\} < (Z_m+\alpha)$$

i.e. $(B-\beta) < (Z_m+Z_b)$

or, since Z_b is approximately equal to zero, $(B-\beta) < Z_m$. In words, the air–bone gap of the non-tested ear should be less than the interaural attenuation of the masking noise.

must be used whenever bon conduction thresholds are measured. When measuring air-conduction thresholds, masking by a graduated masking procedure must be used if either:

(1) the hearing loss (unilateral or bilateral) is purely sensorineural and there is a difference between the thresholds for the two sides of more than 40 dB at a frequency of 500 Hz and above; or

(2) the nature of the hearing loss has not been determined and the threshold of either side at the frequency in question is greater than 40 dB.

Measurement of the threshold of hearing, either by bone or by air conduction, is conveniently performed by *Békésy audiometry*; this implies automatic, continuous-frequency self-recorded audiometry. The advantages of this technique over manual audiometry are:

(1) It excludes experimenter (audiometrician) error.

(2) It affords a ready means of validating responses; if it is not available, some audiologists have recommended that a routine audiometric Stenger test be performed to validate the results of manual audiometry [6].

(3) By using a glide test tone, the audio-frequency range (from 100 Hz to 10 000 Hz) can be swept to include every frequency in that band, instead of a maximum of ten frequencies with manual audiometry.

(4) In using a quasi-continuous intensity range, Békésy-type audiometry can detect smaller ranges in threshold than can be detected with manual audiometry, which uses 5 dB steps.

(5) An automatic write out of the results is provided (Fig. 1.4).

(6) By using different, i.e. continuous (sustained) or intermittent (pulsed) test tones, further information may be obtained, e.g. whether there is a non-organic component in the hearing loss (Fig. 1.5), and whether there is evidence of abnormal auditory adaptation or loudness recruitment. (On the basis of the different patterns of tracings with continuous and intermittent test tones, Jerger [11] classified Békésy audiograms into four types, the type V of non-organic hearing loss being reported later [8].)

Measurement of auditory adaptation

An elevation in the measured threshold of hearing as a function of time, or a difference between

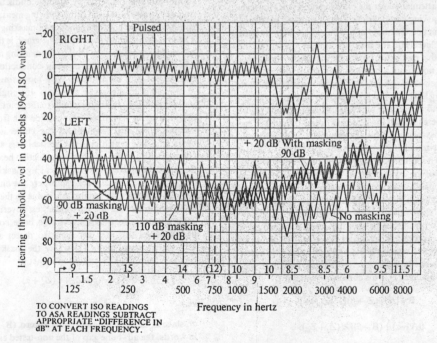

FIG. 1.4. An example of a sweep frequency Békésy audiogram recorded with a pulsed (intermittent) test tone. The threshold for the right ear is normal: that for the left shows a moderately severe hearing loss. (After Hinchcliffe [10].)

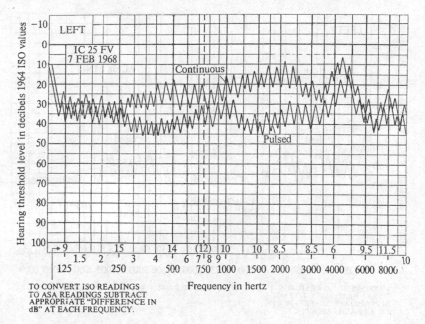

FIG. 1.5. An example of a type V Békésy tracing, i.e. where the continuous test tone threshold is lower than the pulsed tone threshold at one or more frequencies; this pattern characterizes a non-organic hearing loss.

thresholds measured with continuous and intermittent test tones, with better thresholds in response to the intermittent tones, is called auditory adaptation. If the effect is appreciable, it is called 'abnormal'. The magnitude of the effect considered to be abnormal depends on the method of testing. The simplest is Carhart's [12] 'tone decay' test (a misnomer since it is the sensation, and not the tone, that decays). After measuring the threshold of hearing in the normal way, the tester determines the minimal level necessary for the subject to hear a sustained tone for 1 minute. Since adaptation measured by this test is not considered abnormal unless there is a difference of at least 20 dB between the measured threshold and the 1-minute threshold, the test should be started at 20 dB SL [13]. Using this procedure nineteen out of twenty patients with vestibulocochlear nerve tumours showed auditory adaptation of 35 dB or more [13]. This modified Carhart test can be used as a convenient screening procedure, beginning at a frequency of 4000 Hz; however, at this frequency its sensitivity is such that subjects not suffering from tumours or demyelinating disorders may show abnormal auditory adaptation.

Patients exhibiting abnormal auditory adaptation with the Carhart test can be examined in more detail with Békésy audiometry using both sweep frequency and fixed frequency tones. An example of abnormal auditory adaptation with fixed frequency recordings is shown in Fig. 1.6, and with sweep frequency recordings in Fig. 1.7.

Measurement of loudness recruitment

Patients with hearing losses due to certain cochlear lesions characteristically exhibit a growth in the sensation of loudness with increasing stimulus intensity that is more rapid than in normal subjects. This phenomenon is termed *loudness recruitment*. The clinico-pathological significance of the phenomenon was clarified by Dix and her colleagues in 1948 [14]. The phenomenon can be accounted for by the loss of the 'tips' of the frequency-threshold (tuning) curves of individual cochlear neurones [15].

Loudness recruitment is traditionally measured by the subject performing alternate binaural loudness balances. fig. 1.8 shows an example of a hearing loss with loudness recruitment and Fig. 1.9 one without it.

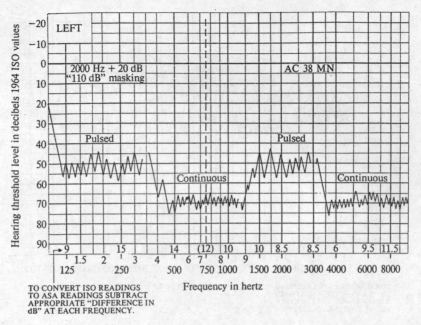

Fig. 1.6. Abnormal auditory adaptation at threshold demonstrated with fixed frequency Békésy audiometry. Since the stimulus has a fixed frequency (2000 Hz), the correct labelling of the horizontal axis should be in units of elapsed time (the horizontal span of the graph covers about 8 minutes). (After Hinchcliffe [10].)

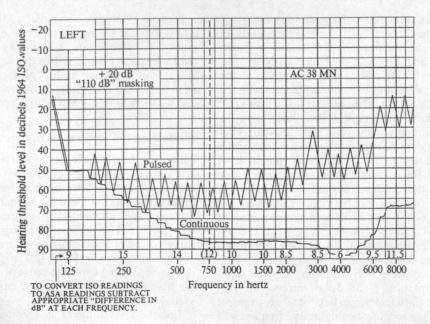

Fig. 1.7. Abnormal auditory adaptation at threshold demonstrated with sweep frequency Békésy audiometry. Note the marked separation of the threshold for a pulsed test tone from that for a continuous test tone; actually there is no measurable hearing with the latter signal; the path which has been tracked is that of the upper limit of the audiometer's output. (After Hinchcliffe [10].)

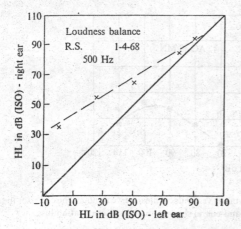

FIG. 1.8. Alternate binaural loudness matching (Fowler's test). The interrupted line is fitted to the points (x) which indicate 500 Hz sounds that are considered by the subject to be equally loud at the two ears. The diagonal in the graph is the point of equal loudness for normally hearing subjects. (After Hinchcliffe [16].)

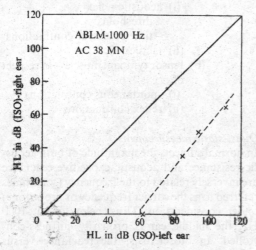

FIG. 1.9. Similar graph for a patient who does not exhibit loudness recruitment.

Speech audiometry

Whereas pure tone audiometry tests the ability to hear tones, speech audiometry tests the ability to hear speech sounds. The test material may be recorded on discs or on magnetic tape. It consists of either phonetically-balanced (PB) or iso-phonemic monosyllabic or spondaic (equally accented disyllabic) words. Phonetically-balanced lists are those in which each phoneme in the list appears in proportion to its frequency of occurrence in natural language; isophonemic lists are those in which a phoneme occurs once only in each list, as in those of Boothroyd [17] where each list consists of 10 CVC (consonant–vowel–consonant) items. The latter are gaining in popularity partly because of their shorter lengths and partly because a single occurrence of each phoneme in each list makes an analysis of error responses much easier.

A normal speech audiometric curve is shown on the left-hand side in Fig. 1.10; an abnormal curve is shown on the right-hand side. Abnormally hearing ears may show one or more of four changes in the curve, i.e.:

(1) a shift of the curve to the right (speech hearing loss);

(2) a failure to achieve a score of 100% or thereabouts (discrimination loss);

(3) a reversal of the direction of the curve (rollover); and

(4) a decreasing slope of the rising segment of the curve.

All these four features are seen in the curve on the right-hand side of Fig. 1.10. Shifts of the curve to the right, unassociated with the other three changes, are characteristic of pure conductive hearing losses of any magnitude and of cochlear impairments with speech hearing losses less than 31 dB [18]. Neuronal hearing losses, especially those due to vestibulocochlear nerve tumours, are characterized by a marked discrimination loss.

Acoustic admittance and impedance

Acoustic admittance (Y_A) defines the ease with which the flow of sound energy can be accomplished, and *acoustic impedance* (Z_A) the corresponding difficulty. Thus acoustic impedance is the reciprocal of acoustic admittance. Acoustic admittance and impedance are analogous to electrical admittance and impedance. Consequently, it is convenient to discuss the flow of acoustical energy by analogy to the flow of electrical energy in an alternating current circuit.

As with the electrical analogues, acoustic admittance and acoustic impedance each have two principal component measures. Thus, acoustic conductance (G_A) and acoustic susceptance (B_A) are components of acoustic admittance, and acoustic resistance (R_A) together with acoustic

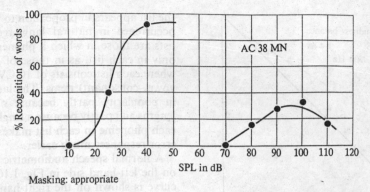

FIG. 1.10. Speech audiogram of a 38-year-old man with a diagnosis of left vestibulocochlear nerve tumour. The curve for the right ear (left-hand curve) is normal; that for the left ear (right-hand curve) shows a marked discrimination loss.

reactance (X_A) are components of acoustic impedance. Moreover, acoustic susceptance and acoustic reactance are themselves composed of two measures, i.e. on the one hand capacitive susceptance (B_C) and inductive susceptance (B_L), and, on the other hand, capacitive reactance (X_C) and inductive reactance (X_L).

Acoustic admittance and impedance in audiology

The function of the external and middle ears is to facilitate the transmission of an airborne acoustic signal to the internal ear by matching the high acoustic impedance of the cochlear fluid to the low acoustic impedance of air. This impedance matching is primarily achieved by a pressure transformation which is achieved by a disparity of the areas of the tympanic membrane and of the base of the stapes. Since impedances are usually complex, i.e. possess both resistive and reactive components, and real transformers cannot be made without mass and elasticity, a consideration of frequency is of paramount importance. It follows that studies of the acoustic admittance or impedance of the ear should provide information of diagnostic value in respect of middle ear function.

In clinical practice, acoustic admittance/impedance techniques can be used for:
A. Quasi-static measurements*
B. Dynamic measurements
   (1) as a function of time
   (2) as a function of changes in intrameatal

*'Quasi-static' is preferable to the term 'static' because sound, by its very nature, cannot be static.

pressure (tympanometry), and this perhaps as a function of frequency
(3) as an index of tympanic muscle contractions
   (a) stapedius muscle – in respect of
      (i) acoustic reflex
         – thresholds
         – time course of contractions
      (ii) tactile reflex
   (b) tensor tympani muscle – in respect of
      (i) spontaneous contractions
      (ii) reflex contractions

Quasi-static measurements

In normal subjects the magnitude of both acoustic resistance and acoustic capacitive reactance are inversely related to the frequency (sometimes referred to as the carrier frequency or probe tone) under consideration. Thus, below about 1000 Hz, the middle ear is primarily stiffness-controlled. In otosclerosis, the reactance versus frequency curve is shifted in the direction of greater acoustic capacitive reactance and greater acoustic resistance; in conditions of ossicular chain disruption, the converse occurs. With instruments measuring acoustic admittance, otosclerosis causes a decrease in acoustic capacitive susceptance, and ossicular chain disruption shows an increase in acoustic capacitive susceptance. Unfortunately, because of considerable overlap between the distributions of the component admittance and impedance measures for normal subjects and for subjects with ossicular disorders, these measurements often prove too insensitive to have diagnostic value.

Admittance impedance as a function of time
Fluctuation of admittance measures may be seen in *tensor tympani* disorders and in patients with a *patulous auditory tube*, where large fluctuations are seen synchronous with the respiratory cycle.

Admittance as a function of intrameatal pressure
The study of admittance changes as a function of intrameatal pressure changes is known as *tympanometry* (Fig. 1.11).

Tympanometry is valuable for detecting fluid in the middle ear. The presence of fluid in the middle ear is characterized by three changes in the tympanogram:

(1) the curve is displaced to the left (corresponding to negative middle ear pressures)

(2) a decrease in acoustic compliance (or acoustic capacitive susceptance) is measured, and

(3) there is a reduction in the peakiness of the curve [19].

Of these three changes, the last is the most sensitive index of intra-tympanic fluid. Tympanometry is thus a valuable diagnostic tool for detecting secretory otitis media in children.

Acoustic stapedius muscle reflex (ASR)
The ASR is a consensual (bilateral) reflex. Studies of the response of the contralateral stapedius muscle to acoustic stimulation of the ear have shown that, over the frequency range 250–4000 Hz, the acoustic stapedius reflex threshold (ASRT) is about 80 dB HL [20]. Acoustic impedance changes produced by stapedius muscle contraction are not only an indication of such a contraction but are also a measure of the magnitude of the contraction. The recording of the response to contralateral stimulation depends upon the integrity of a reflex arc which depends on the integrity of the auditory afferent pathway, the brain stem, the ipsilateral facial nerve, the nerve to stapedius, the stapedius

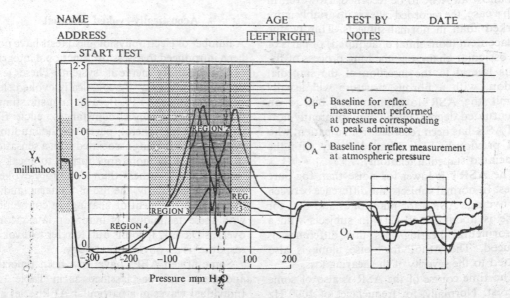

FIG. 1.11. Automatic tympanogram recorded on an otologically normal subject. The middle of the three peaked curves was the first to be recorded; it shows a slight negative middle ear pressure (this is normal) and an admittance of 1·4 siemens (millimhos); the peaked curve to the left was recorded after swallowing with the nose pinched (this aspirates some air from the middle ear cleft); the curve to the right, which shows a peak at about +600 Pa (labelled '+60 mm H₂O' on the graph) has been produced after a Valsalva manoeuvre; this inflates the middle ear cleft and slightly increases the middle ear pressure. The continuation of the tympanograms to the right produces two successive depressions in the tracing; these are two consecutive recordings of the ipsilateral acoustic stapedius reflex.

muscle, and the tympano-ossicular mechanism. The reflex, including its threshold, will therefore be impaired in hearing defects in the opposite ear to that in which the stapedius muscle is being tested and in brain stem lesions as well as in facial nerve palsies, stapedius muscle dysfunctions, or tympano-ossicular disorders on the side examined. Thus, inability to elicit the reflex from an ear with a hearing loss in the presence of normal hearing on the stimulated (contralateral) side indicates a conductive hearing loss on that side. Conversely, eliciting a normal ASR should exclude a conductive loss. Four points, however, should be made. First, if there is a recruiting hearing loss on the side on which the test tone is administered, normal ASRTs may be obtained. Thus, the ability to demonstrate normal ASRTs in patients who record an impaired threshold of hearing to conventional audiometry implies that the recorded loss is either recruiting and/or is non-organic. Secondly, disruption of the ossicular chain, e.g. fracture of the limbs of the stapes medial to the insertion of the stapedial tendon will allow an ASR to be recorded. However, in such a case, the recorded reflex is invariably more marked than in normal subjects. Thirdly, the replacement (congenital or acquired) of parts of the ossicular chain, e.g. the long process of the incus lateral to the insertion of the stapedial tendon, with a fibrous structure will usually permit the ASR to be manifest, but to an accentuated degree. Finally, an apparently normal ASR has been recorded from a patient who had previously had a stapedectomy with the associated stapedial tenotomy.

The ASRT is lower for noise than for pure tones. In normal subjects, the difference between the average ASRT for pure tones and that for noise is about 30 dB [21]. In subjects with a sensorineural hearing loss this difference is reduced. The ASRT for noise alone is also related to the severity of the hearing loss.

The time course of the ASR is also of some interest. Normally, for frequencies of 1000 Hz and below, the ASR maintains a plateau of contraction for stimuli presented at 10 dB above the reflex threshold and for at least 10 seconds. At 2000 Hz and above, the reflex 'decays' to about 50% or more over that 10-second period. Although one speaks of the 'decay' of this reflex,

the mechanism is one of suprathreshold adaptation in respect of the auditory input. Marked 'decay', i.e. abnormal suprathreshold auditory adaptation, occurs in tumours of, or compressing, the vestibulocochlear nerve [22].

A *tactile stapedius reflex* (TSR) may be produced by a puff of air to the walls of the external meatus opposite to the side on which the stapedius is examined, or by touching the skin of the anterior part of the auricle with a twist of cotton wool. The afferent part of this reflex is the trigeminal nerve; the efferent part is the same as that which has just been described for the ASR, i.e. via the facial nerve. Thus, the TSR can be used to determine whether the inability to elicit an ASR is due to an interruption of the afferent pathway or the efferent pathway. An *electro-cutaneous stapedius reflex* (EST) uses the same pathway as the TSR, and, like the TSR and the ASR, it is a consensual reflex. The ESR has the additional advantage over the TSR in that it can be quantified more easily but has the disadvantage that it is more uncomfortable.

Acoustically-evoked potentials

A number of electrophysiological tests have now been introduced to assess the functional integrity of the auditory nervous system. These tests depend on a variety of acoustically-evoked electrical potentials (AEP). Because acoustic stimuli may, under certain circumstances, elicit EPs from more peripheral parts of the auditory system without being associated with a sensation of hearing, it is more appropriate to speak of 'acoustically-' rather than 'auditory-evoked' potentials. Similarly, the use of the term 'audiometry' (measurement of hearing) in connection with these techniques is inappropriate. Moreover, as Davis [23] points out, to refer to 'evoked response' is an obvious tautology.

Some fifteen AEPs have now been reported and these may be classified as in Table 1.2. Individual waves in a particular AEP series are usually (but not always) referenced by an alphanumeric code, which consists of an initial capital letter, P or N, to designate whether the wave is positive or negative, and a subscripted number after the latter. Unfortunately, there is, as yet, no uniformity in the use of this number. In some

TABLE 1.2. A classification of the various auditory evoked potentials. (After Davis [23])

Probable source			Designation	Latency (ms)	Best response
Vertex Potentials	Cortex		Contingent negative variation	DC Shift	
			Expectancy wave	250–600	P_{300}
			Slow cortical (asleep)	200–800	$P_{200}-N_{300}:N_{600}\rightarrow P$
			Slow cortical (awake)	40–300	$N_{90}-P_{180}-N_{250}$
			Neurogenic	10–40	P_{35}
	Muscle		Myogenic	10–75	P_{12}
	Brain stem		Brain stem	2–10	P_6
			Frequency following		
ECochG	Cochlea	AP		1–4	N_1
		CM		0.1	
		SP			

(Between Cortex/Neurogenic and the lower rows the table is labelled vertically LATE / MIDDLE / EARLY)

instances, it may refer to the order in which the particular wave occurs in the series, or it may refer to the latency of that wave in milliseconds. The disadvantage of the latter method of numbering is that latency is invariably a function of one or more stimulus parameter. It would, perhaps, be more convenient to define the latency used for identifying a wave as the average latency, to the nearest integer, that is found in normally hearing subjects at a given sound level, e.g. 60 dB SL (sensation level). Fortunately, what the subscripted number refers to is usually clear from the context.

Cortical evoked potentials

The slow cortical response for awake subjects shows a maximum voltage at, or very near, the vertex (hence reference to it as the vertex (or V-) potential). With the reference electrode on the chin, lobule of the auricle, mastoid or neck, it is typically triphasic, with vertex-negative peaks for clicks at about 90 ms (N_1) and 250 ms (N_2) and a vertex-positive peak at about 180 ms (P_2) (Fig. 1.12). In older children and adults, the AEP threshold agrees very well, on average, with the subjective threshold of hearing [24]. In preschool children, the measured threshold using the V-potential is about 20 dB poorer than the

behavioural threshold, and, in infants, it may be as much as 40 dB poorer.

The latencies of the waves of the V-potential are stable with respect of intensity down to about 30 dB SL;* below that level they are progressively prolonged.

In clinical practice, the use of this EP is invaluable in determining the threshold of hearing where non-organic hearing loss is suspected or there is a non-auditory handicap, e.g. blindness, interfering with the use of conventional audiometry.

Brain stem evoked potentials

To date, two types of brain stem AEPs have been demonstrated, i.e. Jewett's fast waves and the frequency following response (FFR). Jewett & Williston [25] and Picton and his colleagues [26] identified a fast series of vertex EPs in the latency range 2–12 ms. These EPs comprise a series of about six positive waves at about 1 ms intervals which are recorded with electrodes on the vertex and on the lobule of the ear. With lower frequency (<30 Hz) cut-offs these responses are

* Throughout the AEP literature there is a tendency to use SL (sensation level) and HL (hearing level) interchangeably; strictly speaking, SL should be used when the reference level is the threshold of hearing for the particular subject under consideration.

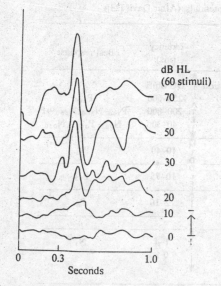

dB HL
(60 stimuli)

— 70

— 50

— 30

— 20

— 10

— 0

0   0.3   1.0
Seconds

Fig. 1.12. An example of a well-marked slow vertex potential on an awake normal subject; stimuli presented in descending order of intensity. (Reproduced by courtesy of H. A. Beagley, Esq., FRCS.)

superimposed upon a gradual vertex-positive shift of the base line, at least as far as the fifth wave.

The value of this AEP is not so much for measuring auditory threshold, but for detecting lesions involving the auditory nervous system, particularly vestibulocochlear nerve tumours and multiple sclerosis.

Electrocochleography (ECochG)

Electrocochleography refers to the recording of AEPs from the cochlea.

A variety of electrode placements have been used for the ECochG, but the most popular at the moment is a permeatal transtympanic electrode in contact with the promontory, which was introduced some 10 years ago [27, 28].

The Bordeaux group have subsequently reviewed the subject both in English [29] and in French [30]. The reader should also consult the monograph by Eggermont and his colleagues [31] and the report of a recent conference by Ruben and his colleagues [32].

Three distinct EPs may be recorded with ECochG, i.e.:

(1) the *cochlear microphonic potential*;

(2) the *summating potential*; and

(3) the *vestibulocochlear nerve compound action potential*.

Cochlear microphonic potential

The cochlear microphonic potential (CM) is an a.c. response generated in the cochlea. For a sinusoidal a.c. signal the CM faithfully follows the sinusoid with a one-to-one frequency. Complex acoustic patterns are, however, not reproduced with an unaltered waveform, because individual frequency components sustain varying amounts of attenuation and relative phase shift in their passage through the middle and internal ears; for a wide band click, the CM shows as a damped oscillation which, however, may in part be due to the 'ringing' which results from resonance in the earphone. The CM shows a negligible latency; in fact, in response to transients, a CM can be recorded in the guinea-pig cochlea with a delay of only 50 μs.

There is no 'all-or-none' threshold for the CM; measured thresholds depend upon the noise in the organism, the measuring equipment and the surroundings. In terms of voltage, CM output grows linearly with the input of the acoustic stimulus until relatively high levels (greater than 90 dB HL) are reached.

In clinical recordings of the CM, every single hair cell in the cochlea contributes to the recorded potential, and each with differing magnitude and phase, with relatively less effect the more distant they are from the recording electrode. Thus, with the recording electrode on the promontory, the CM will be the vectorial sum of the outputs of the several hundred hair cells in the adjacent basal turn.

Experimental studies have shown that impairment of CM parallels loss of hair cells in the spiral organ.

Summating potential (SP)

The SP is the sum of various components, although only two are emphasized, i.e. a positive SP and a negative SP [33]. The former is more pronounced at relatively low sound pressure levels; the latter increases in magnitude with increasing sound pressure of the stimulus, but, unlike the CM, it does not reach a limiting value.

In the normal cochlea, the SP$^+$, like the CM, is primarily produced by the outer hair cells.

In practice, the AP is separated from the SP by using the property of the AP to decrease in magnitude with increasing rates of stimulation; this property of the AP was discovered by Derbyshire & Davis [34] who referred to it as equilibration (subsequently termed adaptation). The immunity of the SP from exhibiting this decline is attributed to it being a presynaptic potential [31].

Possibly relevant to considering the results obtained in clinical electrocochleography is the observation that the polarity of the SP may be reversed either by increasing the hydrostatic pressure in the cochlea or by asphyxia. All but one of twenty-two patients with Ménière's disease showed a negative SP with a well-marked input–output function [31].

Vestibulocochlear nerve compound action potential

Unlike the CM, the vestibulocochlear nerve compound action potential (AP) exhibits an 'all-or-none' response. Since the form of the AP is independent of the polarity of the stimulus, alternating the polarity of the AC stimulus should cancel out the CM and leave the AP unaffected. However, precise superimposition of alternate APs does not occur, since the latency of the AP is shorter for rarefaction than for condensation clicks, at least for high stimulus levels.

If earphones have been used to deliver the stimulus, the observed AP may be contaminated by electrical artifacts since the shortest AP latencies are of the order of 1 millisecond. This can be remedied by achieving an acoustic delay of 2 ms more by using a loudspeaker as the signal source.

In contrast to single unit action potentials which are diphasic, the AP is normally essentially monophasic (Fig. 1.13).

In its fullest expression, an AP is characterized by three negative deflections, termed N_1, N_2 and N_3. The three are separated by about 1 ms intervals, and N_1 has a latency of just over 1 ms at high intensities, e.g. click levels of 90 dB SL. Normally, with decreasing magnitude of the a.c. stimulus, the latency of N_1 increases; N_1 eventually disappears from the recorded response and

N_2 appears, gradually increasing in latency as threshold is approached. The response pattern in the intermediate levels (about 65 dB SL), where N_1 and N_2 coexist, is sometimes referred to as a W-response. Associated with this normal change in the AP configuration as a function of the magnitude of the stimulus, there is a point of

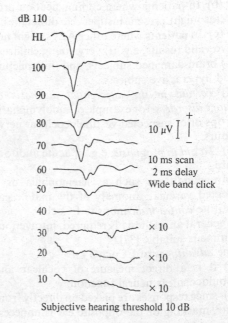

FIG. 1.13. Electrocochleography. Normal ear. Typical AP response as a function of stimulus level. (Reproduced by courtesy of H. A. Beagley, Esq., FRCS.)

inflexion in the input–output amplitude function around 50 dB SL; one may therefore consider this function as having two limbs, i.e. the L (low intensity) and H (high intensity) curves of Yoshie [35]. Consequently, it has been suggested that the pattern of AP responses provides evidence for two populations of hair cells. Initially it was thought that these two populations were those of the inner and outer hair cells. Recent animal work [31], and human studies [36], point to these two populations, i.e. those corresponding to low intensity responses and those corresponding to high intensity responses, being the hair cells of the middle and basal turns of the cochlea respectively.

Clinical use of ECochG

The *indications* for the use of ECochG in clinical practice are:

(1) *To obtain a measure of auditory function*

(a) In patients who would not be sufficiently co-operative without the use of anaesthesia, e.g. frightened or emotionally disturbed children;

(b) In patients where communication problems might present insuperable difficulties;

(c) In patients where other AEPs might not give valid results, e.g. (i) very young children, (ii) brain-damaged subjects, and (iii) epileptic and hyperactive subjects.

(2) *To aid in the differential diagnosis of auditory disorders*, for example of endolymphatic hydrops or of suspected vestibulocochlear nerve tumours.

(3) *To aid in prognosis*, e.g. of acute auditory failure.

Rare conditions such as haemophilia or a suspected vascular anomaly of the middle ear constitute *contra-indications* to ECochG.

If general anaesthesia is required, intravenous ketamine is suitable [37].

The *advantages* of ECochG are:

(1) it is a direct measure of cochlear and vestibulocochlear neural function;

(2) since responses are picked up directly from an ear, masking of the opposite ear is unnecessary;

(3) results are highly reproducible;

(4) responses are unaffected by anaesthesia.

The *disadvantages* are:

(1) it is relatively costly when one considers the medical and scientific staff required, let alone the equipment necessary;

(2) it is a hospital procedure;

(3) anaesthesia – either local or general – is required;

(4) it requires at least some medical skill to place the electrode;

(5) trauma, almost invariably minimal, is entailed in the customary transtympanic procedure; although many thousands of cases have been done without sequelae, one case of temporary vertigo, probably due to the local anaesthetic, and one case of mild middle ear infection have been reported [38]; a persisting perilymph leak has also developed in one child who had a congenital anomaly of the internal ear;

(6) wide band clicks, which are the most effective stimuli, provide little frequency information; it is, however, possible to obtain a measure of the auditory threshold as a function of frequency, with varying degrees of success, by (a) using filtered clicks [31], (b) using high pass masking [31] or (c) using certain computerized signal processing methods, e.g. deconvolution [36].

In the *interpretation* of ECochG, attention should be given to:

(1) the presence or absence of each of the following: AP, CM, SP;

(2) the pattern of the APs;

(3) the input–output function of the APs;

(4) the size and polarity of the SM; and

(5) the relationship of the AP, CM, and subjective thresholds to one another.

None of the three EPs are present in an ear that has been destroyed, for example, by an acute purulent labyrinthitis. The presence of a CM with an absent AP indicates a lesion of the vestibulocochlear nerve, whilst the presence of an AP, in the absence of a CM, indicates an auditory lesion restricted to the outer hair cells.

A prominent positive deflection immediately following the N_1 deflection produces a diphasic pattern; this is associated with ears exhibiting loudness recruitment, e.g. in endolymphatic hydrops. Aran and Portmann [29] relate amplitude and latency input–output function patterns ('normal', 'dissociated' and 'recruiting') to particular types of cochlear disorders.

A broad, trough-like AP with delayed recovery to the prestimulus level is seen in vestibulocochlear nerve tumours. Unfortunately, this sign is not pathognomonic. The 'most difficult group to distinguish from the tumours using ECochG proved to be patients with Ménière's syndrome' [39]; this, of course, is precisely where differential diagnosis is frequently required. A diagnosis of a vestibulocochlear nerve tumour is likely if three criteria are met:

(1) broadening of the AP,

(2) presence of a clear CM and

(3) preservation of the AP even when using stimulus intensities that are not audible to the

patient [40]. One would also anticipate, by analogy to the results for the audiometric examination for abnormal auditory adaptation, that vestibulocochlear tumours might show more marked adaptation of the AP [41].

The broad negative responses (3–8 ms) in Ménière's disorder are considered to be a function of the severity of the preceding episode of the disorder [29].

Management of auditory disorders

There is much that can now be done in the way of medical treatment for patients with auditory disorders. However, there remains a large population of patients who require rehabilitation. Rehabilitation should be aimed not only at the restoration of normal auditory function with prosthetic and other devices, but also, by fulfilling Maslow's [42] hierarchy of needs, at the restoration of the patient as a social being. Psychotherapy can be of immense value in the overall management of patients with auditory disorders, including tinnitus. In the UK, a residential centre (LINK) provides rehabilitation for subjects with acute bilateral deafness [43].

The cornerstone in the auditory rehabilitative process [44] is provided by one or other auditory prosthesis [45]. Even with conductive hearing losses, only a small proportion (of the order of 1%) of patients require bone conduction hearing aids. Since the usual aid is equivalent to a sound amplifying system, it can only reduce the sound attenuation that is produced by a hearing loss; it cannot improve on the maximum discrimination score shown by the speech audiogram. Thus the maximum discrimination score sets the limits of what can be achieved by a hearing aid. In cochlear disorders, there are a variety of major distortions of the acoustical signal [46]. It is thus not surprising that patients with sensorineural hearing losses have a greater discrimination loss in noise compared to patients with conductive losses, and this effect is accentuated when wearing hearing aids [47]. The impairment of speech discrimination with current hearing aids is such that patients with mild sensorineural hearing losses will not be benefited by an aid. Because of this effect of ambient noise, hearing aid assessments should be conducted with free-field speech audiometry in a background of noise to simulate everyday speech perception [48].

Apart from the amplification of sound, other advantages may accrue from hearing aids, e.g. the masking of tinnitus and improved sound localization. Good sound localization is, however, by no means certain, even with binaural ear-level aids. This is partly because there is a breakdown in the *masking level difference* (MLD) effect (colloquially termed the *cocktail party effect*) in both cochlear lesions and the degenerative changes in the central nervous system which are associated with presbyacusis. The MLD effect is a phenomenon whereby the discrimination of a signal in noise may improve by up to about 15 dB by changes in the interaural phase relations of the signal and the noise. Nevertheless, a study of the auditory directionalization ability of hearing-impaired subjects using various hearing aid systems has shown that binaural postaural aid systems are the best [49]. This finding should be borne in mind when fitting hearing aids to the blind. Similarly, a *contralateral routing of signals* (CROS) system may be of value in the rehabilitation of blind subjects with a profound unilateral hearing loss [50]. The CROS system, first reported by Hartford & Barry [51], has subsequently been expanded and the full range of the system is indicated by Martin [45].

References

[1] DAVIS H. (1970) Abnormal hearing and deafness. In *Hearing and Deafness*, eds. Davis H. & Silverman S. R., 3rd Ed., Chap. 4, New York: Holt, Rinehart & Winston.

[2] COLES. R. R. A., SNASHALL, S. E. & STEPHENS S. D. G. (1975) Some varieties of objective tinnitus. *British Journal of Audiology* 9, 1.

[3] GLANVILLE J. D., COLES R. R. A. & SULLIVAN B. M. (1971) A family with high-tonal objective tinnitus. *Journal of Laryngology* 85, 1.

[4] MARTIN M. C. (1976) In *Scientific Foundations of Otolaryngology*, eds. Hinchcliffe R. & Harrison D. F. N., Chap. 56. London: Heinemann.

[5] KNIGHT J. J. (1976) Audiometry. In *Scientific Foundations of Otolaryngology*, eds. Hinchcliffe R. & Harrison D. F. N., Chap. 57. London: Heinemann.

[6] COLES R. R. A. & PRIEDE V. M. (1971) Nonorganic

overlay in noise-induced hearing loss. *Proceedings of the Royal Society of Medicine* 64, 194.

[7] HINCHCLIFFE R. & LITTLER T. S. (1958) Methodology of air conduction audiometry for hearing surveys. *Annals of Occupational Hygiene* 1, 114.

[8] JERGER J. & HERER G.(1961) Unexpected dividend in Békésy audiometry. *Journal of Speech and Hearing Disorders* 26, 390.

[9] CHEESMAN A. D. & STEPHENS S. D. G. (1965) A new method for the detection of functional hearing loss. *Charing Cross Hospital Gazette* pp. vii–xii.

[10] HINCHCLIFFE R. (1971) Examen otoneurologique pour le diagnostic des neurinomes acoustiques. *Acta oto rhino. – laryngol., belg.* 25, 770.

[11] JERGER J. (1960) Békésy audiometry in the analysis of auditory disorders. *Journal of Speech and Hearing Research* 3, 275.

[12] CARHART R. (1957) Clinical determination of abnormal auditory adaptation. *Archives of Otolaryngology* 65, 32.

[13] OLSEN W. O. & NOFFSINGER D. (1974) Comparison of one new and three old tests of auditory adaptation. *Archives of Otolaryngology* 99, 94.

[14] DIX M. R., HALLPIKE C. S. & HOOD J. D. (1948) Observations upon the loudness recruitment phenomenon with especial reference to the differential diagnosis of disorders of the internal ear and VIII nerves. *Proceedings of the Royal Society of Medicine* 14, 516.

[15] EVANS E. F. (1975) The sharpening of cochlear frequency selectivity in the normal and abnormal cochlea. *Audiology* 14, 419.

[16] HINCHCLIFFE R. (1970) Hearing loss due to physical agents. *British Journal of Hospital Medicine* 4, 303.

[17] BOOTHROYD A. (1968) Developments in speech audiometry. *Sound* 2, 3.

[18] HOOD J. D. & POOLE J. P. (1971) Speech audiometry in conductive and sensorineural hearing loss. *Sound* 5, 30.

[19] BROOKS D. N. (1976) Acoustic impedance. In *Scientific Foundations of Otolaryngology*, eds. Hinchcliffe R. & Harrison D. F. N., Chap. 19. London: Heinemann.

[20] JEPSEN O. (1955) *Studies on the Acoustic Strapedius Reflex in Man.* Aarhus: Universitetsforlaget.

[21] NIEMEYER W. & SESTERHENN G. (1974) Calculating the hearing threshold from the stapedius reflex threshold for different sound stimuli. *Audiology* 13, 421.

[22] ANDERSON H., BARR B. & WEDENBERG E. (1970) The early detection of acoustic tumours by the stapedius reflex test. In *Sensorineural Hearing Loss*, eds. Wolstenholme G. E. W. & Knight Julie. Ciba Foundation Symposium. London: Churchill.

[23] DAVIS H. (1976) Principles of electric response audiometry. *Annals of Otology, Rhinology and Laryngology* Suppl. 28.

[24] BEAGLEY H. A. & KELLOGG SUSAN E. (1969) A comparison of evoked responses and subjective auditory thresholds. *International Audiology* 8, 345.

[25] JEWETT D. L. & WILLISTON J. S. (1971) Auditory evoked far-fields averaged from the scalp of humans. *Brain* 94, 681.

[26] PICTON T. W., HILLYARD S. A., KRAUSZ H. & GALAMBOS R. (1974) Human auditory evoked potentials. *EEG Clinical Neurophysiology* 36, 179.

[27] PORTMANN M., LE BERT G. & ARAN J.-M. (1967) Potentiels cochléaires obtenues chez l'homme en dehors de toute intervention chirurgicale. *Revue d'Otorhinolaryngologie (Bordeaux)* 88, 157.

[28] YOSHIE N., OHASHI T. & SUZUKI T. (1967) Non-surgical recording of auditory nerve action potentials in man. *Laryngoscope* 77, 76.

[29] ARAN J.-M. & PORTMANN M. (1976) Applied cochlear electrophysiology. In *Scientific Foundations of Otolaryngology*, eds. Hinchcliffe R. & Harrison D. F. N., Chap. 21. London: Heinemann.

[30] ARAN J. M. (1971) L'electrocochléogramme. *Les Cahiers de la C.F.A. 12, 13, 14.* Compagnie Française d'Audiologie.

[31] EGGERMONT J. J., ODENTHAL D. W., SCHMIDT P. H. & SPOOR A. (1974) Electrocochleograhy. Basic principles and clinical application. *Acta Otolaryngologica (Stockh.) Suppl.* 316.

[32] RUBEN R. J., ELBERLING C. & SALOMON G. (1976) Electrocochleography. *Proceedings of Conference on Electrocochleography*, New York, 1974.

[33] DAVIS H., DEATHERAGE B. H., ELDREDGE D. H. & SMITH C. A. (1958) Summating potentials of the cochlea. *American Journal of Physiology* 195, 251.

[34] DERBYSHIRE A. J. & DAVIS H. (1935) The action potentials of the auditory nerve. *American Journal of Physiology* 113, 476.

[35] YOSHIE N. (1968) Auditory nerve action potential responses to clicks in man. *Laryngoscope* 78, 198.

[36] ELBERLING C. (1976) Deconvolution of action potentials recorded from the ear canal in man. In *Disorders of Auditory Function II*, ed. Stephens S. D. G. London: Academic Press.

[37] HUTTON J. N. T. (1976) Anaesthesia for electrocochleography. *Clinical Otolaryngology* 1, 39.

[38] SCHMIDT P. H. & SPOOR A. (1974) The place of electrocochleography in clinical audiometry. *Acta Otolaryngology (Stockh.) Suppl.* 316, 5.

[39] GIBSON W.P. R. & BEAGLEY H. A. (1975) *Electro-cochleography in the diagnosis of acoustic neuroma.* Paper read at *Section of Otology, Royal Society of Medicine*, London, February.

[40] MORRISON A. W., GIBSON W. P. R. & BEAGLEY H. A. (1976) Transtympanic electrocochleography in the diagnosis of retrocochlear tumours. *Clinical Otolaryngology* 1, 153.

[41] YOSHIE N. & OHASHI T. (1971) Abnormal adaptation of human cochlear nerve action potential responses: clinical observations by non-surgical recording. *Revue d'Otorhinolaryngologie (Bordeaux) Suppl.* 92, 673.

[42] MASLOW A. H. (1970) *Motivation and Personality.* New York: Harper and Row.

[43] McCALL ROSEMARY (1971) Link – a centre for the newly deafened. *Hearing* 26, 120.

[44] OYER H. J. & FRANKMANN JUDITH P. (1975) *Aural*

Rehabilitation Process. A Conceptual Framework Analysis. New York: Holt, Rinehart & Winston.

[45] MARTIN M. C. (1976) Auditory prostheses. In *Scientific Foundations of Otolaryngology*, eds. Hinchcliffe R. & Harrison D. F. N., Chap. 59. London: Heinemann.

[46] STEPHENS S. D. G. (1976) The input for a damaged cochlea: a brief review. *British Journal of Audiology* 10, 97.

[47] CARHART R. (170) *Principles of Competing Message Speech Audiometry. Proceedings of the Second DANA-VOX Symposium, Denmark.*

[48] NIEMEYER W. (1976) Speech audiometry. *Audiology* 15, 421.

[49] HEYES A. D. & FERRIS A. J. (1975) Auditory localisation using hearing aids. *British Journal of Audiology* 9, 102.

[50] RINTELMANN W., HARFORD E. & BURCHFIELD S. (1970) A special case of auditory localisation. *Archives of Otolaryngology* 91, 284.

[51] HARFORD E. & BARRY J. (1965) A rehabilitative approach to the problems of unilateral hearing impairments: the contralateral routing of signals (CROS). *Journal of Speech and Hearing Disorders* 30, 121.

CHAPTER 2

Investigation of Vertigo ╱

Disorders of balance can occur at all ages but most commonly in the middle-aged and elderly. Few persons living the normal life span fail to experience a disorder of balance at some time. This may be a transient phenomenon associated with weakness after a severe illness, anaemia, a viral infection, alcohol, hypertension, head trauma, motion sickness, etc. It may be recurrent associated with migraine, psychosomatic stress or inner ear disorders, or it may be a continuing disorder associated with certain diseases of the inner ear or central nervous system.

Although a clear-cut cause may be present in an individual patient this is not always the case. Often the balance disorder results from a summation of subliminal effects or from a combination of events, especially in the older age groups where the threshold of vertigo, or imbalance, is lowered by one or more diseases, so that further and often minor illnesses, fatigue, stress, anaemia, etc., tip the balance. Therefore, investigation of any balance disorder must be broadly based and must include the psychological effects [1]. The cause is more often medical than surgical and if one considers the whole cross-section of people with such a disorder it is remarkable how seldom surgery is required.

Primary inner ear disorders such as Menière's disease are relatively uncommon in a general ENT practice and acoustic neurinomata are distinctly rare.

The investigation of inner ear disorders has now reached a degree of precision which is extremely valuable, especially in relation to auditory defects. There is still much room for improvement in the differential diagnosis of vestibular disorders. Whatever methods of vestibular analysis develop now or in the future they must clearly be based upon preliminary expert audiological assessment.

History

History taking is both an art and a science. The science comes in knowing what questions to ask and the art in knowing how to ask these questions of any particular patient, and in interpreting the answers.

Much useful information is usually obtained from an exact description of the first attack of imbalance or vertigo; whether this occurred when seated, standing, walking, driving, swimming, diving, lying in bed, or in an aircraft. The time of onset, precipitating factors, the duration of the attack, the presence of headache, tinnitus, deafness, nausea, vomiting, or loss of consciousness must be carefully ascertained. The effect of head movement on the vertigo should be enquired into.

The past medical history is also essential, particularly previous ear disease, deafness and tinnitus, cardiovascular disease, migraine, peripheral vascular instability or disease, previous ototoxic drugs, head or neck trauma, cervical arthritis and diseases of the central nervous system.

The pattern of the attacks must also be discovered; their frequency, duration, regularity and severity and any difficulties in walking, turning, lying or turning over in bed, coming downstairs, crossing the road, etc., between the attacks.

The personal habits of the patient particularly in relation to alcohol and tobacco are important, as are his present and past occupations. A history of acoustic trauma must be excluded. Past and present drug treatment may have to be gone into in detail, particularly in long-standing cases. When we have completed this part of the history we know something of the patient and his background but we need to know more about his previous ear, nose, and throat problems and must ask specific questions about deafness and tinnitus. These may be unilateral or bilateral, fluctuant or frankly intermittent, or constant, associated with noise intolerance or with diplacusis, slight or severe; the pitch of the tinnitus may also give useful information. Typical groups of symptoms often occur and the experienced physician will have a 'pattern' of the common disorders in mind as he questions the patient and records the replies. The history is the main source of information upon which specialized and time-consuming tests are decided. These must be used wisely and unnecessary testing must not be started when the history taking has been inadequate.

Clinical examination

The clinical examination of a patient with vertigo begins the moment he enters the consulting room. The appearance of the patient, the way he walks and sits down should all be noted. Special attention should be given to pallor, tremor, hypo- or hyperthyroidism and excessive anxiety.

The physical examination should be approached systematically. Start by feeling the neck to see if the carotid artery pulses are equal, then put the head through a full range of neck movements to detect cervical spine disease or spasm of the posterior cervical muscles – these are all best done from behind the patient who should be sitting in a straight-backed chair. Move to the front of the patient and test for gaze nystagmus, discobolos and past pointing – then check the cranial nerves. Follow this by a routine ENT examination finishing with the ears and the hearing. Then check the blood pressure; this should preferably be done in both arms and with the patient sitting and lying down.

Finally, perform simple clinical balance tests, which can be done in the consulting room if this is of a fair size. It is helpful to have a white line 4 or 5 m long down the centre of the floor. The tests should include the Romberg test, standing on each leg with eyes open, heel-toe walking, turning quickly to right and left, walking with eyes closed and a sudden upset of the patient's balance to test for 'the defence of equilibrium'.

The last test can give valuable information but should be used with discretion especially in the elderly or in those with previous back trouble. Central disturbances tend to affect performance adversely especially in heel-toe walking, turning in both directions and in poor defence of equilibrium. Acute peripheral lesions may affect eyes-closed standing and walking, single leg standing especially when standing on the contralateral leg, and turning to the contralateral side. A quick and reliable test to establish that balance is normal at the time of the investigation is for the patient to stand on one leg with both arms outstretched forwards and the hands supinated; if he can then maintain his position for a few seconds after closing his eyes there can be little wrong with his balance. Peitersen's [2] stepping test is also useful.

If special blood, serological, radiological and electroencephalographic investigations as well as a full auditory and vestibular analysis are considered essential many of these can be done as an out-patient, but it may be more convenient for the patient and for the investigating team if short-term admission to hospital is arranged.

Interpretation
Vestibular analysis forms part of clinical assessment in which the history, clinical examination and auditory findings are essential. These preliminary examinations may, in some cases, be all that is required to make a diagnosis.

Examples of this are an acute labyrinthitis, or a chronic ear infection with labyrinthine involvement and a positive fistula sign, or a post-operative labyrinthine lesion.

Balance is upset during the acute stage of a labyrinthine upset but is usually perfectly normal between attacks. It is also affected in vertebro-basilar disease, after injury to the head and neck and after ototoxic damage to the vestibular apparatus.

In acute labyrinthitis the patient tends to fall to the side of the lesion and cannot stand or walk with the eyes closed.

In vertebro-basilar disease (where the sensori-neural hearing loss is commonly symmetrical and largely confined to the middle and higher frequencies) the main difficulty is often in heel-toe walking.

Following head injury different clinical pictures emerge depending on the site of the lesion but difficulty in standing or walking with the eyes closed and in turning quickly is common.

Whip-lash injuries of the neck causing petechial haemorrhages in the brain stem often produce difficulty with balance when the eyes are closed and failure in the defence of the patient's equilibrium when this is suddenly upset.

Severe dysequilibrium is common also in ototoxic vestibular damage and again is most apparent when the eyes are closed. These patients may have severe and dangerous vestibular disorientation when they go from light to darkness or when swimming.

Vestibular analysis

A single hearing test, under variable conditions, cannot give an accurate estimation of an individual's threshold of hearing as well as information as to the site of the lesion. Equally, a single vestibular test cannot give enough information to lead to an intelligent differential diagnosis in vertigo but for many years the caloric test has been expected to do just this, and the advent of electronystagmography further obscured the fundamental underlying problem. Although the caloric test gives information, and the bithermal caloric test more than some of the other variants, it suffers from several drawbacks.

(1) It can be difficult to irrigate some ears for mechanical reasons;

(2) the stimulus (whether hot or cold) is relatively large and unpleasant;

(3) there are considerable problems in registering and interpreting the results, which electronystagmography has increased;

(4) caloric tests are not suitable for ears with a perforated tympanic membrane or a mastoid cavity.

The main problem in testing the vestibular system is to select a reliable method of registering vestibular function and dysfunction. Unlike cochlear function where we give an auditory signal and record an auditory response, vestibular function has to be estimated through its connections with other organs. Such connections are part of the central nervous system, so that we are testing a complicated neuronal system which can have faults at several levels. When studying the induced eye movements various problems have to be overcome, many of them technical as well as those of interpretation.

The reliance placed upon the caloric test up to now has also obscured a very important aspect of vestibular function – its extreme sensitivity. We try to test auditory function with great finesse, recognizing that the ear can differentiate between sounds varying only 1 or 2 dB in loudness but we expect to get equal information from a massive vestibular stimulus delivered at one level only. The vestibular system must therefore be tested by a number of different stimuli of different intensity.

There is a wide range of auditory tests, several of which are of fundamental importance and which have been almost universally adopted and standardized. Unfortunately we have not yet reached this point in vestibular testing where the whole process is much more complex and time consuming. There is a growing appreciation that vestibular analysis must be extended and standardized.

The vestibular apparatus consists of the semicircular canals and the otolith organs and their central connections; all of these require investigation. The effect of related afferent nervous impulses which may adversely affect vestibular function must also be studied.

The semicircular canals can be tested by inducing thermal currents within a particular canal. In the traditional caloric test the head is in such a position that the horizontal canal is vertical and thermal effects are maximal. The horizontal canals can also be tested by a measured angular acceleration with the head positioned to keep these paired canals truly horizontal as in rotational testing. The torsion swing may also be used to produce deceleration and acceleration in the horizontal plane.

The otolith organ can be tested by positional tests and by the parallel swing which produces linear accelerations.

The vestibulo-optic pathways can be tested by optokinetic tests and by the study of gaze nystagmus.

The effects of cervical muscle and spinal afferents upon vestibular reflexes can be tested by neck torsion tests [3].

Electronystagmography (ENG)

Before considering the various tests in detail we must understand the technical and human problems involved in the recording of nystagmus. Before testing a patient it is important to give him a brief account of the test, emphasizing its simplicity, and reassuring and encouraging him. Stable intelligible nystagmus cannot be recorded in an anxious patient. The technician must provide the right milieu but he cannot do this if he is given insufficient time for each patient.

The subject must provide a steady eye gaze and a uniform head position (a head-rest is less efficient than a head-clamp but also less alarming). He should also suppress the blink reflex, especially with eyes open in the dark testing techniques, as blinking distorts nystagmus. Mental arousal takes the subject's mind off the test, suppresses central inhibitory factors and helps to maintain optimal conditions for testing. The exact technique of mental arousal used is probably unimportant; simple serial 7 subtraction is often satisfactory.

Patients who are tired, sleepy, uninterested or depressed do not perform well as they often make spontaneous eye and head movements which may mask nystagmus, especially of small amplitude. Attention to detail is therefore vital in performing tests at or near threshold level. At bigger stimulations producing nystagmus of greater amplitude this aspect is less critical. True ocular instability does of course also occur and must be recognized.

Other sources of interference may need to be eliminated such as static electrical charges on nylon or synthetic clothing, and electrical induction from neighbouring power cables.

The presence of congenital strabismus, congenital nystagmus and powerful latent spontaneous nystagmus (nystagmus not visible to the naked eye but which appears on electronystagmographic recordings under certain conditions) all interfere with the recording of induced nystagmus whichever stimulus is employed [4].

Preparation and fitting of electrodes

Using a modern AC ENG and a high impedance input, the exact position of each electrode is not very important provided they are fitted in the correct plane. If the electrode is too far from the signal source the signal becomes weak and artefacts will tend to dominate if amplification is increased to compensate for the weak signal. Placing the electrodes too near the eye also causes problems, e.g. paste in the eyelashes, and low frequency electrode movement, due to movement of the eyelids and peri-orbital muscles, plus the effect of tears, etc., causing instability of the tracing.

Electrode connections may be checked using an ohmmeter, but in practice a clear stable recorded base line plus precise voluntary eye movements (i.e. calibrated eye movements) are sufficient to demonstrate successful connections. Poor connections result in unwanted signals.

The *polarity* of electrodes is very important as the direction of nystagmus must be recorded in a standard way. The electrodes therefore must be placed in such a way as to conform to a conventional standard, i.e. quick phase *left* = downward deflection on recording paper; quick phase *right* = upward deflection. Different instruments use different electrode lead codes, but symbols, letters or colour codes are usually provided.

It is essential to carry out a pre-test calibration of the electrodes so that eye displacement measured in millimetres can be converted into degrees.

Types of amplification

Direct current (DC) amplification is desirable if information regarding the precise position of the eye is required, i.e. the exact part of the eye movement range in which the nystagmus is beating. DC amplification requires more care with fitting the electrodes and skin cleansing. This system is also more liable to pen drift in response to low frequency inputs, e.g. gentle head movements, or electrode lead movement and peri-orbital skin and muscle movements. Using the electrodes for more than 30 minutes increases the problems, due to body heat drying up the electrode paste and increasing the skin–electrode resistance.

An alternative to DC amplification is alternating current (AC) with a stabilizing factor known as a time constant which centralizes the pen, following a change of potential, in a pre-determined time. The longer the time constant the more the response becomes like that of DC amplification and generally the more problematic the instrument is. Conversely, the use of shorter time constants, e.g. 3–5 seconds, improve markedly the stability of the equipment, maintaining a constant tendency to centre the pen so that recorded information is written straight down the centre of the recording chart.

AC amplifiers with time constants therefore provide an excellent means of recording nystagmus and present the result in a stable way. If a time constant of 3 seconds is used, nystagmus of a frequency not less than 1 in 3 seconds will be recorded faithfully, both quick and slow phases as in pure DC recording.

AC recorded nystagmus can therefore be always interpreted provided the time constant is known and is not so short that return of the pen simulates the slow phase of nystagmus. The recording of gaze nystagmus is most faithfully recorded by DC amplification [5] but AC recording can also be used provided the time constant factor is understood.

Positional tests

These are usually performed as described by Dix & Hallpike [6]. The induced nystagmus is observed visually with the eyes open and fixed on a reference point, or by ENG with the eyes shut. The value of this test is to show whether nystagmus can be induced by position change; the result can be recorded by ENG but this seldom adds to the value of the test.

Marked nystagmus is usually peripheral in origin, is fatiguable and may sometimes be accompanied by vertigo violent enough to make visual observation difficult and ENG impossible. A vertical component is often present in positional nystagmus.

This test has the disadvantage that a certain amount of neck torsion is produced in each head-down position. Suitable tilting tables have been used to produce the same head positions without neck torsion. In some patients neck torsion is responsible for the nystagmus rather than the actual head position in space [7]; ENG is almost obligatory with such tilting equipment.

Interpretation

Head positioning produces a fatiguable nys-

tagmus in many patients with idiopathic positional nystagmus thought to be due to a benign otolith disturbance following many head injuries, and in some patients with vertigo where multiple factors appear to be operating and no clear diagnosis emerges.

A non-fatiguable positional nystagmus is associated with central lesions. Direction changing nystagmus of this type is associated with brain stem lesions. Direction fixed persistent nystagmus may also occur in brain stem lesions or in peripheral lesions in approximately equal numbers. Transient positional nystagmus may also occur in peripheral and brain stem lesions [8, 9].

Caloric tests

The bithermal caloric test with water at 30° and 44° C is standard practice in most units in the United Kingdom. The hot tests alone are probably sufficient to give all the requisite information [10] but this has not been widely adopted.

Attention to detail in the test is important. The water must be at the correct temperature, the irrigating nozzle must enter but not obstruct the external auditory canal and the patient's head must be correctly positioned.

If the nystagmus is observed visually the patient must fix his eyes on a spot directly in front of him; the duration of the nystagmus is measured as accurately as possible by the observer. If ENG is used the patient's eyes are closed for the duration of each thermal test.

This test has marked limitations. It was designed to give a moderate stimulus to each ear separately when little was known of vestibular response threshold, so that patients with a very low threshold may experience sweating, nausea and vomiting: in those with a moderate threshold the test is unpleasant, and the test is only tolerated in those with a naturally high or pathologically raised threshold. It is not a delicate test, and 'normal' caloric reactions are frequently obtained (by both visual and ENG recordings) in patients with vestibular symptoms and audiological abnormalities. Conversely 'abnormal' reactions often occur in patients with normal hearing and no vestibular symptoms.

Interpretation

In most patients requiring caloric tests, auditory clues will be of paramount importance. A unilateral sensorineural deafness is present in patients with Menière's disease, acoustic neuromata and perilymph fistula; it fluctuates in Menière's disease and perilymph fistula; recruitment may be present in all three (although least likely in an acoustic neurinoma), but tone decay is present only in acoustic neuroma. Balance is usually normal in all three conditions and the head positional tests, neck torsion tests and optokinetic tests are negative. While a clear-cut canal paresis or marked directional preponderance gives definite information, in the vast majority of patients with imbalance or vertigo the results of the caloric test are inconclusive and often almost meaningless.

The advent of ENG was hailed as a great step forward. Instead of 'we will do a caloric test' it became 'we will do an ENG' as if such an examination was equivalent scientifically to an ECG or EEG. On the contrary, ENG introduced many new problems without solving any of the old ones and without increasing the differential diagnostic potential of the test.

Using the normal bithermal technique and recording by ENG we must be able to interpret our recordings. First, we find that the duration of the reaction is at least 1 minute longer than with the eyes open technique. Secondly, the left cold and right hot water stimuli produce nystagmus beating quickly to the *right* and the right cold and left hot produce quick nystagmus to the *left*.

Apart from the duration of the reaction, which with ENG may be of little importance, the frequency, the amplitude, the 'character' and other parameters relating to the nystagmus should also be studied.

The maximum frequency is considered at the height of the reaction over a 10 or 20 second period. The paper speed is known and as calibrated paper is normally used it is simple to work out the beats per second. Similar portions of each trace can be measured and the differences compared.

Amplitude is measured by previous calibration of the pen movements in relation to known horizontal eye movements. The average maximum amplitude over the same time intervals of each trace can then be estimated.

The speed of the slow component in nystagmus produced by DC recording or with AC recordings using a long time constant can be estimated. This is related to the total eye activity and has been used by many investigators to represent the vestibular reaction to thermal tests [11, 12].

With AC recording another representative figure can be calculated: the 'average eye shift per second' over the maximum reaction period, which is the sum of all the individual amplitudes divided by the time [13].

This is a relatively simple and practical expression of the eye activity. It obviates the need for accurate calculation of the speed of the slow phase of nystagmus for which the less robust DC recording equipment is required.

Normally all these parameters should be similar on both sides and in relation to both hot and cold stimuli. In patients with canal paresis the average eye shift is reduced on the affected side because both amplitude and frequency are reduced, but the duration of the reaction may not be significantly abnormal.

Nystagmic traces may be affected by the presence of latent spontaneous nystagmus. This often appears while testing with the eyes closed or open in the dark. It must not be confused with gaze nystagmus.

When a minor degree of latent spontaneous nystagmus is present (e.g. to the right) we find that the left cold and right hot reactions which produce right beating nystagmus are enhanced and that the left beating nystagmus produced by the opposite tests may be reduced, but if a strong latent spontaneous nystagmus is present, such as may occur soon after vestibular neuronitis, the picture may be quite different [14]. Here the nystagmus beats in the same direction in three of the four traces, accentuated or reduced on the 'active' side and unaffected on the inactive side; in effect a canal paresis masked by the spontaneous nystagmus. To determine the 'duration' or end-point of the nystagmus we must study the reaction carefully noting the diminution of the amplitude and the reduction in frequency. Frequently we find a slight reactionary (or counterswing) nystagmus in the opposite direction just after the end of the true reaction, and this helps in localizing the end-point. Usually this can be localized within 1–3 seconds. In addition to frequency, amplitude, direction and duration we can also study the character of the nystagmus. It may be rhythmical or dysrhythmical, well or poorly shaped, disproportionately large or small in relation to the calibration, and of exceptionally high frequency. In short, with ENG recording of caloric nystagmus we can demonstrate qualitative as well as quantitative changes.

To summarize: clear-cut findings are the exception rather than the rule in caloric testing. With a unilateral peripheral lesion a canal paresis on that side is found which may present as a total paralysis in an advanced lesion, or as a relatively minor loss of function in early cases. Directional preponderance of the nystagmus to the opposite side is also often present in a peripheral lesion and may co-exist with canal paresis.

If directional preponderance only is present this may be caused by a nuclear or supranuclear lesion on the same side. Minor degrees of directional preponderance are commonly found in normal individuals [15].

The caloric test may be similar in Ménière's disease, perilymph fistula and an early acoustic neuroma, but when the acoustic neuroma is more advanced there is a canal paresis on this side.

Rotation tests

Balance is not a unilateral function nor is it entirely comparable to the special senses of hearing, sight, taste and smell, all of which are relatively pure special senses. Balance depends upon many afferent nervous impulses from various parts of the body and the function is largely a computerized one, with the central nervous system playing the vital role. Faulty or altered afferent impulses can affect the system, just as unilateral labyrinthine disease can upset the harmony between the two sides. Disease in the vestibular nuclei can also interfere in what should be a balanced pattern. Therefore, if we confine our vestibular testing to unilateral tests much valuable information about the state of the vestibular system generally is lost.

A person with a non-functioning vestibular apparatus in one ear may have perfect balance and be symptom free because of central compensation. Conversely, a patient may have normal caloric test results but be suffering from vertiginous attacks or from chronic imbalance. In the latter case we assume that the peripheral mechanism is little affected whereas the central controlling mechanism is faulty.

Real progress in rotational testing was not made until sophisticated rotational equipment and ENG became available. Initially the turning equipment was used in much the same way as with thermal stimuli to give a relatively massive stimulus. This formed the basis of *cupulometry*, where a stop stimulus was applied after a constant speed of rotation had been achieved. Different grades of stimulus could be used [16] allowing the first attempts to plot stimuli against nystagmic reactions. This was a big step forward but the majority of the stimuli were still relatively large, so that it was difficult to demonstrate slight or early vestibular lesions. As technology advanced it became clear that accurate and finely adjustable turning equipment, combined with ENG, provided sources of information unobtainable with thermal unilateral tests. Graded series of stimulations can be used and the effects of turning clockwise or anti-clockwise compared.

The true threshold of vestibular function can be estimated by a simple standardized [17] technique using a low intensity acceleratory stimulus. Large stimuli can also be given and the equipment can also be used for cupulometry.

If the nystagmus induced by all these stimuli is measured it can be plotted against the stimulus so that comparisons can be made between clockwise and anti-clockwise function and between the response to low, medium and strong stimuli. There is an almost direct correlation between eye movement and stimulus in normal people, but not in certain diseases.

Other parameters can also be measured. For instance, the normal semicircular canal responds to a very small acceleratory stimulus with virtually no latent period but a damaged vestibular system, especially after certain head injuries, may show considerable increase in the latent period even with large stimuli. Similarly, if we have a latent spontaneous nystagmus to one side, we can measure the 'strength' of this nystagmus by finding the rotational stimulus in the opposite direction which just overcomes it. With varied stimuli the 'character' of the nystagmus may give information which is not readily translated into a conventional figure such as 'speed of slow component', 'duration', 'eye shift per second' or 'frequency'.

Interpretation

The chief values of rotational tests in interpretation of the clinical picture are in plotting the nystagmic reaction against the stimulus, in observing the presence or absence of latent spontaneous nystagmus and in measuring its strength and in noting the character changes of the nystagmus in response to the different grades of stimulus.

Rotational activity is grossly diminished by ototoxic drugs like streptomycin and neomycin [18], when frequency and amplitude of nystagmus are both affected. Gross asymmetry of reaction is the common finding in recent cases of vestibular neuronitis; this is usually associated with a strong latent spontaneous nystagmus to one side only [14].

In Menière's disease activity is also reduced but in an unusual manner, the frequency of beating being often within the normal range but amplitude is down to one-half or one-third of normal; this usually occurs on both sides even if the hearing loss is unilateral [19]. Rotational tests used in this way can also estimate function before and after drug therapy [20]. They can similarly be used to assess the results of diagnostic procedures such as cervical sympathetic block or the glycerol test or a histamine drip; and/or therapeutic procedures such as drainage of the endolymphatic sac, division of the vestibular branch of the eighth cranial nerve and cervical sympathectomy.

In brief, rotational tests and/or torsion swing tests provide valuable differential diagnostic information complementary to that provided by thermal tests.

Neck torsion tests

Nystagmus produced by disease of the cervical spine or muscles is usually fine and difficult to detect visually so that ENG should be used. The neck can be extended, flexed, twisted or tilted to either side; either the eyes should be kept shut or the test can be performed in a darkened chamber with the eyes open.

The induced nystagmus may occur with one type of movement of the neck only and always be in the same direction, or it may occur with different neck movements and may sometimes be to one side and sometimes to the other. A vertical component is again sometimes found. The value of the test is to demonstrate that cervical factors may be causing, or contributing to, vertigo. 'Cervical' vertigo is common and is a very satisfactory form of imbalance to treat [3].

Interpretation

Neck torsion, commonly to one side only, produces a fine, usually fatiguable, nystagmus if the cervical spine or musculature appears to be the source of afferent nerve disturbance of the vestibular nuclear function. It can do so in patients with cervical arthritis, with or without evidence of vertebro-basilar insufficiency and after trauma to the head and neck.

Gaze nystagmus tests

The equipment and technique for studying this type of spontaneous nystagmus has been described by Hood [5] who emphasizes the necessity for DC recording.

Interpretation

Gaze nystagmus is present in peripheral labyrinthine lesions when it is increased by eye closure, in lesions of the eighth nerve where it is decreased by eye closure and in central lesions where it is abolished by eye closure [5].

Optokinetic tests

Many methods of delivering optokinetic stimuli have been devised but for clinical purposes a simple drum with a suitable ball-bearing axle is sufficient. This can be placed at a fixed distance from the patient's eyes and is revolved horizontally or vertically to provoke the appropriate type of nystagmus. Black and white stripes are usually used on the drum, but for children other more interesting visual stimuli, such as animal paintings, can be used. In more refined equipment the optokinetic stimulus revolves around the patient, or the patient rotates while the stimulus remains stationary [21].

Visual observation of the induced horizontal nystagmus differentiates gross inequalities to right and left, but ENG allows more accurate study. Horizontal rotation of the drum to the patient's left produces nystagmus with the quick phase to the right and vice versa. If the drum rotates at the same speed in opposite directions the nystagmus should be equal and symmetrical. Vertical rotation of the drum upwards, and downwards in front of the patient, produces vertical optokinetic nystagmus which should be equal and symmetrical in the two directions.

Interpretation

While markedly deficient optokinetic nystagmus to one side usually denotes a central brain stem lesion [22], lesser abnormalities are not confined to central lesions. For instance when there is clear dominance of function to one side on rotation testing it is common to find a similar predominance on optokinetic testing. In many such cases the clinical and audiological findings suggest a peripheral lesion.

Optokinetic asymmetry is marked in central disorders of the vestibulo-optic system [21] but it can and frequently does occur to a more limited extent in any case where there is a pronounced LSN to one side, where there is a positive gaze nystagmus, or where there is a pronounced preponderance of induced nystagmus on semicircular canal testing procedures.

The majority of temporo-parietal cerebral lesions are associated with abnormal or absent horizontal optic nystagmus on the contralateral side: in brain stem lesions this is characteristically on the same side while in lesions of the pons or mesencephalon the changes are on both sides [22]. Vertical optic nystagmus changes are present in about 75% of cases where the horizontal nystagmus is abnormal. This is true in supratentorial lesions in which cases 50% show changes in both vertical directions. In brain stem lesions the proportion falls to 68% of whom 30% get changes in both vertical directions. In almost all lesions of the pons or mesencephalon vertical changes in both directions are found.

It should be noted that all vertigo due to disease of the peripheral organ or the vestibular nuclei is exacerbated by head movement.

Eye tracking test

This test consists of the recording of eye movements in response to a visual pendular stimulus which produces a sinusoidal curve tracing, which indicates the quality of eye movement. Four patterns are described [23]:

(1) sinusoidal;

(2) sinusoidal with superimposed non-nystagmic movements;

(3) sinusoidal with superimposed nystagmic or saccadic movements;

(4) non-sinusoidal.

The first two patterns are normal. Non-sinusoidal is always due to central changes while sinusoidal with superimposed nystagmic movements can occur in peripheral lesions (33%) or in central lesions (67%).

Torsion swing tests

The basic equipment consists of a chair suspended by two chains or a single high tension wire; the bottom of the chair can be fixed to the floor in such a way that the movements of the chair and degree of swing are limited.

The chair executes sinusoidal movements provoking positive and negative angular accelerations and the stimulus progressively declines. The chair must be weighted so that the movements are standard irrespective of the weight of the patient. This is a valid scientific method of testing which provides accurate repeatable nystagmus throughout a range of stimuli. Electronystagmography is essential [24].

Parallel swing tests

Again the equipment is uncomplicated [25]. A platform (or stretcher) is suspended by four cables and the movement is again a sinusoidal one but this time inducing a linear acceleration and not an angular one. Gravity and the linear horizontal accelerations, forwards and backwards, act together and produce both vestibular sensations and reflex eye movements. The latter are not nystagmus but are compensatory movements which follow the movements of the swing.

Sono-ocular test

All normal people probably have a threshold at which acoustic stimuli produce nystagmus, but some have an abnormally low threshold which may account for certain cases of noise-linked vertigo. Direct contact between the stapes base and the membranous labyrinth may be the responsible factor [26, 27].

Galvanic test

A constant current of 0·5 milli-amps adjustable from 0–25 volts, with the direction controlled by a foot switch, is applied to a blindfolded subject standing in the Romberg position. First a negative charge is applied to the left mastoid and then a positive charge; the same test is then applied to the right mastoid. The time measured before the patient loses balance and the reactions on the two sides are compared. The test is seldom used.

Special investigations

Cervical sympathetic block

Although the precise role of the autonomic nervous system in relation to inner ear function is not known, cochlear function is certainly affected by local changes in blood supply [28], particularly in sensorineural hearing loss when the low tones are predominantly affected and spontaneous fluctuations of hearing occur. Sympathetic release in these cases frequently causes hearing gains within 20–30 minutes, and diminution of the tinnitus. A sympathetic block has also been used successfully in the treatment of acute episodes of vertigo in Menière's disease [29, 30].

Infiltration of the stellate ganglion itself is unnecessary, the local anaesthetic should be injected just anterior to the pre-vertebral fascia in the region of the sixth cervical vertebra on the appropriate side and with the patient lying on a couch with the head slightly extended and turned a little to the opposite side. After injection the patient should sit up vertically to allow the anaesthetic to gravitate down to the stellate ganglion; a Horner's syndrome should develop within a few minutes.

The test is of therapeutic as well as diagnostic value. If the hearing improves and tinnitus diminishes, or vertigo is abolished, this is immediately apparent to the patient, and confirms the reversibility or partial reversibility of the lesion.

Such reversibility is also of diagnostic value to the investigator. It occurs particularly in true Menière's disease without severe hearing impairment, and can be very important if both ears are involved and bilateral cervical sympathectomy [28] is being considered as part of the management. The injection can be given on each side at the same time by anyone skilled in the technique.

Glycerol test

This is designed to cause a chemically-induced hypotension of the inner ear [31]. It is an efficient and reliable test and frequently produces improvements in hearing threshold in patients with endolymphatic hydrops and fluctuating hearing. No effect occurs in more advanced cases with non-fluctuating hearing loss or in perceptive deafness of less specific types. It can therefore be used to differentiate between reversible and irreversible cases of Menière's disease and from other cases of perceptive deafness without endolymphatic hydrops. There are two minor disadvantages; it cannot be used selectively on one ear and it usually produces an unpleasant temporary headache.

Blood and cerebrospinal fluid tests

Syphilitic involvement of the inner ear often causes inner ear symptoms although cochlear loss is usually the main finding. Congenital syphilis is the main culprit and can cause Menière-like symptoms, especially in the 40–60-year-old age group.

The most reliable serological test is the fluorescent treponemal antibody absorption test which is often positive long after the Wassermann test has become negative [32].

Serum cholesterol estimation can be valuable. Tinnitus and deafness are often present in atherosclerotic cerebrovascular degenerative disease and the vestibule may also be involved.

Serum osmolality estimation before and after the administration of oral glycerol can give valuable information. In those with endolymphatic hydrops there is a pronounced rise in the osmolality, which does not occur in normal individuals or in those without hydrops [33].

Cerebrospinal fluid protein is elevated in an advanced acoustic neuroma but is usually normal in cases confined to the internal auditory meatus.

Radiology

Although radiology has been used to demonstrate a labyrinthine fistula and abnormalities of the endolymphatic sac its main use is in delineating the auditory meatus and in the diagnosis of acoustic neuromata. This may be achieved by top quality straight skull radiography using careful positioning of the head and tube, or by tomography. But the majority of these tumours are finally defined by radiopaque fluid myelography. The normal internal auditory meatus should, with suitable positioning, fill with the fluid and a filling defect on the side of a suspected neuroma is significant. Such filling defects occur even in early cases. This technique is described further in Chapter 4.

The development of brain stem scanning techniques using radioactive isotopes injected into the cerebral circulation is also of significance in relation to vertigo. Petechial haemorrhages occur in brain stem injuries even in the absence of serious skull damage and of neurological signs. Such injuries appear to induce vascular spasm in the area affected causing relative ischaemia of the brain stem vestibular nuclei, and possibly permanent impairment of balance.

Electroencephalography

While never a primary investigation, this may form part of the neurological or neurosurgical assessment if a space-occupying cerebral lesion is suspected.

References

[1] HINCHCLIFFE R. (1967) Personality profile in Menière's disease. *Journal of Laryngology and Otology* 81, 447.

[2] PEITERSEN E. (1967) Vestibulo-spinal reflexes. *Archives of Otolaryngology* 85, 192.

[3] JONGKEES L. B. W. (1969) Cervical vertigo. *The Laryngoscope* 79, 1473.

[4] COATES A. C. (1968) Central and peripheral optokinetic asymmetry. *Annals of Otology* 77, 938.

[5] HOOD J. D. (1968) Electronystagmography. *Journal of Laryngology and Otology* 82, 167.

[6] DIX M. R. & HALLPIKE C. S. (1952) The pathology, symptoms, and diagnosis of certain common disorders of the vestibular system. *Annals of Otology* 61, 987.

[7] BARBER H. O. (1964) Positional nystagmus testing and interpretation. *Annals of Otology* 73, 838.

[8] BARBER H. O. (1964) Positional nystagmus especially after brain injury. *The Laryngoscope* 74, 891.

[9] DOLOWITZ D. (1972) Cristo-ocular and cristo-spinal reflexes – a review after 1000 cases of vertigo. *The Laryngoscope* 82, 1410.

[10] HINCHCLIFFE R. (1967) Validity of measures of caloric test response. *Acta Oto-Laryngologica (Stockh.)* 63, 69.

[11] COATS A. C. (1965) Electronystagmographic examination history, technique and interpretation. *Medical Records Annal (Houston)* 58, 48.

[12] BLAUERT J. (1972) The electronystagmometer. A new aid in quantitative vestibulometry. *Journal of Laryngology and Rhinology* 51–52, 110.

[13] LINTHICUM F. H. & CHURCHILL D. (1968) Vestibular test results in acoustic tumour cases. *Archives of Otolaryngology* 88, 604.

[14] WILMOT T. J. (1973) Vestibular analysis in vestibular neuronitis. *Journal of Laryngology and Otology* 87, 239.

[15] MILOJEVIC B. (1965) Vestibular asymmetrics in right and left handed people. *Acta Oto-Laryngologica (Stockh.)* 60, 322.

[16] VAN EGMOND A. L. J., GROEN J. J. & JONGKEES L. B. W. (1948) The turning test with small regulable stimuli. *Journal of Laryngology and Otology* 62, 63.

[17] DITTRICH F. L. & WILMOT T. J. (1965) Threshold testing of vestibular function. *Journal of Laryngology and Otology* 79, 888.

[18] WILMOT T. J. (1973) Vestibular analysis in streptomycin ototoxicity. *Journal of Laryngology and Otology* 87, 235.

[19] WILMOT T. J. (1973) Vestibular analysis in Menière's disease. *Journal of Laryngology and Otology* 88, 295.

[20] WILMOT T. J. (1971) An objective study of the effect of betahistine hydrochloride on hearing and vestibular function tests in patients with Menière's disease. *Journal of Laryngology and Otology* 85, 369.

[21] HOOD J. D. (1967) Observations upon the neurological mechanism of opto-kinetic nystagmus with special reference to the contribution of peripheral vision. *Acta Oto-Laryngologica (Stockh.)* 63, 208.

[22] TOS M., ADSER J. & ROSBERG J. (1973) Optokinetic nystagmus in diseases of the central nervous system. *Journal of Laryngology and Otology* 87, 333.

[23] BENITEZ J. T. (1970) Eye-tracking and opto-kinetic tests. Diagnostic significance in peripheral and central disorders. *The Laryngoscope* 80, 834.

[24] JANEKE C. E., JANEKE J. B. & OOSTERVELD W. J. (1971) An improved version of the torsion-swing chair. *Annals of Otology* **80**, 229.

[25] OOSTERVELD W. J. (1970) The parallel-swing. *Archives of Otolaryngology* **91**, 154.

[26] KACKER S. K. & HINCHCLIFFE R. (1970) Unusual Tullio phenomenon. *Journal of Laryngology and Otology* **84**, 155.

[27] STEPHENS S. D. G. & BALLAM H. M. (1974) The sono-ocular test. *Journal of Laryngology and Otology* **88**, 1049.

[28] SEYMOUR J. C. (1960) The aetiology, pathology and conservative treatment of Menière's disease. *Journal of Laryngology and Otology* **74**, 599.

[29] PASSE E. R. G. (1948) Menière's syndrome. Successful treatment by surgery on the sympathetic. *British Medical Journal* **2**, 812.

[30] WILMOT T. J. (1969) Sympathectomy for Menière's disease – long-term review. *Journal of Laryngology and Otology* **83**, 323.

[31] KLOCKHOFF I. (1966) Endolymphatic hydrops revealed by glycerol test. *Acta Oto-Laryngologica (Stockh.)* **61**, 459.

[32] KERR A. G., SMITH G. D. L. & CINNAMOND M. J. (1973) Congenital syphilitic deafness. *Journal of Laryngology and Otology* **87**, 1.

[33] ANGELBORG C., KLOCKHOFF I. & STAHLE J. (1973) Serum osmolality in patients with Menière's disease. *Acta Oto-Laryngologica (Stockh.)* **76**, 450.

CHAPTER 3

Pathology and Treatment of Vertigo

MENIÈRE'S DISEASE

This condition, first described by Prosper Menière in 1861, consists of episodic attacks of vertigo, associated with nausea, vomiting, tinnitus and sensorineural deafness.

Pathology

Despite much research the aetiology is still not fully understood. The most consistent histological finding is of endolymphatic hydrops. Various theories have been advanced to explain this and they fall into two main groups:

(1) Disturbance in the formation of the inner ear fluids, which results in an increase in the endolymphatic compartment; and

(2) Disordered function of the endolymphatic sac, resulting in decreased absorption and, therefore, accumulation of endolymph.

Those concerned with abnormal fluid formation are mainly dependent on the principle of radial flow of inner ear fluids [1]. This suggests that the stria vascularis absorbs the endolymph and that this is derived from surrounding perilymph. Any decrease in the production of perilymph could, therefore, result in an apparent increase of endolymph which later becomes a true increase as electrolyte content in the endolymph increases. Others have thought the basic defect to be one of excess histamine being present in the stria vascularis causing a vasodilatation, increase in capillary permeability, and hydrops [2]. Underlying labyrinthine ischaemia has also been thought for some time to be the basic defect present. One theory suggests that this results in local anoxia and production of a decreased amount of endolymph of high osmolarity [3]. Fluid is then transferred by osmosis from the surrounding perilymph and vascular spaces to the endolymph. There is, however, no theory yet which is universally accepted.

There is also evidence which suggests that the underlying problem is one of malfunction of the endolymphatic sac which, it has been proposed, resorbs the endolymph [4]. This theory has been lent support by experiments where endolymphatic hydrops was reproduced in guinea pigs [5], cats [6], and rabbits [7] by obliterating the endolymphatic duct or by destroying the sac. The microscopic appearance of the endolymphatic sac in animals is similar to that found in structures with an absorptive function [8] and it is thought that loss of this function results in an accumulation of endolymph and, therefore, hydrops [9]. Although this theory has received some support from the results of shunt procedures in man the underlying reason for this dysfunction is not clear.

Other proposals for the aetiology of the disease have included avitaminosis [10], viral infection [11], endocrine disturbance [12], and psychosomatic disorder [13], but none of these have gained wide acceptance.

The histopathological feature of the disease is an increase in volume of the pars inferior, the cochlea and saccule, of the endolymphatic system. Reissner's membrane becomes distorted and displaced into the scala vestibuli. The saccule also becomes dilated early in the disease and in severe cases it displaces the utricle postero-superiorly and lies in contact with the underside of the footplate. Reissner's membrane may be herniated and in some cases this may extend through the helicotrema and into the scala tympani as far as the second turn [14]; complete collapse of the membranous labyrinth may also occur, presumably after rupture. It has been suggested that build-up of pressure causes acute attacks which

34

are relieved by rupture [15]. This hypothesis, however, has not gained general acceptance.

Atrophic changes in the organ of Corti have been described [16] but these were seen in only two out of thirteen ears with Menière's disease. Electronmicroscopy has similarly shown atrophic changes in the cochlea [17], these changes, however, being indistinguishable from those which are attributed to ageing [18].

Clinical features

The classical triad of symptoms associated with Menière's disease is vertigo, deafness, and tinnitus. To these can be added nausea and vomiting during acute attacks. The attacks are episodic in character with intervals of remission, lasting from a few weeks to several years, during which the tinnitus may diminish and the hearing improve. Occasionally the attacks come in clusters. The first of these is often the worst and the subsequent, quickly occurring attacks diminish in severity until they stop.

The disease can occur at any age although it is rare in childhood [19] and it starts most commonly in the fifth and sixth decades. Males are affected slightly more than females. Bilateral involvement occurs in from 10% [20] to 44% [21] the difference between these figures reflecting the time of observation and criteria used.

The acute attack is characterized by the sudden onset of severe vertigo. Some patients may experience prodromal symptoms of fullness in the ear or a dull ache which forewarns them of an attack and allows them to prepare for it. In others the onset of vertigo is immediate, causing the patient to fall or collapse. The vertigo, usually rotatory, but occasionally with linear components or rocking motions, is severe. The patient lies as still as possible with the eyes closed, often holding on to a nearby object for support because any slight movement worsens the vertigo. Nausea and vomiting soon follow. Vagal symptoms of sweating, abdominal pain, and bradycardia may be present, presumably arising from spread of impulses within the brain stem. Diarrhoea also occasionally occurs. The vertigo gradually settles within a few minutes or hours. It is then that the concomitant symptoms of deafness and tinnitus become troublesome.

After an interval of a few hours or a few days the patient's life returns to normal. The anxiety associated with the acute episode settles and the dysequilibrium improves. Injudicious or sudden head movements, however, still can cause unsteadiness and these are avoided.

The deafness present in nearly every case tends to improve between attacks initially but if they become frequent the hearing loss becomes more permanent. The patients complain of distortion of hearing and of diplacusis; intolerance of loud noises due to recruitment may also be present. The low frequencies tend to be affected first in the earlier stages and this is characteristic of Menière's disease. Later all frequencies are affected to produce a flat audiogram or a high tone loss.

Tinnitus is present in most cases, and is of a variable type often described as a persistent background hum; it can be quite distressing and, like deafness, may have been present before the vertiginous episodes commenced.

Variants of the clinical picture have been described where vertigo exists for some time before the deafness develops. In other patients deafness and tinnitus are followed by the later development of vertigo.

The Lermoyez syndrome, sometimes considered a reverse form of Menière's disease, consists of episodes of deafness and tinnitus lasting a few days. This is followed by an episode of vertigo following which the hearing improves.

Investigation

Clinical examination

General examination of the patient is mandatory, particular attention being paid to the cardiovascular system and the central nervous system.

Examination of the ears usually shows normal mobile tympanic membranes but it is performed to rule out other pathological conditions which can mimic the disease. Previous operations such as stapedectomy can give rise to similar symptoms and, of course, evidence of labyrinthine fistula secondary to chronic ear disease should be sought.

In the acute attack examination of the eyes will show a persistent nystagmus directed to either side in early cases but as labyrinthine function is diminished the quick component of the nystagmus is usually towards the opposite ear.

Blood samples should be sent for haemoglobin, blood film, and serological tests for syphilis.

Audiological investigation
Tuning fork tests will, if deafness is present, show a sensorineural deafness. A false negative Rinné test may be found where there is a severe unilateral deafness.

Pure-tone audiometry in early cases will show a sensorineural deafness usually involving the low tones. If the condition is more advanced the curve becomes flatter. Some improvement in thresholds may be seen in early cases between attacks. No particular curve is pathognomonic of the disease.

Good correlation is found between the threshold for speech and the pure tone threshold. Owing to distortion there is diminished speech discrimination but this is not as severe as in neural lesions. Loudness balance, when it can be performed, demonstrates complete or over recruitment but there is no tone decay and Békésy audiometry will usually show a type II response.

Vestibular tests
In early cases caloric tests may show little or no abnormality but later may show a reduced function on the affected side. This may be demonstrated by a canal paresis on that side, a directional preponderance to the other side, or a combination of both [22]. Normal caloric tests put the diagnosis in doubt.

Electronystagmography should be done when possible. Latent spontaneous nystagmus will often be seen after an acute attack when it cannot be seen with the naked eye. There is no positional nystagmus and caloric testing may confirm the hypofunction of the affected side. Hypofunction of the other side raises the possibility of bilateral involvement.

Radiology
Views of the petrous bones should be taken, careful attention being paid to the internal auditory meatus. Tomography of the vestibular aqueduct has been advocated to demonstrate its patency as sufferers from Menière's disease were said to show stenosis or obliteration [23]. This has been challenged, however, by the consistent finding in temporal bones of normal vestibular aqueducts with narrower than normal endolymphatic ducts [24, 25]. The vestibular aqueducts are said to be consistently shorter and straighter than in normal subjects [24].

Special tests
The *glycerol test* can be a valuable diagnostic aid. Transient hearing improvement occurs after a measured dose of glycerol [26, 27] in some patients. This is said to indicate that a good result will be obtained from saccus surgery [28]. If the hearing does not improve saccus surgery is not indicated.

Electrocochleography may prove useful in diagnosis. Studies carried out so far have shown an increased negative summation potential thought to be due to the displacement of Reissner's membrane in the disease [29]. There may also be widening of the action potential and summation potential wave form with a reduced cochlear microphonic [30].

Treatment

The principles of treatment have been based on the supposed aetiologies and, therefore, have varied widely throughout the years. Because of the characteristic remissions, exacerbations, and spontaneous cures, assessment of treatment has been difficult. Long term follow-up is often not possible and there is as yet no treatment which has been shown to give consistently good long term benefit.

The acute attack is treated by confining the patient to bed. Sedation should be adequate and good relief is obtained using any one of a number of sedatives with anti-emetic activity. Among those used are promethazine hydrochloride (Phenergan), chlorpromazine hydrochloride (Largactil), and dimenhydrinate (Dramamine). In severe episodes intra-muscular preparations may be required – Hyoscine is often useful.

In the remission phase treatment can be medical or surgical. Most would agree that a good trial of medical treatment is always worthwhile and that surgery should only be performed if the disease is progressing.

Medical treatment

Medical treatment can be classified into the following groups:
(1) Vasodilators.
(2) Vestibular suppressants.
(3) Vestibular decompressants.
(4) Miscellaneous drugs.

Vasodilators

The use of these drugs is based on the theory of labyrinthine ischaemia causing Menière's disease. Various preparations have been used over the years, notably nicotinic acid, buphenamine hydrochloride and tolazoline hydrochloride, and thymoxamine. Of these thymoxamine (Opilon) appears to be most effective. Vasodilators appear only to be effective when the hearing loss is of low tone type and fluctuating. There have, however, been no therapeutic trials which have convincingly shown their efficacy [31].

It has been postulated [32] that histamine is an intrinsic microcirculatory dilator and this has helped reinforce the rationale for using histaminics as vasodilators. The oral histamine analogue, betahistine, has been the subject of at least three double blind trials and has been shown in all of them to be more effective than a placebo in control of vertigo [33–35]. There was also a statistically significant improvement in hearing and reduction in tinnitus in one trial [35]. It seems, therefore, that there is both theoretical and clinical justification for the continuance of this drug in the treatment of the disorder.

Vestibular suppressants

Prochlorperazine and cinnarizine are useful in controlling vertigo and are widely used. They are, however, only symptomatic treatment.

Streptomycin therapy has been utilized, more particularly in the United States, to destroy the vestibular labyrinth. Its results are less predictable than surgical treatment and carry a greater risk of cochlear damage. There may be a place for this treatment in younger people with bilateral disease who refuse operative intervention. It should never be used in older patients.

Vestibular decompressants

Alterations in the electrolyte content of the body fluids has been implicated in the aetiology of the disease [36, 37] and various regimes of salt and water restriction and diuretic agents have been tried with varying effect.

In some centres a diuretic regime is adopted vigorously in all cases with reported good results [38].

Miscellaneous drugs

Glucocorticoids and mineralocorticoids have been reported as effective agents in the disorder [31]. Their action and effect, like other drugs is, however, rather empirical and they are rarely used.

Surgical treatment

This can be classified into the following main groups:
(1) Decompression procedures.
(2) Destructive procedures.
(3) Vasodilation procedures.
(4) Miscellaneous.

Decompression procedures

Based on the premise that the effects of Menière's disease are caused by increased volume of endolymph and, therefore, increased pressure in the endolymphatic system, various techniques have been evolved in an attempt to diminish this pressure.

(a) *Decompression of the saccule*. First described in 1964 by Fick and modified by others [39], this procedure consists of inserting a small steel tack through the footplate and leaving it in position. The distended saccule comes into contact with this and automatically bursts and decompresses the endolymphatic hydrops. Further accumulation results in further dilation of the saccule and further decompression. Relief of vertigo in up to 95% of patients was claimed with, however, significant hearing loss in 18%. The flaw in this technique is that in some cases the cochlear duct becomes so dilated that it is in contact with the footplate and cochlear damage results. The operation has never achieved universal acceptance and is now rarely carried out.

(b) *Decompression of the endolymphatic sac*. The

first decompression of the endolymphatic sac was described by Portmann in 1927 [40] who made a small incision in the sac. Since then various modifications of the procedure have been described with only small differences in results.

Decompression by insertion of a Teflon endolymphatic subarachnoid shunt [41, 42] has been reported as giving relief from vertigo in 75–91% with improvement of tinnitus in about 50% and improved hearing in 11–55%.

Decompression by an incision in the external wall of the sac which is kept patent by a Teflon sheet or muscle flap gives similar results [43, 44].

Overall, two-thirds of the patients are helped by the procedure. Best results are obtained in those with a short history and a true fluctuating hearing loss with a bone and speech conduction threshold of no more than 70 dB. Caloric tests and glycerol dehydration tests may be useful in helping select the patients [28].

Destructive procedures
These techniques are all designed to relieve vertigo by destroying the end organ or its neural connections.

(a) *Ultrasonic labyrinthectomy.* The aim of this procedure is to destroy the vestibular sensory elements while leaving the cochlear component unaffected. The mode of action may be a selective destruction of the neuro-epithelium of the vestibule but alteration in the electrolyte content of the endolymph has been shown to occur in guinea pigs [45]. Results over a number of years show relief of vertigo in 70–85% of patients with, however, cochlear damage in up to 40% [46, 47]. As a conservative operation designed to stop vertigo and preserve hearing its results are not as good as saccus surgery but it can be repeated and the only complication reported is transient facial paralysis.

(b) *Vestibular neurectomy.* This technique was pioneered by Dandy in 1928 using a posterior fossa route. Many prominent otologists today now regard this operation, using a middle cranial fossa approach, as the operation of choice [44, 48, 49]. Relief of vertigo in over 90% of cases is achieved with improvement of hearing in a varying number. The reason for the cochlear improvement is not understood and long-term fol-

low-up shows a deterioration in hearing [50]. This one would expect, as the operation is purely symptomatic and not designed to relieve endolymphatic hydrops. Those advocating this procedure claim it is safe and useful as it preserves hearing, at least temporarily. The only stipulation is that the hearing loss should be no greater than 70 dB with 50% speech discrimination.

(c) *Labyrinthectomy.* This is the final procedure done when there is persistent vertigo with little or no hearing present. It is not performed in bilateral disease unless absolutely necessary and it is only performed in unilateral cases as a last resort.

The approach can be transmeatal, exposing the oval window and removing the vestibular contents by suction and dissection, but the destruction may be incomplete. The transmastoid approach involves exposing and removing all the semicircular canals, removing the vestibular contents, and in some centres vestibular neurectomy. This will destroy any cochlear function and will rid the patient of vertigo in virtually every case. Tinnitus may not be affected.

Vasodilation procedures
In an attempt to improve the microcirculation of the labyrinth and reverse the suspected underlying sympathetic vasospasm, cervical sympathectomy has been advocated [51]. Although successful reduction in vertigo with improvement in hearing has been reported from several centres the operation has not fulfilled its earlier promise and is now rarely performed [52].

Miscellaneous procedures
Several other procedures have been advocated in the past. These include insertion of a grommet into the tympanic membrane [53] and insertion of sodium chloride into the middle ear [54]. Although encouraging results were reported by the authors their effectiveness has not been verified by subsequent investigators.

Summary of treatment

Since an undetermined number of cases become bilateral conservatism is essential. A trial of medical measures, consisting of vasodilators, betahistine, or vestibular suppressants, should be carried out on all patients. If this fails to control the vertigo even after as little as 3 months a surgical procedure is required. If the hearing loss is fluctuating and responds well to glycerol dehydration a saccus drainage procedure should be tried. In the others with residual hearing a vestibular neurectomy should be done. Finally, after all else fails to control a distressing vertigo with no residual hearing, a transmastoid labyrinthectomy with or without vestibular neurectomy should be performed.

VESTIBULAR NEURONITIS

This condition was first recognized and investigated in the late 1940s [55]. It consists essentially of a sudden and often severe unilateral vestibular failure. Other names for the condition include 'epidemic vertigo' and 'epidemic labyrinthitis'. A chronic form also exists.

Pathology

The aetiology is still obscure. Viral studies have failed to reveal any viral agent [56] but the often epidemic nature of attacks suggest an infective aetiology. In many cases there is a mild febrile illness or upper respiratory tract infection associated with the condition. The sexes are equally involved with the majority of cases occurring between the ages of 30 and 50 years.

The site of involvement has not yet been established. Cochlear involvement does not occur and there are no brain stem symptoms, which would be expected if the lesion occurred there. The consensus of opinion is that the lesion is in the vestibular nerve between the labyrinth and the vestibular nuclei. Electronystagmographic studies seem to support this as does the lack of pathological findings in the labyrinth [57, 58].

Clinical features

There is a sudden onset of vertigo in some cases severe enough to cause drop attacks. Nausea and vomiting are usually present and can be severe. Head movements tend to exacerbate the vertigo and the patient lies still. The vertigo is paroxysmal and gradually settles. This can take from a few days to weeks as compensation occurs. Older people tend to take longer to recover from the vertigo and can remain unsteady for some months after the attack. There are no cochlear symptoms and no other neurological disturbances.

Investigations

Clinical examination

If seen during an acute episode there is spontaneous nystagmus. If seen after the acute attack has settled there is no nystagmus but the patient may still be obviously unsteady, with Rombergism present. No other neurological signs are seen. The tympanic membranes are entirely normal.

Audiometry

Audiograms are within the normal limits for the age groups.

Vestibulometry

There is always evidence of vestibular dysfunction on the affected side. This consists of partial or complete canal paresis, in some cases combined with a directional preponderance to the other side.

Treatment

This is purely symptomatic. The patient is confined to bed and labyrinthine sedatives are administered. Except in older patients full recovery can be anticipated in 3–4 weeks. The vestibular responses remain abnormal.

Chronic vestibular neuronitis

This is a rarer and less severe disease than acute vestibular neuronitis. The age group affected and associated upper respiratory tract infection are similar. The pathological basis for the disease is tenuous but the clinical picture suggests a lesion of the vestibular nerve. The attacks of vertigo are less severe and shorter than the acute variety but they tend to recur over a number of years [59]. Many, although not all patients, have evidence of vestibular dysfunction in one or both ears.

There are no cochlear signs or symptoms.

Treatment is symptomatic and it is important to reassure the patient as to the benign nature of the disease.

BENIGN PAROXYSMAL POSITIONAL NYSTAGMUS

This condition, first described in 1921 [60], is also known as postural vertigo or cupulolithiasis.

It consists of attacks of vertigo usually of short duration precipitated by head movements. Its features are possibly explained by the finding of inorganic deposits on the cupulae of the posterior canals of affected individuals.

Pathology

The disease affects the sexes equally, occurring most commonly in the fifth to seventh decades. There is often a history of a recent upper respiratory tract illness. In a few patients there are also definite causative factors of which head injury is the commonest. Positional vertigo has been described in 47% of patients with longitudinal fractures of the temporal bone and 20·8% of severe head injuries without fractures [61].

Evidence of otitis media, either previous or present, has been found in 25% of cases [62]. Where only one ear is affected positional nystagmus is elicited by placing this ear undermost during testing. Positional vertigo may also be seen rarely after footplate surgery, presumably due to disruption of the utricular macula. Finally a positional vertigo may often follow an attack of severe vertigo very similar to that found in vestibular neuronitis. This suggests that the original lesion may in fact have been a thrombosis of the anterior vestibular artery.

Two main histological groups have been described:

(1) Degeneration of the utricular macula with degeneration of the cristae of the superior and lateral semicircular canals in association with degeneration of the superior vestibular nerve [62–64]. These are the findings identified with thrombosis of the anterior vestibular artery and this may be a separate disease entity.

(2) Deposits of inorganic material on the cupula of the posterior semicircular canal [65].

Although small deposits have been described in nearly 40% of 391 normal temporal bones, none were as big as the deposits in those suffering from postural vertigo [66].

It is not clear where these deposits originate but degeneration of otolithic membranes with loosening of the otoconia has been demonstrated in cats following section of the anterior vestibular nerve [67]. Similarly otoconial material has been dislodged from the macula during acceleration studies [68]. It seems possible that loose particles could gravitate to the most dependent part of the labyrinth. In the erect position this is the ampulla of the posterior canal. Thus, when the head is moved from the erect position to a position where the cupula of the posterior canal is uppermost then the effect of the material on the cupula may be to pull it towards the utricle. This would result in nystagmus. Once the particles have been displaced or the cupula has returned to its previous position the nystagmus settles.

Clinical features

The history is usually very suggestive of the disease. There may be an antecedent event such as head injury or acute vestibular upset but the principle complaint is of a vertigo precipitated by placing the head in a certain position. The symptoms may be brought on in bed by twisting the head to one position or by sudden movements, usually a result of horizontal rotation; it is occasionally found with neck extension or flexion. The vertigo may be severe but is usually short-lived and settles quickly. In severe cases there may be nausea or vomiting. If the patient adopts the same position shortly afterwards the vertigo, if present, is very much less severe. There are no cochlear symptoms or evidence of any other disorders in the majority of patients.

Investigations

Clinical examination
The diagnostic feature of this disorder is a positive provocation test.

The patient is positioned on a couch and his head is turned 30–40° to one side. He is instructed to keep his eyes open all the time. The examiner then grasps the head in both hands and quickly lowers the head and the trunk till the patient's head is hanging over the couch below the horizontal. After a latent period of several seconds, if the test is positive, the patient complains of intense vertigo and struggles to get upright and a nystagmus is observed by the examiner. It is usually rotatory in character, anticlockwise if the head is to the right and clockwise if the head is to the left. Horizontal nystagmus towards the undermost ear may also be observed. After a variable period the nystagmus settles. The patient is then brought back to the original position when there is vertigo and nystagmus in the reverse direction to that noticed previously but less severe. The test may be repeated but it fatigues quickly and after one or two tests is no longer obtainable.

Some patients with a history of positional vertigo do not respond to the test and it is sometimes necessary to see them on several occasions before the test becomes positive.

Audiometry

This is normal unless there is other disease present.

Vestibular tests

Caloric tests are normal in about half the cases. In others there may be canal paresis of the affected ear or a directional preponderance or a combination. It is sometimes useful in doubtful cases to carry out the test procedure at the start of an electronystagmographic test. The test can, therefore, be done with the eyes closed and the nystagmus if present enhanced. A true rotatory nystagmus however may not be recordable by this method.

Treatment

Although the disease is labelled benign not all cases settle spontaneously and some, especially those following head injury, can persist for years. Others, however, do settle and their symptoms gradually become less troublesome over a period from a few weeks to several months. It is important to reassure the patient and instruct him to avoid the provoking position. Many intelligent patients have already deduced this but others,

especially older people, may need several reminders.

DYSEQUILIBRIUM OF AGEING

In all clinics dealing with vertiginous patients there are a large number of patients past middle age who present with vague and often confused stories of dizziness or imbalance, staggering, or being unable to move quickly because of unsteadiness. Some of these patients have vertebrobasilar ischaemia or some other definitive pathology but in a large proportion objective signs of disease are absent. A diagnosis of chronic ischaemia or just old age is usually made.

Pathology

Ageing is associated with degeneration of tissues and the vestibular apparatus is no exception. The basic underlying cause may be chronic arterial insufficiency and anoxia though histological proof of this is lacking. Certain changes, however, have been identified in the temporal bones of old people. Cupulolithiasis (q.v.) has been described and degeneration of the sensory epithelia of both the cristae and the maculae have been demonstrated in temporal bones of old people [14, 69–71].

The unsteadiness associated with walking may be due to degeneration in the central connections of the vestibular nuclei but again histological verification is lacking.

Clinical features

The patients are usually elderly, over the age of 60. The types of symptoms described by them are varied. In some there is unsteadiness on head movements either to the side or in extension or flexion. The imbalance, sometimes vertiginous and sometimes merely a lightheaded feeling, is momentary and there are no other associated symptoms. Occasionally there is vertigo sufficient to cause the patient to fall and in aged individuals this can cause considerable problems. In others there is imbalance on getting up from a recumbent or sitting position. The patient has to remain still for a minute or two until the unsteadiness settles. These symptoms may be short-lived but in the older patients they tend to be long lasting and often permanent.

Investigation

Clinical examination
Other causes of vertigo must be excluded. Full otological examination reveals no gross abnormality. Neurological examination is normal. Similarly the cardiovascular system may be normal. If there are signs of arterial disease elsewhere then a diagnosis of chronic ischaemia is usually made.

Audiometry
Pure tone and speech audiograms are usually normal for the age although in some of those diagnosed as being of ischaemic origin the change may be more pronounced.

Vestibular tests
Normal vestibular function for the age is usually found. Occasionally there are bilateral depressed caloric responses. Some of those with a definite positional element may show up a brief nystagmus on electronystagmography.

Treatment

This is basically supportive. The patient should be reassured and given an explanation of the symptoms. Any other condition, of course, such as anaemia or mature onset diabetes should be corrected. Occasionally vestibular suppressants may be of value in cases where the vertigo is severe. In those with a definite positional element a cervical collar is sometimes useful for a short time as it helps steady the head and prevents undue movement of the neck.

DISORDERS OF CIRCULATION

Vertebro-basilar ischaemia

Vertebro-basilar ischaemia commonly presents as transient episodes of vertigo which are always associated with other signs of brain stem disturbance, if not at first then usually within a few days of the onset of the vertigo [72]. These episodes are often the precursors of more major ischaemic attacks and appropriate steps should be taken to prevent recurrence [73].

Pathology

Most transient ischaemic attacks are thought to be due to micro-emboli lodging in small vessels of the brain stem. Occasionally they may be due to incipient thrombosis of major vessels. The emboli probably originate from atheromatous plaques on the vertebral arteries and they are more likely to occur, therefore, in people with advanced vascular disease. There is also usually atheromatous involvement of the carotid system and irregular and abnormal flow patterns in the cerebral blood vessels which can lead to localized ischaemia. Kinking of an atheromatous vertebral artery with associated cervical spondylosis can give rise to transient brain stem ischaemia but this is much less common [74]. Other disorders such as anaemia, polycythaemia, and cardiac arrhythmias are occasionally implicated.

Transient brain stem ischaemia may also be a result of the *subclavian steal syndrome*. Here there is severe atheroma of the innominate or subclavian artery proximal to the origin of the vertebral arteries. When the upper limb on that side is exercised its blood supply is increased as the arteries dilate and since the subclavian artery cannot meet this demand backflow occurs along the vertebral artery and thus produces ischaemia.

Clinical features

The patients are usually middle-aged or elderly and commonly have evidence of generalized arteriosclerosis. They complain of transient attacks of vertigo which can be precipitated by neck movements. There may be mental confusion and occasionally loss of consciousness. Other symptoms which commonly present include transient diplopia, dysarthria, staggering, ataxia, and paraesthesiae of any of the limbs, sometimes with muscle weakness; nausea and vomiting are unusual symptoms. In those patients with the subclavian steal syndrome the episodes of vertigo are always related to exercise of one of the upper limbs.

Investigations

Clinical examination

If seen during an attack the patient may show a few or many signs of brain stem ischaemia. There may be spontaneous nystagmus, dysarthria, ataxia, confusion, and occasional ocular or limb paresis. Cochlear involvement is rare.

Between attacks there may be no localizing signs but evidence of arterial disease in the coronary, cranial, or peripheral vessels. Occasionally bruits are noted in the neck over the carotid vessels. Hypertension may coexist.

Audiometry

This shows only the audiogram expected for the age.

Vestibular tests

These are generally unhelpful and are usually normal. Spontaneous nystagmus may be seen in the acute attacks.

Radiology

Radiographs of the cervical spine will inevitably show some degree of cervical spondylosis and its significance is doubtful.

Vertebral angiograms are rarely justified but they will reveal areas of narrowing due to atheroma and due to cervical osteophytes. These often coincide.

Treatment

The disorder is primarily a cardiovascular one and should be referred to an internal medicine specialist. Correction of hypertension, anaemia, cardiac arrhythmias, and anticoagulation may be necessary as many cases go on to larger emboli or thrombosis. Surgery is not possible except in the subclavian steal syndrome when an endarterectomy may be possible. Occasionally in mild cases associated with neck movements a cervical collar may be beneficial for a short time.

Lateral medullary syndrome

Also known as *Wallenberg's syndrome*, this disorder results from occlusion of the posterior inferior cerebellar artery or more commonly the vertebral artery by thrombosis or embolus [75].

Pathology

The area of brain affected is the inferior surface of the cerebellum and the lateral part of the medulla oblongata involving the descending vestibular nuclei. Other tracts sometimes involved are the descending spinal tract of the trigeminal nerve, crossed spinothalamic tracts from the trunk and limbs, nucleus ambiguus involving the ninth and tenth nerves, and sympathetic fibres in the reticular formation.

Clinical features

The onset may be gradual or sudden. Initially there is severe vertigo with vomiting, headache, and facial pain. Other symptoms soon develop. These include ipsilateral analgesia, ipsilateral paralysis of the soft palate, larynx, and pharynx giving rise to dysphagia and dysphonia and contralateral anaesthesia of the limbs and trunk. Other findings include an ipsilateral involvement of the sixth, seventh, and eighth cranial nerves. Consciousness is usually maintained. Audiometry if carried out usually shows normal hearing. Vestibulometry may show a directional preponderance to the opposite ear [76].

Treatment

This should be carried out by internal medicine specialists with a view to preventing further thrombosis or emboli.

Occlusion of the anterior inferior cerebellar artery

Clinical features

This presents as a sudden attack of vertigo with nausea and vomiting. Consciousness is usually maintained and the diagnosis becomes evident with the onset of facial paralysis, deafness, cerebellar disturbance, and sensory disorders. The area of brain stem and cerebellum involved results in degenerative changes in the auditory and vestibular nuclei along with the nearby spinal tracts and nuclei. There may also, therefore, be loss of pain and temperature on that side of the face due to involvement of the trigeminal spinal tract and nucleus.

Treatment

Symptomatic treatment should be started and the patient then referred to an internal medicine specialist for further investigation.

Occlusion of the anterior vestibular artery

Clinical features

This syndrome, described in 1956 [77], consists of sudden severe vertigo with no cochlear signs, followed by gradual recovery. After some weeks the patient then develops a positional vertigo which can persist for weeks or years. It is thought to be due to occlusion of the anterior cerebellar artery and degenerative changes have been noted in the utricular macula and the cristae of the lateral and superior semicircular canals in the temporal bone of a patient with this history.

Treatment

This is symptomatic with referral to an internal medicine specialist if generalized arterial disease is suspected.

Labyrinthine vascular accident

Clinical features

Haemorrhage into the labyrinth usually occurs after a head injury or during the course of a haemorrhagic diathesis. Leukaemia has been frequently cited [78] but other haemorrhagic diseases almost certainly can cause this too. It is improbable that spontaneous haemorrhage occurs in normal healthy individuals except possibly following a blow to the head (q.v.).

The disturbance of the labyrinth caused by the blood results in vertigo and deafness and this is probably due to biochemical upset in the perilymphatic and endolymphatic fluids although varying degrees of degenerative changes in the sensory receptors have been seen [78].

Treatment

This consists of treatment of the underlying condition.

Basilar artery migraine

This is a functional disorder found most commonly in adolescent girls [79]. Thought to be due to a migrainous disturbance involving the basilar artery the syndrome consists of visual disturbances such as loss of vision, followed by vertigo and staggering. There may also be dysarthria and paraesthesiae of hands and feet. The symptoms last for 10–30 seconds and are usually followed by occipital headaches and drowsiness or loss of consciousness.

Should this disease be suspected the patient should be referred to a medical neurologist.

NEUROLOGICAL CAUSES OF VERTIGO

Apart from vascular disturbance of the CNS causing vertigo there are several other conditions which sometimes present as vertiginous problems.

Disseminated sclerosis

An episode of dysequilibrium or vertigo is common in those suffering from disseminated sclerosis [80]. The attack may come on during the course of established disease. In those cases the diagnosis is self-evident and the vertigo evidence of a further episode of demyelination involving the vestibular connections. In other cases an episode of vertigo occurring in an otherwise healthy individual and which settles spontaneously is taken to be an attack of vestibular neuronitis and it is only later that the true cause is revealed when other nerves become involved.

Pathology

Disseminated sclerosis is a disease of demyelination. The foci of demyelination can occur throughout the central nervous system but are commonest in the posterior cranial fossa and spinal column and it is only when the vestibular nuclei or other central connections are involved that vertigo becomes apparent.

Clinical features

A common presentation is a single severe attack

of rotatory vertigo similar in many respects to vestibular neuronitis. Also common are repeated less severe attacks. Very occasionally there is cochlear involvement causing sudden deafness presumably by spread of the demyelination within the brain stem.

Investigations

Clinical examination

In established disease the diagnosis is obvious and there may be a plethora of signs present. In others there are no other signs of disease and examination is normal. Spontaneous nystagmus is sometimes seen and others demonstrate a positional nystagmus of the central type when tested.

Positional nystagmus

The procedure is the same as for benign paroxysmal postural nystagmus but the following differences in the result are seen:

(1) The nystagmus elicited occurs immediately on positioning the head.

(2) It is non-fatiguable.

(3) The fast component is directed away from the lowermost ear.

(4) There is no reversal of the nystagmus on sitting up.

(5) The nystagmus is often seen to be changing from moment to moment.

Audiometry

This is usually normal.

Vestibulometry

Spontaneous nystagmus is often present and often distorts caloric tests which, however, are always abnormal. They may show any combination of directional preponderance or canal paresis, or show bilateral abnormalities.

Treatment

Referral to a neurologist is necessary for those with other signs. In patients presenting with vertigo and a picture indistinguishable from vestibular neuronitis it is best to pursue an expectant policy.

Intracranial neoplasms

Many neoplasms, whether primary or metastatic, give rise to giddiness. This can result from direct pressure of an expanding mass or cyst on the vestibular nerve, nuclei, or brain stem connections. Raised intracranial pressure from tumour or other causes may also cause vertigo. Clinical examination will reveal the presence of other neurological abnormalities and a central type of positional nystagmus may be present.

Urgent referral to a surgical or medical neurologist is necessary.

Intracranial infections

Brain abscess especially in the cerebellum or temporal lobe may cause rotatory vertigo or ataxia from pressure on the intracranial vestibular pathways. The origin may be otogenic.

Epilepsy

Vertigo is occasionally present in the aura which precedes an epileptiform attack. If severe and associated with loss of consciousness it may be difficult to identify an epilepsy unless a careful history is taken. Occasionally in such patients there is other evidence of temporal lobe involvement by infection or tumour and the vertigo is thought to be due to disturbance of the cortical connections of the vestibular tracts. In others the feeling is more of general imbalance and not localizable to any specific area.

Referral to a neurologist is necessary.

Psychogenic causes

There are certain people who give histories of vertigo in whom no abnormality can be found on repeated examination and assessment. In addition their descriptions of attacks and sometimes bizarre ways of expressing their symptoms leads one to suspect a functional overlay. Their symptoms, however, may seem real to them and despite reassurance they still complain of them.

If it is possible to exclude other diseases then the patient, if still complaining of vertigo, should be referred to a psychiatrist for further evaluation.

Miscellaneous

There are several other conditions which give rise to feelings of giddiness sometimes indistinguishable from vertigo.

Anaemia

This is a not uncommon cause of dizzy turns. There may be coexistent vascular disease and the two combined cause sufficient hypoxia of the brain to give rise to symptoms. A routine haematological screening should be performed in every case and if anaemia is detected it should be investigated and treated by the appropriate specialist.

Hypotension

Diminution in oxygen supply to the brain because of hypotension is a very common cause of dizziness. True vertigo may also be present. Postural hypotension occurs as a result of rising from a sitting or recumbent position. The cardiovascular system is unable to compensate quickly enough to prevent a transitory fall in blood pressure to the brain and a feeling of dizziness results. Some anti-hypertensive drugs have this side effect.

Hypotension can also result from cardiac disease. Arrhythmias such as paroxysmal tachycardia or heart block may present as transitory imbalance.

In extreme cases syncope results and vertigo is often present just before the patient loses consciousness.

Diabetes

Sensorineural deafness and vestibular dysfunction may be seen in diabetes as a result of the microangiopathy of the disease. There are no specific features present and the treatment is that of the underlying cause.

Acoustic neuroma, see Chapter 4.

Labyrinthine trauma, see Chapter 9.

Labyrinthitis, see Chapter 13.

Differential diagnoses of vertigo

There are, therefore, many diseases which can give rise to vertigo and it is important to differentiate them. They may be divided into two groups, one in which there is vertigo but no other aural symptoms and the other in which deafness and tinnitus may also occur. In both groups there may be other symptoms present.

Group I. Vertigo

(a) Vestibular neuronitis

The onset is often associated with an upper respiratory tract illness but the vertigo can be as severe as Menière's disease. The confirming feature is that there is no hearing impairment or subjective tinnitus.

(b) Benign paroxysmal positional nystagmus

The vertigo in this disorder is always positional in type, usually of short duration. Hearing and caloric tests are normal.

(c) Chronic ischaemia

This occurs in older people and the vertigo is of very short duration. There are no obvious signs of atherosclerosis and hearing is within normal limits for the age of the patient.

(d) Disseminated sclerosis

The onset may be identical to vestibular neuronitis but there are often other signs of brain stem involvement present such as diplopia.

(e) Epilepsy

A vertiginous aura may precede either a grand mal or petit mal attack. A reliable history from a witness will clarify the diagnosis. Audiometry and calorics will be normal.

(f) Migraine

Some migrainous attacks may be preceded by a vertiginous aura. The ensuing headache and vomiting with no associated cochlear signs will establish the diagnosis.

(g) Psychogenic dizziness

The vague history and manner of giving it along with repeatedly negative clinical examination, audiometry, and vestibulometry will give the diagnosis. Care should be taken, however, in making this diagnosis and most patients will require three or more visits and probably repeated investigations.

(h) Anaemia

Fainting attacks or dizzy turns often impossible to differentiate from vertigo can be caused by anaemia. Audiometry and calorics are normal and haematological investigations will delineate the cause.

(i) Thrombosis of posterior inferior cerebellar artery

This gives rise to acute paroxysmal vertigo. There is no hearing loss and the onset of other neurological signs make the diagnosis. Associated paresis may include ninth and tenth nerves as well as the spinothalamic tracts.

(j) Vertebrobasilar ischaemia

The vertigo is of short duration, sometimes positional in type. There are signs of general atherosclerosis and other evidence of brain stem ischaemia is present. Hearing may be normal for the age group. Caloric tests are normal.

Group II. Vertigo, deafness, and tinnitus

(a) Menière's disease

There are recurring episodes of vertigo, deafness and tinnitus, usually with accompanying nausea and vomiting. Initially the hearing may recover between attacks but eventually it becomes permanently affected. Audiometry shows a sensorineural hearing loss which is cochlear in type and there is usually disordered vestibular function.

(b) Infective labyrinthitis

In the acute septic form and serous labyrinthitis there are signs of middle ear infection as well as deafness. In the chronic form the fistula sign is positive even if the middle ear looks healthy. In the viral diseases there are signs of the offending disease with vertigo and tinnitus accompanying the clinical picture.

(c) Toxic labyrinthitis

This may be due to streptomycin but other drugs may be to blame. A history of the drug being administered and an awareness of the possibility of dizziness from them will clarify the diagnosis.

(d) Trauma

There is a history of a head injury with or without evidence of fracture of the temporal bone. The vertigo is less violent than in Menière's disease and usually positional. There is often an accompanying sensorineural loss.

(e) Acoustic neuroma

The vertigo if present is less severe than in Menière's disease and of variable type. There is a sensorineural hearing loss but recruitment is present in a small percentage of patients; there is usually tone decay present and very poor speech discrimination. In large neuromas there may be involvement of the ninth, tenth, and fifth nerves. Radiography including internal auditory meatogram will differentiate these lesions.

(f) CNS neoplasms

Vertigo may be present in lesions involving the cerebellum, brain stem, or mid-brain. There is an irregular nystagmus not enhanced by darkness and usually other signs of intracranial disease.

(g) Syphilis

This can give an acute paroxysmal vertigo like Menière's disease with associated cochlear loss. Serology will be positive and may be the only way of differentiating the condition.

(h) Cogan's disease

This syndrome, of unknown aetiology, consists of sudden vertigo, tinnitus, and rapidly deteriorating hearing with associated ocular symptoms of non-syphilitic interstitial keratitis. It occurs mostly in young adults and may be a collagen disease.

References

[1] NAFTALIN L. & HARRISON M. S. (1958) Circulation of labyrinthine fluids. *Journal of Laryngology and Otology* **72**, 118.

[2] WILLIAMS H. L. (1965) A review of the literature as to the physiological dysfunction of Menière's disease: a new hypothesis as to its fundamental cause. *Laryngoscope* **75**, 1661.

[3] SEYMOUR J. C. (1960) The aetiology, pathology and conservative surgical treatment of Menière's disease. *Journal of Laryngology and Otology* **74**, 599.

[4] BAST, T. H. & ANSON B. J. (1950) Post natal growth and adult structure of the otic (endolymphatic) sac. *Annals of Otology, Rhinology and Laryngology* **59**, 1088.

[5] NAITO T. (1955) Clinical and pathological studies of Menière's disease. *Sixtieth Annual Meeting of the Otorhino-laryngological Society of Japan, Tokyo.*

[6] KIMURA R. & SCHUKNECHT H. (1965) Membranous hydrops in the inner ear of the guinea pig after obliteration of the endolymphatic sac. *Practica oto-rhino-laryngologica* **27**, 343.

[7] BEAL D. (1968) Effect of endolymphatic sac ablation in the rabbit and cat. *Acta oto-laryngologica* **66**, 333.

[8] LUNDQUIST P. G., KIMURA R. & WERSALL J. (1964) Ultrastructural organisation of the epithelial lining in the endolymphatic duct and sac in the guinea pig. *Acta oto-laryngologica* **57**, 65.

[9] ARENBERG I., MAROVITZ W. & SHAMBAUGH G. JR. (1970) The role of the endolymphatic sac in the pathogenesis of endolymphatic hydrops in man. *Acta oto-laryngologica* Supplement **275.**

[10] SELFRIDGE G. (1940) A survey of the relation between nutrition and the ear. *Annals of Otology, Rhinology and Laryngology* **72**, 687.

[11] LEMPERT J., WOLFF D., RAMBO J., WEVER E. & LAWRENCE M. (1952) New theory for the correlation of the pathology and the symptomatology of Menière's disease. *Annals of Otology, Rhinology and Laryngology* **61**, 717.

[12] GOLDMAN H. B. (1962) Hypoadrenocorticism and endocrinologic treatment of Menière's disease. *New York Journal of Medicine* **63**, 377.

[13] WATSON C., BARNES C., DONALDSON J. & KLETT W. (1967) Psychosomatic aspects of Menière's disease. *Archives of Otolaryngology* **86**, 543.

[14] SCHUKNECHT H. F. (1974) *Pathology of the Ear.* Cambridge, Mass.: Harvard University Press.

[15] LINDSAY J. R. (1960) Hydrops of the labyrinth. *Archives of Otolaryngology* **71**, 500.

[16] LINDSAY J., KOHUT R. & SCIARRA P. (1967) Menière's disease; pathology and manifestations. *Annals of Otology, Rhinology and Laryngology* **76**, 1.

[17] LITTON W. & LAWRENCE M. (1961) Electronmicroscopy in Menière's disease. *Archives of Otolaryngology* **74**, 32.

[18] KIMURA R & SCHUKNECHT H. (1970) The ultrastructure of the human stria vascularis. *Acta oto-laryngologica* **69**, 415.

[19] PARVING A. (1976) Menière's disease in childhood. *Journal of Laryngology and Otology* **90**, 817.

[20] CAWTHORNE T. (1969) Choice of labyrinthine surgery for hydrops. *Archives of Otolaryngology* **89**, 108.

[21] GOLDING-WOOD P. H. (1960) Menière's disease and its pathological mechanism. *Journal of Laryngology and Otology* **74**, 803.

[22] CAWTHORNE T. & HEWLETT A. B. (1954) Menière's disease. *Proceedings of the Royal Society of Medicine* **487**, 663.

[23] SCANLAN R. L. & GRAHAM M. D. Radiological findings of the endolymphatic and perilymphatic ducts in Menière's disease. *Proceedings of the Fourth Extraordinary Barany Society Meeting in Los Angeles.* To be published.

[24] ARENBERG I. K., RASK-ANDERSON H., WELBRAND, H. & STAHLE J. (1977) The surgical anatomy of the endolymphatic sac. *Archives of Otolaryngology* **103**, 1.

[25] YUEN S. S. & SCHUKNECHT H. F. (1972) Vestibular aqueduct and endolymphatic duct in Menière's disease. *Archives of Otolaryngology* **96**, 553.

[26] KLOCKHOFF I. & LINDBLOM V. (1967) Glycerol test in Menière's disease. *Acta oto-laryngologica* Supplement **224**, 450.

[27] KLOCKHOFF I. (1975) Effect of glycerin on fluctuant hearing loss. *Otolaryngological Clinics of North America* **8.2**, 345.

[28] ARENBERG I. K. & SPECTOR G. J. (1977) Endolymphatic sac surgery for hearing conservation in Menière's disease. *Archives of Otolaryngology* **103**, 268.

[29] EGGERMONT J. J., ODENTHAL D. W., SCHMIDT P. H. & SPOOR A. (1974) Study of Menière's disease by electrocochleography. *Acta oto-laryngologica* Supplement **316**, 75.

[30] GIBSON W. P. R., MOFFAT D. A. & RAMSDEN R. T. (1977) Clinical electrocochleography in the diagnosis and management of Menière's disorder. *Audiology* **16**, 389.

[31] HINCHCLIFFE R. (1972) Review of treatment of Menière's syndrome. *Acta oto-laryngologica* Supplement **305**, 10.

[32] SCHAYER R. W. (1964) Histamine and autonomous responses of the microcirculation; relationship to glucocorticoid action. *Annals of the New York Academy of Science* **116**, 891.

[33] ELIA J. C. (1966) Double blind evaluation of a new treatment for Menière's syndrome. *Journal of the American Medical Association* **196**, 187.

[34] HICKS J. J., HICKS J. N. & COOLEY, H. N. (1967)

Menière's disease. *Archives of Otolaryngology* 86, 810.

[35] WILMOT T. J. & MENON G. N. (1976) Betahistine in Menière's disease. *Journal of Laryngology and Otology* 90, 833.

[36] MYGIND S. H. (1926) Affections labyrinthiques d'origine endocreinienne. *Acta oto-laryngologica* 10, 561.

[37] HARRISON M. S. & NAFTALIN L. (1968) Menière's disease. Springfield, Illinois: Chas. C. Thomson.

[38] KLOCKHOFF I., LINDBLOM U. & STAHLE J. (1974) Diuretic treatment of Menière's disease. *Archives of Otolaryngology* 100, 262.

[39] CODY D. T. R., SIMONTON, K. M. & HALLBERG O. E. (1967) Automatic repetitive decompression of the saccule in endolymphatic hydrops. *Laryngoscope* 77, 1480.

[40] PORTMANN G. (1972) Vertigo. Surgical treatment by opening the saccus endolymphaticus. *Archives of Otolaryngology* 6, 309.

[41] HOUSE W. F. (1964) Sub-arachnoid shunt drainage of hydrops. *Archives of Otolaryngology* 79, 338.

[42] AUSTIN D. F. (1968) The endolymphatic shunt operation. *Otolaryngological Clinics of North America* 1, 589.

[43] SHAMBAUGH G. E. (1975) Effect of endolymphatic sac decompression on fluctuant hearing loss. *Otolaryngological Clinics of North America*, 8, 537.

[44] FISCH U. (1976) Surgical treatment of vertigo. In *Proceedings of the Fourth British Academic Conference in Otolaryngology. Journal of Laryngology and Otology* 90, 75.

[45] JAMES J. A. FREUNDLICH H. F., BULLEN M. A., WELLS P. N. T. & WILLIAMS D. C. F. (1964) The physical and biological properties of ultrasound and clinical experience. *Acta oto-laryngologica* Supplement 192, 143.

[46] STAHLE J. (1976) Ultrasound treatment of Menière's disease. *Acta oto-laryngologica* 81, 120.

[47] JAMES J. A. (1969) Menière's disease: a present status of ultrasonic therapy. *Archives of Otolaryngology* 89, 95.

[48] SYMTH G. D. L., KERR, A. G., & GORDON, D. S. (1976) Vestibular nerve section for Menière's disease. *Journal of Laryngology and Otology* 90, 823.

[49] PALVA T., KARJA J. & PALVA A. (1976) Surgical treatment of Menière's disease. *Acta oto-laryngologica* 82, 303.

[50] GREEN R. E. (1959) Surgical treatment of vertigo. *Clinical Neurosurgery* 6, 141.

[51] PASSE E. & SEYMOUR J. (1948) Menière's syndrome: successful treatment by surgery on the sympathetic. *British Medical Journal* 2, 812.

[52] CLEMIS J. D. (1969) Medical management of Menière's disorder. *Archives of Otolaryngology* 89, 90.

[53] TUMARKIN A. (1966) Thoughts on the treatment of labyrinthopathy. *Journal of Laryngology and Otology* 80, 1041.

[54] ARSLAN M. (1972) Symposium on Menière's disease: IV. Treatment of Menière's disease by apposition of sodium chloride crystals on the round window. *Laryngoscope* 82, 1736.

[55] HALLPIKE C. S. (1949) *Proceedings of the IV International Congress on Otolaryngology*, Vol. 2, p. 514. London: British Medical Association.

[56] MERIFIELD D. (1965) Self-limited idiopathic vertigo (epidemic vertigo). *Archives of Otolaryngology* 81, 335.

[57] PFALTZ C. (1955) Diagnose und Therapie der vestibularen Neuronitis. *Practica oto-rhino-laryngologica* 17, 454.

[58] MARSHALL J. (1955) Epidemic vertigo. *Lancet* 1, 458.

[59] HARRISON M. (1962) Epidemic vertigo – vestibular neuronitis, a clinical study. *Brain* 85, 613.

[60] BARANY R. (1921) Diagnose von Krahkheitsercheinungen in Bereiche des otolithenapparates. *Acta oto-laryngologica* 2, 434.

[61] BARBER H. (1964) Positional nystagmus; testing and interpretation. *Annals of Otology, Rhinology and Laryngology* 73, 838.

[62] DIX M. & HALLPIKE C. (1952) The pathology, symptomatology and diagnosis of certain disorders of the vestibular system. *Annals of Otology, Rhinology and Laryngology* 61, 687.

[63] CAWTHORNE T. & HALLPIKE C. (1957) A study of the clinical features and pathological changes within the temporal bones, brain stem and cerebellum of an early case of positional nystagmus of the so-called benign paroxysmal type. *Acta oto-laryngologica* 48, 89.

[64] LINDSAY J. & HEMENWAY W. (1956) Postural vertigo due to unilateral sudden partial loss of vestibular function. *Annals of Otology, Rhinology and Laryngology* 65, 692.

[65] SCHUKNECHT H. (1969) Cupulolithiasis. *Archives of Otolaryngology* 90, 765.

[66] SCHUKNECHT H. & RUBY R. (1973) Cupulolithiasis. *Advances in Oto-rhino-laryngology* 20, 434.

[67] SCHUKNECHT H. (1962) Positional vertigo: clinical and experimental observations. *Transactions of the American Academy of Ophthalmology and Otolaryngology* 66, 319.

[68] PARKER D., COVELL W. & GIERKE H. VON (1968) Exploration of vestibular damage in guinea pigs following mechanical stimulation. *Acta oto-laryngologica* Supplement 239.

[69] ISHII T., MUKARAMI Y., KIMURA R. & BALOGH K. JR. (1967) Electronmicroscopic and histochemical identification of lipofuscin in the human inner ear. *Acta oto-laryngologica* 64, 17.

[70] SCHUKNECHT H. F., IGARASHI M. & GACEK R. (1965) The pathological types of cochlea-saccular degeneration. *Acta oto-laryngologica* 59, 114.

[71] JOHNSSON L. (1971) Degenerative changes and anomalies of the vestibular system in man. *Laryngoscope* 81, 1682.

[72] BARBER H. & DIONNE J. (1971) Vestibular findings in vertebro-basilar ischaemia. *Annals of Otology, Rhinology and Laryngology* 80, 805.

[73] ADAMS R. D. (1977) *Harrison's Principles of Internal Medicine*, 8th ed., p. 1849. New York: McGraw-Hill.

[74] MEYER J. S. (1970) New concepts of cerebral vascular disease. *Medical Clinics of North America* 352.

[75] FISHER C., KARNES W. & KEIBIK C. (1961) Lateral medullary infarction – the pattern of vascular occlusion. *Journal of Neuropathology and Experimental Neurology* **20**, 323.

[76] HALLPIKE C. (1965) Clinical otoneurology and its contribution to theory and practice. *Proceedings of the Royal Society of Medicine* **58**, 185.

[77] LINDSAY J. & HEMMENWAY W. (1956) Postural vertigo due to unilateral sudden partial loss of vestibular function. *Annals of Otology, Rhinology and Laryngology* **65**, 692.

[78] FRASER J. (1928) Affectations of the labyrinth and eighth nerve in leukemia. *Annals of Otology, Rhinology and Laryngology* **37**, 361.

[79] BICKERSTAFF E. R. (1962) The basilar artery and the migraine–epilepsy syndrome. *Proceedings of the Royal Society of Medicine* **55**, 167.

[80] EDWARDS C. P. (1973) *Neurology of Ear, Nose and Throat Disease*, p. 158. London: Butterworths.

CHAPTER 4

Acoustic Neuroma

Most patients with an acoustic neuroma first present to the otologist with the chief complaints of unilateral progressive hearing loss, tinnitus and dizziness. While this has always been the case, it is only in the past 20 years or so that the otologist has been able to meet the challenge of acoustic neuroma successfully. Armed with advanced methods of early diagnosis, modern anatomic approaches and microsurgical techniques, the otologist is able to reduce significantly the operative morbidity and mortality to levels never known before. Removal of small tumours with preservation or even improvement of hearing became possible.

The surgical removal of acoustic neuroma is related to its size. Small tumours, in the past, were difficult to detect. The evolution of the current surgical technique was therefore linked to the development of more accurate and sensitive audiometric, vestibular and radiologic methods of investigation which are able to detect small tumours. However, the most important role in early diagnosis still remains with the clinician. His acquaintance with the early symptoms of small tumours, along with a high index of suspicion will ensure a correct and early diagnosis.

The improved results with acoustic tumour surgery could not have been possible without teamwork. Close cooperation with the diagnostic services, and with a team consisting of a neurosurgeon, anaesthetist, physician and ophthalmologist, is essential.

PATHOLOGY

The term 'acoustic neuroma' is inaccurate for two reasons. These tumours do not arise from nervous tissue, but from the neurilemma or Schwann cell sheath which has a supporting function in covering the axon. Furthermore, the great majority arise from the vestibular rather than the cochlear nerve. Rarely, tumours are encountered which at surgery prove to be truly 'acoustic' in origin. Thus, 'vestibular Schwannoma' or 'vestibular neurilemmoma' would really describe the condition more appropriately, although it seems unlikely that these terms will ever replace 'acoustic neuroma', sanctified as it is by long usage. The eighth cranial nerve, as it leaves the brain stem in the region of the lower pons, is covered by a loose stroma of glial tissue and does not acquire a neurilemmal covering until it enters the internal acoustic meatus. The glial-neurilemmal junction is thought to be the site of origin of most acoustic neuromas, and thus most tumours arise within the internal auditory meatus. Growth is therefore initially intrameatal, and pressure effects may be produced relatively early on the contents of the meatus, the cochlear division of the eighth nerve, the vestibular nerves, the facial nerve with the nervus intermedius and the branches of the internal acoustic artery supplying the cochlea and labyrinth. The veins which drain the inner ear, however, do not for the most part run in the internal meatus, so that the important derangements of cochlear circulation which may accompany acoustic neuroma are probably due to arterial obstruction.

With further increase in size, the tumour enlarges from the porus acusticus into the cerebellopontine angle and may begin to erode the walls of the internal meatus superiorly, inferiorly and posteriorly, creating a funnelling of the porus which may be detectable radiologically. Freed of the restraints of the bony canal, the tumour can now continue to expand in three main directions, medially, anterosuperiorly and posteroinferiorly. As growth proceeds in a medial direction, the tumour eventually approaches and indents the brain stem in the region of the pons. By this stage the neuroma will be approximately 2·5 cm in diameter and may be in intimate relationship with the anterior inferior cerebellar artery on its medial surface. This is a most important artery which is responsible for the blood supply of the lateral portion of the pons and medulla. Meticulous separation of it from the tumour is one of the most vital parts of acoustic neuroma surgery. Further medial enlargement of the growth causes gradual compression and distortion of the pons and the aqueduct, producing both localizing brain stem signs and obstructive hydrocephalus.

Expansion of the tumour in an anterosuperior direction causes displacement of the facial nerve before it, with thinning and stretching of that structure over the surface of the tumour. The neuroma may become firmly adherent to the facial nerve, but does not usually envelop the nerve, so that even with very large neuromas the facial nerve can be separated from the tumour. With further extension of the mass forward and upward, the trigeminal nerve is commonly involved. The Gasserian ganglion occupies a diverticulum of dura called Meckel's cave, situated on and grooving the middle fossa surface of the apex of the petrous temporal bone. The tumour usually lifts the nerve up from below and the fibres which are most sensitive to this distortion are those subserving the afferent part of the corneal reflex. Fifth nerve involvement is a very common occurrence in medium sized (under 3 cm in diameter) and large (more than 3 cm in diameter) tumours. Extensive medial extension may on occasion involve the abducent nerve.

Growth in a posteroinferior direction may cause compression of the middle cerebellar peduncle and the cerebellum. The ninth, tenth and eleventh nerves may be stretched as the lower pole approaches the foramen magnum. The majority of acoustic neuromas grow intracisternally, i.e. within the subarachnoid space, the part of which lateral to the tumour may become isolated from the rest of the cistern, with the formation of a pseudocyst containing a yellow protein-rich fluid.

A small percentage of Schwannomas arise in the cerebellopontine angle, medial to the porus acusticus, reflecting, no doubt, the variability in the point at which the eighth nerve acquires its Schwann cell covering. Because there is no early intrameatal expansion, these tumours may achieve considerable size before they are identified. Many of their clinical, audiological and radiological features are atypical.

Acoustic neuromas have always been regarded as slow-growing tumours, and this assumption was essential to the philosophy of non-interference to which the great neurosurgeons of the earlier part of the century adhered. One estimate of the rate of their expansion suggests 0·5 cm per year. There is no doubt, however, that there are variations in the growth rate between patients and at different times in the same patient. Expansion may be particularly rapid in the young adult, whereas several series have confirmed the coincidental postmortem finding of small asymptomatic tumours in the elderly (incidence about 1%). Haemorrhage or cyst formation within the substance of the tumour may cause a rapid increase in the size of a hitherto slowly growing neuroma.

The importance of the degenerative changes in the cochlea and labyrinth which may accompany a space-occupying lesion of the internal meatus have to a great extent been ignored. It seems likely, however, that they will attract increasing attention as workers in the field of electric response audiometry look for pathological changes to explain the abnormalities of the cochlear and eighth nerve potentials which occur with high consistency in acoustic neuroma. For the anatomical reasons mentioned earlier, an expanding mass in the internal meatus may occlude the arterial supply to the internal ear, but is unlikely to have much effect on the venous drainage (Fig. 4.1). The resultant changes in the cochlea and labyrinth are biochemical alterations of the inner ear fluids and destruction of the sense organs themselves. It has been known for many years that an acidophil precipitate is commonly present in the perilymphatic spaces, and occasionally in the cochlear duct of ears harbouring acoustic neuromas. Perilymph removed through the lateral semicircular canal at the time of translabyrinthine surgery has an extremely high concentration of protein. Micro-

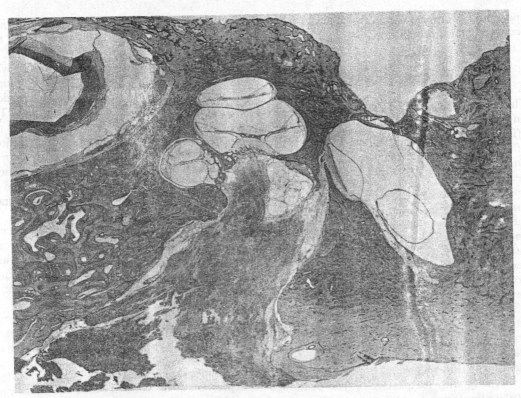

FIG. 4.1. Low power micrograph of acoustic neuroma arising from the inferior vestibular nerve, projecting toward the basal turn of the cochlea. The tumour fills the entire internal auditory canal.

scopically the stria vascularis and the spiral ligament appear to be the most grossly disorganized structures, with severe degeneration and cyst and vacuole formation. The hair cells of the organ of Corti often remain fairly normal on light microscopy even in regions of the cochlea where strial and spiral ganglion degeneration is advanced.

Macroscopically, the neuroma takes the form of a well-defined, fleshy lobulated mass. It may be soft and cystic in places and is relatively avascular although circumscribed areas of old haemorrhage may be present and these may give rise to a variegated appearance. Small white patches of calcification are frequently present. The histological picture is characterized by two patterns, Type A or fasciculated pattern and Type B or reticular pattern. Type A tumours are characterized by an orderly regimentation of nuclei, the spindle-shaped cells in places being arranged parallel to one another in interlacing

bundles which alternate with reticular fibres. In the Type B pattern, the tumour appears less cellular and more vacuolated and the cell pattern is less organized. As yet, there appears to be little correlation between the histological picture and clinical behaviour.

Von Recklinghausen's disease or familial neurofibromatosis is a generalized hamartomatous dysplasia of nerve sheath tissue which may be transmitted as an autosomal dominant characteristic. Neurofibromas are found on peripheral cutaneous nerves, as well as on spinal and cranial nerves. Meningiomas, angiomas and ependymomas occur less frequently. Areas of skin pigmentation (café-au-lait spots) are a common finding. Patients with this disorder are very likely to develop acoustic nerve neurofibromas, which are usually bilateral. Their behaviour differs from that of the 'normal' acoustic neuroma in that they tend to invade the cochlea through the cribrose area; indeed they may arise and remain confined within the cochlea ('intra-cochlear neurofibromatosis').

CLINICAL FEATURES

The patient is usually in the fourth or fifth decade on presentation (50%) but all age groups can be affected. There may be a slight sex bias in favour of women. Among those patients seen at the Otologic Medical Group the first symptom was hearing loss in 73% [1], tinnitus in 11% [2] and unsteadiness in 8·2%. Most patients have more than one of these symptoms when they consult their physicians. The hearing loss is usually unilateral and slowly progressive (in 40% of patients for 1–3 years), and may eventually become complete. The loss of speech discrimination, which is characteristic of retrocochlear pathology, may be volunteered by the patient who finds that he cannot make out conversation, particularly on the telephone. Tinnitus usually begins at the same time as the hearing loss, but may precede it by months or years and may remain the only symptom. It usually progresses in intensity with the passage of time. Although most patients present with a gradually progressive history, it is of the greatest importance to realize that some 15% have a sudden onset of hearing loss which may lead to the mistaken incrimination of viral or vascular aetiologies.

A common pitfall in the diagnosis of acoustic neuroma may be encountered in patients presenting with *bilateral* hearing loss, most commonly presbycusis, in whom the unilaterality of the tumour symptom complex is masked by the hearing loss in the other ear. Careful attention must be paid to these patients' history concerning *any* localizing ear symptoms (asymmetry of hearing loss progression, tinnitus) or asymmetrical results of diagnostic tests (asymmetry of hearing level or speech discrimination score) or reduced vestibular response that can yield clinical clues to the presence of acoustic neuroma.

Disturbance of balance is rarely severe. The slow growth of the neuroma means that loss of peripheral function is accompanied by a continuous process of compensation by the contralateral ear. Transient unsteadiness may occur, however, in association with sudden changes in position or with head movement. Sometimes imbalance may occur early in the course of the disease to disappear and be forgotten later. In roughly 30% of patients there is true vertigo with a sense of rotation, nausea and vomiting; Menière's disease may be misdiagnosed, particularly if there is a fluctuating hearing loss. The end-organ nature of these symptoms reflects the inner ear changes seen in temporal bone sections and described above. Spontaneous nystagmus should be sought and its presence may be more readily detected if optical fixation is abolished by the use of Frenzl's glasses and by electronystagmography.

Otalgia is a frequent symptom present even when the tumour is still small. It is most commonly a deep ache within the ear or mastoid and may be due to pressure on the nervus intermedius. Tension neck pain on the same side is common.

The first neurologic manifestation of an acoustic neuroma other than seventh and eighth nerve involvement is usually sensory trigeminal involvement. While obvious facial numbness may sometimes be present it is more likely that depression of the corneal reflex will be the only evidence, and must be deliberately sought by the clinician. Bouts of devastating facial pain, tic douloureux, occur occasionally (0·4%). Motor fibres, on the other hand, withstand compression with little adverse effect. It is rare to find weakness of the muscles of mastication or the facial nerve. Although it is closely applied to the surface of the tumour, obvious weakness of the muscles of facial expression is seldom seen. The fibres which run in the nervus intermedius, however, are more vulnerable. These are the pre-ganglionic parasympathetic secretomotor fibres bound for, among other sites, the lacrimal gland and those fibres which subserve taste on the anterior two-thirds of the tongue. It is rare for the patient to complain of altered taste, but an elevation of the threshold of electrogustometry is possible. A difference of more than 20 μA between the two sides is considered significant. Decreased lacrimation may be detected using Schirmer's test. The combination of decreased corneal sensation, delayed blink reflex and decreased tear production may give rise to a variety of eye symptoms, particularly dryness or grittiness. One may encounter the occasional patient who volunteers that a contact lens is better tolerated in the affected eye. The sensory branch of the facial nerve supplies the postero-superior part of the external auditory meatus and a decreased sensation in this area is a physical sign often present but rarely sought.

Involvement of other cranial nerves implies a large tumour. Diplopia on looking to the side of the lesion is due to pressure on the abducent nerve and is seen occasionally. Pharyngeal and laryngeal symptoms caused by stretching of the glossopharyngeal and vagus nerves are rare. Pressure on the cerebellum and brain stem is common with large tumours and such involve-ment usually means that the tumour is at least 3 cm in diameter. Spontaneous direction changing nystagmus is a very consistent and reliable indicator of central involvement. It is coarse and is usually slower when the patient looks to the side of the tumour. Ataxia is more marked in the lower limbs than the arms and may manifest as a disturbance of gait. Headache, loss of vision and papilloedema occur late.

INVESTIGATIONS

Short of positive contrast radiology, there is no test which taken individually is diagnostic of acoustic neuroma. It is the consideration of the overall picture that leads one to suspect the condition and to embark finally for confirmation on definitive neuroradiological techniques, such as computerized cranial tomography and myelo-graphy.

Audiologic tests

The recognition of retrocochlear pathology on the basis of conventional speech discrimination, auditory fatigue and loudness function tests are so well known as to need little elaboration.

Pure tone audiometry shows no typical diagnostic pattern. If any hearing remains there is a unila-teral sensorineural hearing loss which often shows a sharp high tone drop (66%), but flat (13%), low tone (9%) or trough-shaped (12%) audiograms may be seen.

Speech discrimination with neuronal lesions is typically poorer than one might expect from consideration of the pure tone audiogram because words, being more complex than pure tones, require more intact neurons for their transmission. Although 56% of patients with acoustic neuromas have speech discrimination scores of under 30%, a high score does not exclude a tumour since 26% of confirmed cases show scores of 62–100%.

Auditory fatigue tests study the amount of adap-tation that occurs during exposure to a con-tinuous sound presented just above threshold. Patients with retrocochlear pathology often exhibit this tendency to an exaggerated degree. The phenomenon is known as tone decay, and the tests most frequently employed to detect it are Carhart's test, the modified tone decay test (MTDT) and Békésy audiometry.

Loudness function tests such as Fowler's alternate binaural loudness balance test (ABLB) and the short increment sensitivity index (SISI) fail to demonstrate recruitment in most cases of acous-tic neuroma. Indeed, 'decruitment' may be pre-sent. Since, however, 23% of confirmed neur-omas show complete recruitment on ABLB and 34% on SISI these tests cannot by themselves be considered as diagnostic.

Acoustic reflex measurements are of great value, and provide objective information about loud-ness function and auditory fatigue, assuming that the middle ear is normal. If the ear is recruiting, the gap between the pure tone thresh-old and the acoustic reflex threshold (ART) will be considerably less than the normal of about 80 dB, whereas with the same hearing loss caused by a neuronal lesion, recruitment is absent and the gap between the pure tone and acoustic reflex thresholds is normal. Indeed, if the hearing loss is profound then the acoustic reflex may not be obtainable due to limitations in the output of the audiometer.

The acoustic reflex decay test can provide an early audiometric evidence of neuronal disease. In the normal ear and the ear with cochlear disease, there is no relaxation of the stapedius during suprathreshold reflex stimulation, particularly at frequencies below 2 kHz. With retrocochlear pathology the reflex decays to about half its original magnitude within 5 seconds. The reflex interferes with the afferent (eighth nerve) part of the reflex rather than the efferent fibres (seventh nerve).

Electrocochleography (ECoG) provides objective information about the electrical events in the cochlea and eighth nerve following acoustic stimulation. The recordings are usually made with minimal discomfort from a transtympanic promontory electrode. Certain features occur consistently in the presence of acoustic neuroma:

(1) The compound eighth nerve action potential (AP) is widened, usually to greater than 4 ms (normal–1·5 ms).

(2) The cochlear microphonic (CM) is normal in patients with no impairment of blood supply to the cochlea.

(3) In large medially placed tumours causing brain stem compression, the objective threshold on cochleography may be better than the psychoacoustic threshold on pure tone audiometry.

About 90% of neuromas may be successfully identified by this method.

Brain Stem Electric Response Audiometry (BERA) is the latest and very promising electro-physiologic audiometric test based on the assumption that mechanical pressure applied on the acoustic nerve, as by an acoustic neuroma, tends to delay the propagation of the auditory electric response through the nerve from the sound-stimulated cochlea to the auditory nuclei in the brain stem [3].

Auditory potentials are generated by the cochlea in response to a series of clicks presented to the ear by earphones or free field. These minute potentials are picked up by scalp surface electrodes, then amplified and recorded on an oscilloscope. Random background electric signals from the brain, heart and voluntary muscles are cancelled out by an averaging computer synchronized with the stimulating sound. Broadband masking noise is applied to the non-tested ear.

Excitation of the cochlear nerve and the auditory nuclei along the central auditory pathways in the brain stem produces a chain of six positive peaks on the recorded brain stem electric response (Jewett waves) (Fig. 4.2). The most prominent and consistent is the fifth wave (P5) which is related to the excitation of the inferior colliculi. Each peak wave has a characteristic latency, the time interval between the sound stimulation of the cochlea and the arrival of the

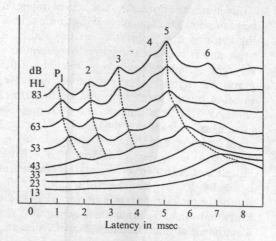

Fig. 4.2. Electric responses from a normal ear, showing the first six peaks described by Jewett *et al.* Parameter is stimulus intensity. Dotted lines show latency-intensity function. Cochlear delay is noted in the low intensity clicks (there is a delay in P1 – cochlear nerve action potential) whereas the latency relations of the various peaks remain constant as the neural propagation rate does not change. High intensity clicks at 83 dB are clinically used. Reproduced with permission from Selters & Brackmann [3].

propagative response to the relays in the brain stem. Normally, the latencies of P5 in both ears are equal (interaural latency, ITS), the difference does not exceed 0·2 ms. If an acoustic neuroma is present the latency of P5 on the affected side is prolonged and ITS is greater than 0·4 ms. The increase in ITS is related to the size of the tumour (Fig. 4.3).

Large acoustic tumours causing pressure on the brain stem with displacement of the fourth ventricle increase the latency of P5 on the contralateral side as well. Pressure on the brain stem can, therefore, be diagnosed by this test. Removal of the tumour relieves the pressure on the brain stem and causes the P5 latency on the contralateral side to return to normal.

Brain stem audiometry has proved to be highly accurate (97%) and probably the most reliable test in the whole audiometric battery.

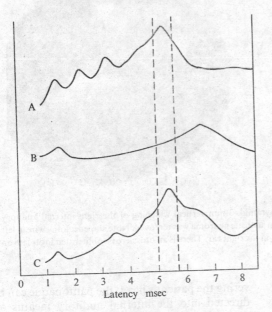

FIG. 4.3. Electric responses from three pathologic ears. Vertical dotted lines mark the latency range in twenty normal ears.

A. Ménière's disease, flat 35 dB sensorineural hearing loss. T5 of 5·2 m is normal as cochlear lesions result in normal neural latencies.

B. 3-cm acoustic neuroma with 35 dB flat sensorineural hearing loss and 80% speech discrimination. Normal P1 of 1·5 m is followed by 5 m gap and large P5 at 6·6 m P2–P4 disappeared. The delayed P5 is consistent with increased neural latency.

C. 1-cm intracanalicular acoustic neuroma. Latency of P5 is normal. Some flattening of P2–P4. Reproduced with permission from Selters & Brackmann [3].

Vestibular tests

Vestibular tests are an integral part of the evaluation of inner ear function. As part of the test battery for detecting acoustic neuromas, the vestibular response to various stimulations contributes to the assessment of the vestibular peripheral end-organ function and the integrity of its central connections. While no clear-cut indications of the site of the lesion can be obtained a distorted pendulum track test can point to a central lesion.

Spontaneous nystagmus and induced nystagmus as a response to positional and bilateral bithermal caloric stimulation are recorded and analysed by electronystamography (ENG). Of patients with proved acoustic neuromas 87% were found to have a reduced vestibular response (RVR) (30% or more) to caloric stimulation on the affected side. The degree of RVR is usually quantitatively related to the size of the tumour.

Vestibular RVR is a non-specific response and as such, is not diagnostic of acoustic neuroma. Its significance must be weighed in accordance with other localizing clues derived from the clinical examination and other tests. The amount of postoperative dizziness after removal of a tumour can be predicted by the determination of the preoperative RVR. The more advanced the loss of vestibular function, the fewer symptoms will the patient have.

No clinical test is available to stimulate the posterior semicircular canal which is connected centrally through the inferior vestibular nerve, the site of origin for 50% of acoustic neuromas.

Radiologic investigation

Plain radiography of the petrous pyramid of the temporal bone is diagnostic in 90% of the cases. Technically adequate transorbital, Stenvers, Towne and skull base views demonstrate asymmetric widening and bony erosion of the internal auditory canal.

Linear or hypocycloidal tomography of the temporal bone provides a reliable and non-invasive method for the diagnosis of acoustic neuroma. Enlargement of the internal auditory meatus is demonstrated in 90% of patients (Fig. 4.4).

The criteria for abnormality proposed by Valvassori are:

(1) Vertical enlargement of 2 mm or more of any portion compared with the opposite side.

(2) Shortening of the posterior wall by at least 3 mm compared with the normal side.

(3) The position of the crista falciformis differs by at least 2 mm compared to the normal side.

The range of normal values for the dimensions of the internal meatus is quite wide and a certain asymmetry may be normal. The height of the normal meatus may lie between 2 and 8 mm, and

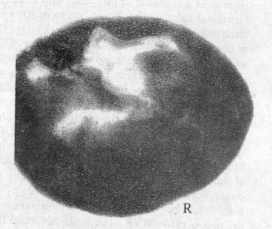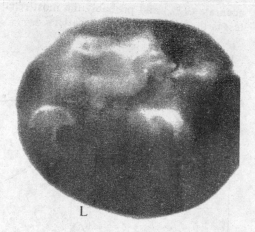

R   L

FIG. 4.4. Bilateral anteroposterior polytome of petrous pyramid. 3-mm vertical widening of the right internal auditory canal. The margins are funnelled and demineralized. A 3-cm acoustic neuroma was removed. Note stapedectomy wire in left middle ear, performed prior to the discovery of the tumour in the right ear. There is an otosclerotic obliterated footplate on the right.

an asymmetry of up to 1 mm in this measurement is acceptable. A common source of error in interpreting these films may be the presence of a large petrous apex air cell which on some cuts may mimic erosion. The 10% of negative X-rays occur with very early neuromas and also with some large tumors if they arose medially in the cerebellopontine angle rather than within the meatus.

Meatocysternography provides the final and most definitive diagnostic test for acoustic neuroma and is the best method of detecting intracanalicular tumour. At the Otologic Medical Group in Los Angeles a pantopaque contrast study combined with polytomography of the temporal bone is preferred in all cases to pneumoencephalography. This test is performed on an out-patient basis. After a complete oto-neurologic examination (including fundoscopy to rule out papilloedema) a lumbar puncture is done with the patient in a seated position. Through a 22-gauge spinal needle, approximately 1·0 ml of cerebrospinal fluid is removed for protein analysis. Pantopaque 1–1·25 ml is then slowly introduced into the subarachnoid space and the needle is withdrawn. By tilting the patient's body head down, the contrast material is run into the posterior fossa without fluoroscopy. By manoeu-

vering the patient's head, the pantopaque can be directed into the internal auditory meatus on each side separately. Polytomography is then carried out. If the internal auditory canal is free of tumour, excellent delineation of its bony borders and the transverse crest can be achieved (Fig. 4.5). If a space-occupying lesion is present, the meatus will not fill or will only fill partially, demonstrating a filling defect (Fig. 4.6).

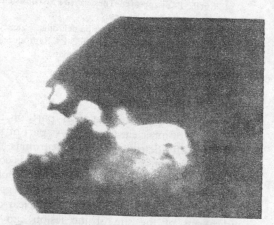

FIG. 4.5. Polytome pantopaque myelogram which shows good filling of the left internal auditory canal. Note the filling defect of the fifth nerve ganglion on the upper medial portion of the petrous ridge.

With lesions protruding into the cerebellopontine angle, this investigation may help to differentiate acoustic neuroma from meningioma and cholesteatoma. A neuroma usually has a smooth rounded medial surface whereas meningiomas and cholesteatomas often present an irregular, scalloped, or fragmented appearance.

The out-patient procedure of small aliquot polytome pantopaque has the following advantages:

(1) After completion of the test the patient is able to be discharged home.

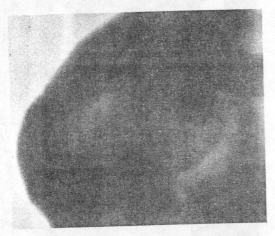

FIG. 4.6. Polytome pantopaque myelogram which shows a 4·5-cm right acoustic neuroma. There is marked vertical widening of the internal auditory canal with bony destruction. Contrast material is pooling in the cerebellopontine angle and delineating the medial border of the tumour with no filling of the internal auditory canal.

(2) By performing this test on an out-patient basis, hospitalization is avoided, thus cutting down on the medical expenses of the medical care.

Large dose myelography is performed in the hospital by the neuroradiologist and the neurosurgeon in selected cases:

(1) Patients with history of spinal injury or spinal surgery.

(2) Patients with von Recklinghausen's disease who usually have spinal cord tumours concomitantly with their acoustic neuromas. The use of large bolus contrast material provides spinal myelography in addition to posterior fossa myelography. The presence of spinal tumours may alter the indication for removal of acoustic neuroma.

(3) Rarely, on patients on whom the small bolus contrast material study had failed technically.

(4) In patients with a clinical suspicion of large tumours, not shown by computerized cranial tomography.

In either technique, the residual amount of contrast material left in the subarachnoid space tends to accumulate asymptomatically in the sacral region and can be re-run into the posterior fossa at a later date (up to a few years) without the necessity of repeating the lumbar puncture. The amount of residual contrast material available can be checked by a scout film of the sacral region. The use of small bored spinal needles has lowered the incidence of headache and backache following these tests.

Computerized Cranial Tomography (CCT) has revolutionized diagnostic neurology. A new era was launched in diagnostic neuroradiology, adding new dimensions to the diagnosis of intracranial pathology.

The incomparable diagnostic usefulness of CCT scanning of the head is due to its ability to depict intracranial and cranial anatomical structures accurately. This is possible by highly sensitive differentiation between various tissues according to their relative density and the amount of X-ray absorption in the tomographic cross section. The density of water has been given the reading of zero. Fat and air are less dense, while cerebrospinal fluid, blood, brain tissue, calcification and bone are of higher density. The diagnostic effectiveness was further increased by adding an angiographic effect. Intravenous injection of iodinated contrast material causes increases the density of vascular lesions compared to the density of normal brain tissue. Thus, vascular tumours are depicted as radio-opaque masses after intravenous injection of contrast material (enhancement phenomenon) (Figs. 4.7 and 4.8). By adjusting the sensitivity of the scan, bony structures of the skull will become more prominent. The porus of the internal auditory canal can be seen by this method and pathologic widening or destruction can be detected.

Acoustic neuromas, being relatively vascular lesions with a density close to that of brain tissue, are usually demonstrated only by the enhancement technique. These tumours appear on the tumours larger than 2–2·5 cm are seen; intracanalicular tumours cannot be seen. From our experience up to 16% of tumours are not diagnosed by CCT.

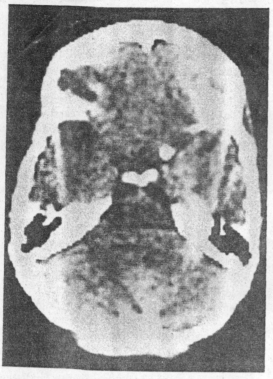

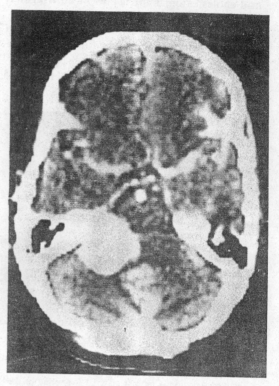

FIG. 4.7. Figs 4.7, 4.8 and 4.9 concern a 30-year-old female, epileptic with normal hearing, asymptomatic. CCT scan, posterior fossa level. Note clear delineation of petrous pyramids and mastoid air cells. No lesion is seen in the posterior fossa.

FIG. 4.8. Same CCT scan of the posterior fossa as Fig. 4.7, with intravenous injection of iodinated contrast material. An approximately 3·5-cm acoustic neuroma is demonstrated on the left, approaching the midline.

scan as a round or oval mass medial to the porus of the internal auditory canal and the size of the tumour can be estimated. The ventricular system is well demonstrated, yielding most vital information about its size and location. Obstructive hydrocephalus due to pressure of the tumour on the aqueduct appears as dilation of the ventricular system (Fig. 4.9). Pressure on the brain stem will be demonstrated by a shift of the fourth ventricle to the contralateral side. Information about the size of the cisterns and the cerebral blood supply can also be obtained.

Detection of small acoustic neuromas of 1 cm in diameter has been reported, but usually only

The details obtainable by CCT provide enough information for differential diagnosis of the posterior fossa lesions. Congenital cholesteatomas appear as low density lesions with smooth borders, not enhanceable. Meningiomas will appear as an irregular dense mass before enhancement associated with pronounced bony destruction. Postoperative cranial complications can also be diagnosed, as haematomas, hydrocephalus and abscesses. Repeated CCT allows accurate postoperative follow-up of these complications.

The non-interventional nature of this unique, innovative technique, combined with its high

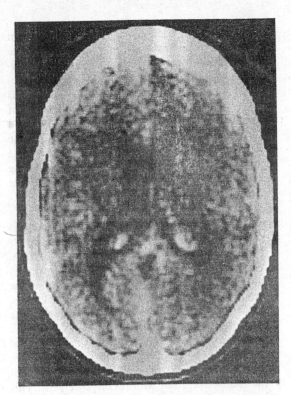

FIG. 4.9. Same patient as in Figs. 4.7 and 4.8. This shows marked dilation of the ventricular system and obstructive hydrocephalus secondary to a large left acoustic neuroma.

yield of accurate information, justified its prominent role in neurodiagnosis.

Current practice

The test battery as practised at the Otologic Medical Group is composed of informative and non-invasive tests grouped as a *basic screening test battery*.

(1) *Audiometric tests*

Pure tone air and bone conduction thresholds.

Speech reception threshold (SRT) and speech discrimination score.

Impedance audiometry to determine the presence of acoustic reflexes and acoustic reflex decay.

Modified tone decay test.

(2) *Vestibular tests*

Using electronystagmography, spontaneous, positional and bilateral bi-thermal caloric induced nystagmus is recorded and analysed.

(3) *Radiology*

Plain radiography of the petrous pyramids, or polytomography.

In 1975, the clinical use of Békésy and SISI tests was discontinued at the Otologic Medical Group and has been rarely performed since. Impedance audiometry has inherited the role of testing both the auditory fatigue and loudness function. Impedance audiometry is feasible at hearing levels of 75 dB or better at 500–1000 Hz.

Absence or decay of acoustic reflexes were diagnosed in 82% of proven acoustic neuromas [4], compared with an accuracy of 60% for Békésy and 68% for SISI. Brain stem evoked response audiometry (BERA) has become the most accurate audiometric test for acoustic neuroma. It is currently performed after obtaining some positive results from the basic screening tests, or when a strong clinical suspicion is not matched with positive results of those tests.

Any positive result obtained from the basic screening tests further strengthens the clinical diagnosis of acoustic neuroma and definite radiological studies should be used: CCT scan and/or angle myelography (polytome pantopaque). Negative basic screening tests allow the clinician to follow his patient closely and watch for further development of new symptoms with periodic retesting. Proceeding with the definitive radiologic tests should not be discouraged if it is felt that the symptoms warrant it.

A CCT scan should precede angle myelography because:

(1) A positive CCT scan eliminates the need for myelography, thus saving the patient an invasive procedure.

(2) Residual contrast material in the posterior fossa following an angle myelography shows as artefacts on CCT scan.

It should be kept in mind that the CCT scan will usually demonstrate fairly large extracanalicular tumors (2 cm and larger) with a false negative rate of 16%. Angle myelography should be performed, therefore, on patients with a negative CCT scan. Patients with clinical suspicion of a small tumour should have angle myelography following the basic screening tests without a CCT scan.

The rational approach to the use of the various diagnostic tests will assure prompt and accurate diagnosis with minimal morbidity and cost.

MANAGEMENT

The ultimate goal of the treatment of acoustic neuroma is total surgical removal without further neurologic deficit. Achievement of this goal is inversely related to tumour size. The progress made in acoustic neuroma surgery in the past two decades was intimately linked to the simultaneous major developments in the diagnostic methods, with refinement of the surgical approaches and techniques.

Advances in surgical instrumentation

Microsurgery. The introduction of the otomicroscope to neuro-otology provided unprecedented illumination and magnification that enabled fine and controlled dissection with newly designed micro-instruments to be carried out. Complete control of the operative field became possible. The ability to establish subarachnoid avascular planes around the tumour with positive identification and preservation of neural and vascular structures increased the surgeon's ability to reduce surgical morbidity and mortality.

Continuous irrigation–suction. The use of this technique as an adjunct to the bony and soft tissue dissection added efficiency and safety to the surgical technique. The drilling burr and the bone are kept cool, thus preventing thermal damage to the adjacent neural tissue (facial nerve). Floating bone dust is easily removed by suction, keeping the drilling site clear. Blood clots around soft tissue are washed out and removed with the aid of a fenestrated irrigation–suction device that diminishes the amount of negative pressure applied on delicate neural and vascular tissue (Brackmann suction).

Bipolar electro-coagulation. The temporal bone is surrounded by a large number of major arteries

and veins. Vital arterial supply to the brain stem is frequently encountered during dissection in the cerebellopontine angle and in the internal auditory canal. Control of bleeding throughout surgery is necessary in order to reduce blood loss and to keep the operative field clear. The use of bipolar electro-coagulation provides a quick and reliable method of haemostasis. It affords precise local application of electrical current between the poles, without the spread of the coagulating current along the vessel that can cause retrograde thrombosis beyond the bleeding point.

House–Urban dissector. Tumour exposure is started by progressive blunt dissection along its borders in subarachnoidal avascular planes. Manipulation of the tumour in any direction is harmful and should be avoided. It can cause compression and kinking of the major arteries, pressure on the brain stem and damage to the facial nerve by stretching it.

The principle of tumour dissection is gradual intracapsular piecemeal enucleation of its core from the centre centrifugally allowing collapse of the tumour on itself without displacement. This is executed with the aid of the House–Urban rotatory suction dissector. Constant suction through the opening of a rotating blade feeds the tumour into the blade and the cut pieces are eliminated by the suction. The capsule of the tumour is then separated from adjacent tissue.

Anatomic surgical approaches to acoustic neuroma

The better access to the deep structures of the temporal bone with the aid of the oto-microscope and improved instrumentation lead to the concept of direct transtemporal approaches to the internal auditory canal and the cerebellopontine angle. Through these approaches to the internal auditory canal the preservation of the facial nerve has become a reality. In contrast to the suboccipital craniectomy, the new transtemporal approaches helped to reduce surgical morbidity and mortality:

(1) by avoiding retraction or resection of the cerebellum,

(2) by positioning the patient supine instead of in the hazardous seated position, and

(3) by a direct access to the tumour bed in case of postoperative haemorrhage.

Middle fossa approach

Access to the internal auditory canal is obtained through a craniectomy in the squamous portion of the temporal bone. By the extradural retraction of the temporal lobe medially, positive identification of the geniculate ganglion and the facial nerve on the skull base leads to the internal auditory canal by removal of bone from its roof. The facial nerve, the cochlear division of the eighth nerve and the internal auditory vessels can be preserved during tumour dissection. This approach is limited to patients with intracanalicular tumour and serviceable hearing on the affected side (3·4% of cases). Preservation of hearing was achieved in 60% of these patients. Application of this approach to tumour with extension into the cerebellopontine angle carries a higher risk of damage to the facial and cochlear nerves and the internal auditory artery.

Translabyrinthine approach

This is the approach of choice to extracanalicular tumours. Through a complete mastoidectomy and labyrinthectomy the internal auditory canal is exposed to around 270° of its superior, lateral and inferior circumference. Excellent exposure of the facial nerve along its entire course is afforded. The cerebellopontine angle is reached directly through the posterior fossa dura in front of the cerebellum without retracting it.

Combined translabyrinthine and suboccipital approach

The translabyrinthine approach can be extended posteriorly as a combined translabyrinthine and suboccipital approach. Extension of the operative field posteriorly is achieved by wide removal of occipital bone extradurally. This approach is used to remove large tumours associated with increased intracranial pressure or fifth nerve findings. It allows excellent decompression of the posterior fossa.

Transcochlear approach

The translabyrinthine approach can be extended forward as a transcochlear approach [5]. Removal of the cochlea in combination with the translabyrinthine approach allows exposure of the apex of the petrous pyramid and the clivus of the skull base anterior to the internal auditory canal. The anterior border of the operative field is then the internal carotid artery. The facial nerve is rerouted posteriorly after freeing the geniculate ganglion from the greater superficial petrosal nerve. This approach has been used for tumours of the petrous pyramid apex and clivus, mostly meningiomas and cholesteatomas.

Retrolabyrinthine approach

This approach allows exploration of the cerebellopontine angle and its neural and vascular content, with preservation of the labyrinth. Through a complete mastoidectomy, the sigmoid sinus is retracted posteriorly and the cerebellopontine angle is penetrated through an incision in the posterior fossa dura between the sigmoid sinus and the medial aspect of the labyrinth. The fifth to the ninth cranial nerves are fully exposed. This approach has been used mostly for selective section of the posterior root of the fifth nerve for trigeminal neuralgia and tic doloureux. Newer indications for the use of this approach include [6]:

(1) Exploration of the cerebellopontine angle for biopsy and removal of otherwise unidentifiable tumours. This is done without damage to the labyrinth.

(2) Treatment of hemifacial spasm and selective section of cranial nerves for neuralgias. It is used primarily for fifth nerve section.

Conservative surgical treatment of acoustic neuroma

Any procedure short of total removal is a compromise of the ideal treatment.

Forced partial removal. The indication for the intraoperative decision of partial removal is repeated sudden severe changes in vital signs during dissection. If repeated attempts to resume the surgical dissection will persistently induce vital sign changes, the operation is terminated, while the residual tumour is left intact. After complete healing and recovery, a further attempt to remove the tumour is made after 3–4 months.

Bony decompression with preservation of hearing. This conservative surgical approach is usually performed on the only hearing ear of a patient with bilateral acoustic neuromas, after the removal of a tumour on one side. Bony decompression allows further tumour growth, with preservation of hearing, as long as a definite surgical procedure can be postponed under close observation and follow-up. This can be accomplished by two approaches:

(1) *Middle fossa approach.* With extensive decompression of the internal auditory canal and petrous ridge. The acoustic nerve is left intact.

(2) *Suboccipital approach.* Bony decompression of the posterior fossa, extradurally.

Partial removal of acoustic neuroma without preservation of hearing. This is used in the management of elderly patients or patients who are considered a poor surgical risk. Partial tumour removal through a translabyrinthine approach is carried out in a fast procedure. The vestibular nerves are cut to alleviate dizziness.

A review of the 495 cases of acoustic neuroma operated at the Otologic Medical Group over a 7-year period (22 March 1968 to 31 January 1975) revealed that twenty-nine cases underwent partial removal (5·9%). (Thirteen of these cases eventually underwent total removal.) Twenty-five were considered large tumours. Four were considered medium sized tumours. In seventeen cases (3·4%) fragments of tumour were left. Ten were large tumours and seven were medium-sized tumours. As experience with acoustic neuroma surgery was gained, the percentage of patients undergoing partial removal constantly decreased, from 44% of the first fifty cases in 1964 to 14% of cases 151–200 in 1968.

Treatment policy

At the Otologic Medical Group a system of surgical management has been evolved, depending on the classification of patients into six categories.

(1) Intracanalicular tumour (up to 8 mm in diameter) in patients with useful hearing. The treatment indicated here is a middle fossa approach which allows preservation of the facial and cochlear nerves. Hearing can be preserved in 60% of patients and there has been no mortality.

(2) Intracanalicular tumours in patients without useful hearing. Surgical removal is via the translabyrinthine approach. The risks to facial nerve and to life are minimal.

(3) Medium sized tumours (2·5–3 cm in diameter) with or without fifth nerve involvement but without increase in intracranial pressure, long tract or cerebellar signs. Translabyrinthine removal is the treatment of choice. The facial nerve is usually well seen throughout and the mortality is low (less than 2%).

(4) Large tumours (larger than 3 cm in diameter) with fifth nerve involvement and evidence of raised intracranial pressure, cerebellar and brain stem compression. Treatment is by the combined suboccipital petrosal or transsigmoid approach. The mortality rate is 7%.

(5) Medium to large tumours in the only hearing ear. This situation is usually encountered in patients with von Recklinghausen's disease with bilateral neuromas in whom the hearing is already lost on one side. Surgical treatment is conservative. Bony decompression through a middle fossa or suboccipital approach will enable further growth of tumour without producing elevated intracranial pressure, thus delaying total surgical removal.

(6) Any other tumour in a high-risk patient with disabling symptoms. A translabyrinthine partial removal takes little time and denervating the vestibular end organ abolishes the distressing symptoms.

References

[1] JOHNSON E. W. (1977) Auditory test results in 500 cases of acoustic neuroma. *Archives of Otolaryngology* **103**, 152.
[2] HOUSE W. F. *Acoustic Neuroma.* To be published.
[3] SELTERS W. A. & BRACKMANN D. E. (1977) Acoustic tumor detection with brainstem electric response audiometry. *Archives of Otolaryngology* **103**, 181.
[4] SHEEHY J. L. & INZER B. E. (1976) Acoustic reflex test in neuro-otologic diagnosis. *Archives of Otolaryngology* **102**, 647.
[5] HOUSE W. F. & HITSELBERGER W. E. (1976) The transcochlear approach to the skull base. *Archives of Otolaryngology* **102**, 334.
[6] BRACKMANN D. E. & HITSELBERGER W. E. *Retrolabyrinthine Approach Technique and New Indications.* To be published.

CHAPTER 5

Facial Paralysis

The disfigurement caused by a permanently paralysed face is so gross that the attending physician must have both accurate diagnostic tests for early prognosis and effective therapeutic measures for cases with bad prognosis.

Laumans & Jongkccs must bc crcditcd for having recognized the clinical value of percutaneous electrical stimulation of the facial nerve (the so-called nerve excitability test) in establishing the severity of intratemporal nerve injury [1]. With the nerve excitability test it became possible to determine as early as 3 days after the onset of the palsy whether the observed paralysis of the face was due to a reversible block of impulse conduction (neuropraxia) or to Wallerian degeneration (axonotmesis, neurotmesis). Maximal rather than minimal stimulation improves the reliability of electrodiagnosis and shortens the delay between denervation and observation [2]. The advantage of maximal stimulation is due to the fact that a minimal stimulus used for the nerve excitability test will produce the same visible twitch of the facial muscles as long as a sufficient number of residual nerve fibres is still available for stimulation. In contrast to that, all fibres capable of firing will respond after application of a maximal stimulus. Esslen recorded the potentials evoked by maximal nerve stimulation in a representative number of facial muscles using bipolar surface electrodes [3]. With this method, called electroneuronography (ENoG), quantitative analysis of the evoked integrated action of the facial muscles can be obtained as early as 24 hours following onset of an intratemporal facial palsy [4]. ENoG is to date the most precise, comprehensive and timely electrodiagnostic test and has determined our therapeutic approach to intratemporal facial nerve lesions.

The development of the middle cranial fossa and the translabyrinthine approaches for the most hidden intrameatal and intralabyrinthine segments of the facial nerve [5, 6, 7] and the refinements of oto-microsurgical techniques for nerve anastomosis have also revolutionized the surgical repair of facial nerve lesions [8].

INCIDENCE AND AETIOLOGY OF INTRATEMPORAL FACIAL PALSY

The incidence of the most common form of intratemporal facial palsy, i.e. Bell's palsy, varies in Europe between 11·5 and 18·8 patients per 100 000 per year. Higher figures are reported from countries like Egypt, Columbia and India. A recent survey in Australia has demonstrated that 75% of general practitioners see one to three cases of Bell's palsy a year, 37% see less than one case a year, and 6% see between four and ten cases per year [9].

In order of frequency the most common forms of intratemporal facial palsy are:
(1) idiopathic or Bell's palsy (39·7%);
(2) trauma (24·7%);
(3) tumours (12·5%);
(4) herpes zoster oticus (6·8%);
(5) acute and chronic otitis media (5·5%).

As seen in Table 5.1, Bell's palsy and traumatic palsy are evenly distributed in children and adults. Palsies due to acute middle ear infections predominate in children, whereas herpetic lesions characteristically occur in the adult. Tumours originating from the facial nerve (neurinomas, haemangiomas) or involving the seventh nerve (glomus jugulare tumours, meningiomas, epidermoids) are mostly found in adults.

DIAGNOSIS OF FACIAL PALSY

Careful history, precise clinical examination and

65

TABLE 5.1. Aetiology and frequency of facial palsy in 365 patients (75 children and 290 adults)

Aetiology	Children		Adults		Total	
	Number of patients	%	Number of patients	%	Number of patients	%
Congenital	13	17·5	—	—	13	3·6
Bell's palsy	27	36	118	40·6	145	39·7
Trauma	19	25·4	71	24·5	90	24·7
Herpes zoster	—	—	25	8·7	25	6·8
Acute otitis media	7	9·4	8	2·8	15	4·1
Chronic otitis media	2	2·6	3	1	5	1·4
Tumour	2	2·6	44	15	46	12·6
Other	·5	6·5	21	7·4	26	7·1
Total	75	100	290	100	365	100

electrodiagnosis are the prerequisites for the successful management of facial palsy.

Clinical features

The evolution of the palsy (sudden or progressive onset, delay after injury, etc.) is of prime diagnostic importance and can only be established by a careful history. The essential differentiation between a palsy of the upper or lower motor neuron is made according to the clinical evaluation of mobility in the upper portion of the face (particularly the forehead). The complete absence of voluntary facial movements (complete paralysis) has a different prognostic value than the retention of some voluntary movements (paresis). The tone of facial tissues, which depends upon constitution, age and general condition of the patient, strongly influences the asymmetry of the paralysed face and may create difficulties in evaluating the completeness of a palsy. This is particularly true in young children and in the presence of fresh injuries. ENoG has shown that normal facial movements may occur in the presence of 70% degenerated nerve fibres. Therefore, one should be very careful and rely upon electrodiagnosis when there is the slightest doubt in the clinical evaluation of facial movements. Associated lesions such as herpetic vesicles and involvement of other cranial nerves (particularly cochlear and vestibular deficien-

cies) should be investigated. Radiographs (Stenvers projections and polytomography) are required to rule out a tumour when the palsy is recurrent or of slow onset. The same should be done when no return of facial movements is observed 6 months after a so-called 'idiopathic' palsy.

Electrodiagnosis

Electrical tests should be used as soon as facial paralysis is diagnosed. They are the only techniques available to collect objective information on the condition of the seventh nerve in the absence of voluntary facial movements. Adequate management of the paralysed face is impossible without electrodiagnosis.

The percutaneous electrical tests used for the diagnosis of intratemporal facial palsy (nerve excitability test, maximal stimulation test and ENoG) are based on the observations that:

(1) preservation of nerve conduction distal to the site of injury indicates reversible damage (neuropraxia) with very good prognosis; and

(2) absence of nerve conduction distal from the site of injury indicates degeneration due to severe damage of the axons (axonotmesis) or nerve fibres (neurotmesis) and indicates a bad prognosis (Fig. 5.1).

Electroneuronography

ENoG is the best electrodiagnostic test because it

gives objective quantitative information on the evolution of degeneration as early as 24 hours after the onset of an intratemporal facial palsy. The principle of ENoG is shown in Fig. 5.2. The same bipolar electrodes having a diameter of 7 mm and placed 50 mm apart are used for both stimulation and recording. Square wave impulses of 0·2 msec duration, 50–150 volt amplitude, and a frequency of 1/sec are used for maximal stimulation of the facial nerve. The

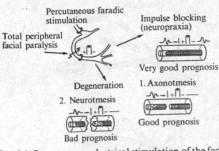

FIG. 5.1. Percutaneous electrical stimulation of the facial nerve. Preservation of nerve conduction distal from the site of injury indicates reversible damage (neuropraxia) with very good prognosis. Absence of nerve conduction distal from the site of injury indicates degeneration due to either damage of the axons (axonotmesis) with good prognosis or severe damage of the endoneural tubes (neurotmesis) with bad prognosis. Note that it is impossible to distinguish by electrodiagnosis between axonotmesis and neurotmesis.

stimulation is performed outside the stylomastoid foramen in front of the tragus. The recording electrodes are firmly applied in the nasolabial fold. For practical purposes recording of the summating potentials of the peroral muscles has been found satisfactory although other facial muscles can also be tested separately. A fibreoptic cathode ray oscilloscope provides direct recording of the summating potentials on daylight developing paper. The amplitude of the evoked summating potentials of the intact and involved side of the face are measured peak-to-peak (Fig. 5.3). The number of degenerated fibres is given by the difference in amplitude of the measured summating potentials. Latency measurements are possible, but have not proven of practical value. The great advantage of ENoG versus the simple observation of facial movements – May's maximal stimulation test [2] – is the quantitative analysis of recorded evoked

responses (Fig. 5.3). Of course, the variability of skin resistance as well as that of pressure and localization of recording and stimulating electrodes may induce artefacts that can only be avoided by experience. In experienced hands the

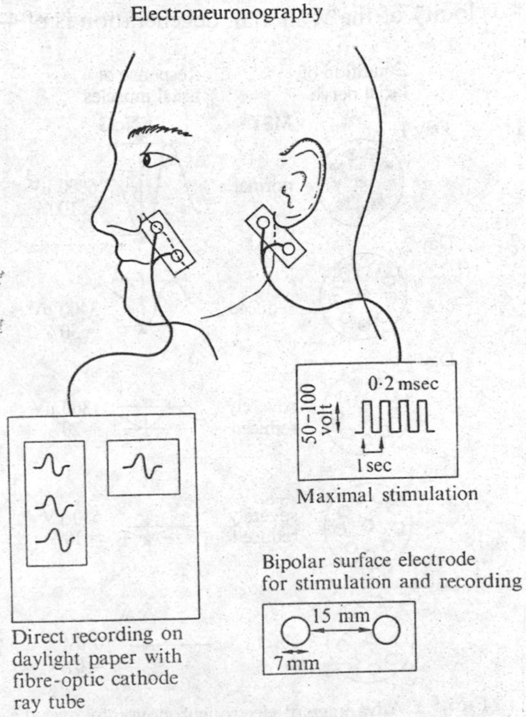

Electroneuronography

Maximal stimulation

Bipolar surface electrode for stimulation and recording

Direct recording on daylight paper with fibre-optic cathode ray tube

FIG. 5.2. Electroneuronography is based upon recording of the evoked summating potentials of the facial muscles with bipolar surface electrodes.

error occurring in repeated measurements of the summating potentials of the intact side of the face does not exceed 5% [3]. An experienced examiner obtains reliable measurements even when degeneration reaches the 97 or 98% level (potentials of 50–100 mV). Difficulties in interpreting electroneuronographic results do occur when desynchronization of stimulated nerve fibres is present. The asynchronous firing of stimulated fibres may produce a considerable drop in the evoked summating potentials. This phenomenon occurs particularly during early deblocking or beginning regeneration.

The information given by electroneuronography on intratemporal facial nerve lesions has a delay of 24 hours. This delay is due to the time needed by Wallerian degeneration to progress from the site of injury (inside the temporal bone) to the site of electrical stimulation (outside the stylomastoid foramen). Assuming that the facial nerve has been injured at the entrance of the Fallopian canal and that the average centrifugal velocity of the Wallerian degeneration is of 4–6

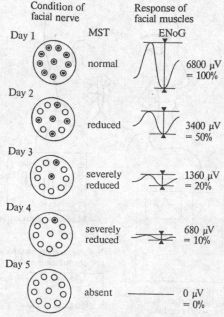

Condition of facial nerve		MST	Response of facial muscles ENoG	
Day 1		normal		6800 µV = 100%
Day 2		reduced		3400 µV = 50%
Day 3		severely reduced		1360 µV = 20%
Day 4		severely reduced		680 µV = 10%
Day 5		absent		0 µV = 0%

Fig. 5.3. Advantage of electroneuronography over the maximal stimulation test. It is not possible to distinguish visually between the response obtained after maximal stimulation by day 3 and day 4. The recorded summating potentials of the facial muscles show that degeneration has progressed from 80 to 90% in these 2 days.

cm per day [10], degeneration will not reach the point of electrical stimulation – about 4 cm distal to the site of lesion – until 24 hours after the injury (Fig. 5.4). This delay must be considered when evaluating the results of treatment. A progression of degeneration occurring 24 hours after total intratemporal decompression for Bell's palsy is not due to a failure of the operation but to the normal distal progression of Wallerian degeneration.

The evolution of degeneration at the stimulating point not only depends on the distance from the actual site of the lesion, but also upon the extent and duration of the injury itself. This is

why both the amount and the evolution of degeneration must be considered in order to make accurate electrodiagnostic assessments. The maximal value of degeneration as well as the time needed to reach the maximal value of degeneration should always be known when results of treatment are compared.

Another often disregarded limitation of electrodiagnosis is the inability to distinguish with

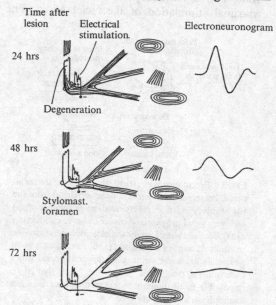

Fig. 5.4. The information given by electroneuronography on intratemporal facial lesions has a delay of at least 24 hours due to the time needed by Wallerian degeneration to progress from the site of injury (inside the temporal bone) to the site of electrical stimulation (outside the stylomastoid foramen).

electrical stimulation between injuries limited to the axons (axonotmesis) and those involving the connective tissue surrounding the axons, the endoneural tubes (neurotmesis). Conduction of nerve impulses is lost following both types of lesions, those limited to the axons and those involving axons and endoneural tubes (Fig. 5.1). However, axonotmesis carries a good prognosis since the intact endoneural tube will guide the regenerating axons to their original place, whereas neurotmesis has a bad prognosis because it is always followed by the intermingling of regenerating axons and, therefore, by disturbing mass movements of the face (synkinesis).

This is why electrodiagnosis can be used to assess the extent of degeneration of a motor nerve fibre population but cannot be used, *per se*, to predict the precise outcome of functional restitution. For this purpose the evolution of degeneration, as determined by repeated electroneuronographic tests, must be related both to the type of injury and to the natural course of restitution after that injury.

Only this combined information will permit valid prognostications. This is why prognosis based on electrodiagnosis still remains subject to statistical errors. The extent of such errors should be kept in mind when evaluating results of treatment of intratemporal facial paralysis. In Bell's palsy degeneration of more than 95% of the motor nerve fibres within 2 weeks from the onset of the palsy indicates neurotmesis with insufficient return of function in 50% of the patients. This means that one out of two patients with more than 95% degenerated nerve fibres has a bad prognosis. The fact that one out of two patients with a bad prognosis may end up with sufficient spontaneous restitution of facial movements does not signify an error in electrodiagnostic assessment but points to the undetected presence of a high degree of axonotmesis. The impossibility of estimating by electrical stimulation the number of intact endoneural tubes when total degeneration is present explains why double blind prospective statistical studies are necessary for evaluation of the results of therapy in facial paralysis.

Electromyography
Electromyography is of no use in the acute phase of most intratemporal facial palsies since denervation potentials are not recorded with this method before 14 days after onset of the palsy. The electromyogram can be, however, of value:

(1) in showing activity of residual motor units when early deblocking of motor fibres occurs with questionable return of facial movements; and

(2) in showing signs of re-innervation before clinical detection of facial movements.

Early deblocking is a sign of good prognosis in Bell's palsy even when it occurs in the presence of extensive degeneration. An electromyogram showing reinnervation potentials may induce re-evaluation of proposed surgery when spontaneous recovery fails to appear clinically at the expected time.

Topographic diagnosis

Measurements of *taste, stapedius reflex* and *lacrimation* have been used to determine the anatomical level of the lesion, particularly since the work of Tschiassny [11]. It has been our experience that contradictory results may be obtained with topographical investigation throughout the evolution of an intratemporal palsy. This apparent contradiction can be explained by:

(1) the different distribution of pathology across the entire nerve fibre population; and

(2) the variable number of nerve fibres which must be affected in order to suppress the stapedial reflex, taste or lacrimation.

Lacrimation
In spite of the above mentioned limitations lacrimation is of particular value because of its surgical implication. Trans- or suprageniculate facial nerve lesions must be approached through the middle cranial fossa or the labyrinth, whereas infrageniculate lesions are handled through a transcanal or transmastoid approach. Only quantitative measurements of lacrimal secretion are useful. Expressions such as that of a 'dry eye' are meaningless. For the quantitative evaluation of lacrimation we use two strips of blotting paper 0·1 mm thick, 50 mm long and 5 mm wide. One end of each strip is bent over a length of 5 mm and carefully placed into the lower conjunctival fornix of the patient. The introduction of the blotting paper in the non-anaesthetized conjunctival sac is not painful and acts as a sufficient stimulus for lacrimal secretion. The amount of lacrimation is determined by the length of paper which has become wet by tearing in 5 minutes.

Lacrimation is abnormal when

(1) the difference between the lacrimal flow of both eyes exceeds 30% of the total bilateral lacrimation; and

(2) the sum of the secretion of both eyes does not reach 25 mm of blotting paper (Fig. 5.5). It is important to realize that unilateral transgeniculate lesions may produce bilateral symmetric

reduction of lacrimation. This latter phenomenon is observed in 69% of the patients submitted to unilateral geniculate ganglionectomy
because of petrosal neuralgia [12]. Although a
similar bilateral effect of parasympathetic denervation has been reported after unilateral vidian
neurectomy, its significance in evaluating lacrimation was completely disregarded in the past.

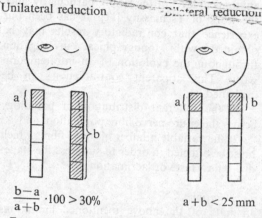

$$\frac{b-a}{a+b} \cdot 100 > 30\%$$

$$a+b < 25\,mm$$

FIG. 5.5. Quantitative evaluation of Schirmer's test.
Lacrimation is abnormal when (1) the difference
between the lacrimal flow of both eyes exceeds 30% of
total bilateral lacrimation (unilateral reduction) and (2)
the sum of the secretion of both eyes does not reach 25
mm of blotting paper (bilateral reduction).

Abnormal Schirmer's test values were
recorded in 92% of patients with traumatic
palsies and in all patients with idiopathic and
herpetic palsy having more than 90% maximal
degeneration. These data indicate that abnormal
lacrimation can be used as a sign of poor
prognosis. Disturbances of the salivary flow are
also useful prognostic indicators since they
become reduced early in patients likely to
develop denervation [13].

In contrast to lacrimation and salivary flow,
taste and stapedial reflex do not correlate with
the maximal degree of degeneration. A normal
stapedial reflex can be measured in 20% of the
patients having more than 90% maximal degeneration in Bell's palsy. Taste and stapedial
reflex can therefore, not be used for prognostic
implications.

Topographical diagnostic tests, including lacrimation, are unreliable in presence of facial

nerve tumours, particularly neurinomas. Normal taste, stapedius reflex and lacrimation have
been repeatedly found in the presence of large
neurinomas originating from the geniculate
ganglion.

Intraoperative evoked electromyography
This test is used for localizing the site of the lesion
when the nerve is surgically exposed. The test can
only be used if at operation 3–5% blocked motor
nerve fibres are still present. The same equipment
is used as for ENoG. One or two EMG needles

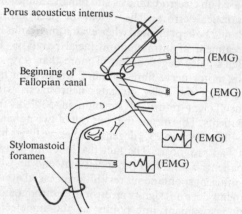

FIG. 5.6. Intraoperative evoked electromyography in
Bell's palsy. Ninety-three per cent of the motor nerve
fibres are degenerated, 7% blocked. Stimulation performed above the lesion (internal auditory meatus and
proximal labyrinthine segment) will not evoke potentials
from the facial muscles. Evoked potentials do appear as
soon as the stimulating electrodes have reached a point
distal to the lesion (genu of the facial nerve, mastoid
segment). The lesion can be localized between the
entrance of the Fallopian canal and the geniculate
ganglion.

are introduced into the facial muscles still re-
sponding to percutaneous stimulation before
inducing general anaesthesia. The exposed nerve
is then stimulated with bipolar forceps. Stimulation performed above the lesion will not evoke
potentials from the facial muscles. However, as
soon as the stimulating electrode reaches a point
distal to the lesion, potentials will be recorded
from the corresponding facial muscles (Fig. 5.6).

Intraoperative evoked electromyography
should be recommended for objective localization of the lesion in intratemporal facial paralysis. The use of this method will stop endless

discussions concerning subjective evaluations of intraoperative pathology (such as swellings, oedema, discolorations, etc.) and open the place for objective comparison of electrophysiological data.

MANAGEMENT OF INTRA-TEMPORAL FACIAL PARALYSIS

Temporal bone fractures

Clinical features

Facial paralysis is observed in 40% of transverse fractures and in 20% of longitudinal fractures of the petrous pyramid. Traffic accidents are the usual cause. Young adults between 20 and 25 years of age and children between 8 and 10 years are most frequently involved. Longitudinal fractures occur more often than transverse fractures. Therefore, patients with facial paralysis following longitudinal fractures are seen six times more frequently than those with the same lesion after transverse fracture. Mixed fractures may occur. For practical purposes they can be disregarded since a transverse fracture which does not affect the inner ear, must be considered a longitudinal one.

Pathology

Longitudinal fractures usually begin in the temporal squama, extend through the postero-superior external bony canal wall and run across the roof of the middle ear, close to the labyrinthine capsule, to end in the middle cranial fossa near the carotid canal and the foramen spinosum (Fig. 5.7). The clinical symptoms of a longitudinal fracture are

(1) bleeding and eventually CSF otorrhoea;
(2) visible fracture in the posterosuperior bony canal wall; and
(3) conductive deafness.

Longitudinal fractures generally occur in highly pneumatized temporal bones and injure the facial nerve by stretching it along a line parallel to its tympanic segment and to the greater superficial petrosal nerve (Figs. 5.7 and 5.12). The following main types of lesions are observed:

(1) impression of a bony fragment into the Fallopian canal (18%);
(2) complete severance of the facial nerve (28·5%); and
(3) intraneural haematoma (53·5%). One-third of the intraneural haematomas present with associated lacerations of the greater superficial petrosal nerve. Ninety-three per cent of the facial nerve lesions occurring after longitudinal fractures are localized just distal to the geniculate ganglion. This confirms earlier histological

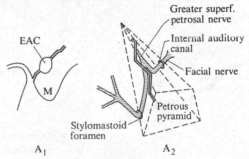

FIG. 5.7. Typical longitudinal fracture producing facial paralysis. A1, Runström II view; A2, The fracture line runs across the roof of the middle ear close to the labyrinthine capsule.

observations [14] which have been ignored for years. The fibrosis resulting from untreated intraneural haematomas prevents the regenerating nerve fibres from following their normal path to the middle ear and forces them to grow along the greater superficial petrosal nerve (Fig. 5.8). This abnormal regeneration pattern explains the bad results observed when surgical revisions limited to the mastoid and tympanic segments of the nerve failed to reveal significant pathology [7].

Transverse fractures extend across the labyrinthine capsule of the temporal bone and usually involve the jugular foramen, the vestibule and eventually the internal acoustic meatus (Fig. 5.9). The fracture line is frequently Y-shaped and breaks out a triangular piece of bone which includes portions of the lateral vestibular wall. The Fallopian canal is injured in its proximal labyrinthine segment and/or along the medial wall of the middle ear.

The clinical symptoms of a transverse fracture are

(1) haematotympanum; and
(2) total sensorineural deafness as well as total loss of vestibular function of the involved side.

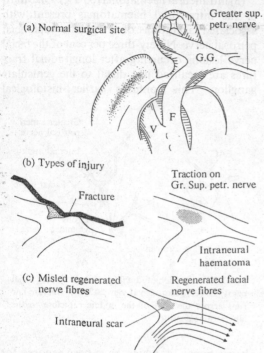

(a) Normal surgical site

Greater sup. petr. nerve

G.G.

V   F

(b) Types of injury

Fracture

Traction on Gr. Sup. petr. nerve

Intraneural haematoma

(c) Misled regenerated nerve fibres

Regenerated facial nerve fibres

Intraneural scar

FIG. 5.8. Intraneural fibrosis resulting from untreated lacerations or intraneural haematomas distal to the geniculate ganglion prevents the regenerating motor nerve fibres from reaching the middle ear and forces them to grow along the greater superficial petrosal nerve.

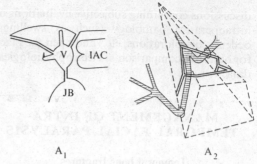

A_1 A_2

FIG. 5.9. Typical transverse fracture producing facial paralysis. A1, Stenvers view; A2, Y-shaped fracture line breaking out a triangular piece of bone which includes the lateral wall of the vestibule.

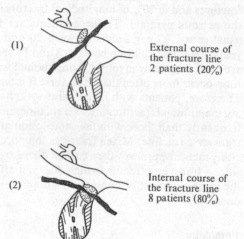

(1)   External course of the fracture line 2 patients (20%)

(2)   Internal course of the fracture line 8 patients (80%)

FIG. 5.10. Types of injury in transverse fractures of the petrous bone.

Transverse fractures injure the facial nerve in its proximal labyrinthine segment (80% of the cases) and in its tympanic segment (20% of the cases) (Fig. 5.10). Both types of lesions may occur in combination. In all instances complete or nearly complete severance of the facial nerve is present.

Mixed fractures are classified according to their symptoms (particularly the type of hearing loss) into either one of the two above-mentioned main types.

Radiology

Radiology (Runström II and Stenvers views, polytomography) is of relative value in establishing the precise site of traumatic facial nerve lesions. In our hands correct radiological localization of the lesion was possible in 45% of the transverse and only in 5% of the longitudinal fractures. The difficulty in localizing the facial nerve lesion in longitudinal fractures is due to the tortuous course of the fracture line (Fig. 5.7) which eludes the ideal plane for radiological demonstration.

Management

An incomplete traumatic palsy has a good prognosis and is treated conservatively. A complete paralysis should be treated as an emergency. Although in general the prognosis of a paralysis occurring with a delay of a few days following the injury is better than that of a paralysis of immediate onset, the delay between injury and onset of the palsy cannot be taken as a reliable measure of the severity of the lesion [15]. Repeated electroneuronograms performed as soon as permitted by the general condition of the patient are necessary in order to clarify the situation. Animal experiments have demonstrated that severe trauma requiring surgical correction is invariably followed by more than 90% degeneration of facial nerve motor fibres within 6 days of the injury. Surgery is, therefore, indicated when 90% degeneration is reached within 6 days of the onset of the palsy (*not* from the occurrence of the fracture). An immediate facial paralysis reaching 90% degeneration well after the 6 days' limit has a good prognosis and does not require surgical revision. On the other hand, a delayed paralysis showing 90% degeneration within 6 days of onset requires surgery to ensure optimal recovery (Fig. 5.11). According to the above-mentioned electroneuronographic criteria unnecessary surgery has been performed in only 7% of the patients [15].

In temporal bone fractures delayed surgery may also be indicated. Some patients are still referred for evaluation of their palsy weeks or months after the trauma when the absent regeneration 'begins' to concern both the patient and the attending physician. Total degeneration of nerve fibres is usually found at ENoG in these cases. If there are no clinical or electromyographic signs of beginning regeneration, the therapeutic decision is based upon

(1) the clinical and radiological estimation of the extent of the intratemporal lesion; and

(2) the result of the Schirmer's test. Fractures with absent or minimal radiologic injury and a normal Schirmer's test are treated conservatively. Surgery is immediately performed when the radiographs show a severe fracture with abnormal Schirmer's test values. An expectant attitude is taken when in doubt. If regeneration fails to appear 6–8 months after the trauma, surgical revision is carried out. At surgery intraneural scars preventing normal regeneration are excised and replaced by autogenous nerve grafts [8]. To ensure good results, specimens of the proximal stump of the facial nerve must be

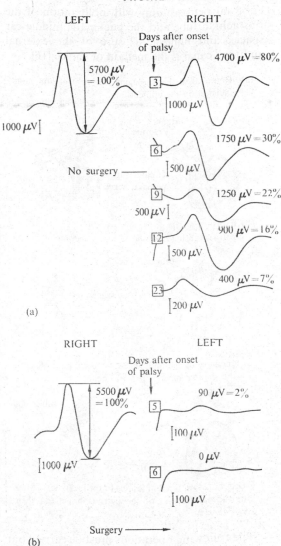

(a)

(b)

FIG. 5.11. Electroneuronograms after immediate (a) and delayed (b) facial paralysis after longitudinal fracture. Surgery is indicated independently from the delay of onset of the palsy when 90% of the motor nerve fibres degenerate within 6 days from onset of the palsy (not from injury).

evaluated by frozen sections during the operation to confirm the presence of normal nerve fibres.

In transverse fractures surgery is not only designed for nerve repair, but also to avoid the permanent threat of meningitis due to the insufficient callus formed by the labyrinthine capsule.

Subtotal petrosectomy with obliteration of the Eustachian tube and the pneumatic middle ear spaces and blindsac closure of the external auditory canal is the method of choice [16].

(a) Removal of the impinging fragment of bone and incision on the epineurium

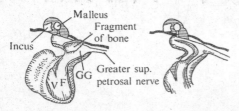

(b) Excision of the geniculate ganglion with rerouting and end-to-end anastomosis

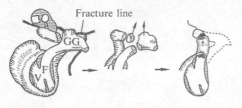

(c) Incision of the epineurium with clipping of the greater superior petrosal nerve

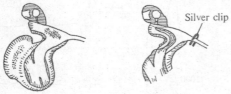

FIG. 5.12. Main types of lesions of the facial nerve after longitudinal fracture of the petrous bone and their surgical repair.

The following operations must be carried out through the middle cranial fossa to rehabilitate the function of the facial nerve in longitudinal fractures (Fig. 5.12):

(1) removal of the impinging fragment of bone with incision of the epineurium of the nerve;

(2) re-routing of the Fallopian canal around the superior ampulla with excision of the geniculum and end-to-end anastomosis (or nerve grafting); and

(3) evacuation of the intraneural haematoma with incision of the epineurium and clipping of the greater superficial petrosal nerve.

The last measure is taken to avoid misdirection of regrowing motor fibres along the greater superficial petrosal nerve.

In transverse fractures surgical repair requires exposure of the entire intratemporal course of the seventh nerve through the translabyrinthine approach. The continuity of the nerve is restored by creating a new bony canal between the stylomastoid foramen and the internal auditory meatus (Fig. 5.13). This meato-mastoidal re-routing permits enough gain in nerve length to perform an end-to-end anastomosis after excision of the traumatized portion of the nerve. Interposition of a graft is, however, indicated whenever the slightest tension is found when approximating the nerve stumps. The recommended techniques of anastomosis are (Fig. 5.13):

(1) removal of the epineurium 3–5 mm from the proposed anastomotic surface;

(2) oblique cutting of the nerve ends; and

(3) use of 10–0 nylon monofilament sutures or collagen splints for fixation of the nerve stumps.

Surgical trauma

Clinical features

Incomplete or complete facial palsy may result from lesions produced inadvertently during middle ear or temporal bone surgery. As in fractures the onset of the palsy can be immediate or delayed. The incidence of inadvertent intraoperative facial nerve lesions varies from 0·6 to 3·7% [17].

Pathology

The most common sites of surgical injury to the facial nerve are, in order of frequency:

(1) the tympanic and mastoid segments, particularly in the region of the oval window niche (mastoidectomy or posterior tympanotomy performed in sclerosed bone or in the presence of extensive cholesteatoma);

(2) the distal portion of the mastoid segment (surgery for agenetic ears);

(3) dehiscences of the Fallopian canal, particularly above the oval window (myringoplasty, stapedectomy ; and

(4) the labyrinthine segment (cholesteatomas

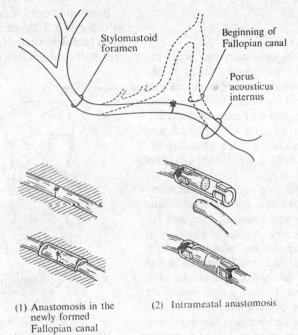

(1) Anastomosis in the newly formed Fallopian canal

(2) Intrameatal anastomosis

FIG. 5.13(a). The translabyrinthine meatomastoid rerouting with an end-to-end anastomosis (or interposition of a nerve graft) is the most common type of repair of transverse fractures of the temporal bone.

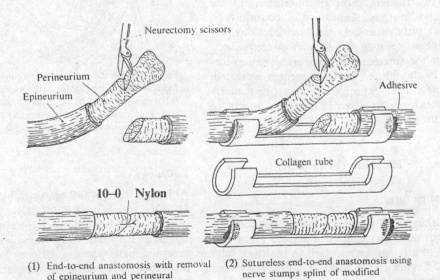

(1) End-to-end anastomosis with removal of epineurium and perineural suture in place

(2) Sutureless end-to-end anastomosis using nerve stumps splint of modified collagen tube

FIG. 5.13(b). Techniques of nerve anastomosis. (1) Removal of epineurium, oblique cutting of the nerve ends and 11–0 nylon monofilament suture. (2) Sutureless end-to-end anastomosis using collagen splints* and adhesive (histoacryl*).

* Braun, Melsungen, West Germany.

of the anterior epitympanic spaces, middle cranial fossa approaches).

Management

If the palsy is incomplete one can await the further evolution of the lesion. When doubt exists about the extent of the palsy, electrical tests should be performed immediately and repeatedly. Immediate surgical revision is indicated

(1) when the extent of the lesion is known; and

(2) in case of an unknown lesion when degeneration reaches the 90% level within 4–6 days following the injury.

Usually the traumatized segment of the nerve is excised and replaced by a graft. The technique of nerve grafting is the same as discussed for lesions due to fractures. A unique situation is created when manipulations around the oval window have produced herniation of the nerve fibres through the lacerated epineurium of a dehiscent facial nerve. In such a case immediate repair with exposure of the Fallopian canal and wide incision of the surrounding epineurium is required in order to equalize the oedematous pressure of the nerve (Fig. 5.14). Failure to do so will result in nerve fibrosis and permanent paralysis [18]. If at revision severe crushing of the nerve without apparent loss of continuity is present, only experience with nerve lesions permits the surgeon to decide whether simple incision of the surrounding epineurium or replacement of the injured nerve segment is indicated. Complete eradication of disease (particularly cholesteatoma) is essential for good return of function [18].

Idiopathic (Bell's palsy)

Clinical picture

Idiopathic palsy is the most common form of isolated facial palsy. It is of sudden onset and occurs at any age, particularly in healthy adults of 20–35 years and children of 6–12 years of age. Exposure to cold, emotional stress, and pain over the mastoid may precede the onset of the lesion.

Although recent observations [19, 20] indicate that viral infections may be the possible cause of the disease, the diagnosis of Bell's palsy remains one of exclusion of any other known cause.

Bilateral idiopathic facial palsy has been noted to occur in 1·5–2% of all Bell's palsies [21] and must be differentiated from alternating or recurrent Bell's palsy which are more common.

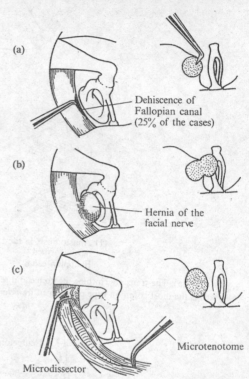

FIG. 5.14. Laceration of the epineurium of a dehiscent facial nerve may produce herniation causing permanent facial paralysis (a and b). Immediate repair of the lesion with wide incision of the surrounding epineurium in order to equalize the oedematous pressure of the nerve (c).

Pathology

Although there is still considerable speculation as to the aetiology of Bell's palsy, strangulation of the swollen nerve along its intraosseous course through the petrous pyramid is the most accepted pathogenesis. Before the advent of modern otoneurosurgical technique, the easily accessible distal mastoid segment of the facial nerve (between the stylomastoid foramen and the branching of the chorda tympani) was considered to be most commonly involved [17]. Following the introduction of techniques permitting the total intratemporal exposure of the facial nerve it was found that morphological changes occur most often proximal to the geniculate ganglion in Bell's palsy. The facial nerve was found to be strangulated at the entrance of the

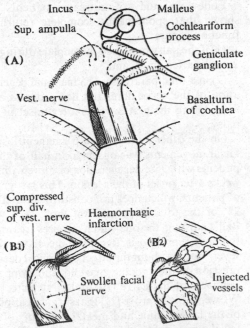

(A)

Incus — Malleus
Sup. ampulla — Cochleariform process
— Geniculate ganglion
Vest. nerve — Basalturn of cochlea

Compressed sup. div. of vest. nerve — Haemorrhagic infarction

(B1) **(B2)**

Swollen facial nerve — Injected vessels

FIG. 5.15. Typical findings after exposure of the labyrinthine and meatal segments of the facial nerve in Bell's palsy (B1) and herpes zoster oticus (B2). The strangulation of the nerve occurs at the entrance of the Fallopian canal. Haemorrhagic infarction is seen at the site of injury in Bell's palsy. Herpetic lesions are characterized by inflammatory vascular injection. The swelling of the facial nerve observed in the distal portion of the internal auditory canal is probably secondary and is due to damming of the axoplasm proximal to the strangulation of the facial nerve.

Fallopian canal in more than 90% of the cases. Haemorrhagic infarction occurred distally while oedematous swelling existed proximal to the site of strangulation (Fig. 5.15). The proximal site of the pathology in Bell's palsy has been confirmed by evoked intraoperative electromyography, meatal cisternography, vestibular testing and by the results of Schirmer's test [22, 23, 4].

Histological measurements (Table 5.2) have demonstrated that the labyrinthine segment is the narrowest portion of the entire Fallopian

canal. The narrowest lumen of the canal is situated at its entrance and measures 0·68 mm in diameter (Fig. 5.16). The facial nerve fibres which are loosely arranged without epineural covering in the internal auditory meatus, are physiologically 'pressed' into the Fallopian canal at the meatal fundus. It is evident that the resulting anatomical bottleneck situation predisposes to strangulation of the nerve if there is

TABLE 5.2. Average diameter of the facial nerve and the Fallopian canal obtained by averaging measurements taken from histological sections of twenty-eight temporal bones of adults

	Facial nerve	Fallopian canal	Difference
Labyrinthine segment	0·85±0·07 mm	1·02±0·08 mm	0·17 mm
Tympanic segment	1·12±0·09 mm	1·53±0·14 mm	0·41 mm
Mastoidal segment	0·94±0·05 mm	1·48±0·12 mm	0·54 mm

oedema. The histopathologic observations obtained during the acute phase of Bell's palsy by Fowler [24] and by Proctor [25] demonstrate degeneration of the myelin sheath and axon cylinders of the seventh nerve occurring in the Fallopian canal proximal to the geniculate ganglion and also in the internal auditory canal. Since it is known that Wallerian degeneration does not progress for more than a few millimetres in a centripetal direction the reported histopathologic information supports our clinical findings concerning the proximal site of the pathology in Bell's palsy. The nerve swelling that we have observed inside the internal auditory meatus is probably the expression of damming of axoplasm in front of the strangulated nerve. Only one of the seventeen operated patients presented with a lesion confined to the mastoid segment at the level of the branching of the chorda tympani nerve. This finding could support May's hypothesis [26] of the possible role of the chorda tympani in initiating retrograde pathology leading to the strangulation of facial nerve fibres in the Fallopian canal.

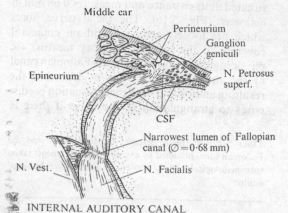

Middle ear

Perineurium

Ganglion
geniculi

Epineurium

N. Petrosus
superf.

CSF

Narrowest lumen of Fallopian
canal (⌀ = 0·68 mm)

N. Vest.

N. Facialis

INTERNAL AUDITORY CANAL

FIG. 5.16. Anatomy of the labyrinthine segment of the facial nerve. Note the narrow lumen of the entrance of the Fallopian canal. The subarachnoidal space extends as far distal as the geniculate ganglion and the greater superficial petrosal nerve in most instances. The ingrowth of connective tissue distal from the geniculate ganglion separates the different facial nerve fasciculi.

Management

Electroneuronographic study of the natural course of Bell's palsy has shown that maximal degeneration is reached in 92% of the patients within 14 days from the onset of the palsy [3, 27]. This observation indicates that the acute phase of the process responsible for nerve degeneration does not last longer than 2 weeks (Fig. 5.17). It is logical, therefore, to conclude that the spontaneous course of degeneration can only be influenced during the first 2 weeks after the onset of a Bell's palsy. There has been experimental confirmation of this assumption [28].

Follow-up study of untreated patients has shown that spontaneous, complete return of function occurs

(1) if the palsy remained incomplete during the 2 weeks after onset; and

(2) in a total paralysis when maximal degeneration of the nerve fibres did not progress over 95% during the first 2 weeks after onset of the palsy.

On the other hand, severe permanent loss of facial movements was observed in half of those patients with 95% degeneration or more within 2 weeks after onset of their lesion. This last group of patients, which does not constitute more than 7% of the total population of those seen with Bell's palsy, is the one which requires treatment to improve prognosis. Recent studies have raised severe doubts about the effect of surgical decompression limited to the mastoid and tympanic segments of the nerve [19] and of steroids [13]. We were able to prove [27] that surgical exposure of the labyrinthine and meatal segments of the facial nerve performed before the critical level of 95% degeneration is reached considerably improved the chances of good recovery (Fig. 5.18).

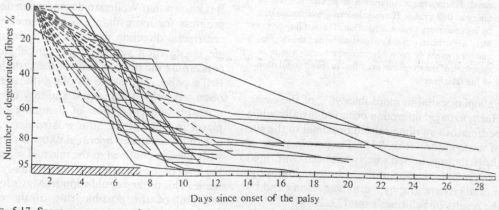

FIG. 5.17. Spontaneous course of degeneration in Bell's palsy as determined by electroneuronography in twenty-five consecutive patients. Note that maximal degeneration is reached with few exceptions within 14 days after onset of the palsy (acute phase of the disease). The critical level of maximal degeneration is of 95%. Patients with less than 95% degeneration at the end of the acute phase of Bell's palsy have a complete spontaneous return of function. Patients with more than 95% degeneration at the end of the acute phase of the disease have a 50% chance to have permanent disfiguring facial paralysis.

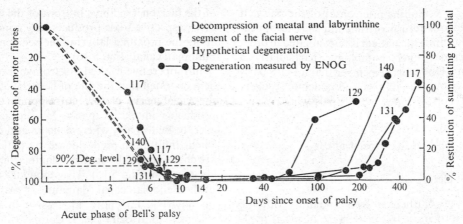

FIG. 5.18. Effect of surgery in idiopathic facial palsy. The decompression of the meatal and labyrinthine segment of the facial nerve was carried out in all four patients, because degeneration reached the 90% level within 2 weeks from onset of the palsy. Complete degeneration occurred only in one patient. Excellent recovery was obtained in all instances.

Experiments performed in cats have also shown that release of circumferential pressure within 12 days of injury prevents disruption of the endoneural tubes despite total degeneration of the motor nerve fibres [28]. We advocate, therefore, immediate proximal decompression of the facial nerve as soon as 90% degeneration is reached within 2 weeks from onset of idiopathic

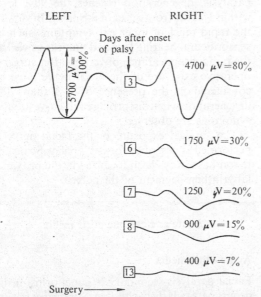

FIG. 5.19. Electroneuronogram of a patient with Bell's palsy and complete facial paralysis. Surgery was performed because degeneration reached 93% within 14 days from onset of the palsy.

palsy (Fig. 5.19). The operation is started from the middle cranial fossa exposing the meatal and labyrinthine segments of the seventh nerve. If the lesion, as it occurs in 94% of the cases, is localized by evoked electromyography at the entrance of the Fallopian canal, the epineurium and the meatal dura are incised over the exposed length of the nerve and the operation is finished. In rare instances where intraoperative evoked electromyography does not confirm the presence of proximal pathology, the operation is continued through a retroauricular incision exposing the tympanic and mastoid segments of the Fallopian canal. The lesion is then localized and the epineurium of the nerve incised.

The only complication observed following middle cranial fossa exposure of the meatal and labyrinthine segments of the facial nerve has been conductive deafness in one of our first cases. Reconstruction of the tegmen tympani with a fragment of the craniotomy bone has avoided this complication [18]. Of course, in view of the non-vital indication for this operation, the age, general health and personal attitude of the patient towards his palsy are respected when making the decision to operate.

Failure to realize the significance of early electrodiagnosis will delay for weeks or months the referral of patients with Bell's palsy for objective evaluation of the lesion. In such cases total degeneration of the nerve fibres is usually found. An expectant attitude is advised for as long as 4–6 months after onset of the palsy. If spontaneous return of function fails to appear after this time, the patient is re-evaluated in order to exclude other pathology (particularly a tumour). One must remember that a Bell's palsy which shows no sign of spontaneous recovery after 6 months is not a Bell's palsy.

Herpes zoster oticus

Clinical picture

Herpes zoster oticus or Ramsay Hunt syndrome is the third most frequent cause of facial paralysis. The disease occurs particularly in adults between 20 and 30, and 50 and 70 years of age. The characteristic herpetic vesicles are found mostly around the auricle, in the external meatus and in the concha. Sometimes the vesicles are confined to the tonsillar fossa or the soft palate and are overlooked if one does not search for them. Usually the disease starts with acute and severe pain about one ear followed over the next few days by the appearance of the typical eruption and the palsy. Sensorineural hearing loss, tinnitus and vertigo may be associated symptoms. An herpetic palsy is usually complete and tends to recover poorly particularly in elderly patients.

Pathology

Herpes zoster is probably a reactivation of a dormant virus left by a previous attack of chicken pox in the nerve ganglion, awaiting a still unknown stimulus which is able to revive it. Ramsay Hunt wrote as early as 1870 that the syndrome is probably explained by a lesion of the geniculate ganglion. Although herpes zoster may produce meningo-encephalomyelitis, facial paralysis is due to viral neuritis. Psammoma bodies found all along the labyrinthine segment of the facial nerve indicate that the subarachnoid space quite often extends as far distal as the geniculate ganglion. Since it is known that the cerebrospinal fluid is reabsorbed along the routes of the spinal nerves, the same may occur along the labyrinthine segment of the seventh nerve. This particular situation may explain why viruses and/or

of the facial nerve fibres in front of the entrance their respective toxic products may concentrate along the proximal labyrinthine segment of the Fallopian canal (Fig. 5.16).

Intraoperative evoked electromyography has demonstrated that the site of herpetic lesions of the facial nerve closely corresponds to those producing idiopathic palsy. In contrast, however, to Bell's palsy where oedema and haemorrhagic infiltration predominate, herpetic lesions are characterized by severe inflammatory vascular injection (Fig. 5.15). The secondary swelling of the Fallopian canal (damming of axoplasmatic flow?) is far more impressive in herpetic lesions than in Bell's palsy. Compression of the vestibular and cochlear nerves by the swollen facial nerve in the distal portion of the meatus has been observed frequently in herpetic palsy.

Management

The acute phase of herpes zoster oticus lasts longer than that of an idiopathic palsy so that electroneuronographic recording must be continued for 3 rather than 2 weeks after onset of the palsy. Surgery is indicated when, in a case of paralysis, degeneration reaches the 90% level within 3 weeks from onset of the palsy. In view of the rapid relief of inner ear symptoms such as sensorineural hearing loss and tinnitus as well as the rapid disappearance of vertigo after surgery, operative exposure of the facial nerve must be considered in the presence of less than 90% degeneration when disturbing cochleo-vestibular symptoms are observed.

The surgical exposure of the facial nerve is performed as described for Bell's palsy. So far the lesion has always been localized in the proximal labyrinthine segment of the nerve.

Acute and chronic otitis media

Acute otitis media

Facial paralysis secondary to acute otitis media occurs particularly in children. Surgical exposure of the facial nerve is indicated when, in spite of paracentesis and antibiotic treatment, 90% of the motor nerve fibres degenerate within 6 days of onset of the palsy. The extent of surgery is determined by the site of the lesion as determined by intraoperative evoked electromyography. So far all lesions produced by acute otitis media have been localized to the level of a dehiscent Fallopian canal, above the oval window or proximal to the cochleariform process. A transmastoid approach was sufficient for surgical exposure of the lesion. The progression of degeneration was stopped and complete restitution of function was obtained in all instances [29].

Chronic otitis media

In chronic otitis media, particularly if complicated by cholesteatoma, decompression is indicated as soon as the palsy becomes clinically visible. Obviously ENoG is of great help in indicating the precise degree of degeneration in the presence of a completely paralysed face.

Tumours

Clinical features

Tumours involving the facial nerve are found at any age with the maximum in the fourth decade of life. Progressive facial nerve palsy is the usual initial symptom. Twitching of the facial nerve may occur before onset of the palsy and is often confused with idiopathic hemifacial spasm. Occasionally the facial paralysis produced by a tumour is of sudden onset and may be confused with Bell's palsy. Every 'idiopathic' palsy showing no signs of recovery after 4–6 months should be carefully investigated in order to rule out the presence of a tumour. Conductive hearing loss is often present when the tumour originates from the tympanic segment of the facial nerve or from the middle ear.

Pathology

Table 5.3 shows the pathology in forty-three intratemporal tumours involving the facial nerve. Most tumours originated in the region of the geniculate ganglion. The complexity of the embryological development and of the structure of the facial nerve predisposes it to neoplastic or hamartoblastomatous formations in this area (Fig. 5.16) [30]. Facial nerve neurinomas frequently involve the labyrinthine segment of the nerve and may extend into the internal auditory meatus (Fig. 5.20). Eighty per cent of congenital cholesteatomas originate close to the geniculate ganglion where they strangulate the facial nerve and produce extensive asymptomatic inner ear fistulas. Haemangiomas belong to the cavernous or to the 'ossified' type (Fig. 5.21). Ossified haemangiomas were described for the first time

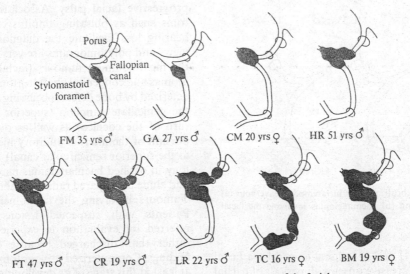

FIG. 5.20. Localization of intratemporal neurinomas of the facial nerve.

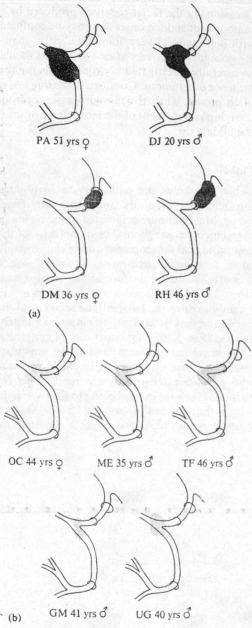

PA 51 yrs ♀   DJ 20 yrs ♂

DM 36 yrs ♀   RH 46 yrs ♂

(a)

OC 44 yrs ♀   ME 35 yrs ♂   TF 46 yrs ♂

(b)   GM 41 yrs ♂   UG 40 yrs ♂

FIG. 5.21. Localization of intratemporal cavernous (a) and ossifying (b) haemangiomas involving the facial nerve.

by Fisch [31] and are characterized by a facial palsy of progressive onset with periods of partial recovery. Meningiomas with facial palsy as the

TABLE 5.3 Intratemporal tumours involving the facial nerve (43 cases = 100%)

I. *Tumours of the facial nerve*		
Neurinoma	9	21%
II. *Tumours of tissues surrounding the facial nerve*		
(A) Benign		
Congenital cholesteatoma		
– Supralabyrinthine	10 }12	28%
– Apex	2 }	
Hemangioma		
–Cavernous	4 }9	21%
– Ossifying	5 }	
Meningioma	3	7%
Glomus jugulare tumours	3	7%
Arachnoidal cyst	1	2%
(B) Malignant		
Squamous cell carcinoma	4	9%
Rhabdomyosarcoma	2	5%

initial symptom may also remain confined to the geniculate ganglion [31].

Management

A complete otoneurological investigation is required to rule out a tumour in the presence of progressive facial palsy. Associated ear symptoms such as pulsating tinnitus or conductive hearing loss facilitate the diagnosis. Stenvers' views and polytomograms are very helpful since the most common tumours (facial nerve neurinomas and congenital cholesteatomas) are characterized by bone defects occurring at the level of the geniculate ganglion (superior to the basal turn of the cochlea) as well as over the distal portion of the internal auditory meatus (medial to the superior semicircular canal). Bone pathology in ossified haemangiomas may be minimal and elude unprepared radiological investigation. Tumours involving the facial nerve are rare. Patients with suspected lesions should be referred for evaluation to experienced centres rather than discharged because of 'negative' findings. Computerized tomography is of no use, at least at this stage of its development, if there is no intracranial invasion. Meatocisternography with a minimal quantity of dye is useful when the tumor has invaded the internal auditory meatus [12]. The size of the intrameatal portion of a tumor should be defined exactly in order to decide whether the middle cranial fossa approach with conservation of hearing or the translabyrinthine approach with sacrifice of the inner ear function has to be used.

Treatment

Tumours involving the facial nerve should be removed surgically as soon as they are diagnosed. Familiarity with modern otoneurosurgical procedures is essential for successful results [32]. Grafting of the facial nerve must be performed quite often after tumour excision [8]. The technique of nerve anastomosis has already been described above. Removal of the epineurium from the nerve stumps is essential to determine the precise area for anastomosis. Quite often the size of the graft shrinks considerably following removal of epineurium so that two grafts rather than one will be used to bridge the defect of the injured nerve. In the mastoid and tympanic segments of the Fallopian canal sutureless perineural approximation, depending upon the natural adhesive properties of the nerve ends is

the procedure of choice [8]. Grafting in the labyrinthine and meatal segments presents particular problems because of the depth of the operative field (middle cranial fossa approach) and the presence of cerebrospinal fluid. Collagen splints and adhesive facilitate fixation of the nerve stumps [8]. Using the above modern otomicrosurgical techniques a 75% return of function is observed in 60% of patients. Less good results of grafting have been observed in patients presenting with a long-standing complete or nearly complete facial paralysis (as, e.g., in ossified haemangiomas).

To achieve the best functional results tumours involving the facial nerve should be operated upon as soon as possible before extensive degeneration of the nerve fibres compromising the return in function has occurred.

Special techniques

Permanent anterior displacement of the facial nerve
Re-routing of the facial nerve outside the temporal bone permits preservation of the seventh nerve when removing large tumours of the intralabyrinthine space (glomus jugulare

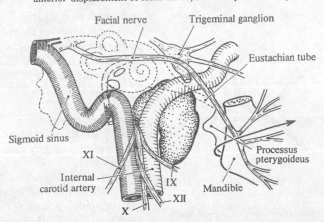

INFRATEMPORAL FOSSA APPROACH: resection of zygomatic arch and mandibular condyle, permanent anterior displacement of facial nerve, subtotal petrosectomy.

Facial nerve — Trigeminal ganglion — Eustachian tube — Sigmoid sinus — XI — Internal carotid artery — IX — XII — X — Mandible — Processus pterygoideus

FIG. 5.22. Rerouting of the facial nerve outside the temporal bone (permanent anterior displacement of the facial nerve). This procedure is usually combined with the obliteration of the pneumatic spaces of the temporal bone (subtotal petrosectomy). The Eustachian tube is obliterated and the external auditory canal closed as a blindsack. The operative cavity is filled with the temporalis muscle or fat from the abdominal wall.

tumours), the apex of the pyramid and the base of the skull (clivus chordomas, meningiomas, clivus chondromas, etc. [30]. This procedure is usually combined with obliteration of the pneumatic spaces of the temporal bone (subtotal petrosectomy). For this latter purpose obliteration of the Eustachian tube and blindsac closure of the external auditory canal are required. Primary wound healing is then obtained in 8–10 days. The conductive hearing loss is permanent (Fig. 5.22).

Substitution operations

In the few cases in which the proximal stump of the nerve cannot be reached (intracranial degeneration following head trauma, extensive

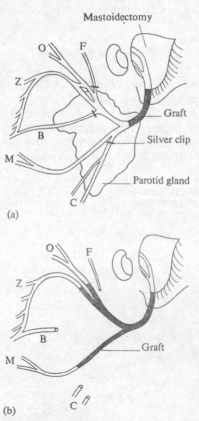

FIG. 5.23. Directed regeneration in extratemporal facial nerve grafting. The same procedure with clipping of the unnecessary facial nerve fibres is used to concentrate the movements in important areas of the face in facial hypoglossal anastomosis.

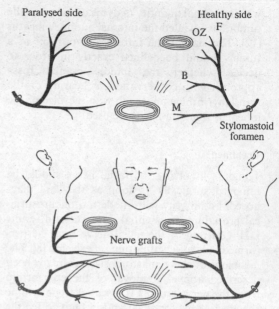

FIG. 5.24. Technique of cross-face grafting in unilateral facial paralysis.

intracranial extension of temporal bone tumours), facial-hypoglossal as well as cross-face anastomosis are performed.

Facial-hypoglossal anastomosis

In spite of criticism due to the lack of emotional expression, the hypoglossal cross-over operation still is one of the most simple and reliable substitution operations for the seventh nerve. Besides progress of the microtechniques, anastomosis with clipping of unnecessary branches in the parotid area (Fig. 5.23) has contributed to improve the quality of the facial movements and to reduce synkinesis [8].

Cross-face anastomosis

This is the most modern development in nerve substitution surgery for restoration of facial movements. The operation consists of anastomosing all unimportant buccal and zygomatic branches of the healthy side to the mandibular and orbicular branches of the paralysed side of the face (Fig. 5.24). The facial nerve is exposed on both sides as for a conventional lateral parotidectomy. Two skin incisions in the nasolabial folds are necessary to create a supralabial tunnel for the sural nerve grafts (Fig. 5.24). The main advantage of the cross-face anastomosis is the preservation of the emotional expression of facial muscles. The operation requires considerable time and skill. Due to the long delay of reinnervation the results are still questionable. The best results have been observed so far by combining facial hypoglossial cross-over with a subsequent cross-face anastomosis.

References

[1] LAUMANS E. P. S. & JONGKEES L. B. W. (1963) On the prognosis of peripheral facial paralysis of endotemporal origin. *Annals of Otology, Rhinology and Laryngology* **72**, 307.

[2] MAY M., HARVEY J. E., MAROVITZ W. F. & STROUD M. (1971) The prognostic accuracy of the maximal stimulation test compared with that of the nerve excitability test in Bell's palsy. *Laryngoscope* **81**, 931.

[3] ESSLEN E. (1973) Electrodiagnosis of facial palsy. In *Surgery of the Facial Nerve*, 2nd edn, ed. Miehlke A. Munich: Urban & Schwarzenberg.

[4] FISCH U. (1977) Diagnostic studies on idiopathic facial palsy. In *Proceedings of the Shambaugh Fifth International Workshop on Middle Ear Microsurgery and Fluctuant Hearing Loss.* Huntsville, Alabama, USA: The Strode Publisher, Inc.

[5] HOUSE W. F. (1963) Middle cranial fossa approach to the petrous pyramid. *Archives of Otolaryngology* **78**, 460.

[6] PULEC J. L. (1966) Total decompression of the facial nerve. *Laryngoscope* **76**, 1015.

[7] FISCH U. (1973) Operations on the facial nerve in its labyrinthine and meatal course. In *Surgery of the Facial Nerve*, ed. Miehlke A., pp. 175–205. Munich: Urban & Schwarzenberg.

[8] FISCH U. (1974) Facial nerve grafting. *Otolaryngology Clinics of North America.* **7**, 517.

[9] SEYMOUR J. (1977) Incidence and management of Bell's palsy. In *Proceedings of the Third International Symposium on Facial Nerve Surgery*, pp. 331, 333. Birmingham, Alabama, USA: Aesculapius Publishing Co.

[10] LUNDBORG G. (1970) Ischemic nerve injury. *Scandanavian Journal of Plastic Reconstructive Surgery (Stockh.)*, Suppl. 6.

[11] TSCHIASSNY K. (1953) Eight syndromes of facial paralysis and their significance in locating the lesion. *Annals of Otology* **62**, 677.

[12] FISCH U. P., NEDZELSKI J. & WELLAUER J. (1975) Diagnostic value of meato-cisternography. *Archives of Otolaryngology* **101**, 339.

[13] MAY M., HARDIN W. B. JR., SULLIVAN J. & WETTE R. (1976) Natural history of Bell's palsy: the salivary flow test and other prognostic indicators. *Laryngoscope* **86**, 704.

[14] ULRICH K. (1926) *Verletzungen des Gehörorgans bei Schädelbasisfrakturen.* Helsingfors: Habilitationsschrift.

[15] FISCH U. (1974) Facial paralysis in fractures of the petrous bone. *Laryngoscope* **84**, 2141.

[16] FISCH U. (1977) Die Microchirurgie des Felsenbeines. HNO **25**, 193.

[17] MIEHLKE A. (1973) *Surgery of the facial nerve.* Munich: Urban & Schwarzenberg.

[18] FISCH U. (1976) Chirurgie im inneren Gehörgang und an benachbarten Strukturen. In *Kopf-und Halschirurgie Bd Bd 3: Ohrregion*, ed. Naumann H. H., pp. 457–544. Stuttgart: Thieme.

[19] ADOUR K. K. (1973) Electronystagmographic comparison of acute idiopathic and herpes zoster facial paralysis. *Laryngoscope* **83**, 2029.

[20] DJUPESLAND G., BERDAL P. & JOHANNESSEN T. A. (1976) Viral infection as a cause of acute peripheral facial palsy. *Archives of Otolaryngology* **102**, 403.

[21] RONTAL E. & SIGEL M. E. (1972) Bilateral facial paralysis. *Laryngoscope* **82**, 607.

[22] FISCH U. & ESSLEN E. (1972) Total intratemporal exposure of the facial nerve. *Archives of Otolaryngology* **95**, 335.

[23] LAEMMLI K. & FISCH U. (1974) Vestibular symptoms in idiopathic facial palsy. *Acta Otolaryngologica* **78**, 15.

[24] FOWLER E. P. JR. (1963) The pathologic findings in a case of facial paralysis. *Transactions of the American Academy of Ophthalmology and Otolaryngology* **67**, 187.

[25] PROCTOR B., CORGILL D. A. & PROUD G. (1976) The pathology of Bell's palsy. *Transactions of the American Academy of Otolaryngology* **82**, 70.

[26] MAY M. (1977) Etiology and pathogenesis of Bell's palsy. In *Proceedings of the Third International Symposium on Facial Nerve Surgery*, p. 371. Birmingham, Alabama, USA: Aesculapius Publishing Co.

[27] FISCH U. (1977) Total facial nerve decompression and electroneuronography. In *Neurological Surgery of the Ear*, Birmingham, Alabama, USA: Aesculapius Publishing Co.

[28] YAMAMOTO E. & FISCH U. (1975) Experimentally induced facial nerve compression in cats. *Acta Otolaryngologica* **79**, 390.

[29] HOF E. (1977) Facial palsy of infectious origin in children. In *Proceedings of the Third International Symposium on Facial Nerve Surgery*, pp. 414–418. Birmingham, Alabama, USA: Aesculapius Publishing Co.

[30] FISCH U. (1977) Surgery of temporal bone tumors. In *Neurological Surgery of the Ear.* Birmingham, Alabama, USA: Aesculapius Publishing Co.

[31] FISCH U. & RUETTNER J. (1977) Pathology of intratemporal tumors involving the facial nerve. In *Proceedings of the Third Symposium on Facial Nerve Surgery*, pp. 448–456. Birmingham, Alabama, USA: Aesculapius Publishing Co.

[32] FISCH U. (1976) The middle fossa approach to the internal auditory meatus. In *Operative Surgery*, 3rd edn, pp. 179–92. London: Butterworth.

CHAPTER 6

Deafness of Ageing

The term presbycusis implies hearing loss resulting from the degenerative changes of ageing. Functional losses of the auditory system are as consistent a part of the ageing process as those affecting any other system of the body. The durability of the auditory mechanism is determined by genetic influence and by the physical stress to which it is subjected during a lifetime. The age of onset and the rate of progression of presbycusis vary widely. When the losses occur early in life a clear distinction between hereditary influence and early presbycusis cannot be made. Superimposed upon the inherited processes is the gradual accumulation of errors in DNA which probably causes a decline in the normal mechanisms of repair. Ageing of the whole body, and of specific organs, proceeds unevenly, occurring sooner in some cells and later in others. It is known that with increasing age there is a decreased ability of certain cell systems to undergo mitosis, there are decreases in nuclear proteins, accumulations of pigment and other insoluble compounds in cytoplasm, and chemical changes in the intercellular fluid.

It is quite clear that ageing cannot be accounted for on the basis of changes in one system alone, for example, the cardiovascular system. Although there is a popular cliche, 'that a man is as old as his arteries', there is no satisfactory parallel between vascular age and senility. The study of ageing changes in individual cells is difficult because the cellular populations of many organs are replaced during life, and it is difficult to distinguish the normal changes of ageing from alterations caused by injury and disease.

On a clinical as well as histological basis, it is possible to identify four types of presbycusis. These types are caused by selective atrophy of different cochlear structures which may be in-

volved individually or in combination. The hearing losses are symmetrical in the two ears and progress slowly [1].

Sensory presbycusis

This disorder is characterized functionally by abrupt high tone hearing losses and histologically by atrophy of the organ of Corti in the basal end of the cochlea. The degenerative change usually begins in middle age but can have its onset in childhood. Its progression is so slow that even in advanced age, the lesion frequently is limited to a few millimetres at the basal end of the cochlea and may, therefore, have no significant effect on the hearing of speech frequencies. In the early stages, there is slight distortion and flattening of the organ of Corti. This is followed by loss of supporting and sensory cells, and eventually the organ of Corti may appear as an epithelial mound or may completely disappear leaving a totally denuded basilar membrane (Figs. 6.1 and 6.2).

Neural presbycusis

Neural presbycusis may begin at any age. It has little or no effect on hearing until late in life when the population of neural units falls below that required for effective transmission, integration and decoding of the neural patterns. The temporal bones of affected individuals show a diffuse loss of population of cochlear neurones which is usually more severe in the basal turn. Neurones are probably lost also in the higher auditory pathways, but this has not yet been confirmed histologically.

The classical clinical picture is a loss of speech

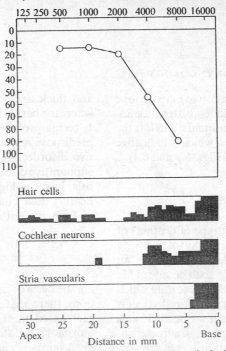

Hair cells

Cochlear neurons

Stria vascularis

FIG. 6.1. Audiogram and cochlear charts of the right ear of a 70-year-old man who had a bilateral symmetrical high tone hearing loss, classical for the sensory type of presbycusis. The loss of hair cells is most pronounced at the basal end of the cochlea. The loss of spiral ganglion cells at the basal end is judged to be caused by changes in the supporting cells of the organ of Corti.

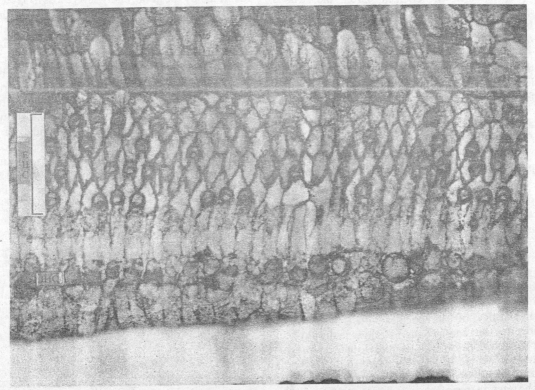

FIG. 6.2. Surface preparation of the organ of Corti taken from the basal turn of a 67-year-old woman showing sensory presbycusis. There is a diffuse, scattered, partial loss of external hair cells (EHC). The population of internal hair cells (IHC) is normal. Silver stain. Courtesy of Watanuki.

discrimination out of proportion to the pure tone threshold loss. There is no consistent audiometric loss for pure tone thresholds, and it is the loss of speech discrimination which is indicative of the neural degeneration (Figs. 6.3 and 6.4).

Strial presbycusis

Probably the most common type of deafness of ageing is that caused by atrophy of the stria vascularis. Typically, the hearing loss has an insidious onset in the third to sixth decade of life and progresses slowly. The clinical feature which distinguishes it from other types of presbycusis is the flat audiometric pattern associated with excellent speech discrimination. Characteristically, the speech discrimination scores are normal until the threshold elevation exceeds 50 dB. Histological studies show a patchy atrophy of the stria vascularis which is most severe in the apical half of the cochlea. Often the stria is replaced by cystic structures and occasionally by basophilic deposits. This is associated with loss of all three cell layers of the stria vascularis. It is presumed that atrophy of the strial cells affects the quality of endolymph throughout the cochlear duct, thus accounting for a loss of hearing for all frequencies (Figs. 6.5 and 6.6).

Cochlear conductive presbycusis

Although not yet a proven pathological entity, cochlear conductive presbycusis seems an appropriate explanation for that type of hearing loss which is characterized by symmetrical descending audiometric patterns. This type of deafness first becomes evident in middle age. Histological studies usually show no morphological changes in the sensorineural structures to explain the hearing losses. It is proposed, therefore, that hearing loss is due to a disorder in the motion mechanics of the cochlear duct. The theory implies that ageing causes changes in the physical characteristics of the cochlear duct, the magnitude of which is directly related to the thickness and width of the basilar membrane. Thus, the changes in physical response are greater in the basal turn where the basilar membrane is narrow

and thick and less severe in the apical region where the basilar membrane is wider and thinner. It seems probable that some otologic diseases predispose and aggravate the cochlear conductive disorder. For example, ears with chronic suppurative disease, Paget's disease and otosclerosis have a high incidence of sensorineural hearing loss characterized by the descending audiometric patterns (Figs. 6.7 and 6.8).

Summary

On the basis of clinical and histological observations, there are four types of deafness of ageing, each based on degenerative changes in a specific morphological structure in the inner ear. Sensory presbycusis is characterized by an abrupt high tone hearing loss which is caused by degeneration of the organ of Corti most severe in the basal turn of the cochlea. Neural presbycusis can be identified by the abnormally severe loss in speech discrimination and is the result of loss in the population of cochlear neurones, and possibly neurones of the higher auditory centres. Strial presbycusis shows a distinct flat audiometric pattern with excellent speech discrimination. The histological correlate is atrophy of the stria vascularis most severe in the apical half of the cochlea. Cochlear conductive presbycusis shows the descending audiometric pattern and is presumed to be caused by alterations in the physical characteristics of the cochlear duct. The resulting alteration in motion mechanics is most severe at the basal end of the cochlea where the basilar membrane is narrow and thick and less severe in the apical region where it is wider and thinner.

The time of onset and magnitude of the degenerative changes vary widely and are determined, in great part, by genetic factors. The losses are slowly progressive and symmetrical in the two ears. There is no known medical treatment which will delay the onset or alter the course of these ageing changes in the inner ear.

Reference

[1] SCHUKNECHT H. F. (1974) *Pathology of the Ear*. Cambridge, Massachusetts: Harvard University Press.

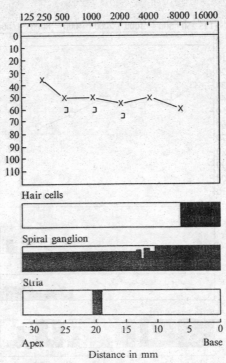

Hair cells

Spiral ganglion

Stria

| 30 | 25 | 20 | 15 | 10 | 5 | 0 |

Apex   Base

Distance in mm

FIG. 6.3. Audiogram and cochlear chart of the left ear of a 63-year-old woman who had a bilateral symmetrical hearing loss of 7 years' duration. The principle pathological change is a severe loss of cochlear neurones, classical for the neural type of presbycusis. See also Fig. 6.4.

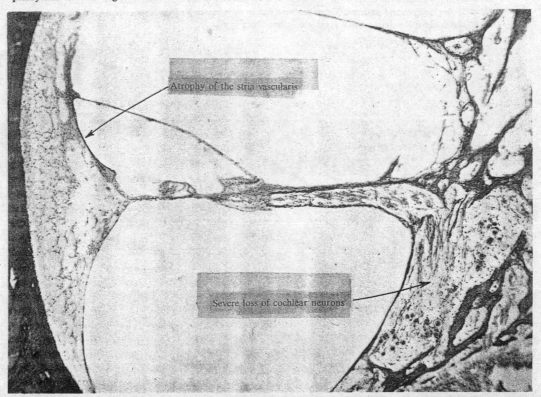

Atrophy of the stria vascularis

Severe loss of cochlear neurons

FIG. 6.4. Photomicrograph from the 20 mm region of the same ear shown in Fig. 6.3. The severe loss of cochlear neurons is typical for neural presbycusis. The small isolated area of strial atrophy is probably of no functional significance. The organ of Corti is normal.

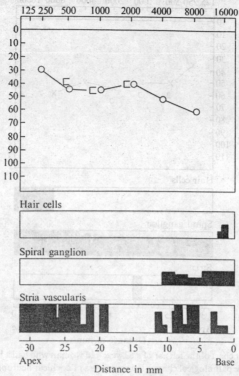

Hair cells

Spiral ganglion

Stria vascularis

| 30 | 25 | 20 | 15 | 10 | 5 | 0 |
| Apex | | | | | | Base |

Distance in mm

FIG. 6.5. Audiogram and cochlear chart of the right ear of a 77-year-old woman with bilateral symmetrical hearing loss characterized by flat audiometric patterns. There is severe patchy degeneration of the stria vascularis most severe in the apical region, classical for the strial type of presbycusis. See also Fig. 6.6.

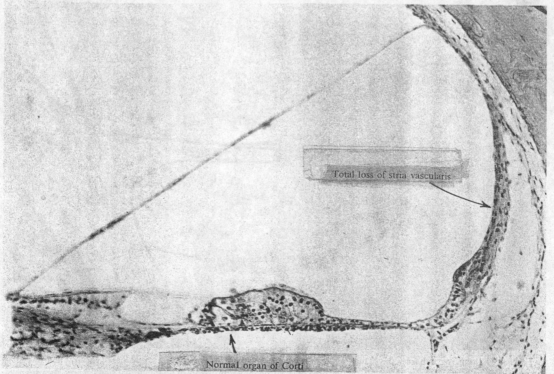

Total loss of stria vascularis

Normal organ of Corti

FIG. 6.6. Photomicrograph from the 19 mm area of the same ear shown in Fig. 6.5. In this area, there is a total loss of strial tissue, typical for strial presbycusis. The organ of Corti is normal.

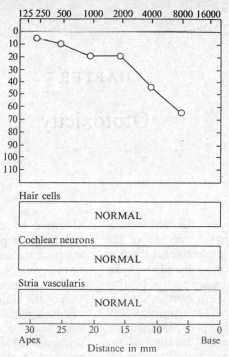

Hair cells

NORMAL

Cochlear neurons

NORMAL

Stria vascularis

NORMAL

FIG. 6.7. Audiogram and cochlear chart of the right ear of a 53-year-old man with bilateral symmetrical hearing loss characterized by descending audiometric patterns. Light microscopy fails to show a pathological basis for the hearing loss. It is theorized that the loss may be caused by an interference with cochlear motion mechanics, in other words, an inner ear conductive deafness. See also Fig. 6.8.

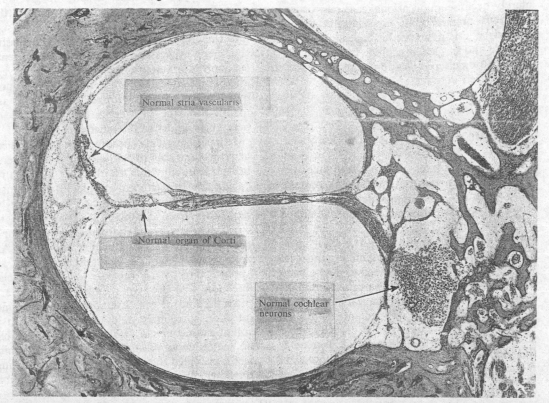

FIG. 6.8. Photomicrograph from the 10 mm area of the same ear shown in Fig. 6.7. This area of the cochlea serves the 4 kHz region of the auditory spectrum, for which there was a 45 dB hearing loss. The organ of Corti, cochlear neurones, and stria vascularis appear normal. Changes in the spiral ligament are normal for age. In the absence of significant morphological

CHAPTER 7

Ototoxicity

Some valuable drugs, including the antibiotics of the aminoglycoside group and certain of the newer diuretics, can exert a selective toxic action on the sensory cells of the cochlear and vestibular end organs. The resulting impairment of hearing or disturbance of postural equilibrium may be transient or permanent. The symptoms can range from slight to disabling, depending upon the drug used, the dose, the duration of the treatment, and other factors not always under the physician's control. The otolaryngologist must be thoroughly familiar with ototoxicity and the types of drugs that exhibit this property, not merely because an occasional case may occur in his own practice, but especially because he should be able to advise his colleagues in other medical and surgical disciplines in which unforeseen ototoxic complications are more often encountered.

THE AMINOGLYCOSIDES

The aminoglycosides are basic molecules containing aminosugars obtained by fermentation from various species of *Streptomyces* and other genera of soil-dwelling micro-organisms. A good example is the antibiotic kanamycin, whose formula is shown in Fig. 7.1a. It consists of the aminocyclitol 2-deoxystreptamine and two aminohexoses, which are joined to it by glycosidic linkage. Other clinically important aminoglycosides closely related in chemical structure are tobramycin, neomycin, and gentamicin. Streptomycin (Fig. 7.1b) contains the guanidocyclitol streptidine, linked to a disaccharide formed by the pentose streptose and the aminohexose *N*-methyl-L-glucosamine.

Since the aminoglycosides are not readily absorbed by the intestinal mucosa, they are usually given parenterally. After intramuscular injection the concentration in the blood plasma rises rapidly, reaches a peak between 1 and 2 hours, and then declines gradually due to excretion by the kidneys. Only glomerular filtration is involved, without tubular secretion or reabsorption, and the antibiotic appears in the urine unchanged. The half-life of kanamycin (the time required for the concentration to fall to half its peak value) is 4–6 hours in the adult, but may be more than twice that long in the infant.

Aminoglycosides must usually be given repeatedly over a period of days (or weeks in the streptomycin treatment of tuberculosis) to sustain the concentrations required for successful treatment of systemic infections. When renal function is impaired excretion may be delayed, and plasma concentrations tend to be higher and more persistent. The longer such levels are maintained, the greater is the likelihood of permanent injury to the inner ear [1].

In meningitis it may become necessary to inject gentamicin or tobramycin directly into the cerebrospinal fluid by the intrathecal or intraventricular route. In peritoneal and pleural infections a local injection into the affected cavity may be required. Neomycin may be given orally to sterilize the gut before abdominal operation, or it may be used to wash out an infected bladder. An aminoglycoside-containing ointment may be applied directly to the site of a superficial infection, and drops containing neomycin are often used in the ear. Stubborn cases of wound infection sometimes yield to irrigation with a solution of neomycin. Ototoxic injury is possible no matter how an aminoglycoside is administered, provided the amount eventually reaching the inner ear, whether by way of the circulation or otherwise, is sufficiently great.

Cochlear toxicity

The ototoxic action of kanamycin, and especially that of neomycin, affects the cochlea almost exclusively. The first indication of ototoxicity is usually an elevation of auditory thresholds for the higher frequencies. In clinical audiometry this initial shift can be observed at 8 or 10 kHz, but experimental studies in non-human primates indicate that the very highest audible frequencies

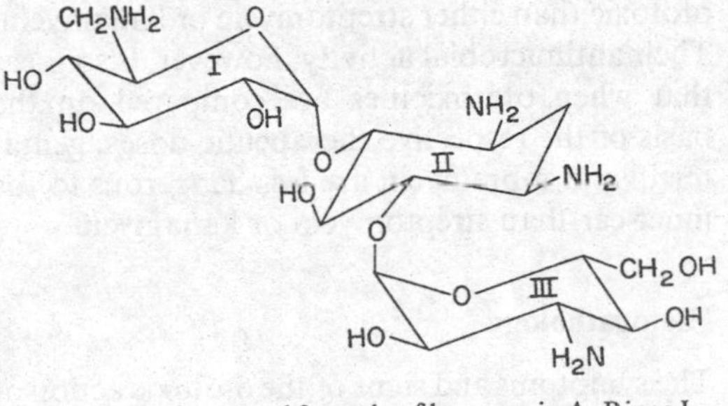

FIG. 7.1(a). Structural formula of kanamycin A. Rings I and III are 6-glucosamine and 3-glucosamine, respectively. Ring II is the base 2-deoxystreptamine, common to neomycin, gentamicin, and tobramycin as well.

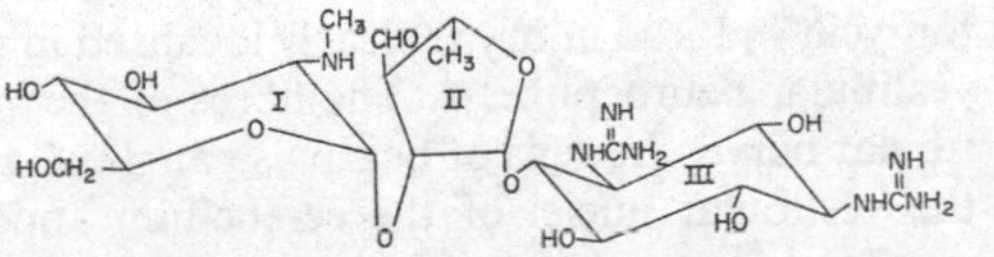

FIG. 7.1(b). Structural formula of streptomycin. Ring I is N-methyl-L-glucosamine, ring II streptose; together they make up the disaccharide streptobiosamine. Ring III is the base streptidine.

(about 45 kHz in the monkey, or 20 kHz in man) are the first to be affected. The patient may experience a high-pitched tinnitus, but this warning symptom is not always present. In these early stages hearing for speech shows little or no change, but if treatment is continued, the hearing loss progresses to involve the speech frequencies (i.e. the three octaves from 4 kHz down to 0·5 kHz) and eventually still lower frequencies, by which time the patient is severely deaf. If the antibiotic is stopped, further deterioration of the hearing can often be halted, at least so long as renal function remains normal.

A distressing exception was dihydrostreptomycin, once widely used for prolonged treatment of tuberculosis. An insignificant hearing loss appearing during dihydrostreptomycin therapy sometimes progressed to a severe deafness after the antibiotic had been discontinued. Neomycin has been known to produce similar disasters much more suddenly, especially because its excretion is often impaired by its own nephrotoxic action on the renal tubules. Because of their insidious tendency to cause hearing loss, even after a few doses, approval for the clinical use of dihydrostreptomycin was withdrawn years ago, and parenteral administration of neomycin has long been considered unjustified.

With gentamicin and tobramycin, as with kanamycin, cochlear ototoxicity can usually be avoided or at least minimized by keeping the dose levels as low and the duration of treatment as short as may be compatible with a successful therapeutic result. When renal insufficiency is present, the blood levels of any aminoglycoside must be carefully monitored and the dose adjusted to avoid cochlear injury. Vancomycin also is toxic for both the cochlea and the kidney (Table 7.1).

TABLE 7.1. Toxicity of aminoglycosides and other basic antibiotics

OTOTOXICITY		
Cochlear	*Vestibulo-cochlear*	
Neomycin	Dihydrostreptomycin	
Kanamycin	Viomycin	
Vancomycin	Gentamicin	
Amikacin	Tobramycin	
Sissomicin		
Vestibular		
Streptomycin		

NEPHROTOXICITY		
Neomycin	Gentamicin	Viomycin
Kanamycin	Tobramycin	Vancomycin

Vestibular toxicity

Streptomycin, the first of the aminoglycosides to be discovered, exerts its ototoxic action mainly, although not exclusively, on the vestibular end organs. Vestibular toxicity is exhibited also by gentamicin and tobramycin, and by the polycationic but non-aminoglycosidic antibiotic viomycin.

Streptomycin was introduced immediately after World War II, and was given initially in large doses (up to 3 gm daily, i.m.) in the treatment of tuberculosis. Almost all patients receiving streptomycin for more than 30 days developed what was described as 'a peculiar disturbance of equilibrium', or 'a most unusual type of dizziness'. Their initial complaint was of oscillopsia, i.e. a blurring of vision when reading, or of an inability to fix the gaze. Objects in the field of vision tended to 'jump', or to become 'jumbled'. They also experienced vertigo, or a sense of continued rotation, after turning the head or turning over in bed. Ambulatory patients became ataxic, and had difficulty walking in the dark, on uneven ground, or on mattresses that had been placed in hospital corridors to protect unsteady strollers from bumps and bruises. The 'mattress test' came to be recommended as a sensitive indicator of streptomycin-induced inco-ordination. Spontaneous nystagmus was seldom if ever seen, but caloric tests showed a reduction or absence of nystagmus, and many patients were described as having 'dead labyrinths'. Galvanic stimulation on the other hand could cause nystagmus, indicating that the vestibular nerve and its central connections were still intact. These effects, which differed sharply from the symptoms of Menière's disease or of other familiar vestibular disorders, were in fact similar to those previously observed in patients whose vestibular nerves had been divided to relieve the symptoms of Menière's disease. They represented an acute loss of vestibular function rather than vestibular hypersensitivity or overstimulation and emphasized the extent to which man still depends upon his vestibular system for the normal control of posture, gait, and eye movements [2].

The symptoms of streptomycin intoxication often subsided even while treatment was continued, but patients still tended to walk with a wide base. Compensation for the vestibular deficit was usually more rapid in children than in adults. Occasionally at least partial recovery of vestibular function was noted, but in elderly patients there was often neither recovery nor compensation. Instead, the handicap was severe and permanent.

When viomycin has been given in the pro-

longed treatment of tuberculosis, the effects on the vestibular system have resembled those of streptomycin. Because gentamicin and tobramycin are generally given in relatively short courses to seriously-ill patients, they have caused few cases of dramatic loss of vestibular function. Animal experiments have shown that they are both capable of producing the same type and degree of vestibular disturbance as streptomycin. On a weight-for-weight basis they are more ototoxic than either streptomycin or kanamycin. Their antimicrobial activity, however, is so great that when ototoxicities are compared on the basis of the respective therapeutic doses, gentamicin and tobramycin are less dangerous to the inner ear than streptomycin or kanamycin.

Histopathology

The symptoms and signs of the ototoxic action of streptomycin suggested to early investigators that they might reflect damage to central vestibular neurones rather than to the peripheral end organs. Histopathological studies in experimental animals have shown, however, that the streptomycin-induced injury is clearly localized in the vestibular neuroepithelia. The fibres of the vestibular nerve, the cells of Scarpa's ganglion, and the vestibular nuclei of the cerebellum appear unaffected, regardless of the severity of the disturbance of function.

Degeneration and disappearance of hair cells are the most striking features of the lesion. Both the globular cells of Type I with their nerve chalices and the cylindrical cells of Type II may be lost, especially the Type I cells along the upper surface of the crista. Cells on the slopes of the crista tend to persist longer, but they often show changes in mitochondria, Golgi apparatus, and other cytoplasmic organelles. The sensory hairs of many surviving cells become fused, but wide areas of the neuroepithelium appear completely bald when examined under the scanning electron microscope (Fig. 7.2). By transmission electronmicroscopy (EM) cross-sections of the tissue show widespread degeneration of hair cells, but the supporting cells remain. The dark cells at the base of the ampullar crista also show extensive damage, and the epithelium of the planum semilunatum appears shrunken [2].

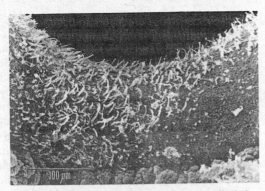

FIG. 7.2. Clumping and loss of stereocilia from the hair cells of the ampullar crista of the horizontal semicircular canal after streptomycin treatment. Arrows indicate the areas most severely affected. S, secretory epithelium. Scanning electron micrograph, squirrel monkey.

In the cochlea the initial loss of hair cells is confined to the most basal portion of the organ of Corti, in keeping with the hearing loss for the highest audible frequencies. After kanamycin treatment the guinea-pig shows a selective loss of outer hair cells, especially those of the first row, throughout the basal turn (Fig. 7.3). The corresponding inner hair cells are usually still present and appear to be intact, but transmission EM reveals incipient changes in their stereocilia and subcuticular organelles [3]. In other species the inner hair cells of the basal turn may also disappear. In the apical turn they are likely to be more susceptible than the outer hair cells. When the hair cells degenerate the potential gap in the reticular lamina is closed by growth of the phalangeal plates of the supporting cells to form a phalangeal scar. After kanamycin the mosaic pattern of the reticular lamina is usually well preserved, but after neomycin the scarring may be highly irregular (Fig. 7.4). Many supporting

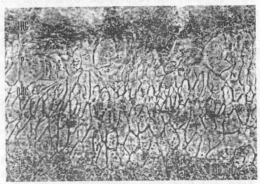

FIG. 7.4. Loss of almost all inner and outer hair cells (IHC, OHC) from the upper part of turn 2 in a 12-year-old patient who had shown a 60-dB hearing loss after receiving neomycin during renal transplantation. The irregular scarring of the reticular lamina, including the pillar cells (P) is characteristic of neomycin ototoxicity. H, Hensen cells. Reproduced with permission from Hawkins J. E. (1976) Drug ototoxicity. In *Handbook of Sensory Physiology*, Vol. 3, p. 725. Heidelberg: Springer-Verlag.

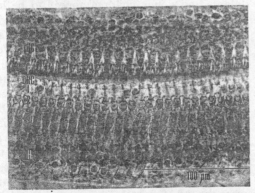

FIG. 7.3. Loss of outer hair cells (OHC), especially from row 1, after kanamycin treatment. The arrow indicates two recent phalangeal scars replacing outer hair cells of row 2. Inner hair cells (IHC) and outer hair cells of row 3 are still present. P, pillar cells. H, Hensen cells. Guinea-pig, third turn. OsO₄, phase contrast. Reproduced with permission from Hawkins J. E. (1976) Drug ototoxicity. In *Handbook of Sensory Physiology*, Vol. 3, p. 724. Heidelberg: Springer-Verlag.

cells also degenerate and disappear, so that portions of Corti's organ may be entirely absent, leaving the basilar membrane covered only by an undifferentiated epithelium consisting of large, flat cells of irregular shape. In such areas the myelinated fibres of the cochlear nerve also degenerate. Even in patients with profound ototoxic deafness, some myelinated fibres may persist for many years in the apical turn, despite the extensive destruction of the organ of Corti.

Degenerative changes have also been described in Reissner's membrane, in the stria vascularis, and in the suprastrial spiral ligament, tissues which control the microhomeostasis of the endolymph and perilymph. The temporal and possibly causal relationships between injury to these tissues and the degeneration of the hair cells remain uncertain. The stria vascularis may become atrophic, or it may recover from ototoxic injury. Even some degree of irregular regeneration of unmyelinated nerve fibres has occasionally been observed, but there is no regeneration or replacement of lost hair cells. The entire process of dissolution of cochlear tissues caused by ototoxic drugs closely resembles the slowly progressive cochlear changes that occur with ageing, which also begin in the lower basal turn. Ototoxic hearing loss may therefore be likened to an accelerated presbyacusis in which both sensory and metabolic aspects are combined.

Mechanisms of action

The remarkable selectivity of the aminoglycosides in exerting their toxic action on two organs of the body, the inner ear and the kidney, appears to be related to their persistence in the labyrinthine fluids and in the renal tissue after they have been cleared from the blood [4]. The membranous labyrinth and the renal tubular epithelia are exposed to higher concentrations for longer periods than other tissues. No direct correlation between serum levels and perilymph levels has been established, since the perilymph concentration shows neither the sharp peak nor the rapid fall characteristic of the typical curve for serum concentration. Binding to tissue proteins, which is known to occur in the kidney, may help to account for the slow removal of aminoglycosides from the perilymph.

Delayed excretion, as a result of kidney failure due to nephrotoxicity, infection, or other disease, causes higher and longer-lasting serum levels, and further accumulation in the inner ear. When patients with renal insufficiency need an aminoglycoside the dose and frequency of administration must be adjusted to keep the serum level within bounds. By careful monitoring of serum creatinine levels the dosage should be regulated to individual needs. Safe upper limits cannot be specified with confidence, but ototoxic manifestations are likely to occur above aminoglycoside levels of 10–12 μg/ml. If the patient's renal status changes and the aminoglycoside level becomes dangerously high, ototoxic injury may be forestalled by haemodialysis to remove the excess drug [5].

Until recently it was assumed that the aminoglycosides interfere with the same metabolic processes in mammalian tissues as in susceptible micro-organisms. Their antimicrobial effect depends upon inhibition of protein synthesis by interaction with the 30S ribosomal subunit. In mammalian tissues, however, recent investigation has revealed an interference with the lipids of the cell membrane rather than with protein synthesis. Structure and function of the cell membrane depend upon the metabolism of the phosphoinositides, including their binding of calcium ions. Neomycin disrupts these processes, so that the cell can no longer function and eventually dies. It is not yet clear why neomycin and kanamycin affect the cochlear hair cells primarily, and streptomycin, gentamicin, and tobramycin the vestibular end organs. Differences in susceptibility of the respective secretory tissues (e.g. stria vascularis and dark cells) may be involved. Local differences in concentrations of the aminoglycosides in the endolymph and perilymph of different portions of the labyrinth are conceivable, but they have not been demonstrated.

Clinical considerations

Infants and young children appear to be less susceptible to ototoxic complications than adolescents and adults. Used with appropriate restraint, kanamycin, gentamicin, and tobramycin have proved of inestimable value in treating neonatal infections, but special caution seems necessary with premature infants because excretory function is not yet fully developed. Oral neomycin has a place in the treatment of diarrhoea in infants, but it too must be used with caution. Enough of it can be absorbed by the inflamed intestinal mucosa to cause severe hearing loss, which may be discovered only later when the child fails to develop normal speech [5].

Whatever the route by which neomycin is administered, its special potential for ototoxic mischief must be kept in mind. Profound deafness has been caused when neomycin has been given orally, topically on ulcerated skin, or as an aerosol for treating pulmonary infections [1, 5]. Although wound irrigation with neomycin may bring persistent infections under control, the amount absorbed systemically is often sufficient to produce total loss of hearing.

Neomycin has long been a major component of various preparations for local administration in the form of ear drops. The possibility of ototoxic complications as a result of such use has bothered many otologists, but there have been virtually no reports of measurable hearing losses clearly attributable to it. Some of the high-frequency sensorineural loss that can occur as a result of otitis media may possibly be due to extensive use of such neomycin-containing drops in the ear. Intratympanic administration of aminoglycosides in minute amounts to experimental animals produces dramatic injury to both the cochlea and the vestibular end organs as a result of absorption into the perilymph through the round window membrane. In intractable Menière's disease streptomycin has been given by the intratympanic route as well as parenterally to abolish labyrinthine function. Except for such deliberate destruction, aminoglycosides must not be introduced into the middle ear [1, 5].

THE DIURETICS

An acute ototoxic action can be exerted by the natriuretic agents ethacrynic acid and frusemide (Lasix). Although the two compounds are entirely different in chemical structure [6], both act on the renal tubules to inhibit the reabsorption of water in the proximal limb of the loop of Henle. In patients treated for oliguria they frequently produce a severe but transient hearing loss, with complete recovery within a few hours. Unfortunately the loss is not always reversible. Several cases of permanent deafness have been reported in uraemic patients who had received ethacrynic acid. More recently, irreversible hearing losses have also occurred after frusemide, especially when given rapidly in large intravenous doses. The use of one or other of these diuretics in a patient who is receiving aminoglycoside treatment can be particularly dangerous to the hearing, since there is both clinical and experimental evidence that a true potentiation of ototoxic action can occur [3].

Experimental studies indicate that the primary action of the diuretics is on the stria vascularis, where they can produce a striking oedema. Whether this engorgement of the intercellular spaces represents an increased movement of water and ions or a more or less complete stasis is not clear, but the latter seems the more plausible. Associated with it is a sharp fall or even a reversal of the positive endocochlear potential, which eventually returns to normal, as does the swollen stria itself. Hair cell loss is not usually seen, except when an aminoglycoside is given shortly before or after the diuretic. Their combined ototoxic action may be sufficient to cause extensive destruction of Corti's organ, even though either drug alone would have had no adverse effect.

The biochemical basis for the action of ethacrynic acid and frusemide has been assumed to be the same in the stria vascularis as in the renal tubules, where they inhibit Na^+K^+-ATPase, but cochlear adenyl cyclase is more susceptible to the inhibitory action of ethacrynic acid than the ATPase. The ototoxic effect may therefore involve inhibition of this enzyme.

OTHER OTOTOXIC DRUGS

Among the ototoxic drugs listed as 'Traditional' in Table 7.2, tinnitus and hearing loss have long been associated with quinine as an antimalarial agent and with large doses of salicylates used in treating rheumatoid arthritis. These symptoms usually disappear when the drugs are withdrawn. Audiograms of arthritic patients receiving salicylates often show a flat loss of about 30 dB. Such depressed hearing levels have reverted to normal even after years of treatment with salicylate. Temporal bone studies *post mortem* have revealed no more than typical presbyacusic changes in the organ of Corti. Hair cell loss has seldom been seen in animals after quinine or salicylate poisoning, but narrowed capillaries have been described in the vessels of the spiral ligament and basilar membrane reminiscent of the extreme vasoconstriction produced in the retina. Although interference with various enzyme systems has been suggested, it appears likely that quinine and salicylate ototoxicity represents a prolonged partial and usually reversible ischaemia of inner ear tissues.

Deafness and vestibular dysfunction have been observed after oral administration of oil of chenopodium (American wormseed) as an anthelmintic, and evidence of damage to the end organs by its major constituent, ascaridole, has been found in experimental animals. The arsenicals atoxyl and arsacetin act upon the stria vascularis, causing a hydrops and then collapse of Reissner's membrane with later degeneration of the organ of Corti [3]. These substances are no longer used, but an increasing number of other drugs, including cytotoxic agents such as the nitrogen mustards and a variety of environmental and industrial poisons, have proven or at least suspected ototoxic properties [1, 7]. The otologist, in keeping with his efforts to conserve his patients' hearing, should also maintain and encourage in his medical and surgical colleagues an attitude of cautious reserve toward new drugs

TABLE 7.2. Major groups of ototoxic drugs

Aminoglycosides	Traditional
Streptomycin	Quinine
Dihydrostreptomycin	Salicylates
Neomycin	Chenopodium
Kanamycin	(Ascaridole)
Gentamicin	
Tobramycin	Arsenicals
Amikacin	Atoxyl
Sissomicin	Arsacetin
Diuretics	Cytotoxic agents
Ethacrynic Acid	Nitrogen Mustard
Frusemide	Cis-DDP

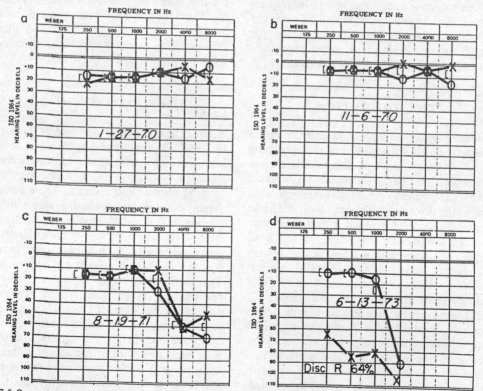

FIG. 7.5. Sensorineural hearing loss, attributable to potentiation of ototoxicity between gentamicin and frusemide in a renal patient who had normal hearing (a, b) before receiving a kidney transplant. Treatment with gentamicin and frusemide during the month following surgery produced a bilateral high-frequency loss (c). Almost 2 years later further treatment with gentamicin, frusemide, and oral neomycin in connection with resection of the aorta for a mycotic aneurism resulted in a severe sensorineural loss in the right ear and almost complete deafness in the left. Reproduced by permission from Quick C. A. (1976) Hearing loss in patients with dialysis and renal transplants. *Annals of Otology, Rhinology and Laryngology* **85**, 776.

until their potential ototoxicity has been evaluated.

Transplacental ototoxicity

Streptomycin has been detected in the fetal blood after it had been administered to the mother, but few convincing cases of ototoxic deafness acquired *in utero* have been recorded. At least one catastrophe has been reported in which both the mother and the child were found to be deaf after the mother had been treated with kanamycin and ethacrynic acid during the 28th week of gestation [2, 5]. The importance of avoiding, if at all possible, the ototoxic drugs during pregnancy should not require special emphasis.

Deafness in renal disease

The relations and similarities between the kidney and the inner ear are so complex and so little understood that unexplained deafness is an all too frequent complication of renal disease treated by dialysis or by renal transplantations. The increased susceptibility of renal patients to the ototoxic action of aminoglycosides as a result of delayed excretion and excessive serum levels has already been stressed. Since diuretics are often required, ototoxic potentiation with aminoglycosides used in treating infections is a further hazard. A cautionary example is seen in a case of hearing loss (Fig. 7.5) attributed to gentamicin and frusemide. The numerous factors which may combine and interact to cause deafness in patients with various types of renal disease have been discussed by Wigand [6] and by Quick [8]. Despite the utmost care on the part of the attending physician in consultation with the otologist, ototoxic drugs carry a risk which cannot always be calculated or avoided.

References

[1] BALLANTYNE J. C. (1973) Ototoxicity: A clinical review. *Audiology* **12**, 325.

[2] HAWKINS J. E. & PRESTON R. E. (1975) Vestibular ototoxicity. In *The Vestibular System*, ed. Naunton R. F., p. 321. New York: Academic Press, Inc.

[3] HAWKINS J. E. (1976) Drug ototoxicity. In *Handbook of Sensory Physiology*, eds. Keidel W. D. & Neff W. D., Vol. V/3, Chap. 16, p. 707. Heidelberg: Springer-Verlag.

[4] STUPP H., KÜPPER K., LAGLER F., SOUS H. & QUANTE M. (1973) Inner ear concentrations and ototoxicity of different antibiotics in local and systemic application. *Audiology* **12**, 350.

[5] HAWKINS J. E. (1975) Drug ototoxicity. In *Differential Diagnosis in Pediatric Otolaryngology*, ed. Strome M., Chap. 4, p. 53. Boston: Little Brown and Company.

[6] WIGAND M. E. (1976) Hearing and equilibrium in renal failure. In *Handbook of Sensory Physiology*, eds. Keidel W. D. & Neff W. D., Vol. V/3, Chap. 6, p. 279. Heidelberg: Springer-Verlag.

[7] AJODHIA J. M. & DIX M. R. (1975) Ototoxic effects of drugs. *Minerva Otolaringologica (Torino)* **25**, 117.

[8] QUICK C. A. (1976) Hearing loss in patients with dialysis and renal transplants. *Annals of Otology, Rhinology and Laryngology* **85**, 776.

CHAPTER 8

Noise Deafness

One of the physical effects of exposure to industrial noise is loss of hearing. That there is a cause–effect relationship between excessive noise and hearing loss has been known for a very long time – 'ears are injured by a perpetual din so that bakers of bread, blacksmiths and coppersmiths become hard of hearing and if they grow old at their work, completely deaf' [1]. Roosa [2] drew attention, in a paper on the aetiology of diseases of the inner ear, to the deafness of telegraph operators, boilermakers and naval officers arising from the nature of their occupations.

Gilbert in 1921 noting the rising noise levels in industry pleaded for an International Board of Physicians to be set up to monitor the resulting hearing losses of factory employees [3]. Jaehn in 1911 [4] in his description of hearing losses in artillery men was the first to recognize the distinction between what he called 'disturbances of hearing occurring immediately after exposure' and 'lasting' injury to the ear. Thus there was the implication in shooting that the deterioration in hearing was permanent and so the phrase 'noise induced permanent threshold shift (NIPTS)' came into use.

Quantitative studies on large numbers of subjects with permanent threshold shifts had to await the development of noise-measuring equipment for noise intensities on the one hand, and instruments for the measurement of hearing to determine hearing losses on the other. Noise measurement proved to be easier than hearing threshold determinations which at first focused on speech evaluation. The speech signal, however, was found to involve problems of spectral and intensity factors and was soon abandoned as a measure of hearing. Then followed an attempt at a 'Social Adequacy Index' made by Davis but this did not survive. Further attempts were made to correlate speech recognition scores (in per-

centages) with a loss for faint sounds (expressed in decibels) but it proved impossible to abstract a single score for impairment from sets of dissimilar measurements [5, 6]. The present practice is to infer impairment for hearing of everyday speech from a five tone audiogram.

To obtain accurate and reproducible data to be used subsequently for comparative research studies, it is necessary to be aware of the techniques of audiometry and to have a working knowledge of the instrumentation [7–10]. A working party of the Industrial Health Advisory Committee (now of the Health and Safety Commission, 1976) has issued a consultative document on audiometry (1978) in which calibration, techniques of recording thresholds, medical history, etc., are discussed. For industrial screening purposes where routine monitoring is desirable, the use of self-recording audiometry is recommended, where the subject himself adjusts the signal intensity to his threshold and a continuous recording of left and right ears is obtained at the selected frequencies recommended by the Code of 0·5, 1, 2, 3, 4 and 6 kHz. These audiometric measurements must be made in a test environment in which the ambient noise levels are known and which must not exceed levels required for 0 dB listening with known headphones (cups and cushions). Furthermore an attempt must be made to ensure a noise-free interval of known duration prior to the test. Noise levels for the test environment are given in the Discussion Document [11].

Temporary and permanent threshold shift

Exposure to intense noise on a sufficient number of occasions or for a certain duration injures the inner ear producing a sensorineural hearing loss.

The injury and the resulting threshold shift may be temporary, lasting for minutes, hours or days after the noise stimulus has ceased. Temporary threshold shift (TTS) is defined as the difference in decibels between post-exposure measurements of auditory sensitivity and pre-exposure measurements for pure tones. When the noise exposure is repeated the injury to the inner ear may produce a permanent hearing loss lasting for the remainder of the life of the subject (Permanent Threshold Shift – PTS). The relationship between TTS and PTS, unfortunately, is not a simple one and it is not possible to predict PTS from known TTS data [12, 13]. It is clear that early hopes for a quick and easy TTS test that would accurately predict an individual's susceptibility to PTS are not likely to be realized. From the early data of Hirsh and Ward [7] there is an initial R-1 phase in the recovery from TTS which occupies 2 minutes after cessation of noise exposure and during which the recovery curves of TTS against time show an irregular shape. The curves thereafter follow a more defined course (R-2 phase). Hence TTS_2, i.e. TTS measured 2 minutes after cessation of noise exposure, is recognized as the conventional TTS measurement. Since 1958 a series of TTS studies [12] has demonstrated an apparent quantitative relationship between TTS_2 and the magnitude of PTS at 4 kHz resulting from 10 years of constant noise exposure: This relationship $TTS_{2m} \simeq PTS_{10y}$ has been accepted as the basis for drawing up Damage Risk Criteria [14] for steady state noise and the basis for defining criteria for impulse noise [15]. It has been shown that TTS from a continuous steady-state noise grows for about 24 hours and then reaches an asymptote. If temporary threshold shifts produced by a fixed level and spectrum of noise truly reach an asymptote, then the threshold shifts at asymptote are an upper boundary on that PTS which can be produced by that sound regardless of the duration of exposure. Further deterioration in PTS will be presbyacusis [16].

Auditory impairment and morphological change in the inner ear

The classical signs and symptoms of sensorineural noise-induced hearing loss are the audiogram shape, the 4 kHz notch, the recruitment, the tinnitus slowly progressive over 10–50 years of industrial exposure and the extent of the hearing loss broadly related to the noise stimulus. In the 1960s and 1970s many fundamental studies of the relationship between the threshold shifts and the morphological changes found in the inner ear were made [17–22].

In the chinchilla histology there were instances of substantial outer hair cell damage with no auditory threshold elevation in the corresponding parts of the frequency range [19]. In noise exposures, in which the total energy was constant but contained different combinations of intensity and duration, the structural damage observed was not always the same. Thus a worrying feature emerging from morphological studies is that noise-induced permanent injury to the inner ear located in the hair cells of the organ of Corti may occur in animals in which no permanent change in hearing threshold is found. A summary of the present position is that [21]:

(1) the mechanisms leading to degeneration of the cells and fibres in a segment of the organ of Corti are still unknown;

(2) outer hair cells are the first to be damaged by noise exposure whereas the inner hair cells are the first to degenerate from ischaemia. It is unlikely that lack of oxygen during noise exposure is the cause of sensory cell degeneration; and

(3) if, as a result of noise exposure, a number of sensory cells degenerate simultaneously, small holes will be left in the reticular lamina. Endolymph can thus enter the fluid spaces of the organ of Corti and the excess of potassium ions will cause isosmotic swelling and rupture of uninjured cells and nerve fibres. If only scattered hair cells have degenerated the time taken to reseal was found to be in the region of 48 hours but, if an entire segment had degenerated, a period between 14 and 30 days was required before a bare portion of the basilar membrane was covered by a layer of epithelial cells [23].

Noise-induced permanent threshold shift (NIPTS)

The term NIPTS implies that an irreversible increase in threshold level has occurred during the interval between two audiometric examinations. Since World War II audiometric data has been obtained mainly from retrospective studies involving audiometric measurements of employees exposed to a known noise level and frequency spectrum for a known exposure time in years. A recent example of the growth of NIPTS over time is shown in Fig. 8.1.

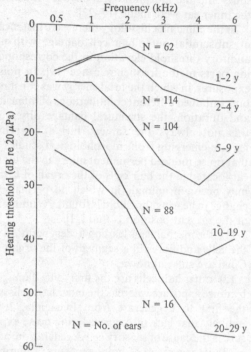

FIG. 8.1. Hearing thresholds of hammer and press operatives excluding pathology and previous noise exposure, by years of exposure. Reproduced from Taylor W., Pelmear P. L. & Kershaw J. G. (1976) Noise levels and hearing thresholds in the drop-forging industry. *Medical Research Council Project Report* G.972/784/C.

In this type of survey uncertainty must always exist concerning the state of hearing prior to noise exposure in the absence of a pre-employment audiogram. The uncertainty is increased if, outside working hours, leisure pursuits involve exposure to excessive noise, e.g. shooting or regular attendance at discotheques. Previous military service, again involving high impact noise levels, complicate the industrial accumulated noise dose. Other important factors inherent in survey audiometry are a history of middle

ear pathology, the use of ototoxic drugs, a history of head injury and finally hearing loss due to age (presbyacusis). There still remains, after subjects found to have any one of the above complications, perhaps the greatest variable in survey work – individual noise susceptibility or biological variation. An example of this is shown in Fig. 8.2 in which all subjects are pure, and those giving a history of any of the above complications have been excluded.

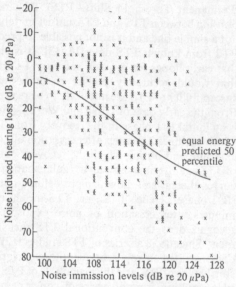

FIG. 8.2. Noise induced hearing loss (individual ears), age corrected, related to noise immission level for 4 kHz frequency. Reproduced from Taylor W., Pelmear P. L. & Kershaw J. G. (1976) Noise levels and hearing thresholds in the drop-forging industry. *Medical Research Council Project Report* G.972/784/C.

The data obtained from industrial NIPTS surveys has established:

(1) The hearing levels of noise-exposed persons increase rapidly in the 3–6 kHz region (and usually at 4 kHz) in the 0–15 years of noise exposure and then the rate of loss is progressively slower and is therefore mainly due to presbyacusis.

(2) The very earliest losses in young subjects exposed to broad-band noise for 1–2 years occur around 6 kHz. With a noise exposure time of 2–5 years, NIPTS slides into the 4 kHz region (the C5 dip or 4 kHz notch) first noted by Fowler in 1927

[24]. With further noise exposure the 4 kHz notch deepens and flattens out to include progressively the 3, 2 and 1 kHz frequencies thus involving the speech range.

(3) Noise-exposed groups show greater inter subject variability than pure non-noise-exposed controls.

(4) With the increasing loss of the high frequencies, noise-exposed subjects experience difficulty first with communication in noisy environments such as cocktail parties. The recruitment of loudness, always present in these cases, leads to distortion of speech and a speech discrimination loss.

(5) With noise exposures of 40–50 years, common in female weavers in textiles exposed to a sound pressure level of 100 dB (loom noise), sign language and lip-reading are adjuncts to severe hearing losses, with, at most, only the 250 and 500 Hz frequencies remaining in the audiogram.

Assessment of noise-induced permanent threshold shift (NIPTS)

For the otologist concerned with noise-induced deafness, a knowledge of his patient's noise environment is essential, in particular the noise level in general terms and the duration of exposure. For simplification, in recent years a single figure measure of noise intensity – dB(A) – has been accepted, where A denotes a weighted scale on a sound level meter in which the less damaging frequencies have been filtered out. This unit has been incorporated in computing the total energy entering the ear (estimated as 'A'-weighted sound energy) [25] and is used to predict hearing impairment. The unit has also been used as the basis for controlling the noise environment in industry. If noise exposure is continued for 8 hours in any 1 day and is a reasonably steady-state sound, the sound level should not exceed 90 dB(A). If the exposure is for a period other than 8 hours or if fluctuating, an equivalent continuous sound level (Leq) is calculated and this value in turn should not exceed 90 dB(A). The methods of measuring and controlling noise exposure are given in detail in the Code of Practice for reducing the exposure of employed persons to noise [26].

In assessing hearing damage however we are concerned with total energy derived from these 'A'-weighted sound measurements. A simple energy relationship has been derived [25] and designated *noise immission level* (NIL). This is the basis of the 'British Standard Method for Estimating the Risk of Hearing Handicap due to Noise Exposure' (BS 5330 : 1976) [27]. In this standard the hearing of a person is deemed impaired sufficiently to cause a handicap if the arithmetic average of the hearing threshold levels of the two ears combined at 1, 2 and 3 kHz is equal to or greater than 30 dB (referred to the audiometric zero of BS 2497). It is assumed that no pathological conditions are involved, that noise and age are the causative factors, and that the hearing levels in the two ears are substantially the same. The hearing handicap is estimated in terms of 'handicap percentage'. The noise exposure is quantified in terms of noise immission.

The equal energy principle postulated by Burns & Robinson [25], which permits sound levels to increase 3 dB each time the daily duration of exposure is halved, has also been applied to high impact noise situations such as hammers and presses in drop forging [28]. In the forging industry there are impact peak sound pressures of 120–145 and Leq's of 106–112 for hammers and 97–100 for presses. In this recent work, where approximately 30 000 audiograms were processed, there was good agreement with the equal energy principle.

Whilst progress is being made developing NIPTS on a scientific basis, there is little evidence that serious efforts are being made to reduce noise at source. It is true that designers of plant and machinery, architects and manufacturers of machinery are becoming aware of the hearing hazard resulting from excessive noise. The introduction of noise legislation in the UK has been slow and has not progressed further than a Voluntary Code. Meanwhile the Health and Safety Commission is considering limiting the noise environment in factories using the general obligations on employers, manufacturers and employees embodied in 'Framing Noise Legislation', a consultative document by the Industrial Health Advisory Sub-Committee on Noise [29]. This report has retained the noise limit of 90 dB(A) Leq. The USA Environmental Protection

Agency has recommended 85 dB(A) but the question of adopting this recommendation or 90 dB(A) has not been settled (1974) [12] for the USA.

Definitions of impairment

Davis [30] has provided useful definitions for impairment, handicap and disability. He defines impairment as a deviation or change in structure or function, handicap as the disadvantage imposed by an impairment sufficient to affect activities of daily living, and disability as interference with one's employment on full wages. By these definitions, it is important to note that significant handicaps in everyday life rarely are handicaps in the work situation which produced the impairment. We have noted the earliest area of impairment in NIPT following noise exposure to be in the 3–6 kHz audiometric range. Many otologists believe that loss of faint sounds in this region is not a handicap in everyday living even in the presence of moderately large losses in this region. It is the understanding of speech which is the important element in everyday life and its impairment is inferred from the measurement of hearing thresholds in the speech frequencies. Consequently the onset of impairment was equated by the American Academy of Ophthalmology and Otolaryngology [31] with an average hearing threshold for the frequencies 0·5, 1 and 2 kHz that was 26 dB less sensitive than the reference zero. Above this 'low fence' level impairment was considered to increase 1·5% per dB up to 100%, there being no allowance for presbyacusis. Those clinicians working with hard of hearing subjects severely criticized this scale on the grounds that speech handicap does not grow in simple proportion to the loss of sensitivity in decibels. Some form of sigmoid relation with handicap first increasing slowly, then more rapidly and finally slowing down fits the clinical history. The British Association of Otolaryngologists (1973) proposed the average of the pure tone losses in the better ear measured over the 1, 2 and 3 kHz frequencies. The point on this scale where loss of hearing begins to result in disablement is 40 dB. Using reception thresholds (SRT) in addition to pure-tone hearing threshold levels, it has been found that an index of 2 kHz + ½(6

kHz – 4 kHz) was better than 0·5, 1 and 2 kHz or than 1, 2 and 3 kHz averages. Normal hearing was associated with an average level of 25 dB and 25–35 dB was still in the lower range of normality [32].

In 1973 the Industrial Injuries Advisory Council issued their Report on Occupational Deafness (HMSO) and concluded that occupational deafness satisfied the conditions of Section 56(2) of the Industrial Injuries Act for Prescription as an Industrial Disease for compensation purposes [33]. The point of entry at which 1% compensation would be paid was fixed at 50 dB, the average of the hearing losses in the better ear over 1, 2 and 3 kHz frequencies representing an assessment of 20%. A presbyacusis correction was included by means of 0·5% for each year over 65.

The role of the otologist

The otologist is concerned in this scheme in two areas, the assessment of the deafness and the differential diagnosis.

There are no signs or symptoms specific to noise-induced deafness apart from the characteristic shape of the audiogram showing typically the greatest loss at or around the 4 kHz frequency. It is necessary to take a careful occupational history relating the NIPTS to the total dosage. There are obvious difficulties for the otologist in arriving at detailed noise parameters such as Leq's and noise immission levels, but a knowledge of the noise intensity and frequency of common occupational noises is an advantage. Accurate noise environment measurements will be necessary to predict hearing losses from the British Standard [27].

The deafness due to noise is sensorineural. The presence and extent of any accompanying conductive loss resulting from ear pathology must be assessed. In addition, the possibility of other forms of sensorineural loss will require consideration since infection involving the inner ear, ototoxic drugs, head injuries, acoustic nerve tumours and Ménière's disease will contribute to the total loss. A common symptom found in occupational deafness cases is tinnitus which when measured for pitch is found to be at or near the maximum hearing loss. In many cases the symptom arises long after exposure to excessive noise has ceased.

Finally there is the difficult question of non-organic functional hearing loss (psychogenic deafness) arising from anxiety states and feigned or simulated deafness. A test for malingerers is essential and these cases are usually found to have an overlay or exaggeration of an organic hearing loss which adds to the difficulties (see Chapter 1).

Noise and the law

The Department of Employment has estimated that some 600 000 workers in the UK are at present exposed to the risk of occupational deafness, with a further 2 million employed in industries where noise levels exceed the accepted 90 dB(A) damage risk criterion for part of the 8 hour shift. Yet compensation claims against employers have been relatively few. Up to 1976, ten cases involving eleven plaintiffs have been heard in the High Court and damages totalling about £51 000 awarded [34]. In the past loud noise has been accepted as a part of industrial life, indeed in boilermakers as a badge of office, and the resulting deafness as an unavoidable consequence of growing old. The industrial environment was never thought of as a source of physical injury. Furthermore there is a long-term growth of hearing loss measured in years where there is a gradual deterioration of clarity and word discrimination with recruitment, both leading to communication difficulties.

With the changing attitudes to hazards at work, legal claims for noise-induced deafness are increasing and substantial damages are being paid by employers. In some cases where claims have been accepted under the National Insurance (Industrial Injuries) Act 1965, the same evidence is being used for a Common Law claim against the employer.

In considering negligence, the crucial questions are how much a reasonable employer is expected to know of the risk involved and from what date. In 1960, 'Noise in Factories' was published by the Department of Scientific and Industrial Research [35]. It was an enlightened document clearly outlining the effects of excessive noise on welfare, safety and work efficiency.

This was followed by the Wilson Report [36] which unfortunately was indefinite on the risk of injury from noise but did emphasize the risk of permanent threshold shift above the 90 dB(A) noise level. Of more significance was 'Noise and the Worker', a Ministry of Labour, Health and Welfare booklet first published in 1963 [37], revised in 1971. In April 1972 the Department of Employment issued the 'Code of Practice for reducing the exposure of employed persons to noise' [26]. Following this publication, if any employer continues to run noisy processes without the provision of approved hearing protectors he is thereby negligent. He would be wise to ensure that the hearing devices meet the claimed attenuation [11]. Recent cases highlight other problems for management. Two recent claims settled out of court could not be defended since excessive noise exposures had occurred between the period 1963–68, during which time the firm was implementing noise reduction procedures and hearing conservation programmes. In two other cases employers were held negligent because in the first case no attempt had been made to size the ear inserts or instruct their employees in their use and in the second case only one form of ear protection, ear muffs, was made available.

Finally, under the Health and Safety at Work Act (1974), a civil claim for damages may be raised for breach of statutory duty under the Factories Act 1961 for ear injury. This action for breach of statutory duty stands alongside negligence in the area of industrial injury and recent claims in Scotland have been raised under both heads.

Hearing conservation programmes

It is clear from recent Government publications that an employer's duty is first to reduce noise levels in his factory below the accepted noise criteria (an engineering responsibility) and secondly, where it is impractical for economic reasons to reduce noise, he has to mount a hearing conservation programme. This calls for more than the issue of ear protective devices – ear muffs, glass down or moulded silicone rubber inserts. It will be necessary to organize a programme of training, education and maintenance of protectors and a noise awareness from the managing director to the shop floor employee. It is not a single initial collaborative effort between engineers, the medical team and the employees but requires constant pressure and application over years to maintain the programme.

The place in such a programme of monitoring audiometry is at present a debatable issue. The advocates of audiometry argue that

(1) audiometry will detect cases specially sensitive to noise damage, 'the susceptibles';

(2) routine monitoring will prove the efficiency of the protective hearing devices;

(3) measuring the hearing thresholds of individuals means contact with the works surgery. The knowledge imparted on the state of their hearing increases the voluntary response rate for hearing protection; and

(4) pre-employment audiometry protects the employer from claims arising from hearing loss incurred in previous noisy employments.

For the medical officer interested in otology there is always the satisfaction of the care and treatment of ear pathology discovered during monitoring programmes. In one legal case in 1973 the judge was prepared to hold the employer negligent for not having carried out audiometric tests which would have indicated that the plaintiff in the case was specially sensitive to noise. On the other hand the opponents of audiometry emphasize the variation in threshold testing, the large cost to firms with factories scattered over wide areas, the non-availability of trained staff and finally that the problem should be tackled from source by placing the emphasis on noise reduction and control [38, 39].

References

[1] RAMAZZINI B. (1713) De morbis Artificium Diatriba.

[2] ROOSA D. B. ST. JOHN (1874) A contribution to the aetiology of diseases of the internal ear. American Journal of Medical Science 68, 377.

[3] GILBERT D. (1921) Origin and development of the factory medical service in Belgium. Journal of Industrial Hygiene and Toxicology 2, 353.

[4] JAEHN A. (1911) Untersuchungen über Hörstörungen bei Fussartilleristen. Zeitschrift für Ohrenheilkunde 62, 111.

[5] DAVIS H. (1948) The articulation area and the social adequacy index for hearing. Laryngoscope 58, 761.

[6] SILVERMAN S. R. & HIRSH I. J. (1955) Problems related to the use of speech in clinical audiometry. Annals of Otology, Rhinology & Laryngology 64, 1234.

[7] HIRSH I. J. (1952) The Measurement of Hearing, Chap. 5. New York: McGraw-Hill.

[8] HINCHCLIFFE R. & LITTLER T. S. (1958) Methodology of air conduction audiometry for hearing surveys. American Occupational Hygiene 1, 114.

[9] LITTLER J. S. (1962) Techniques of industrial audiometry. National Physical Laboratory Symposium, No. 12. London: Her Majesty's Stationery Office.

[10] ROBINSON D. W. (1971) A review of audiometry. Physics in Medicine and Biology 16, 1.

[11] HEALTH AND SAFETY EXECUTIVE (1978) Audiometry in industry. Discussion Document. London: Her Majesty's Stationery Office.

[12] WARD W. D. (1974) Susceptibility to TTS and PTS. In Proceedings of the International Congress on Noise as a Public Health Problem. US Environmental Protection Agency Report, 550/9-73-008. Washington, D.C.: US Government Printing Office.

[13] WARD W. D. (1976) Susceptibility and the Damaged Ear Theory. Hearing and Davis. Essays Honoring Hallowell Davis, eds. Hush S., Eldredge D. H., Hirsh I. J. & Silverman S. R. St. Louis: Washington University Press.

[14] KRYTER K. D., WARD W. D., MILLER J. D. & ELDREDGE D. H. (1966) Hazardous exposure to intermittent and steady state noise. Journal of the Acoustical Society of America 39, 451.

[15] COLES R. R. A., GARINTHER G. R., HODGE D. C. & RICE C. G. (1968) Hazardous exposure to impulse noise. Journal of the Acoustical Society of America 43, 336, 343.

[16] MILLS J. H. (1976) Individual Differences in Noise-Induced Hearing Losses. Hearing and Davis. Essays Honoring Hallowell Davis, eds. Hush S., Eldredge D. H., Hirsh I. J. & Silverman S. R. St. Louis: Washington University Press.

[17] ELDREDGE D. H. & MILLER J. D. (1969) Acceptable noise exposures – damage risk criteria. Noise as a Public Health Hazard. eds. Ward W. D. & Fricke J. B., pp. 110–20. Washington, D.C.: American Speech and Hearing Association.

[18] MILLER J. D., ROTHENBERG S. J. & ELDREDGE D. H. (1971) Preliminary observations on the effects of exposure to noise for seven days on the hearing and inner ear of the chinchilla. Journal of the Acoustical Society of America 50, 1199.

[19] WARD W. D. & DUVALL A. J. (1971) Behavioural and ultra structural correlates of acoustic trauma. Annals of Otology, Rhinology and Laryngology 80, 881.

[20] HENDERSON D., HAMERNIK R. P. & SITLER W. (1972) Comparisons between hair cell losses and permanent threshold shifts produced by three levels of impulse noise. Paper J8, 83rd Meeting of the Acoustical Society of America, Buffalo, 1972.

[21] BOHNE B. A. (1976) Mechanisms of noise damage in the inner ear. In *Effects of Noise on Hearing*, eds. Henderson D., Hammernik R. P., Dosanjh D. S. & Mills J. New York: Raven Press.

[22] BREDBERG G. (1968) Cellular pattern and nerve supply of the human organ of Corti. *Acta oto-laryngologica* Suppl 236.

[23] BOHNE B. A. (1976) *Healing of the Noise-Damaged Inner Ear.* Hearing and Davis. Essays Honoring Hallowell Davis, eds. Hush S., Eldredge D. H., Hirsh I. J. and Silverman S. R. St. Louis: Washington University Press.

[24] FOWLER E. P. (1927) New tests for hearing. *Laryngoscope* 37, 285.

[25] BURNS W. & ROBINSON D. W., eds. (1970) *Hearing and Noise in Industry*. London: Her Majesty's Stationery Office.

[26] CODE OF PRACTICE for reducing the exposure of employed persons to noise (1972) London: Her Majesty's Stationery Office.

[27] ESTIMATING THE RISK OF HEARING HANDICAP DUE TO NOISE EXPOSURE (1976) British Standards Institution (BS 5330: 1976).

[28] KERSHAW J. G. (1976) Noise levels and hearing thresholds in the drop-forging industry. In *Disorders of Auditory Function II*, ed. Stephens S. D. G. London: Academic Press.

[29] FRAMING NOISE LEGISLATION (1975) Report by the Industrial Health Advisory Sub-Committee on Noise, Health and Safety Executive. London: Her Majesty's Stationery Office.

[30] DAVIS H. (1965) Guide for the classification and evaluation of hearing handicap in relation to the international audiometric zero. *Transactions of the American Academy of Ophthalmology and Otolaryngology* 69, 740.

[31] AMERICAN ACADEMY OF OPHTHALMOLOGY AND OTOLARYNGOLOGY (1959) Guide for the classification and evaluation of hearing handicap in relation to the international audiometric zero. *Transactons of the American Academy of Ophthalmology and Otolaryngology* 69, 740.

[32] PEARSON J. C. G., KELL R. L., ACTON W. I. & TAYLOR W. (1971) Social effects of hearing loss due to weaving noise. *Occupational Hearing Loss*, ed. Robinson D. W., pp. 179–91. London: Academic Press.

[33] OCCUPATIONAL DEAFNESS (1973) Report by the Industrial Injuries Advisory Council. Cmnd. 5461. London: Her Majesty's Stationery Office.

[34] INDUSTRIAL NOISE (1976) The Conduct of the Reasonable and Prudent Employer. The Wolfson Unit for Noise and Vibration Control, University of Southampton.

[35] ALDERSLEY-WILLIAMS A. G., ed. (1960) *Noise in Factories*. Building Research Station Factory Building Studies No. 6. Department of Scientific and Industrial Research. London: Her Majesty's Stationery Office.

[36] NOISE FINAL REPORT (1963) Committee on the problem of noise. The Wilson Committee Report.

[37] NOISE AND THE WORKER (1963) Ministry of Labour, Safety, Health and Welfare No. 25, Her Majesty's Stationery Office. (Revised 1971.)

[38] ATHERLEY G. R. C. (1973) The value of audiometry in industry. *Journal of Social Occupational Medicine* 23, 19.

[39] PELMEAR P. L. (1973) Hearing conservation. *Journal of Social Occupational Medicine* 23, 22.

CHAPTER 9

Ear Trauma

The incidence of aural trauma is rising. Increasing violence in society, increasing use of guns and explosives by terrorists, and increasing numbers of road and other accidents are leading to more frequent and more varied injuries to the ear.

The lesions may range from simple haematoma or laceration of the pinna without any loss of tissue, through simple rupture of the tympanic membrane, to transverse fracture of the petrous temporal bone with complete loss of inner ear and facial nerve function. The improved management of those with severe head or other injuries also contributes to the greater numbers of patients surviving to require treatment of aural trauma.

EXTERNAL EAR TRAUMA

Haematoma auris

In a *haematoma* of the pinna, blood collects between the perichondrium and the cartilage. This usually results from sports injuries, as in boxing or other physical contact games, but also can occur from violence in less controlled situations. These injuries should be adequately dealt with as otherwise the extravasated blood becomes organized, with the development of an ugly deformity generally know as 'cauliflower ear' or 'wrestler's ear'.

Treatment
It is important that the efforts to avoid a cauliflower ear are not rewarded by the potentially more deforming sequella of perichondritis. Evacuation of the haematoma can be done under local anaesthesia but it is essential that strict aseptic precautions are taken. An incision is made over the most dependent part of the

haematoma and all the blood clot is evacuated. Usually a small incision is adequate but if evacuation cannot be completed through this, it must be extended. A pressure dressing should be applied to prevent recurrence. If there is no discomfort the dressing may be left on for 2 or 3 days; if the ear becomes painful, suggesting perichondritis, it must be inspected. If infection is developing appropriate antibiotic treatment must be begun.

Lacerations

Trivial injuries of the outer ear commonly follow the use of a hair clip or similar implement in attempts to remove wax or soothe an itching meatus. Apart from causing pain and perhaps bleeding, these injuries are of little significance.

Lacerations of the pinna are potentially more serious than simple haematoma formation because of the likelihood of contamination of the wound, with the attendant risks of perichondritis. It is important that the wounds are cleaned thoroughly and sutured as required. Adequate systemic antibiotic treatment should be given and, if appropriate, tetanus prophylaxis prescribed.

The situation is complicated further when there is loss of tissue. As secondary cosmetic surgery to reconstruct the pinna is difficult and often unrewarding, all viable tissue must be preserved. If the pinna is partially amputated an attempt should be made to reconstruct it; such an attempt is often successful, although vigorous attempts must be made to prevent infection.

Simple lacerations and tears involving the meatal skin can be expected to heal without complication, but when the greater part of the circumference is involved there is a risk of meatal stenosis. In such cases excessive production of granulation tissue should be dealt with and an obturator inserted, such as a small piece of the appropriate size Portex rubber tube, to prevent the development of stenosis. The possibility of this complication persists long after the laceration has healed.

TYMPANIC MEMBRANE AND MIDDLE EAR TRAUMA

Traumatic perforations of the tympanic membrane

Rupture of the tympanic membrane may be caused by changes in air pressure, by fluids or by solid objects.

Pathogenesis

Air pressure changes. Sudden forceful blows on the ear which seal the external auditory meatus can result in sufficient increase in the air pressure in the ear canal to rupture the tympanic membrane. This most often results from blows on the ear with the open hand, as in water polo, or from a ball, as in tennis or squash. A fall on water, as in water skiing or high diving, can have similar consequences.

Blast injury of the ear frequently, and barotrauma infrequently, cause damage to the tympanic membrane. These will be considered later in the chapter.

Eustachian tube inflation, either by the patient or by use of a Eustachian catheter, rarely results in perforation of a normal healthy tympanic membrane but can rupture one weakened by previous disease. Lightning, with the associated air pressure changes, has resulted in perforation of the tympanic membrane.

Fluid. In syringing, it is important to ensure, not only that the fluid is at body temperature but also that the full force of the jet is not directed on to the tympanic membrane. By directing the main force of the jet on to the posterior meatal wall the likelihood of rupture of the tympanic membrane is considerably reduced. Caloric tests in patients with gossamer thin tympanic membranes must be undertaken with considerable caution. In skin diving it is possible for, perforation of the tympanic membrane to occur not only from air pressure differentials but also from fluid pressure in the ear canal.

Solid objects. Although the usual foreign bodies occurring in children rarely themselves rupture the tympanic membrane, match sticks or hair clips used to remove wax or relieve itching in the ear canal sometimes cause damage to the tympanic membrane.

Sparks of hot metal, especially in welders, can perforate the tympanic membrane by burning through it.

Management

Traumatic perforations tend to occur in the healthy members of the community; generally the prognosis is excellent. The two main factors leading to failure of the perforation to heal are loss of tissue and secondary infection; the prognosis is therefore worse in welding injuries. Small perforations are more likely to close spontaneously than large ones. None the less the membrane usually heals and the function of the ear returns to normal.

The most effective management is to do nothing. Because of the risk of introducing infection, the ear should not be cleaned out unless contaminating material is found in the meatus or there is evidence of active infection. Antibiotic ear drops, in the absence of infection, are of no value and may well introduce organisms. Systemic antibiotics also should not be prescribed in the absence of overt infection unless there is good reason to believe that the ear has been contaminated.

There are many advocates of an active approach to the tympanic membrane following trauma. They recommend examination under a microscope with eversion of the edges of the perforation. This approach is reasonable so long as it is carried out by a competent person under aseptic conditions and, in fact, could well be regarded as the ideal. If infection is not introduced it is unlikely that any harm will be done; furthermore, inverted edges are undesirable.

However, immediate surgical repair with grafting is not indicated because the perforation will usually close spontaneously; even subtotal perforations often heal with an excellent end result. If the perforation fails to close spontaneously in 3–6 months surgical closure is indicated.

Complications

The most common complication of a traumatic perforation is secondary infection of the middle ear. The development of squamous epithelial cysts in the middle ear has been seen following perforations caused by blast, and is due to implantation or inversion of squamous epithelium. Depending on the force of the injury causing the perforation there may be ossicular displacement with conductive deafness or inner ear damage, with sensorineural deafness and tinnitus.

Otitic barotrauma (aerotitis)

Pathogenesis

Otitic barotrauma is due to the development of a negative pressure in the middle ear cleft, relative to the environment. Thus, it may occur during descent from altitudes, as in flying, during underwater descent, as in diving, or with abnormal extra tympanic pressure increase, as in a hyperbaric chamber.

For normal function, middle ear pressure should be at or about environmental atmospheric pressure. This equilibrium is maintained by the Eustachian tube. There are no Eustachian tube reflexes, and primitive terrestial man rarely encountered Eustachian tube problems as a result of atmospheric pressure changes, and then only with considerable change in altitude. Modern man, who descends to the bed of the ocean and ascends high into the skies has created yet another problem for himself.

Normally, when the pressure in the middle ear rises in relation to surrounding air pressure, as occurs during ascent in an aeroplane, there is passive escape of air from the middle ear cleft, through the Eustachian tube. Armstrong & Heim [1] estimated that the Eustachian tube opens once for about every 500 feet of ascent.

This equalization of air pressure is a passive process and does not involve any active opening of the Eustachian tube.

In the opposite situation, when the pressure in the middle ear cleft is negative in relation to the environment, the mechanism is quite different. Active opening of the Eustachian tube is essential for equalization of pressures and occurs either by the use of the tensor palati, levator palati, and salpingo-pharyngeus muscles as in swallowing or yawning, or by autoinflation by the Valsalva or Frenzel manoeuvres. Failure to relieve negative middle ear pressure results in in-drawing of the tympanic membrane; further reduction in pressure occurs as the remaining air is absorbed and, when the pressure differential exceeds 90 mmHg, the muscles which normally open the Eustachian tube are rendered impotent.

Failure of the Eustachian tube to open and the persistence of negative pressure causes increasing retraction of the tympanic membrane, oedema and ecchymoses of the middle ear mucosa, transudate of fluid from intact vessels, and if these rupture, bleeding into the middle ear. Rupture of the pars tensa has been reported when the pressure changes have been sudden and intense.

Otitic barotrauma occurs most often following air travel, and even pressurization of modern aircraft has not entirely eliminated the problem. The Eustachian tube is the key to the condition. This may be normal, but simply not in use during descent, as when the passenger has a dry mouth or is asleep. The Eustachian tube may be oedematous from an acute cause such as a cold, or there may be chronic abnormalities of tubal function.

Clinical features

Deafness and discomfort are constant symptoms of this otitic barotrauma. The impairment of hearing may range from nothing more than the sensation of 'blockage' in the ear to a moderate degree of deafness. Discomfort may increase to mild to moderate pain, later becoming extremely severe. This usually subsides in a matter of hours as the high negative pressure is reduced by the production of transudate. Tinnitus also may be present.

The findings will depend on the time of examination and the severity of the symptoms. Initially, there is simply hyperaemia of the tympanic membrane, which becomes retracted and may show ecchymoses. Fluid later develops in the middle ear and may be accompanied by blood staining or frank bleeding. Rupture of the tympanic membrane is rare and precludes the development of the transudate. Sensorineural hearing loss in barotrauma has been reported; it is much more common in underwater diving than with altitude change.

Management

Chronic nasal conditions predisposing to Eustachian tube problems should be dealt with before flying, especially in someone who has had previous trouble with barotrauma. Acute nasal congestion can be reduced by vasoconstricting nasal sprays or systemic decongestant drugs. Sleeping should be avoided during descent, even in pressurized aircraft, and sucking a sweet or chewing gum encourages swallowing. Patients with a history of this condition also should be advised to autoinflate repeatedly by the Valsalva manoeuvre during descent.

If these measures fail and the deafness and pain increase, the otologist may be requested to relieve the symptoms as a matter of urgency. Eustachian tube catheterization, or if this fails, puncturing the tympanic membrane will relieve the negative pressure and the pain instantly. Often pain has settled before the otologist is consulted. If symptoms persist, treatment should be aimed at reaeration by autoinflation, by the use of vasoconstricting nasal sprays and systemic decongestant drugs. If these fail, myringotomy will be required. Many cases resolve spontaneously without the patient seeking medical advice.

Otitic barotrauma in divers

Similar difficulties occur in underwater divers as in those who fly, although the active changes in middle ear air pressure must be made on descent. Failure to achieve these usually demands an immediate return to the surface and elimination of the problem.

Blast injury

Explosive material changes suddenly from solid to gaseous form with a massive increase in volume and pressure, resulting in a blast wave spreading outwards from the seat of the explosion. There is a short-lived positive pressure phase, usually of the order of a few milliseconds and a longer and less marked negative phase, always less than atmospheric pressure and of the order of tens of milliseconds. The amount of energy in each phase of the wave is approximately equal. The front of the blast wave is irregular and damage may be caused in a capricious fashion. The factors influencing such damage are:

(1) the rise time, that is, the speed with which the pressure builds up;

(2) the intensity or height of the peak pressure; and

(3) the duration of the positive pressure wave.

Some people close to the bomb escape ear damage while others, further away, may be severely deafened.

Exposure to blast can result in damage to both middle and inner ears. There may be hyperaemia, or even subepithelial bleeding in the tympanic membrane. Perforation due to the blast occurs in the pars tensa and the ear facing the bomb tends to be more seriously damaged than the ear away from the bomb. Perforations are probably caused by the positive phase of the blast as indicated by the findings of squamous epithelium in the middle ear in postmortem specimens and the formation of epithelial pearls in tympanic membranes that have healed spontaneously. Everted edges are often seen following blast injury but are probably caused secondarily by the suction effect of the negative phase. Most blast injuries of the tympanic membrane heal spontaneously with conservative treatment.

Surgical trauma

The chorda tympanic nerve

In theory, disorders of taste and salivary secretion should follow every instance of surgical trauma to this structure.

In practice, although the nerve is frequently stretched, manipulated, dehydrated and even cut, dysgeusia is an uncommon complaint after stapedectomy and hardly ever occurs following tympanoplasty.

Notwithstanding, because disorders of taste do occur following ear surgery and can considerably diminish the pleasures of the table, sometimes for many months, the surgeon should always handle the chorda tympani with care.

The jugular bulb

This structure is occasionally dehiscent in the posteroinferior quadrant of the mesotympanum when it is at risk, as the annulus fibrosus is elevated from the sulcus tympanicus in creating a tympanomeatal flap during stapedectomy and transcanal tympanoplasty. Brisk venous bleeding at this stage can usually be controlled by promptly replacing the tympanic membrane and its annulus and applying a small pack. If the bleeding area is then avoided, it is usually possible to complete the procedure with only limited inconvenience.

The facial nerve

In all middle ear surgery, especially for chronic suppurative disease, the safety of the facial nerve will depend upon knowledge of several important landmarks.

In a mesotympanum which is completely filled with granulations or cholesteatoma, it is best to find the landmark which is more resistant to disease than all others – the Eustachian tube. From there it is safe to dissect posteriorly over the promontory as far as the grooves for the tympanic plexus. These grooves can then be followed superiorly to the base of the cochleariform process which marks the junction of the labyrinthine and tympanic segments of the nerve. When the process has been destroyed, a useful alternative guide is the muscle belly of tensor tympani, which is usually exposed in such cases.

Dissection can then proceed posteriorly following the osseous canal of the tympanic segment of the nerve. In transcanal tympanoplasty, if any doubts develop about the anatomy of the seventh nerve it is always wise to increase exposure of the area by converting the procedure into a combined approach tympanoplasty (CAT). This permits dissection inferiorly over the medial epitympanic wall and the anterior half of the lateral semicircular canal, exposing the tympanic segment of the nerve from its superior aspect where its bony covering is least likely to be deficient. Once the characteristic pink rounded bone overlying the nerve is compared with the ivory-white labyrinthine bone, the position of the nerve will be apparent, and dissection can proceed over it in all directions.

It should be remembered that there are several possible abnormalities of the facial nerve in this region which may give rise to confusion and possibly disaster if they are not known. The most common of these is the facial nerve which is overlying the footplate of the stapes. For this reason, it is important to identify the facial nerve positively in its normal horizontal canal before removing soft tissue from the surface of the footplate.

In the mastoid segment the following landmarks are of service; the lateral semicircular canal, the fossa incudis, and the digastric ridge. The posterior semicircular canal lies on the medial aspect of the mastoid segment of the nerve. In performing a mastoidectomy or CAT the first landmark is the mastoid antrum. Korner's septum may give rise to confusion and lead the surgeon in an inferior and anterior route into the mastoid segment of the facial nerve. This can be avoided by

(1) awareness of the risk; and
(2) noting the level of the tympanic membrane as compared with the medial wall of the 'false antrum'.

In CAT, posterior tympanotomy is performed by cutting a groove downwards from the tip of the short process of incus towards the mastoid tip. The groove should be parallel to the expected course of the facial nerve, and the bone should be thinned gradually with diamond burrs so that the facial nerve can be seen before it is uncovered. Once the facial sinus has been entered, further enlargement of the posterior tympanotomy is carried out by removing bone inferiorly and laterally. For this, the position of the chordal eminence and the chordal ridge should be known and understood. Exposure of the hypotympanum requires removal of the styloid eminence.

Abnormalities of the facial nerve rarely occur in this area but they should be known. The most common of these is the nerve that passes posteriorly, but bifid facial nerves below the genu have been reported. The digastric ridge and the position of the chorda tympani nerve can be used as guides to the facial nerve when required.

Treatment

Surgical trauma to the facial nerve in temporal bone surgery may result in loss of continuity of the nerve and loss of nerve substance. In these situations, direct anastomosis does not necessarily produce the best result and it is now agreed that grafting with a piece of the great auricular nerve is the preferential method in most instances. The results are better when tension can be avoided and a grafting technique is carried out with the use of magnification from the operating microscope. Excessive proliferation of connective tissue in an anastomotic area can be reduced by the removal of several millimetres of epineurium from the stumps. The ends of the stumps should be approximated after they have been cut in an oblique direction in order to increase the surface areas in contact. Foreign body reaction with connective tissue proliferation is reduced by the avoidance of suturing material. The natural self-adherence of the nerve tissue is often sufficient to retain the position of the nerve graft in the mastoid and tympanic segments.

In conclusion, avoidance of facial nerve trauma in advanced chronic middle ear disease will be enormously enhanced by the recognition of important landmarks such as the cochleariform process, the lateral semicircular canal and the oval window. The great importance of surgical skill, anatomical knowledge and knowledge of variations in normal anatomy, were summed up by Fowler [2] when he said: 'Although traumatic facial palsy is more likely to occur when a surgeon is inexperienced, it can and does occur with the most skilful and experienced otologic surgeon, especially when the course of the nerve is anomalous'.

TEMPORAL BONE TRAUMA
Fractures

The clinical features of fractures of the temporal bone can only be understood by considering their anatomy and pathology. Fractures involving the temporal bone can be classified into longitudinal, transverse and mixed, depending on the relationship of the fracture line to the long axis of the petrous temporal bone. In many the lesion is confined to the squamous temporal, in which case it could be regarded as an incomplete or partial longitudinal fracture. Often the diagnosis is made purely on clinical grounds as the fractures do not always show on routine skull radiographs.

Pathology

Longitudinal fractures. Eighty per cent of temporal bone fractures are longitudinal and usually result from blows to the temporal or parietal areas [3]. The fracture begins in the squamous temporal bone and extends along the roof of the bony external auditory meatus, tearing the tympanic membrane, and crossing the roof of the middle ear into the petrous temporal bone. It then runs anterior to the labyrinthine capsule, through the carotid canal, to end near the foramen spinosum or foramen lacerum (Fig 9.1).

The skin of the external auditory meatus and the tympanic membrane are frequently torn with bleeding from the ear. In the absence of any other obvious cause, bleeding from the ear following a

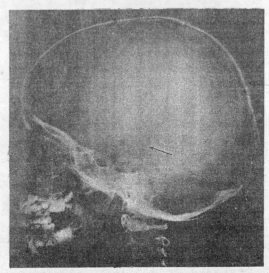

Fig. 9.1. Longitudinal fracture of temporal bone.

head injury can be presumed to indicate a fracture of the base of the skull, usually longitudinal, despite negative X-ray findings. Displacement of the bone is very rare but a gap may be present at the fracture line.

The middle ear structures are always involved in longitudinal factures but in most cases this is not serious and healing occurs spontaneously without residual conductive deafness. However, should there be persistent conductive deafness the possibility of ossicular dislocation must be considered.

Because a longitudinal fracture line usually runs anterior to the hard bone of the labyrinthine capsule, only rarely is the inner ear directly involved, but there may well be concomitant inner ear concussion with high tone sensorineural hearing loss. Facial nerve injuries are uncommon in longitudinal fractures and when they occur usually are delayed in onset.

Transverse fractures. Transverse fractures, usually resulting from frontal or occipital blows, account for approximately 20% of temporal bone fractures [3]. The fracture line extends transversely across the petrous pyramid, passing through the vestibule of the inner ear. Although the fracture can be demonstrated radiologically in about 50% of cases, the diagnosis is essentially clinical (Fig. 9.2). In a pure transverse fracture there is a haemotympanum but no bleeding from the ear. The severe general injuries of the patient may dominate the clinical picture, but, if sought for, there is evidence of severe or complete sensorineural deafness on the affected side, usually accompanied by tinnitus. The deafness is permanent.

Very severe rotatory vertigo with nausea and vomiting, due to severe damage to the vestibular apparatus on the affected side, occurs initially. Nystagmus is usually present with the quick component to the opposite side. Unfortunately, the significance of the severe dizziness, vomiting and nystagmus is often missed by those responsible for the management of the head injury. It may not become apparent that the patient has vestibular damage until he is allowed out of bed a week or two after the injury. The patient then is surprised to find that he is extremely unsteady and unable to walk without support. Central compensation develops in the subsequent weeks and months. Facial nerve injuries occur in about 50% of these patients and the onset is usually immediate.

Mixed fractures. In severe head injuries there may be a combination of longitudinal and transverse fractures.

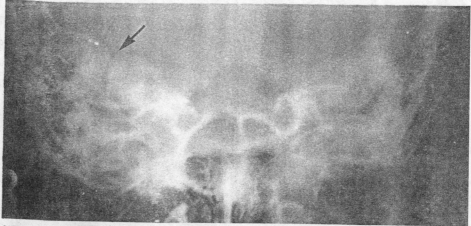

FIG. 9.2. Transverse fracture of temporal bone. P.McG., aged 14, received a blow from a stone on the right occipitomastoid region. There was a short period of unconsciousness. When seen 2 hours later he was complaining of right deafness and tinnitus, was very dizzy and was vomiting; there was blood in the right middle ear behind an intact tympanic membrane and he had horizontal nystagmus to the left. Audiogram showed profound right deafness. He made an unusually rapid recovery from his dizziness and was walking well 10 days later. His deafness is permanent.

Management

The importance of avoiding the introduction of infection into the middle ear cannot be overemphasized and, unless there are signs of active infection, it is better to leave any blood clot in the external auditory meatus untouched. A cerebrospinal fluid leak must be treated by sulphonamides and an antibiotic. The management of the head injury usually takes preference and indeed it may be some days before the otolaryngologist is asked to see the patient.

Cerebrospinal fluid leak

Most cerebrospinal fluid leaks close spontaneously within 7–10 days. If this does not occur more active treatment will be necessary. While the introduction of a spinal drain at this time may well be all that is required to allow the leak to close, many neurosurgeons are unhappy about this approach. They feel that although closure by this method may be sufficient at the time, some leaks will recur later, or, even without a recurrence of the fluid leak, there may be an ascending intracranial infection from a subsequent otitis media. If the leak is profuse or if it fails to close promptly after spinal drainage, exploration and surgical closure is indicated. These leaks usually arise from the middle cranial fossa and the help of a neurosurgeon is desirable in this situation. The middle cranial fossa is explored, the dura elevated and, after exposure of the tear, the defect is covered with a graft of fascia lata or temporalis fascia.

Meatal damage

Tears in the meatal skin may heal with the formation of fibrous bands in the depths of the meatus, resulting in pockets which collect epithelial debris. If these cannot be cleaned adequately and effectively via the meatus or if repeated cleaning will be necessary over many years, surgical removal of these bands, perhaps with grafting of the tympanic membrane, may be required.

A wide fracture line predisposes to invasion of the middle ear cleft by squamous epithelium and, indeed, cholesteatoma development has been reported. However, the vast majority of cholesteatomata diagnosed for the first time after a head injury are not caused by the trauma. Medico-legal problems can arise, but in the absence of a wide fracture line the cholesteatoma can reasonably be presumed to have been present before the injury.

Deafness

The conductive deafness which follows longitudinal fractures almost always recovers spontaneously. Failure to regain normal middle ear transmission is usually due to the formation of adhesions or dislocation of the ossicles. Ossicular damage also can result from head injury in the absence of a skull fracture.

The most commonly affected ossicle is the incus as the malleus and stapes are relatively more stable; the most common defect is a dislocation of the incudostapedial joint [4]. All other lesions are uncommon. These include fracture of the stapedial crura, dislocation of the stapes footplate, total dislocation of the incus, dislocation of the malleus and fixation of the malleus head in the epitympanum by fibrous tissue or bone. Delayed necrosis of the long process of the incus has been described.

In these cases there is usually a conductive deafness with an air–bone gap of 30–40 dB. Exploration of the middle ear is indicated and the prognosis is very good.

The sensorineural deafness caused by head injuries is unfortunately untreatable. Although there may be some spontaneous recovery of the high tone sensorineural loss that often accompanies longitudinal fractures, there is no likelihood of recovery of any useful hearing following transverse fractures.

Although fractures of the temporal bone may be diagnosed on clinical grounds without any radiological confirmation, labyrinthine damage can occur without any clinical or radiological evidence of temporal bone fracture. In these cases it is presumed that labyrinthine concussion is responsible for any associated auditory or vestibular symptoms.

Deafness in these cases affects the high frequencies and, although it is often permanent, there usually is some recovery in the first few weeks or months after the injury. Generally speaking, an injury insufficiently severe to cause loss of consciousness does not damage the hearing; but beware of falling into the trap of believing that such an injury never causes deafness.

Vertigo

Vertigo is common following head injuries and, as with deafness, can occur without a skull fracture. The most common form is that associated with the post-concussional syndrome. These patients tend to have vague unsteadiness, especially when getting up from sitting and usually associated with frequent severe headaches. This symptom tends to settle down in a matter of 6–12 months and when it is prolonged beyond this time the question of a post-concussional neurosis must be considered.

Following transverse fracture of the temporal bone there is severe incapacitating vertigo making it impossible for the patient to walk unaided for a length of time which varies from 1–4 weeks, depending on such factors as the age and motivation of the patient. In the immediate period after head injury the symptoms can be relieved by labyrinthine sedative drugs. There tends to be a slow but gradual improvement; young patients recover to fairly normal balance in a matter of weeks and elderly patients in months. However, the convalescence is often complicated by other injuries and, especially in the elderly, associated brain damage may prevent full compensation.

Benign positional vertigo may follow as a complication of head injuries, with or without fracture of the temporal bone. Schuknecht [5] has postulated that this results from damage to the utricle with disruption of the otolithic membrane, the otoconia of which become adherent to the cupula of the posterior semicircular canal. This is then stimulated by movement of the head, especially when the affected ear is placed undermost. The dizziness is short-lived, associated with transient and fatiguable rotatory nystagmus and always precipitated by head movement; between these induced episodes the patient is perfectly steady. This is a self-limiting condition although it often takes up to 2 years before the vertigo settles.

Perilymph fistulae may also be a cause of post-traumatic vertigo and will be discussed later.

Facial paralysis

Facial paralyses following fracture of the temporal bone are classified broadly into two groups – immediate and delayed. Immediate paralysis usually indicates tearing of the facial nerve in transverse fractures or impaling of the facial nerve by bone in longitudinal fractures. In either case early surgical exploration is indicated if there is to be any reasonable prospect of good functional recovery.

Delayed onset of facial paralysis confirms that, anatomically, the facial nerve is intact, that there is oedema secondary to the injury, and that there has not been any gross trauma directly to the nerve. The management of delayed traumatic facial paralysis is similar to the management of idiopathic facial paralysis (see Chapter 5).

Perilymph fistulae

Perilymph may leak from the inner ear, either from rupture of the stapediovestibular joint or the round window membrane. This condition most often results from pressure changes involving the middle and inner ears but may result from head injuries. The clinical features are variable and usually include fluctuating sensorineural deafness, tinnitus and unsteadiness, often with a disproportionate degree of ataxia. The dizziness due to direct damage to the vestibular apparatus improves dramatically in a matter of weeks, whereas the dizziness associated with a perilymph fistula often persists until the leak is closed. The amount of leaking fluid is usually small and does not fill up the middle ear. One does not expect, therefore, to see a fluid level on routine clinical examination of the middle ear.

A high index of suspicion is necessary for the diagnosis of a perilymph fistula, which is confirmed by exploration of the middle ear. Even at operation the diagnosis may be difficult and one may have to wait several minutes to observe the accumulation of fluid in the oval or round window. Although a defect may rarely be seen at the oval window, this usually is not the case and Goodhill [6], in his large series of oval and round window fistulae, has never *seen* a hole in the round window membrane. In the normal ear, most of the round window membrane is concealed from view, but, in any event, the leak is usually minute and probably marginal in position.

The fistula can usually be closed by removing the surrounding mucous membrane and placing an autogenous soft tissue graft over the area of the leakage.

Penetrating injuries of the temporal bone

Injuries from bullets, missiles, and explosions may result in lesions involving any part of the body. When the temporal bone is involved almost any lesion can occur. In most cases the other injuries predominate and it may be some time after the injury before the otolaryngologist is asked to see the patient.

The lesions of the temporal bone are difficult to classify because of their variability; the management of each patient depends on the specific circumstances. Often the other injuries necessitate compromise in the otological management.

Patients have been reported who had gunshot left in their temporal bone for many years without any complication. In one patient, as a result of gunshot injury, the tympanic membrane was largely destroyed; gunshot remained in the middle ear cleft and brain herniated through a damaged tegmen tympani into the attic [7]. The patient lived for 40 years after the injury and died from other causes. Despite such cases, if there is gunshot in the middle ear cleft, directly exposed to the exterior and with the possibility of infection, surgical exploration and removal is indicated. If, on the other hand, the gunshot is adequately buried, without any infection or likelihood of infection, and is not causing symptoms, action is not required.

INNER EAR TRAUMA

Blast injury

It has been stated in the past that rupture of the tympanic membrane has a significant protective effect on the inner ear. A recent detailed survey has suggested that this is not the case and that sensorineural deafness is no less severe in those whose tympanic membranes have been ruptured [8].

Sensorineural deafness is maximal immediately after the explosion with a natural tendency to spontaneous improvement. There may be complete, bilateral deafness just after the explosion but there is, in the authors' experience, always some recovery. Initially, the rate of recovery is rapid so that patients, unable to hear at all at the site of the explosion, are able to understand loud speech without difficulty 1 hour later. In some, the hearing may have returned to its former level in 48 hours, and in others, while there is permanent sensorineural deafness, this may continue to show slight improvement for up to 6 months.

In view of the tendency to rapid spontaneous recovery it is difficult to control any trial of treatment for blast-induced sensorineural deafness. Numerous regimes have been advocated including vasodilating drugs, corticosteroids, intravenous low molecular weight dextran and anticoagulants. Other injuries may preclude some or even all of these forms of treatment. As there is doubt about the efficacy of the treatment, it is preferable to leave untreated all cases of mild deafness, to use vasodilating drugs only in moderate cases and to reserve the blunderbuss approach only for severe cases in which there are no contraindications.

Tinnitus is a common complaint in those exposed to blast. The severity of the tinnitus tends to reflect the sensorineural deafness. Initially, the tinnitus may be very severe and although it persists as a big problem to some patients, it tends to decrease. When there is permanent sensorineural deafness the tinnitus may never disappear entirely but usually ceases to be a burden to the patient. In the uncomplicated case where the hearing returns to normal, one can expect complete disappearance of the tinnitus.

Whiplash injury

The term whiplash injury, used in an unpublished paper in 1928, was first recorded in 1945 and has been a source of controversy ever since. Many object to the name but all agree that it implies an acceleration-extension injury of the neck; some also include in the syndrome deceleration injuries and forward or lateral flexion movements. The diverse symptomatology and the prolonged litigation that follows these injuries has led to considerable scepticism about this condition. None the less, it has been shown that many patients continue to have symptoms, sometimes disabling, related to whiplash injuries, not only when other simultaneous severe injuries have become symptom free, but even years after litigation has ended and compensation has been paid [9]. While symptoms can occur following forward and lateral flexion injuries, the vast majority arise from acceleration-extension injuries as occur in rear-end collisions. In many instances the initial injury seems trivial, with severe pain in the neck developing only some hours later.

Clinical features

The most common complaint is pain in the neck, but the otolaryngologist becomes involved when the symptoms include dizziness, tinnitus, deafness and dysphagia.

Most physicians have been prepared to accept dizziness as a genuine symptom, despite opposition from some of their colleagues, but only with the advent of electronystagmography has it become possible to demonstrate labyrinthine abnormalities objectively in the majority of those with this complaint. Unfortunately, however, this does not settle the question entirely, as similar abnormalities have been reported in some normal control subjects. What then does one make of this problem? The authors believe that dizziness can result from neck injuries. Typically these patients complain of unsteadiness, especially in certain neck positions, and have electronystagmographic evidence of labyrinthine abnormality, most marked in the alleged precipitating positions. The cause of the unsteadiness is not completely clear but may be due to abnormal cervical afferent impulses or brain damage resulting from the whiplash injury.

A careful history must be taken to ensure first, that a whiplash injury did occur and secondly, that there was not a concomitant head injury.

Tinnitus is a frequent complaint in the early stages after these injuries but it probably results from the concussive effect on the brain rather than any injury to the neck. Deafness has been reported in some publications on this subject but without much substantiating evidence. It seems likely that deafness does not occur in the absence of an associated head injury and that whiplash injuries of themselves do not result in hearing loss.

Treatment

Many modern car seats are so designed that acceleration-extension injuries cannot occur because the back of the seat extends to head level. Widespread use of such seats should reduce the incidence of this syndrome.

Whiplash injuries are better treated during the acute phase. If the nature of the injury and the patient's symptoms suggest this condition, immediate and adequate splinting of the neck is required, accompanied by bed rest to relieve the neck of the weight of the head. This is the time for a collar, not 6 months later. Heat and massage may make the patient feel more comfortable, but probably do nothing to speed the resolution of the underlying lesion.

Treatment in the chronic phase is difficult. If the patient appears to be developing disabling symptoms due to functional overlay, do not over-treat or over-investigate. There is no evidence that prolonged immobilization is of benefit or that, at this stage, heat and massage do more than imprint the symptoms on the patient's mind. Neck traction and muscle strengthening exercises may be of benefit but must not be instituted until it has been established by flexion and extension radiographs that there is no joint instability. A frank and open discussion with the patient about the possibilities of disordered function is the best approach, once the chronic stage has been reached.

While many patients improve with time, especially after litigation has been settled, this is not always the case; do not be misled into thinking that all these patients are malingerers.

Surgical trauma

Injury to any of the structures which lie within the petrous bone is an inherent risk in every ear operation. Although it is certainly true that the introduction of microsurgical techniques in otology has been followed by a reduction in the formerly large incidence of surgical accidents such as dislocation of the stapes, opening of the labyrinth and damage to the facial nerve, nevertheless, the possibility of postoperative labyrinthine dysfunction after any operation on the ear, including myringoplasty, is still ever-present, even for the most experienced otologic surgeon. Cochlear losses are reported more frequently than imbalance but the two can occur together and indeed vestibular defects might be recognized more often were they routinely sought for.

Although gross trauma to the facial nerve and major blood vessels is always possible if anatomical knowledge and surgical expertise are lacking, nowadays the majority of surgical injuries to the ear affect the labyrinth and follow the creation of a fistula of the oval window, or hydraulic effects on the membranous inner ear. Cellular damage from infection, and circulatory changes and alterations in the dynamics of the inner ear fluids are responsible for most of the functional damage which complicates microsurgery of the ear.

Labyrinthine trauma in tympanoplasty

In tympanoplasty the principal causes of cochlear loss are:

(1) Excessive movement of the stapes footplate whilst removing disease from the oval window or from any part of an intact ossicular chain. Similar risks also pertain during reconstruction of the transmission mechanism and the tympanic membrane.

(2) Incautious removal of granulations, tympanosclerosis or cholesteatoma from the oval window with fracture of the stapes footplate or rupture of its annular ligament creating a fistula between the mesotympanum and the vestibule of the inner ear. Prolonged perilymph loss or labyrinthitis may follow.

(3) Contact between a toothed rotating burr and any part of an intact ossicular chain (most commonly the body of the incus) in combined approach tympanoplasty can cause extensive hair cell damage [10].

In a series of 1680 chronic ear operations, Palva *et al* [11] reported a 4·5% incidence of sensorineural deafness after operation, mainly

limited to the frequency range of 4000–8000 Hz. In 81% the ossicular chain was maintained intact throughout the operation. Smyth [12] reported various degrees of sensorineural hearing loss in 2·5% of 3000 tympanoplasty operations.

Apart from the special risk of cochlear trauma in combined approach tympanoplasty from contact of the burr, transmitted through the intact ossicular chain, which occurred in 5·6% of such ears, labyrinthine trauma did not appear to be related to any particular surgical technique. However, it should be noted that 1·3% of all myringoplasties (transcanal tympanoplasty with an intact chain) were complicated by a depression of greater than 10 dB averaged through the frequencies 500–4000 Hz, or a greater than 10% loss in speech discrimination score.

Trauma arising from the removal of diseased tissue from the isolated stapes was considered to be responsible for one-third of the casualties and of these, in one-third the dissection of tympanosclerotic plaques had been noted to cause overmanipulation or fracture of the stapes footplate. In another third of the damaged inner ears in this series the cause appeared to be excessive movement of the stapes footplate during attempts to reconstruct the ossicular chain.

Labyrinthine trauma in stapedectomy

In stapedectomy the inner ear is most threatened by the events which occur when the oval window is fenestrated. The possible sources of labyrinthine damage are numerous and include those listed below.

(1) *Immediate causes*

(a) Excessive movement of all or part of the stapes, usually during attempts to remove a prematurely mobilized footplate, or prolonged manipulation of an oval window soft tissue or gelfoam graft, both causing an hydraulic effect.

(b) Rupture of the membranous inner ear by attempts to remove pieces of footplate from the vestibule.

(c) Distortion of the membranous inner ear arising out of sudden decompression of the vestibule of the inner ear by rapid loss of perilymph, usually because of injudicious use of suction, but occasionally in ears with an abnormally patent cochlear aqueduct.

(d) Acoustic trauma from instrumentation, usually drilling in obliterative otosclerosis.

(2) *Delayed causes*

(a) Damage to the utricular or sacular macula from impingement of an over-long prosthesis.

(b) Hydrops of the scala media due to prolonged perilymph loss owing to a delay of the oval window fenestration to heal.

Clinical evidence of labyrinthine trauma after stapedectomy ranges from transient minor imbalance and temporary depression of hearing to gross and persistent ataxia with permanent profound deafness. It appears possible that many stapedectomies destroy some inner ear function. Although symptomatic evidence for this is often not striking, nevertheless routine investigation of vestibular and auditory function confirm its existence. Postoperative caloric testing and audiometry during the immediate postoperative weeks have demonstrated abnormal function. If the powers of vestibular compensation are good, as they usually are in the young and middle aged, and provided cochlear damage is confined to the basal turn, the patient may be pleased with a 'good result'. However, there are unfortunately a small number of patients who become so ataxic that they require labyrinthectomy or vestibular nerve section and an appreciable number who lose all auditory function. The reported incidence of 'dead' ears within one month following stapedectomy varies from 0·5% to 4%. Unfortunately, it is not possible to determine from most reports how many 'dead ears' are due to trauma at the time of operation and how many are the result of late complications such as perilymphatic fistulae. Shea [13] reports eventual cochlear losses due to postoperative perilymph fistula in 2% of large fenestra operations with the teflon piston and vein graft technique.

Diagnosis

When technical problems which are known to pose a threat to the labyrinth have arisen during any ear operation, the surgeon will not require complicated tests to confirm the presence of trauma. Spontaneous nystagmus (first, second or third degree), depending upon the severity of the lesion, confirms the suspicion of vestibular disease. Bedside voice tests for discrimination with contralateral masking provide invaluable information about the health of the cochlea and should be confirmed by daily bone conduction audiometry.

Because labyrinthine trauma can complicate any apparently straightforward middle ear operation, the detection of immediate postoperative dysfunction often depends upon a permanent high index of suspicion. The risk should be presumed to be present in all forms of ear surgery and the surgeon should enquire *routinely* about tinnitus and vertigo, and should test eye movements and speech discrimination once daily for at least 4 days. Utricular damage which does not cause nystagmus will be implied by vertigo and demonstrated by simple postural tests. Daily bone conduction tests with adequate masking of the other ear are helpful but it must be remembered that routine testing after uncomplicated stapedectomy and tympanoplasty usually shows an elevation of threshold of as much as 10 dB through the speech frequencies for 5 days.

Treatment

'Prevention is better than cure', was never more apt than in the realm of labyrinthine trauma in ear surgery. In tympanoplasty, excessive stapedial movement, even in the simplest myringoplasty, must always be avoided. In removing squamous epithelium from the malleus when the ossicular chain is intact, the surgeon should dissect with slow movements parallel to the handle of the malleus so that the perilymph has time to pass through the helicotrema towards the round window without causing damage to the organ of Corti.

When the ossicles are intact and are involved in tympanosclerosis, profuse granulations or cholesteatoma or are at risk of trauma from the burr, then the incudo-stapedial joint should be disarticulated early in the operation.

When the removal of diseased tissue from the stapes arch or the footplate proves difficult, it is essential to postpone this part of the operation until a second stage 6 months later.

In cholesteatomatous middle ear disease, the possibility of a labyrinthine fistula should always be borne in mind and tested for before operation. *Before* removing squamous epithelium from the semicircular canals it is vital to examine for signs of erosion visually and by palpation. Should a fistula be suspected, removal of the overlying cholesteatoma matrix should be either postponed until the end of the operation when irrigation and suction are no longer necessary, or deferred to a second operation 6 months later when the ear will be free from infection.

If a perilymph fistula from a semicircular canal or the oval window is caused by the surgeon this should be covered immediately with fascia and all further work in the area avoided. Although a further operation will usually be necessary to complete what is required, the risks to function will be reduced to a minimum.

In stapedectomy, because of what occurs at the moment of footplate fenestration, every care must be taken to:

(1) avoid losing control of an excessively mobile footplate. This is best done by making a small hole in the centre of the footplate before the crura are fractured;

(2) limit perilymph loss by using a small fenestra technique with prompt insertion of a prosthesis which will almost fill the fenestra followed by immediate firm placement of gelfoam around the edges of the fenestra. Only very small suction tips should be used and they should never be put so near the fenestration area as to accelerate perilymph loss;

(3) prevent the entry of blood into the vestibule and the need for suction by delaying fenestration of the footplate until all bleeding in the area has ceased;

(4) avoid dangerous levels of noise in the ear by avoiding suction when the oval window is open and limiting the use of a drill in obliterative cases.

Much more serious consideration than has been usual in the past should be given to the prescription of a hearing-aid in young women with obliterative otosclerosis.

By these means much inner ear trauma can be avoided. When it has already occurred and is detected during the early postoperative period, what can be done? Obviously when a fistula of one of the semicircular canals or the oval window

is suspected in tympanoplasty, the decision is straightforward. Early control of bacterial infection will be decisive to the outcome, and therefore the appropriate antibiotic should be given intravenously or intramuscularly in large enough doses to cross the blood-perilymph barrier. It should be noted that the possibility of labyrinthine complications in any chronic ear operation is more than ample justification for routine preoperative bacterial studies so that knowledge of the organism and its sensitivities will be available should antibiotic therapy be required.

However, in many cases of surgical labyrinthine trauma, not only is there some uncertainty about its cause, but there is also very little exact knowledge about the pathology of these conditions. Pressure changes in the vestibule due to excessive movements of the stapes or sudden loss of perilymph after opening the labyrinth, may cause distortion and tears of the membranous ducts. Mixing of endolymph and perilymph leads to hair cell death and neuronal degeneration [14].

Noise of even relatively low intensity, causes spasm of the spiral vessels in the zona arcuata of the basilar membrane in experimental animals [15], and these ischaemic effects on the hair cells are likely to be increased by greater metabolic need in the presence of noise. Spasm followed by vasodilatation, slowing of the circulation, platelet aggregation, hypercoagulation and thrombosis may follow as part of the tissue response to trauma. Hypoxia will retard the production of cyclic adenosine monophosphate with resultant tissue damage. It seems likely that if noise causes circulatory changes in the inner ear, then also other forms of pressure change such as those arising from manipulation of the stapes and perilymph fistula may do so as well. If the experimental work of Lawrence [15] which relates inner ear vasospasm to noise exposure can be extrapolated to additional forms of energy trauma in tympanoplasty, then it follows that the prime aim of treatment should be to restore the inner ear circulation and also combat the already present effects of anoxia.

The arterial supply of the inner ear, which is derived from the intracranial circulation, does not respond to those drugs which are used to promote the circulation elsewhere in the body. The ability to increase perilymph oxygen tension by carbon dioxide inhalation has recently been reported [16], and on this basis inhalations of 5% carbon dioxide and 95% oxygen are recommended at a flow rate of 5 litres per minute for periods of not less than 1 hour at least three times daily. Nicotinic acid (100 mg orally 6-hourly), Thymoxamine (80 mg orally 6-hourly), stellate ganglion block and intravenous histamine have been recommended by some doctors but so far convincing evidence of their efficacy in man is lacking.

The use of corticosteroids has been proposed for their effect on disordered hair cell metabolism; although there is evidence of inhibition of serous labyrinthitis in stapedectomized animals the value of steroid in man as a means of assisting in the recovery of inner ear dysfunction has not yet been confirmed.

To combat hypercoagulation, platelet aggregation and the inflammatory reaction of inner ear trauma as well as disturbances in lipid metabolism, treatment with adrenocorticotrophic hormone and heparin has been advocated, but again the merits of these medications await confirmation.

Although these various suggested means of treating labyrinthine dysfunction may yet lack adequate statistical support, nevertheless in the face of potential disaster, a decision to deny the patient any therapy which might be of assistance incurs a heavy responsibility.

References

[1] ARMSTRONG H. G. & HEIM J. W. (1937) The effect of flight on the middle ear. *Journal of the American Medical Association* 109, 417.

[2] FOWLER E. P. JR. (1961) Variations in the temporal bone course of the facial nerve. *Laryngoscope* 71, 937.

[3] PROCTOR B., GURDJIAN E. S. & WEBSTER J. E. (1956) The ear in head trauma. *Laryngoscope* 66, 16.

[4] HOUGH J. V. D. (1970) Fractures of the temporal bone and associated middle and inner ear trauma. *Proceedings of the Royal Society of Medicine* 63, 245.

[5] SCHUKNECHT H. F. (1969) Cupulolithiasis. *Archives of Otolaryngology* 90, 765.

[6] GOODHILL V. (1976) *Lecture to Section of Otology*, Royal Society of Medicine, London.

[7] KERR A. G. (1967) Gunshot injury of the temporal bone – a histological report. *Journal of the Irish Medical Association* 60, 446.

[8] KERR A. G. & BYRNE J. E. T. (1975) Concussive effects of bomb blast on the ear. *Journal of Laryngology and Otology* 89, 131.

[9] GOTTEN N. (1956) Survey of 100 cases of whiplash injury after settlement of litigation. *Journal of the American Medical Association* 162, 865.

[10] PAPARELLA M. M. (1962) Acoustic trauma from the bone cutting burr. *Laryngoscope* 72, 116.

[11] PALVA T., KARJA J. & PALVA A. (1973) High-tone sensorineural losses following chronic ear surgery. *Archives of Otolaryngology* 98, 176.

[12] SMYTH G. D. L. Sensorineural hearing loss in chronic ear surgery. *Annals of Otology, Rhinology and Laryngology* (In press).

[13] SHEA J. J. JR. (1971) A 15-year report on fenestration of the oval window. *Transactions, American Academy of Ophthalmology and Otolaryngology*.

[14] SCHUKNECHT H. F. (1974) *Pathology of the Ear*, Chap. 12, p. 462. Cambridge, Massachusetts: Harvard University Press.

[15] LAWRENCE M. (1973) *In vivo* studies of the microcirculation. *Advances in Oto-Rhinolaryngology* 20, 244.

[16] SHEA J. J. & KITABSCHI A. E. (1973) Management of fluctuant hearing loss. *Archives of Otolaryngology* 97, 118.

CHAPTER 10

Pathology of Chronic Middle Ear Disease

The mucoperiosteal lining of the air-containing middle ear cleft is subject to many of the inflammatory disorders of the nasopharynx in childhood by reason of anatomical continuity.

The common precursors of chronic disease of the middle ear cleft are repeated attacks of acute middle ear infection and failure of resolution of the acute inflammatory process, aggravated by constant reinfection from the nose and paranasal sinuses and by inadequate treatment. The seeds of chronic ear disease are thus sown usually in childhood, and the afflicted individual may continue to be disadvantaged throughout his formative years and adult life by a variable degree of conductive hearing impairment, with or without chronic otorrhoea.

In contrast with acute inflammation in which the essential pathological feature is one of rapid exudation over a period of hours or days, the chronic inflammatory process is one in which tissue responses may persist for months or years with periods of regression and repair alternating with inflammation and exudation. The phenomena of inflammation and repair may coexist but it is unusual for them to remain in a finely poised balance. The cellular exudate of chronic inflammatory reactions is varied and is composed of leucocytes of all kinds, especially mononuclear cells such as lymphocytes, plasma cells and macrophages. Chronic inflammation is also accompanied by proliferation of the connective tissues of the affected area so that the reaction is often described as formative or productive. In most forms of chronic inflammation the exudative and proliferative processes are combined in varying proportions.

In an entirely different form of chronic middle ear disease the intrusion of keratinizing stratified squamous epithelium into the middle ear cleft gives rise to an encysted collection of keratin called an aural cholesteatoma or keratoma. This is an insidiously destructive condition that may in rare cases cause the dramatic onset of intracranial complications.

These basic considerations as they apply to the mucoperiosteal lining of the middle ear cleft, together with some of the clinical manifestations of chronic ear disease, form the substance of this chapter.

BASIC STRUCTURE AND FUNCTION OF MIDDLE EAR CLEFT

An understanding of the structure, function and behaviour of the mucous membrane lining of the middle ear cleft and its response to ventilation arrest, infection and ingrowth of keratinizing squamous cell epithelium, together with an appreciation of the pathological changes occurring in bone, is essential to the understanding of the pathogenesis of chronic middle ear disease.

Structure of the Eustachian tube

Detailed descriptions of the anatomy of the Eustachian tube have been provided by several workers [1]. Certain features, however, merit special attention because of the role they play in the pathogenesis of chronic middle ear disease.

The Eustachian tube is formed of two distinct parts, the bony and cartilaginous, linked by a narrow isthmus. The bony part merges into the middle ear cavity and its opening is at a higher level than the hypotympanum. The tube therefore cannot serve as a passively draining pathway from the middle ear.

The normal lining of the cartilaginous portion

123

of the Eustachian tube is formed of pseudo-stratified columnar ciliated epithelium with abundant goblet cells and scattered intraepithelial glands. The latter consist of mucous cells arranged around a lumen and are extremely irregular in distribution, their number decreasing towards the middle ear. Some workers have stated that lymphoid follicles may be found in the well-developed submucosa, chiefly in the region of the nasopharyngeal opening. However, others have denied this, claiming that lymphoid aggregations stop short at the pharyngeal end of the normal tube. Tubulo-acinous submucosal glands are certainly present, however. Although some are present in fetal life, most are developed after birth. These submucosal glands are similar to those of the trachea in having an acinous structure, several tubules and one excretory duct. They have an irregular distribution, being more numerous and larger in the medial wall of the auditory tube. The epithelium of the duct system does not contain cilia and it may be that the contraction of the tubal musculature causes pressure which empties the mucus from the glands. This provides a mucous blanket which is transported towards the nasopharynx by ciliary activity.

The epithelium of the bony portion of the tube is formed by tall pseudo-stratified columnar cells although these become flatter towards the tympanic cavity. Approximately 80% of the epithelial cells are ciliated and the remaining 20% are secretory [2]. There are no tubulo-acinous submucosal glands present [3]. Goblet cells and intraepithelial glands are seen, although they decrease markedly in the direction of the middle ear. The subepithelial connective tissue layer is also much thinner in the osseous part than in the cartilaginous portion of the Eustachian tube.

Function of the Eustachian tube

Most accounts of Eustachian tube function largely relate to the cartilaginous portion of the tube. The part played by the rigid-walled bony section and the isthmus area is not understood. Indeed, it may be that the bony tube should be regarded as a protympanum.

The prime function of the Eustachian tube is to equalize the air pressure on the two sides of the tympanic membrane. The tube is normally closed at rest because of the elastic tissue in the submucosa of the cartilaginous portion and the presence of a thin film of mucus which helps to 'gum' the walls together. The tube is opened by contraction of the tensor palati muscle acting on the membranous lateral wall of the cartilaginous section of the tube in response to swallowing and yawning movements.

In 1869, Politzer set forth his theory that Eustachian obstruction results in the absorption of oxygen from the enclosed air spaces. When the pressure damping capacity of the tympanic membrane has been exceeded, and depending upon the size of the air cell system, continued absorption causes a negative pressure within the rigid-walled system. This leads to hyperaemia, oedema of the mucous membrane and the exudation of fluid from the vessels into the tympanic cavity by a process of sterile transudation. This 'ex vacuo' theory has been challenged by a great number of workers, largely on the grounds that many surgical attempts to occlude the tube produce an associated inflammatory reaction, and because of doubt that hermetic sealing of the tube actually occurs in man, except in cases of severe scarring or neoplasm.

Applying a negative pressure to the air cell system of the healthy ear produces barotrauma [4]. The artificial and highly negative pressure of clinical and experimental barotrauma may lead to the development of an effusion and mucosal changes, but the very much lower negative pressure developed as a result of ventilatory obstruction at atmospheric pressure takes a much longer time to give rise to similar alterations and may not always do so. Oxygen reabsorption does occur from the closed pneumatic system, but the resultant decrease in pressure is probably progressively compensated for by mucosal oedema and effusion. Other factors in addition to oxygen reabsorption may therefore be involved in determining the final result in most cases.

Hypofunction of the Eustachian tube may be caused by inflammation, allergies, mechanical causes such as scarring and tumours, cleft palate where the function of the tensor palati is disturbed, and rapid barometric pressure changes. Posture and venous congestion of the head also have a demonstrable effect on tubal function, as do disturbances of nasal function. Polypoid mucosa, scars, adhesions, and granulation tissue may obstruct the tympanic end of the Eustachian tube following chronic otitis media, as may cholesteatoma if sufficiently extensive.

A second function of the Eustachian tube concerns ciliary action which is powerful and is directed towards the nasopharynx. This may assist in the clearance of secretions from the middle ear, and also in the prevention of ascending infection. In this regard the quantity and viscosity of the effusion, the adhesion of the liquid to the bony walls of the cavity, the surface tension of the liquid and the reduced ciliary efficiency due to mucosal oedema, exudation and epithelial desquamation must also be important factors. These factors may cause stagnation of mucus and interfere with the successful clearance of the middle ear cavity. By the accumulation of viscid mucus in the tube, they will interfere with air pressure equalization and predispose to otitis media. Resultant changes, including an increased density of goblet cells in the tubal mucosa and increased secretion from the submucous glands, further complicate the situation.

Structure of middle ear epithelium

Until recently the middle ear epithelium was generally believed to be comprised of low cuboidal or flat non-ciliated cells without mucus secreting elements.

It is now accepted that the normal middle ear lining is an extension of the Eustachian tube respiratory epithelium and is a true mucosa containing secreting cells and ciliated epithelium. The ciliated lining extends from the Eustachian tube to the tympanum in the form of tracts which line the anterior tympanum, hypotympanum and, to a lesser extent, the promontory [5]. The cilia cover the anteroinferior one-third to two-thirds of the middle ear mucosa. The tympanic membrane is devoid of cilia, and the posterosuperior part of the promontory, posterior attic and aditus comprise a non-functioning area from the point of view of ciliary activity.

The mucus producing region is not confined to the ciliated epithelial area, but extends beyond it posteriorly. Tubular subepithelial glands are occasionally present and goblet cells are present in the area of the Eustachian orifice and hypotympanum. However, neither of these are widespread and, based on fetal studies, it is probable that the glands are not a normal component of middle ear mucosa. The major source of mucus in the normal middle ear is the ciliated and non-ciliated cells which show intracellular mucus droplets.

The ciliated mucosa is known to be able to transport foreign particles. This mucociliary transport system is comprised of ciliated cells, secretory cells, and the mucus blanket. It depends on mucus as the coupler, translating ciliary beat into mechanical transport. The cilia beat in a wave-like or rippling pattern (metachronal rhythm) and must play an active part in evacuating fluid from the middle ear. Ciliary insufficiency and impaired clearance may result from damage to the cilia themselves, or may be due to an excessive viscosity of the middle ear fluid, or to hypersecretion. However, resorption by the mucosa is an important factor as evidenced by the ability of the middle ear epithelium rapidly to resorb radioisotopes (macromolecular transport) with resultant passage into the lymphatic capillaries.

The subepithelial connective tissue of the middle ear is mainly formed by collagen fibres with numerous blood and lymph capillaries and nerve fibres. The cellular components are mainly fibrocytes, but occasional mast cells, macrophages, lymphocytes and plasma cells are found. The mast cell granules are known to contain histamine, serotonin and heparin.

Recent immunochemical studies have demonstrated that the normal middle ear mucosa and Eustachian tube can produce immunoglobulins and lysozyme. In addition to the mucociliary transport system, it therefore appears that the middle ear is also endowed with local immunological and enzymatic defence systems.

Whether the middle ear and mastoid mucosal epithelium is a continuous true respiratory epithelium of endodermal origin has been argued. It has been asserted that the endodermal mucosa only extends to the isthmus of the Eustachian tube [6, 7] and it is also thought that the tympanum is a wide transitional region in which the endodermal respiratory epithelium merges with a mesodermal pseudoendothelium [8, 9]. Certainly the epithelium of the mastoid cavity is quite different from that of the tympanic cavity, being comprised of very flat cells with no ciliated or secretory cells [10] and it may well be that the posterosuperior area of the tympanum represents a gradual or abrupt transition zone between tubotympanic endoderm and the mastoid and attic mesothelium. It is in this special junctional region that cholesteatoma develops, and it is also a non-functioning area from the point of view of ciliary activity.

TYPES OF CHRONIC OTITIS MEDIA

Chronic otitis media is defined as long-standing inflammation of the middle ear cleft in which signs of acute inflammation are characteristically missing. Several entities are included under this collective title, and they are classified according to whether the tympanic membrane is intact or perforated, and whether the infection is specific or non-specific (Table 10.1).

Chronic suppurative otitis media of tubotympanic type

Chronic suppurative otitis media of tubotympanic type is a condition of non-healing central perforation of the tympanic membrane associated with chronic inflammatory changes of the mucoperiosteum of the middle ear cleft resulting in mucoid or mucopurulent otorrhoea.

Clinical features

The clinical features include constant or intermittent discharge (usually odourless) from the ear, conductive hearing impairment of slight to moderate degree and absence of pain. Occasionally granulations or polyps may form within the middle ear and a large aural polyp may occlude the external auditory meatus.

The tympanic membrane perforation is confined to the pars tensa, but may vary in size, shape and position (Fig. 10.1). Usually there is a large central or anterior defect with an intact

annulus fibrosus. The effects of a tympanic membrane perforation are many and varied, and depend on the site and size of the defect. The area for sound pressure collection is decreased, and sound energy enters the middle ear reaching both oval and round windows, reducing the preferential mechanism of sound conduction and exerting a back pressure on the inner surface of the tympanic membrane. In general, the hearing loss

TABLE 10.1 Classification of chronic otitis media

NON-SPECIFIC INFLAMMATORY PROCESSES

(1) Tympanic membrane perforated: chronic suppurative otitis media
   Tubotympanic type
   Attico-antral type, usually associated with aural cholesteatoma
(2) Tympanic membrane intact
   Chronic secretory otitis media
   Idiopathic haemotympanum (blue drum) associated with cholesterol granuloma

SPECIFIC INFLAMMATORY PROCESSES

   Tuberculous otomastoiditis
   Syphilitic otomastoiditis and labyrinthitis
   Actinomycotic otomastoiditis

---

tends to increase with posterior location and with increasing size of the perforation. Thus even when the ossicular chain and windows are functioning normally, a perforation can be associated with variable levels of hearing ranging from normal to about 45 dB (ISO) in the speech range (500–2000 Hz).

The mucosa of the middle ear may appear only slightly altered from normal, or can become velvety pink, thickened and oedematous with occasional polyp formation. Chronic mucosal changes may involve the whole middle ear cleft, but are usually most prominent in or confined to the tubotympanic region. The normal epithelium of the middle ear becomes hypersecreting and hypertrophied. The discharge from the middle ear through the perforation is usually mucoid, non-fetid and scanty (usually with a mixed flora of saprophytes and commensals). It may become profuse and mucopurulent if the patient has an upper respiratory infection, allows entry of water into the ear, or develops an infection of the mastoid air cell system which in this disease is often quite well-developed.

The ossicular chain often remains intact in tubotympanic disease, but, with prolonged inflammation, a rarefying osteitis with bone resorption can damage the long process of the

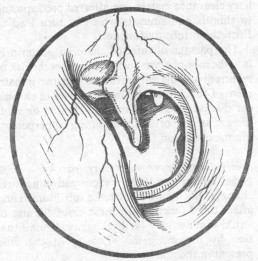

FIG. 10.1. Subtotal defect of left tympanic membrane in chronic tubotympanic disease. The anterior margin of the defect is obscured by a prominent overhang of the anterior canal wall. The annulus fibrosus and peripheral remnant of pars tensa can be seen inferiorly and posteriorly. The handle of the malleus occupies the centre of the field. The tip of the long process of the incus is visible posterosuperiorly and the round window niche posteroinferiorly.

incus, the arch of the stapes, the body of the incus and the manubrium of the malleus. In general, tubotympanic otitis media is a benign form of chronic disease, even when the mastoid segment is involved, because the risk of intracranial suppurative complications is rare.

Pathogenesis

Chronic tubotympanic infection is usually the residue of an acute infection, or rarely of trauma, producing a non-healing defect of the tympanic membrane. It is aggravated by lack of attention or by constant re-infection from the Eustachian

tube or external meatus. Several of the factors that predispose to the chronicity of the mucoperiosteal infection in tubotympanic disease merit further discussion.

Perforation of the tympanic membrane

The tympanic membrane demonstrates a remarkable regenerative capacity so that after spontaneous perforation, as is seen in acute suppurative otitis media or after paracentesis, the opening closes rapidly. Only under special conditions does a perforation fail to heal and become permanent.

The blood supply of the tympanic membrane is in two layers, one on either side of the fibrous layer or lamina propria, anastomosing with each other. Vessels enter the tympanic membrane peripherally, but also run down along the handle of the malleus to the umbo region. The anastomosis between the peripheral and central vessels constitutes a potentially avascular area, and this fact is of importance in the location of central perforations and atrophic changes.

In the pre-antibiotic era, acute otitis media occurred as a complication in about 10% of cases of measles and scarlatina, and the inflammation of the middle ear was often necrotizing with destruction of the tympanic membrane. Inflammatory destruction of the tympanic membrane is still seen, but less commonly, since the introduction of antibiotics. The large size of the perforation and the impaired healing properties after these infections result in a non-healing defect. Permanency is established when the stratified squamous epithelium of the cutaneous layer of the drum grows around the rim of the perforation to meet the mucosal layer of the medial aspect, thus preventing further spontaneous closure.

The healed mucocutaneous junction may lie on the rim of the perforation, occasionally on the lateral aspect of the rim, but usually on the medial aspect. The ingrowth of stratified squamous epithelium onto the medial aspect of the tympanic membrane remnant is usually a limited one that accounts for the relative rarity of middle ear keratoma in cases of central perforation.

Another cause of persistent perforation is trauma by a blow to the ear, by barotrauma, by an explosion, or by entry of a hot welding spark into the ear. In the large ruptures of the tympanic membrane following a blow to the ear healing is prevented by rolling in of the margins of the injured membrane or by absence of bleeding. Welding spark injuries are resistant to healing because of the tissue necrosis and obliteration of local vessels.

The permanent perforation of the tympanic membrane predisposes the tympanic cavity to the risk of recurrent infection carried in through the external meatus (from allowing water to enter the ear during washing or bathing) or spread up the Eustachian tube assisted by nose blowing during acute upper respiratory disease.

Atrophic changes of the tympanic membrane
For the tympanum to become 'atelectatic' it is necessary that there be atrophic segments in the tympanic membrane. These atrophic areas result from the healing of large or small perforations, or from the destruction of the circular and radiating fibres of the membrane by episodes of otitis media or trauma. There may also be vascular changes in the tympanic membrane.

The resultant thin membrane has a stratified squamous epithelium externally and a low cuboidal epithelium medially, with a minimal blood supply. In this situation, should there be malfunction of the Eustachian tube, severe in-drawing and collapse of the atrophic segments will occur causing pocketing of the tympanic membrane, interference with epidermal migration and clearance, and a gross reduction in middle ear volume. This appears to predispose to recurrent episodes of middle ear infection.

Unhealthy tonsils and adenoids
Chronic infection of the tonsils and adenoids favours the spread of infection up the Eustachian tube and along peritubal lymphatics into the middle ear. It is unlikely that either enlarged or diseased tonsils or adenoids cause physical blockage of the Eustachian tube, but large and infected adenoids may cause stasis of secretions in the region of the tubal orifice. This will cause congestion and obstruction and will affect the pressure relationships between the nasopharynx and middle ear during swallowing.

Nasal and sinus disease
Disturbances of nasal airflow patterns as a result of distortions of the nasal septum and turbinates or the presence of nasal lesions, such as polyps, facilitate the deposition of foreign particles, allergens or bacteria and interfere with the air-conditioning function of the nasal mucosa causing congestive changes. The protective mechanisms of the nose, particularly the mucociliary clearance system, are affected predisposing to rhinitis and sinusitis which in turn lead to Eustachian tube dysfunction.

The passage of infected material posteriorly into the nasopharynx further increases the risk of recurrent middle ear infection and the impairment of tubal function. In most cases of chronic ear disease nasal malfunction, rhinitis or sinus disease are important in initiating or perpetuating the condition.

Allergy in the upper respiratory tract
Nasal allergy results in widespread congestive changes which may involve the tubal lumen and affect tubal function. In these cases the use of antihistamines may further aggravate the situation by increasing the viscosity of the fluid present in the middle ear.

Other causes of Eustachian tube malfunction
Neoplasms of the nasopharynx, scars involving the tubal orifice and the condition of cleft palate all frequently cause Eustachian tube malfunction.

Social, geographic and ethnic factors
The frequency of acute upper respiratory tract disease, whether viral or bacterial, and thus the risk of middle ear cleft infection, is increased in infancy and childhood by factors such as substandard nutrition, inadequate hygiene, poor living conditions and overcrowding.

In the late 1960s the prevalence of chronic suppurative otitis media in Great Britain was calculated from general practice statistics as being 2·2–2·8 per 1000 National Health Service patients per year [11] whereas the prevalence of acute otitis media for the same population was 43·8–66·2 per 1000 patients. By contrast, in Australian aboriginal children below the age of fifteen, the prevalence of chronic otitis media with central perforations has been reported as being 100–450 per 1000 [12].

The literature now contains many references to the increased prevalence of chronic suppurative otitis media in certain ethnic groups including Australian aboriginals, Swedish nomad Lapps, south-western Alaskan Eskimos, Navajo Indians in the Colorado Plateau, Maori children in New Zealand, children from Guam, Egypt, and the Vellore area of India. In these groups there is usually an associated high rate of deafness, chronic and recurrent infection of the nasal sinuses, throat and lower respiratory tract together with growth retardation and protein-calorie malnutrition. In other words, the disease which is one of the most common afflictions of mankind seems widespread in under privileged countries and represents a major third-world problem.

Very few causes for the increased prevalence of chronic suppurative otitis media have been suggested other than overcrowding, poor living conditions and inadequate hygiene. Other factors such as deficient immunologic mechanisms or ethnic variations of skull dimensions may be involved. Deficiency of immunoglobulins seems not so far to play a major role, and in Australian aboriginals there have been no abnormally low values. On the contrary, increases of serum immunoglobulins have been present in more than 50% of the cases.

Ethnic anatomical variations of skull dimensions may affect the inter-related mechanics of the nasal cavity, nasopharynx, Eustachian tube, middle ear and mastoid air cells, so that an alteration in the function of one part of this system makes the middle ear cleft prone to develop chronic infective disease.

Climatic factors

Other things being equal, adverse climatic factors may account for the relatively high incidence of actively discharging ears that is encountered in some countries of northern Europe. By contrast, in South Australia with its favourable climatic circumstances, the incidence of frank otorrhoea in cases of chronic tubotympanic disease in the Caucasian population is less than 20% at the time of first consultation.

Pathological changes in middle ear mucosa

Hyperplasia

The mucosa of the middle ear undergoes certain changes following experimental infection of the guinea-pig ear [13]. Ciliated columnar cells and goblet cells increase and gland-like structures appear within 14 days. Studies of human temporal bones and biopsy material have confirmed these findings. The middle ear mucosa reacts by means of a hyperplastic and metaplastic transformation.

Major changes are seen in the submucosa. Inflammatory cells appear, vascular dilation and oedema occurs, new capillaries develop and a proliferation of fibroblasts and collagen fibres is seen, leading to the formation of granulation tissue, with histiocytes, lymphocytes, plasma cells and other mononuclears. Gland-like formations are also noted, the majority being simple tubules with no acini, although branched glands do occur.

There is a marked variation in gland density throughout the middle ear following the inflammatory reaction. The density is highest in the round and oval window niches, in adhesions around the stapes, below the annulus posteriorly and in the hypotympanum posteriorly. It is not until a sufficiently large number of active glands are present that production of mucus increases to a degree that clinical symptoms appear.

The distribution of glands is also irregular, and glands may be seen in either the active phase, when the tubules are narrow and mucous cells predominate, or in the degenerative and inactive phase, when the duct system appears dilated. Transitional stages may be seen between these extremes. The percentage of active glands tends to decrease from the Eustachian tube towards the mastoid process.

Two modes of gland formation have been described. The epithelium may invaginate to form a tube, or the basal cells may divide and grow down into the lamina propria to form a solid cylinder which subsequently becomes canalized. Cells of this cylinder differentiate into ciliated and mucous cells so that the resultant tubules acquire a typical lining of pseudo-stratified ciliated columnar epithelium. The formation of a gland probably takes a month or two and glands do not start producing mucus until a month or two after that.

The epithelium also develops briskly-secreting goblet cells. The goblet cell density is very high compared with the normal middle ear mucosa, the increase in goblet cells taking place before the formation of glands has commenced [14]. The middle ear mucosa of infants is extremely sensitive to minor brief pathological stimuli, but the increase in goblet cell density is reversible after the pathological stimulus has ceased.

Metaplasia

Gland formation and the various epithelial changes in the middle ear are regarded as metaplastic changes rather than due to invasion from the Eustachian tube region. There are many factors which may induce metaplasia, such as friction, hormonal changes, particularly with regard to oestrogens, alterations in vitamin A levels, allergic factors, etc., but the true nature of the inducers which cause alterations in the lining membrane of the middle ear are not known.

Chronic infection, chronic irritation, perhaps by cholesterol crystals, or recurrent infection of the mucosa are certainly among the underlying reasons for the transformation. However, it is not known how long the infection must be present, nor what particular aspect of the infective process induces the changes.

Tissue culture experiments suggest that the induction system may be linked to oxygen and carbon dioxide gradients, or related pH effects, in the middle ear cavity [15]. There is now evidence that in fact there is a higher concentration of carbon dioxide in ears with effusions. This is probably related to tubal dysfunction and impaired middle ear aeration which itself appears to increase the secretory activity of the glands and prevents the transport of mucus to the nasopharynx.

In addition, ventilatory obstruction leads to altered haemodynamics which have also been shown to affect the behaviour of multipotent cells. Any, or all, of these factors may be involved.

Squamous and stratified squamous epithelium has also been observed in the middle ear follow-ing the inflammatory process. It may be of two types [16]. One type appears to be the result of metaplastic change and is generally regarded as non-keratinizing. It may be located side-by-side with columnar epithelium without any cellular or connective tissue reaction. Immigrating squamous epithelium, on the other hand, tends to retain its slight keratinizing properties, but may never actually produce cholesteatoma.

Tympanosclerosis

Tympanosclerosis is an irreversible end product of chronic infection, appearing as whitish firm masses in the middle ear mucosa. From the histological point of view one may see a fibroblastic invasion of the submucosal layers followed by thickening and fusion of the collagenous fibres. Hyaline degeneration follows and produces hyaline masses which form white layers between the epithelium and the bone. Calcification and ossification may occur in these tympanosclerotic plaques. This is discussed further in Chapter 14.

Pathological changes in the petrous air cells

A great volume of literature now exists concerning the common pathological changes occurring within the pneumatic system of the human temporal bone. These effects vary in accordance with the state of development of the system.

Inflammation in the fully-developed pneumatic system

The initial effects are hyperaemia, oedema, thickening and cellular infiltration, which may result in obstruction of the openings of groups of air cells. As more damage occurs, the lining epithelium may be destroyed.

The lining may be converted into a tall columnar, ciliated mucosa with goblet cells and glandular elements [17, 18]. The change has also been noted in bone chips removed at operation [13] but it is still uncertain whether this represents a metaplastic transformation or an extension of the columnar epithelium of the Eustachian tube and middle ear into the pneumatic system.

The islands of bone marrow within the mastoid are also affected. The reticulum swells up, blood-forming elements disappear, fat cells atrophy and degenerate, and the resultant mass of tissue is replaced by granulation tissue.

The lumen of the air cells first fills with a serous transudate which soon becomes purulent and later fibrinized [19, 20] and organized, particularly in the apical cells and in small cells around the antrum. The air spaces are thus partially filled with masses of granulation tissue lined by remnants of epithelium with progressive reduction of the lumen and eventual fibrous obliteration (fibrous sclerosis, fibrocystic sclerosis).

The equilibrium between bone apposition and bone resorption is also disturbed. Resorption dominates when the inflammatory reaction is intense, due to osteoclastic activity, vascularization and halisteresis [19]. Later, however, osteoblastic activity and new bone formation dominates, being greatest in the fibrosed marrow spaces and in the cells which are wholly or largely filled with granulation tissue (fibro-osseous sclerosis). The newly laid down bone may present a reticular, lamellar or mosaic pattern [21].

In chronic or recurring inflammation the pneumatic system may therefore become filled and even obliterated by fibrous tissue and new bone formation, the sclerosis tending to be patchy in distribution with a varying number of cystic cavities remaining [22]. Repneumatization can only occur if the inflammatory reaction has subsided, if tissue proliferation has ceased, and if aeration through natural channels is still possible.

Arrest of pneumatization

A host of theories exists regarding the factors responsible for the primary arrest of air cell development. Most of these are based on theories of pneumatization which have little factual basis. For instance, Wittmaack [23] believed that the pneumatizing capacity of the mucous membrane might be affected by inflammatory changes either due to bacterial infection, meconium or vernix caseosa. On the other hand Eckert-Möbius [24] stated that the inflammatory process prevents bone atrophy, and Krainz [25] considered that arrested pneumatization was due to the formation of scar tissue or new bone formation presenting an unyielding obstacle to the pneumatization process.

One cannot say that the inflammatory theory of pneumatization arrest has been proven. Indeed, it has been claimed that primary sclerosis is determined by genetic and not by purely pathological factors [26, 27] and that the anatomical conditions in the 'infantile' type of temporal bone are factors in producing chronic suppuration and not the result of it [28].

Another possibility is that ventilatory obstruction *per se* plays the major role in pneumatization arrest [29]. Following blockage of aeration, uncomplicated by inflammatory changes, a negative pressure develops in the air space, the subepithelial zone becomes oedematous, existing blood vessels become dilated and congested, new blood vessels and fat cells appear, and new bone is laid down due to osteoblastic activity. These changes appear dependent on alterations in the intraosseous vascular haemodynamics causing passive hyperaemia with its associated high tissue fluid protein. The primary factor is the negative pressure which develops following obstruction of the pathway of ventilation of the air cell system [30, 31].

Despite the exact mechanism involved, the changes in primary pneumatization arrest are of a generalized rather than a patchy nature. The overall size of the system is small and the distance between the anterior boundary of the sigmoid sinus and the osseous posterior meatal wall is reduced. This is different from the anatomical conditions prevailing in secondary sclerosis.

Bone destruction in chronic otitis media

The various theories that have been put forward to explain the mechanism of bone destruction in chronic otitis media include pressure, ischaemia, enzyme activity, hyperaemia and lysosomal activity.

The classical explanation is that the inflammatory process causes thrombosis and that the resultant anoxia leads to bone destruction. The long process of the incus is most commonly affected, but the lenticular process often remains intact in the early stages. It is considered that in chronic ear disease the vessels which come through the attic to reach the shaft and mucosa over the long process become thrombosed. The arteries which pass from the stapes to the lenticular process help to preserve this part, leaving it sitting on the stapes head.

However, granulation tissue is always seen near the region of bone destruction together with an increased blood flow in the capillary proliferations and a marked histiocytosis. It is, therefore, more likely that hyperaemia and lysosomal activity of the histiocytes are the main factors in bone destruction in the middle ear.

Mucus-producing formations may be found in the vascular spaces deep within the bony structure of the affected ossicles. This may be the result of invagination, mesenchymal differentiation, or the migration of stem cells.

Sensorineural hearing impairment in chronic otitis media

Cochlear function can become impaired during chronic otitis media by the absorption of the toxic products of infection and inflammation through the membrane of the round window, through the annular ligament of the stapedio-vestibular joint, or through the endosteum exposed in a 'fistula' of the bony labyrinthine capsule as a result of inflammatory osteoclasis.

The sensory hearing loss may be slight, moderate, profound or total. It is usually of gradual development but may have an abrupt onset as in acute labyrinthitis.

Sensorineural loss may result from the instillation of ototoxic antibiotic ear drops such as neomycin or gentamicin into the tympanum.

Pathological residua of chronic otitis media

The chronic inflammatory disease may eventually become inactive leaving certain pathological residua which are permanent and irreversible, although some of these may be modified by modern otological microsurgery.

These residua or sequelae include:
(1) perforation of the tympanic membrane;
(2) ossicular necrosis with discontinuity of the ossicular chain;
(3) chronic adhesive process and atelectasis of tympanum;

(4) middle ear fibrosis;
(5) tympanosclerosis;
(6) fibro-osseous sclerosis of the mastoid;
(7) stricture of the Eustachian tube;
(8) lipoid granuloma following the therapeutic instillation of oily preparations into the ear.

Epidermoid cholesteatoma, cholesteatosis or aural keratoma

Epidermoid cholesteatoma, cholesteatosis or aural keratoma is a non-malignant destructive ear disease due to the presence within the middle ear cleft of keratinizing stratified squamous epithelium. The keratinizing epithelial layer on a fibrous stroma forms the lining of a cystic structure which continually desquamates its keratinized layers inwards to fill the cyst. This accumulation of exfoliated keratin forms the bulk of the keratoma, and the rapidity of its development is determined to some extent by the degree of associated infection.

The keratoma most commonly occurs in the epitympanum and passes backwards into the mastoid air cell system. It may also pass inferiorly into the middle ear. Rarely is it limited to the middle ear or found behind an intact tympanic membrane.

Pathogenesis

Several theories have been proposed to explain the development of aural cholesteatoma and it now seems probable that individual cholesteatomas have different aetiologies.

Congenital
There is indisputable evidence that epidermoid cell rests may occur in the petrous bone and other intracranial sites. However, these are rare and cannot account for more than the occasional case of cholesteatoma. When found, they are usually behind an intact tympanic membrane in cases with a highly pneumatized mastoid system, and may involve the petrous apex.

Metaplasia
Because histological studies have shown that

squamous metaplasia can occur both in bronchial respiratory lining and also in the lining of the middle ear in the presence of a tympanic perforation, especially when accompanied by infection, it has been presumed that such changes might explain the origin of cholesteatoma. However, keratinization is not seen in cases of bronchial metaplasia and it has not been possible to induce keratinization in the middle ear with oestrogens or suspensions of cholesterol crystals. Until more is known about the factors affecting cellular differentiation and keratinization of the lining of the middle ear and epitympanum, the metaplasia theory must remain in doubt.

Implantation
The physical introduction of squamous epithelium into the middle ear can occur at the time of trauma or surgical intervention, or following a fracture of the temporal bone. The implanted keratinizing epithelium can develop into an epidermoid cyst which may subsequently exhibit all the characteristics of a cholesteatoma.

Direct ingrowth through a tympanic perforation
One long-standing question concerning the aetiology of cholesteatoma is whether a perforation of the tympanic membrane is a prerequisite for its formation. There is no doubt that squamous epithelium from the outer surface of the tympanic membrane can grow into the middle ear through a pre-existent perforation, either central or marginal, replacing or covering the damaged mucous membrane of the middle ear. If desquamation occurs, this leads to the development of the so called 'secondary acquired cholesteatoma'.

Mechanical retraction pocket theory
A popular concept of the genesis of cholesteatoma is based on the presence of chronic tubal dysfunction which leads to a chronic negative pressure within the middle ear with tympanic membrane retraction. As progression occurs, particularly in the posterosuperior quadrant of the tympanic membrane or in Shrapnell's membrane, a blind retraction pocket develops. If this is not self-cleaning, and particularly if there is further irritation from associated inflammation,

the products of desquamation accumulate within the sac which enlarges progressively. The persistence of mesenchyme in the attic and the development of fibrous adhesions between the invaginated sac and the medial wall of the middle ear render the situation irreversible.

The sac opening persists as a pseudo-perforation and clearance from the sac may be further impeded by the formation of obstructive crusts at the opening. On occasions the invaginated sac wall may rupture and facilitate more direct in-growth into the middle ear and air cell system.

Papillary ingrowth theory
This theory is complex and is based on several facts. First, the healthy ears of embryos, newborn children and infants show increased growth tendencies in the nature of hyperkeratosis and acanthosis. This occurs in the epidermis of a well-defined section of external auditory meatus adjoining the tympanic membrane superiorly. It is thought that this tendency is increased in the presence of an inflammatory stimulus and that the basal cells tend to form solid cones which proliferate inwards.

Secondly, the epitympanic space contains persisting embryonal myxomatous tissue in many newborn infants, while in others it may become filled with granulation tissue as a result of an inflammatory process in the attic. In this regard, the drainage of the anterior region of Prussak's space is less free than that of the posterior region. Retention and organization of exudate tends to occur and as the organized tissue contracts it tends to pull Shrapnell's membrane inwards.

Thirdly, there is no lamina propria in Shrapnell's membrane and the layer of differentiated connective tissue under the epidermis, together with the related mucosa, may easily be damaged by attic inflammation.

The composite theory is that basal cells can proliferate inwards and invade the myxomatous or granulation tissue in Prussak's space following fragmentation of the connective tissue and mucosal layers of Shrapnell's membrane. The resultant cores or islands of active epidermis enlarge and, with keratinization and desquamation, form a cholesteatoma, which secondarily perforates through Shrapnell's membrane into the meatus.

Behaviour of cholesteatoma

Very little is known of the mechanism of growth and enlargement of cholesteatoma, of the variations in degree of keratinization, and of the epidermal migration characteristics of cholesteatoma matrix. The relationship of abnormalities of rate, migratory direction and site of epidermal proliferation are important questions with no answers.

The cholesteatoma expands into the pre-formed air pathways of the temporal bone and middle ear, the location and extension being influenced by the anatomical arrangement of the mucosal folds. Curiously, these mucosal folds often remain intact while adjacent bone is resorbed and ossicles destroyed. One concept of the mechanism of bone destruction, namely pressure erosion, is probably an oversimplification.

An alternative view is that the breakdown of underlying bone is the result of enzymic activity of the cholesteatoma matrix. In this regard, Harris [32] found a high concentration of leucine amino peptidase and non-specific esterase in the subepithelial tissues while Abramson *et al.* [33] have shown that the epidermis of a cholesteatoma is rich in collagenase.

Stratified squamous epithelium is never in direct relation to the area of bone destruction, and it can be found lying directly on the bone without any evidence of bone destruction [34]. The conclusion is that cholesteatoma requires infection before it will destroy bone and that the common factor for bone destruction in various types of chronic otitis media, including chole-steatoma, is granulation tissue in regions close to the destroyed bone. The bone erosion in chole-steatoma is thus thought to be caused by inflam-matory hyperaemia and lysosomal activity of the histiocytes.

Finally, it should be mentioned that adults with cholesteatoma usually have hypopneumati-zation of the mastoid air cell system as a result of repeated infection, pneumatic cell obstruction and fibro-osseous sclerosis. In some children, however, the cholesteatoma is often 'invasive', penetrating deeply into the recesses of a relatively highly pneumatized system. One wonders whether the pneumatization process being co-incident with the development of the cholestea-

toma actively facilitates this appearance of inva-sion, or whether there is also a greater degree of mitotic activity in the squamous epithelium in these cases.

Clinical features

In its early stages cholesteatoma is completely asymptomatic and may be compatible with normal hearing and a dry ear. As the keratoma mass expands there is slow destruction of ossicles and a gradual onset of conductive hearing im-pairment which is of slight to moderate degree. Secondary infection of the cholesteatoma acce-lerates its destructive properties and the otor-rhoea is characteristically malodorous and often scanty, but may be profuse. The patient may later become aware of transient vertigo when he changes the position of his head or causes pressure variation in the external auditory meatus, and this is an indication that there is erosion of the bone of the labyrinthine capsule with exposure of endosteum. The fistula test (see Chapter 11), if positive, is an important warning sign that the inner ear is at risk with the possibility of the dangerous complications of labyrinthitis and meningitis.

The congenital aural epidermoid is a rare lesion that occurs deeply within the petrous bone, often in its apical portion. The tympanic membrane may appear completely normal. The symptoms of this condition usually appear in adult life and include unilateral tinnitus, hearing impairment and slowly progressive facial para-lysis. Additional findings such as sensorineural hearing loss, reduced or absent vestibular func-tion and a radiolucent area of bone destruction with a smooth margin in the petrous apex may be confused with those of an acoustic neuroma. In rare cases a primary cholesteatoma presents as a mass behind an intact tympanic membrane which appears opaque, white, full or bulging, and immobile.

The attic keratoma occupying a deep attic retraction pocket may not be obvious at oto-scopic examination because the attic defect or 'pseudo perforation' may be small or sealed over by an innocent-looking dry scab. The removal of these attic crusts under magnification may be difficult but is necessary to expose the diagnostic whitish mass of accumulated keratin within the attic above the short process of the malleus. The pars tensa is intact and may appear completely normal (Fig. 10.2). At a later stage the epitympanic perforation is enlarged by erosion of the notch of Rivinus and destruction of the outer attic wall. The anterior and posterior malleolar folds are prominent and form the inferior margin

canal or to the head of the stapes. In others there is a large slough of the posterior part of the tympanic membrane, with the anterior part of the pars tensa remaining intact. Granulation tissue may be exuberant and a large granulomatous polyp arising from the posterior tympanic ring or ossicles or from the margins of the

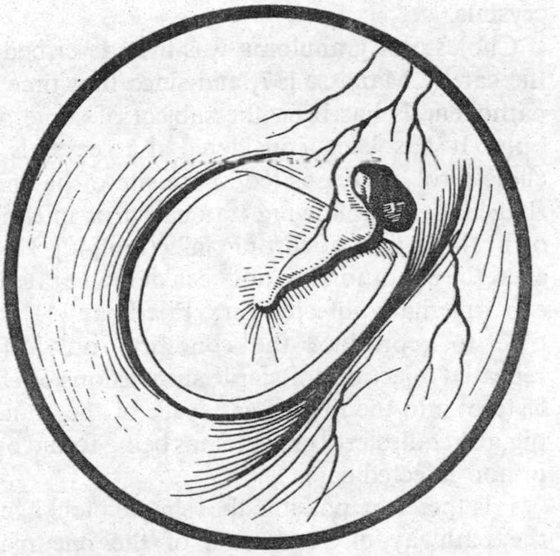

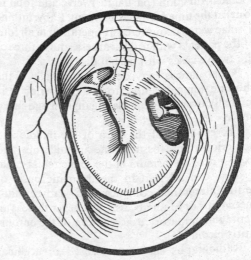

FIG. 10.2. Small attic perforation of right tympanic membrane. The pars tensa is normal.

FIG. 10.3. Posterosuperior marginal perforation of the left tympanic membrane. The incudostapedial articulation, stapedius tendon and round window niche are exposed.

of the perforation which is filled with moist epithelial debris. Attic granulations or a large epitympanic polyp are commonly seen when the lesion is infected, and these may obscure the cholesteatoma.

The other common presentation of cholesteatoma is as a posterosuperior marginal perforation or retraction pocket deep to the tympanic ring (Fig. 10.3). There is usually erosion of bone of the posterosuperior canal wall associated with a subacute inflammatory process and granulation formation. The destruction of the tympanic annulus and the regional atrophy and retraction of the pars tensa allows in-growth of keratinizing squamous epithelium into the middle ear and facial recess – a secondary acquired keratoma. The white pearly sheets of desquamated keratin are readily visible in most cases but may be difficult to see in others. The atrophic membrane of the retraction pocket may be seen adherent to the eroded long process of the incus, to the facial

tympanic windows may completely fill the external auditory meatus. In advanced cases there may be total destruction of the tympanic membrane and ossicles, the middle ear being filled with granulation tissue and moist keratin debris. Enlargement of the keratoma in the attic and mastoid, where it may reach the size of a walnut, produces further bony destruction of the attic and posterior canal walls by an inflammatory osteoclasis so that eventually an appearance resembling a spontaneous radical mastoidectomy cavity lined by matrix may be created.

As the sac grows it follows the path of least resistance into the aditus and mastoid antrum posteriorly or into the facial recess inferiorly. In the narrow aditus the prominent part of the bony lateral semicircular canal may be gradually resorbed so that a fistula of the labyrinth is created in which the perilymphatic space is closed over by a layer of matrix and endosteum.

The superior and posterior semicircular canals can similarly, but less commonly, be destroyed. If the semicircular canal system is destroyed, hearing may be preserved, but a severe or total loss of cochlear function is often found. In a personal series (R.E.G.) of 141 cases of cholesteatoma sixteen patients had severe loss of cochlear function (partial in twelve and total in four) at the time of first assessment. Labyrinthine fistulae were encountered at operation in all four of the patients with total deafness, and in three of the twelve cases with partial deafness.

Facial paresis may develop especially if the cholesteatoma extends from the anterior attic medially over the geniculate ganglion and facial nerve.

The exposure of the dura of the middle and posterior cranial fossae, of the sigmoid sinus, and exposure of endosteum of the semicircular canal system, can all lead to the dramatic onset of septic intracranial complications – labyrinthitis, meningitis or brain abcess – whenever there is an acute inflammatory exacerbation of the chronic otitis media [35].

Radiographs show a sclerosed or acellular mastoid in most cases of cholesteatoma. Signs of bone erosion may be seen in conventional views, but lateral and frontal tomography are required to demonstrate more accurately the extent of this destruction or the presence of a fistula of the lateral semicircular canal.

Non-specific inflammatory processes with intact tympanic membrane

When the tympanic membrane is intact, chronic otitis media is usually referred to as non-suppurative. The commonly accepted types are listed below.

Cholesterol granuloma

Cholesterol granuloma is a separate entity from cholesteatoma. The granuloma initially consists of numerous lens-shaped clefts containing cholesterol crystals embedded in connective tissue, with vessels arranged around the periphery of the clefts. The clefts show no regular pattern of alignment and the connective tissue shows numbers of irregular multinucleate giant cells

and numerous fat-laden foam cells. At a later stage new bone formation occurs and the bone is laid down between the clefts.

In some cases the granulomas form as a reaction to crystals deposited within the tissues following degenerative changes in the mesenchyme. In others, they form by the proliferation of strands of connective tissue into pneumatic spaces which have become filled with cholesterol crystals.

Cholesterol granuloma was first described in the ear by Manasse [37] and since that time its pathogenesis has been the subject of some dispute. It has been considered that crystals of cholesterol are deposited at the site of haemorrhage [38, 39] following trauma, virus infection or in the course of chronic infection [40]. However, the condition has not been demonstrated in experimentally infected ears. Friedman [41] was able to reproduce the condition only after repeated injections of sterile suspensions of cholesterol into the middle ear space of the guinea-pig, the cholesterol granulomas being found only in non-infected ears.

It is therefore possible that simple blockage of the pathway of ventilation of the pneumatic system is the most important factor in the genesis of the condition [42]. Experimental studies on the pneumatized humerus of *Gallus domesticus* indicated that simple prolonged obstruction of ventilation of the air spaces leads to degenerative changes in the lining cells and deeper regions of the mesenchymal tissue with the liberation of fat and cholesterol crystals and the formation of cholesterol granulomas. In later stages new bone is laid down within the granuloma.

Cholesterol granulomas have also been produced in the mastoid cavity of the squirrel monkey by obstruction of the Eustachian tube with silastic sponge [43]. The mechanisms are identical. It remains to be answered conclusively whether haemorrhage precedes or follows cholesterol granuloma formation.

This theory may well explain the frequent association of cholesterol granuloma with cholesteatoma. It is known that cholesteatoma may obstruct the ventilatory pathways to certain mastoid air cell groups and it may be simply this which causes the granuloma to develop in association with other changes such as congestion and oedema of the subepithelial tissues, pathological changes in the lining cells, mesenchymal proliferation with fatty and myeloid changes, and various types of new bone formation.

Chronic secretory otitis media

This is also known as serous otitis, mucoid otitis, glue ear, or seromucinous middle ear catarrh. This is a relatively common condition in which there is accumulation of sterile fluid of variable viscosity, serous or mucoid, within the middle ear cleft, associated with increase of mucus-secreting cells in the lining membrane. This is discussed further in Chapter 41.

Idiopathic haemotympanum (blue drum)

Idiopathic haemotympanum (blue drum) associated with cholesterol granuloma is a relatively uncommon condition in which there is a blue-coloured tympanic membrane due to a collection within the tympanum of sterile, viscid, chocolate-coloured fluid derived from a cholesterol granuloma within the mastoid [36].

Specific inflammatory processes

The infection of tissues with the specific organisms causing tuberculosis, syphilis or actinomycosis sets up chronic inflammation with considerable tissue destruction so that resolution is unlikely and a chronic course is inevitable. All of the following diseases are very rare in economically-developed countries.

(1) Tuberculous otomastoiditis [44].

(2) Syphilitic otomastoiditis and labyrinthitis [45].

(3) Actinomycotic otomastoiditis [46].

Chronic adhesive process and middle ear fibrosis

Chronic adhesive otitis media, chronic adhesive process or middle ear fibrosis are terms denoting the development and end result of a long-standing process of obliteration of the air space of the middle ear by adhesions that have developed as a result of inflammation. Although inflammatory adhesions may develop within the middle ear after suppurative otitis media with perforation of the drumhead, the term 'adhesive otitis media' is traditionally applied only to cases in which the tympanic membrane remains intact [47–51]. Three variants of the condition are seen:

(1) The middle ear air space is obliterated by the formation of granulation tissue which eventually is transformed into a pale, firm, fibrous tissue that immobilizes the tympanic membrane and ossicles (fibrous sclerosis or middle ear fibrosis).

(2) Tubal malfunction and secretory otitis media in association with an atrophic and flaccid tympanic membrane cause severe indrawing and collapse of the thinned membrane on to the promontory of the middle ear, the so called 'atelectasis' of the tympanum. The development of adhesions between the contacting surfaces of the tympanic membrane and walls of middle ear produces an irreversible condition of chronic adhesive process.

(3) Bizarre healing of a central or marginal perforation may lead to adherence of the rim of the tympanic membrane defect to the promontory which then becomes epidermized. Some authors would exclude these residua of middle ear suppuration from the definition of chronic adhesive process.

Pathogenesis

Chronic adhesive otitis media is in most cases due to a neglected and usually mild middle ear inflammation occurring in childhood. The pathological basis for chronic adhesive process and middle ear fibrosis is the organization of exudate within the middle ear cleft. Ojala [48], from histopathological studies of temporal bones from newborn infants and from adults showing signs of otitis, concluded that several factors determined the extensive organization of exudate.

(1) The inflammatory injury had to be of a degree sufficient to destroy some areas of the lining epithelium and produce connective tissue proliferation in the presence of an exudate containing fibrin.

(2) Exudate had to be retained for a sufficient period within the middle ear cleft, and lack of

drainage consequent upon failure of the tympanic membrane to rupture or persistence of tubal obstruction (due to adenoid hypertrophy and infections of the nose and paranasal sinuses) were aggravating factors.

Continuous or recurring inflammation of the mucoperiosteum of the middle ear cleft with connective tissue proliferation is associated with clinical progression of the disease. Middle ear fibrosis thus results from the excessive proliferative and reparative activity of the connective tissue following the vascular and exudative phenomena of inflammation in the middle ear. Some rare cases are considered by Zöllner [52] to be the end result of tuberculous infection. Proliferations of fibroblasts and buds of capillary endothelium grow into the exudate which is replaced by a vascularized red mass of granulation tissue – a process known as organization. The middle ear air space may become completely filled by this highly vascularized connective tissue. When organization is complete, the capillaries decrease in size and number and mostly disappear. The connective tissue shrinks, becomes condensed, develops more collagenous fibres and is transformed from a soft red granulation tissue to a pale, firm fibrous tissue. Shrinkage and contracture produces indrawing and eventually immobility of the tympanic membrane and malleus handle. These changes are accompanied by a progressive deterioration of hearing in contra-distinction to the residua of middle ear suppuration in which the hearing impairment is usually stationary.

The proliferation of fibrous tissue in the middle ear and mastoid (fibrous sclerosis) may be associated with resorption of ossicles and the deposition of hyalinized collagen (tympanosclerosis). Fixation of ossicles is by fibrous tissue, by tympanosclerosis, or by new bone growth. New bone growth, associated with proliferation of fibrous tissue, is common in the pneumatized spaces of the temporal bone (fibro-osseous sclerosis), but is exceptionally rare in the middle ear apart from the oval window niche and the attic. Cystic spaces lined by flat or cuboidal epithelium and filled with fluid containing protein, exfoliated cells and cholesterol are sometimes seen within the fibrous tissue (fibrocystic sclerosis).

In the lesser degrees of severity, the posterior mesotympanum alone is affected, or only a localized area of adhesions, from the organization of fibrinous exudates on opposing mucosal surfaces, forms between the medial aspect of the tympanic membrane and the incus, between the umbo and the promontory, or within the epitympanum.

Clinical features

The condition is often but not necessarily bilateral. At first there is a progressive hearing impairment of conductive type usually commencing in childhood. A preceding episode of mild middle ear inflammation may be recalled in approximately 50% of cases. In the remainder the condition commences insidiously. As the hearing impairment becomes progressively severe it may develop the features of a combined conductive and sensorineural deficit. Tinnitus is common in the affected ear, but paracusis Willisii is not a feature in most cases in contrast to the hearing deficit due to otosclerosis.

The tympanic membrane is intact but is always abnormal in appearance. The most important diagnostic feature is its severely impaired or absent mobility.

In chronic adhesive otitis media associated with tubal malfunction the usual appearance is of an intact, thinned, atrophic membrane collapsed medially on to the promontory and draped over the long process of incus, stapes head and stapedius tendon. The membrane may pass into the round window niche and around the crura of the stapes. The malleus handle may show severe indrawing, with the umbo touching the promontory and the short process protruding prominently. The indrawn membrane forms a diaphragm over the tympanic end of the auditory tube and apart from this area the whole drumhead is adherent and immobile. Certain cases may be incorrectly assessed as a tympanic perforation. The changes of developed chronic adhesive process are permanent and cannot be reversed by Valsalva's procedure, politzerization nor by auditory tube catheterization. In the early stages, however, before adhesions have developed, tubal inflation or the insertion of an artificial ventilation tube through the tympanic membrane may allow the retracted and non-adherent tympanic membrane to return to its normal position.

In middle ear fibrosis, the tympanic membrane appears uniformly opaque and white with some indrawing of the pars tensa and Schrapnell's membrane. The drumhead is immobile or nearly so and aspiration of the ear fails to reveal any fluid. The Eustachian tube is blocked and inflation procedures are of no benefit. Tympanometry produces a curve showing little or no compliance variation with change of pressure in the external auditory meatus. Operative exploration of the middle ear will confirm the filling of the tympanum with fibrous tissue and the absence of an air space. Radiography of the mastoids shows arrested or absent pneumatization in the great majority of cases.

References

[1] GRAVES G. O. & EDWARDS L. F. (1944) The Eustachian tube. *Archives of Otolaryngology* 39, 359.

[2] LIM D. J. (1974) Functional morphology of the lining membrane of the middle ear and Eustachian tube. *The Annals of Otology, Rhinology and Laryngology, Supplement No. 11*, 83, 5.

[3] TOS M (1974) Production of mucus in the middle ear and Eustachian tube. *The Annals of Otology, Rhinology and Laryngology, Supplement No. 11*, 83, 44.

[4] FLISBERG K., INGELSTEDT S. & ORTEGREN U. (1963) On middle ear pressure. *Acta Oto-Laryngologica, Supplement 182*, 43.

[5] SADE J. (1966) Middle ear mucosa. *Archives of Otolaryngology* 84, 137.

[6] SCHWARZBART A. (1958) A re-appraisal of the clinical and morphological classification of the tympanic spaces and Eustachian tube. *The Annals of Otology, Rhinology and Laryngology* 67, 241.

[7] SCHWARZBART A. (1959) Pneumatisation of the temporal bone: a new concept. *The Journal of Laryngology and Otology* 73, 45.

[8] BUCH N. H. & JORGENSEN M. B. (1964) Eustachian tube and middle ear. *Archives of Otolaryngology* 79, 472.

[9] MAROVITZ W. F. & PORUBSKY E. S. (1971) The embryological development of the middle ear space – a new concept. *The Annals of Otology, Rhinology and Laryngology* 80, 384.

[10] BRÉMOND G. & COQUIN A. (1972) Ultrastructure of normal and pathological middle ear mucosa. *The Journal of Laryngology and Otology* 88, 457.

[11] HODGKIN K. (1973) *Towards Earlier Diagnosis*, 3rd edn., p. 280. Edinburgh: Churchill Livingstone.

[12] KAMIEN M. (1974) Ear disease in a part-Aborigine population in New South Wales. *Journal of the Oto-Laryngological Society of Australia* 3, 651.

[13] FRIEDMAN I. (1963) Pathology of secretory otitis media. *Proceedings of the Royal Society of Medicine* 56, 695.

[14] TOS M. & BAK-PEDERSEN K. (1975) Density of goblet cells in chronic secretory otitis media. *Laryngoscope* 75, 377.

[15] SADÉ J. (1972) The mucosa in ear disease. *Otolaryngological Clinics of North America*. 5, 11.

[16] KARMA P. (1972) Middle ear epithelium and chronic ear disease. *Acta Oto-Laryngologica, Supplement 307*.

[17] FRIEDMAN I. (1955) Comparative pathology of otitis media-experimental and human. II. *The Journal of Laryngology and Otology* 69, 588.

[18] SENTURIA B. H., CARR C. D. & AHLVIN R. C. (1972) Middle ear effusions: pathologic changes of the muco-periosteum in the experimental animal. *The Annals of Otology, Rhinology and Laryngology* 71, 632.

[19] STEWART J. P. (1928) The histopathology of mastoiditis. *The Journal of Laryngology and Otology* 43, 689.

[20] OJALA L. (1953) Pathogenesis and histopathology of chronic adhesive otitis. *Archives of Otolaryngology* 57, 378.

[21] FRIEDMAN I. (1957) Pathology of otitis media with particular reference to bone changes. III. *The Journal of Laryngology and Otology* 71, 313.

[22] OJALA L. (1950) Contribution to the physiology and pathology of mastoid air cell formation. *Acta Oto-Laryngologica, Supplement No. 86*.

[23] WITTMAACK K. (1918) *Uber Die Normale und Die Pathologische Pneumatisaion des Schäfenbeines*. Jena: G. Fischer.

[24] ECKERT-MÖBIUS A. (1938) Vergleichend Anatomische Untersuchungen und Pneumatisationslehre. *Acta Oto-Laryngologica* 26, 115.

[25] KRAINZ W. (1924) Uber die Auskleidung der Lufthaltigen Warzenzellen. *Zeitschrift für Hals-Nasen-und Ohrenheilkunde* 8, 46.

[26] ALBRECHT W. (1924) Pneumatisation und Konstitution. *Zeitschrift für Hals-Nasen-und Ohrenheilkunde* 10, 51.

[27] SCHWARZ M. (1929) Die Bedeutung der hereditiären. Anlage für die Pneumatisation der Warzenfortsätze und der Nasennebenhöhlen. *Archiv für Ohren-Nasen-und Kehlkopfheilkunde* 123, 161.

[28] CHEATLE A. H. (1910) The infantile types of the temporal bone and their surgical importance. *Lancet*, i, 491.

[29] BROCK W. (1926) Trommelfellbild und Pneumatisation des Warzenteiles: eine röngenologische studie. *Zeitschrift für Hals-Nasen-und Ohrenheilkunde* 15, 241.

[30] BEAUMONT G. D. (1968) Vascular factors in pneumatisation. *The Journal of Laryngology and Otology* 82, 1067.

[31] BEAUMONT G. D. (1970) Pneumatisation. *Journal of the Oto-Laryngological Society of Australia* 3, 79.

[32] HARRIS A. J. (1962) Cholesteatosis and chronic otitis media. The histopathology of osseous and soft tissues. *Laryngoscope* 72, 954.

[33] ABRAMSON M. & GROSS J. (1971) Further studies on a collagenase in middle ear cholesteatoma. *The Annals of Otology, Rhinology and Laryngology* **80**, 177.

[34] SADÉ J. (1973) Bone destruction in chronic otitis media. *Journal of the Oto-Laryngological Society of Australia* **3**, 495.

[35] SIMPSON D. A. (1957) Cholesteatoma of the petrous apex. *The Journal of Laryngology and Otology* **71**, 548.

[36] BIRRELL J. F. (1958) Idiopathic haemotympanum. *The Journal of Laryngology and Otology* **72**, 769.

[37] MANASSE P. (1917) Die ohrenheilkunde der Gegenwart. *Handbuch der Pathologischen Anatomie des Menschlichen Ohres*, Vol. 9, p. 51. Wiesbaden.

[38] SIMONETTA B. (1949) Chronic cholesteatomatous and chronic cholesterinic otitis. *Acta Oto-Laryngologica* **37**, 509.

[39] ALTES A. J. K. (1966) Cholesterol granuloma in the tympanic cavity. *The Journal of Laryngology and Otology* **80**, 691.

[40] GRIPPAUDO M. (1959) II. Granuloma da Colesterolo, *Valsalva* **35**, 160.

[41] FRIEDMAN I. (1959) Epidermoid cholesteatoma and cholesterol granuloma, experimental and human. *The Annals of Otology, Rhinology and Laryngology* **68**, 57.

[42] BEAUMONT G. D. (1967) Cholesterol granuloma. *Journal of the Oto-Laryngological Society of Australia* **2**, 28.

[43] MAIN T. S. & LIM D. J. (1970) Experimental cholesterol granuloma. *Archives of Otolaryngology* **91**, 356.

[44] BIRRELL J. F. (1973) Aural tuberculosis in children *Proceedings of the Royal Society of Medicine* **66**, 331.

[45] KERR A. G., SMYTH G. D. L. & CINNAMOND M. J. (1973) Congenital syphilic deafness. *Journal of Otolaryngology and Otology* **87**, 1.

[46] LEEK J. H. (1974) Actinomycosis of the tympanomastoid. *Laryngoscope* **84**, 290.

[47] LUMIO J. S. (1951) Contributions to the knowledge of chronic adhesive otitis. *Acta Otolaryngologica* **39**, 196.

[48] OJALA L. (1953) Pathogenesis and histopathology of chronic adhesive otitis. *Archives of Otolaryngology* **57**, 378.

[49] MACNAUGHTAN J. P. J. (1956) Chronic adhesive otitis media. *The Journal of Laryngology and Otology* **70**, 549.

[50] CAWTHORNE T. (1956) Chronic adhesive otitis. *The Journal of Laryngology and Otology* **70**, 559.

[51] SCHUKNECHT H. F. (1974) In *Pathology of the Ear.* Cambridge, Massachusetts: Harvard University Press.

[52] ZÖLLNER F. (1966) *Handbuch Hals-Nasen-Ohrenheilkunde*, eds. Berendes J., Link R. & Zöllner F. Band III/2, p. 1315. Thieme, Verlag Stuttgart.

CHAPTER 11

Management of Chronic Middle Ear Disease

ASSESSMENT

History

Discharge from the ear, deafness, sometimes tinnitus and occasionally bleeding from granulation tissue or a polyp are the usual symptoms of uncomplicated chronic otitis media. The abrupt onset of pain in the ear, facial paresis, vertigo, rigors or headache indicate an impending or developed complication of the chronic ear disease, and will usually require the admission of the patient to hospital without delay for further investigation and treatment.

Examination of upper respiratory tract

In every patient, and particularly in children with active or recurrent tubotympanic disease, the pharynx, nasopharynx, nose and sinuses should be examined for infection.

Otoscopic examination

An accurate diagnosis can only be made by careful otoscopic examination after removal of all wax, discharge and debris preferably with suction apparatus. The advantages of magnification and the brilliant co-axial illumination afforded by the binocular operating microscope are obvious and make this method of examination always desirable. A Siegle's pneumatic otoscope with plain glass lens can be used with the microscope to demonstrate mobility of the tympanic membrane or its remnants or to suck pus from a small perforation hidden under granulation tissue, or to elicit a positive fistula sign. It is a useful practice always to record findings by a sketch. The following observations are particularly to be noted:

(1) the position, colour and mobility of the intact tympanic membrane and the presence of fluid levels or bubbles of air in the middle ear space;

(2) the size, shape and site of any perforation, retraction pocket or deformity of the tympanic membrane;

(3) the presence and location of granulations, discharge or cholesteatoma;

(4) the presence of pulsation which is a sign of active inflammation and loculation of pus. Marked pulsation of profuse purulent otorrhoea suggests an extradural abscess;

(5) the colour and odour of the discharge. Blue-green pus of characteristic sweetish aromatic odour is due to infection with *pseudomonas pyocyanea*. Infection with *Escherichia coli* produces a faecal odour. *Proteus mirabilis* infection has a musty or a putrefactive smell. A malodorous discharge is characteristically found in infected attico-antral disease with bone necrosis and moist keratoma;

(6) inflation of the Eustachian tube by Valsalva's manoeuvre may demonstrate that the tube is patent, that an aerated part of the mesotympanum is sealed off from the diseased area, or that an occult pin-hole perforation exists;

(7) small crusts adherent to the outer attic wall or posterosuperior annulus should be removed gently to ascertain the presence of a retraction pocket or cholesteatoma;

(8) granulations and polypi should be removed and submitted for biopsy to exclude malignancy, tuberculosis or glomus tympanicum tumour;

(9) it is often possible to assess the condition of the exposed tympanic epithelium: whether it is normal; swollen, inflamed and secreting; replaced by an ingrowth of keratinizing squamous

epithelium; or infiltrated by submucosal plaques of tympanosclerosis;

(10) the condition of the incudo-stapedial joint and labyrinthine windows may be visible through a posterior defect of the pars tensa;

(11) a persisting chronic otitis externa may be due to the continuing maceration of canal skin by infected secretions from a chronically draining ear, or to the use of antibiotic ear drops to which the patient has become sensitized.

Fistula test

The bony wall of the labyrinth may be locally eroded by the chronic disease process (usually keratoma) with exposure of endosteum. The presence of this so-called 'fistula' can be detected in some cases by the fistula test. The air pressure in the external canal and middle ear cleft is alternately increased and decreased by compression or release of the bulb of a Siegle's pneumatic otoscope or Politzer bag with adapter fitted to the ear canal. The transmission of these pressure changes to the endosteal membrane bridging the fistula displaces endolymphatic fluid with deflection of the ampullary cupula. This results in a sensation of brief vertigo associated with conjugate deviation of the eyes to one or other side, followed by several nystagmus movements when the pressure change is released. This nystagmus is more accurately recorded by electronystagmography. The 'fistula' is most commonly present in the lateral semicircular canal, and less often in the cochlear wall or labyrinthine windows. A positive test implies a 'fistula' in a functioning vestibular labyrinth and is an indication for elective surgery on that ear as soon as convenient. A negative result does not necessarily exclude the presence of a 'fistula' which could be very small, or exist in a non-functioning labyrinth.

Evaluation of tubal function

The adequacy of tubal function is of great importance to the functional result of middle ear microsurgery. The many elaborate methods that have been described for the assessment of tubal patency before operation are of doubtful value and probably not relevant in practice, because tubal patency may improve after operation when chronic infection is controlled. It seems important only to ascertain that the Eustachian tube is patent before operating by simple tests such as the Valsalva manoeuvre. A negative Valsalva manoeuvre does not contra-indicate tympanoplasty but should draw the surgeon's attention to the condition of the anterior mesotympanum and protympanum [1].

Evaluation of hearing

Modern audiological studies complemented by tuning-fork tests are an essential part of the investigation of hearing and should be carried out after aural toilet is completed. If the ear is actively discharging it is advisable to repeat the tests after an interval of a few weeks when the ear is quiescent.

Basic audiological tests include in all cases the determination of pure-tone thresholds for air conduction (AC) and bone conduction (BC), the assessment of the speech reception threshold (SRT) for spondee words and the maximum discrimination score for a list of phonetically balanced words (PB max.). Accuracy of testing requires an acceptable testing environment, an accurately calibrated audiometer, and a correct and careful testing technique.

Tuning-fork tests (Rinne, Weber and Absolute bone conduction) have in no way been outmoded by the advances of audiology, but have retained their important place in diagnosis. The results of tuning fork tests must be correlated with the audiometric findings, and any discrepancy between these two should bring scrutiny to bear on the audiological test procedure which may require to be repeated after readjustment of masking levels.

A mild to moderate conductive hearing loss is the rule. In the lesser degrees of hearing impairment, a conductive loss with negative Rinne test can only be demonstrated by low frequency tuning forks of 128 and 256 Hz; the higher frequency tuning forks give a Rinne positive response. Assessment of the Rinne response to a series of tuning forks starting at 128 or 256 Hz and continuing by octave intervals until the Rinne test becomes positive is recommended. To prevent the phenomenon of a false negative

Rinne response, due to lateralization of the test tone through the skull to the opposite ear with the better cochlear function, adequate masking noise by a Bárány noise-box must be applied to the ear not under test.

Given normal BC thresholds it is natural to suppose that the position of the AC curve would be an indication of the degree of pathological damage to the sound conducting mechanism. Such an assumption is often correct, but it must also be understood that many factors can influence the patient's hearing. Temporary depression of hearing can result from recent inflammatory mucosal swelling and exudate, when the ossicular chain is intact. On the other hand, excellent hearing can often be maintained through the favourable placement of keratomas, polyps or scars giving rise to a prosthesis effect when the ossicular chain is defective. Some patients note that the hearing is better when the ear is moist than when it is dry, and this is explained by the baffle effect of secretion within the round window niche. In dry ears with central perforations and an intact ossicular chain it is unusual for hearing loss to be greater than 40 dB (ISO). Complete destruction of the ossicular chain and tympanic membrane usually produces a deficit of 50–60 dB.

Prosthesis test

In central perforation of the tympanic membrane the function of the ossicular chain and the two windows can be tested by assessing the effect on hearing of the introduction of a suitable prosthesis (Silastic sheeting) to seal the defect. If there is hearing gain the ossicular chain is probably intact and mobile and the labyrinthine windows are probably normal. If the hearing is unchanged or worse there could be interruption or fixation of the ossicular chain.

Bacteriological investigation

Culture of the secretion from a discharging ear allows identification of the specific microorganisms and determination of their antibiotic sensitivity, providing a guide to the effective control of infection by local or systemic antibiotics. This knowledge is of practical value in chronic otitis media when there is an acute exacerbation of infection with pyogenic organisms particularly in tubotympanic disease.

Attico-antral disease with a moist infected keratoma provides an ideal condition for the growth of opportunistic saprophytes and commensals such as *Pseudomonas pyocyanea*, *Escherichia coli* and *Proteus mirabilis* which are Gram negative bacilli resistant to many antimicrobial agents. The elimination of these organisms depends entirely upon the surgical eradication of the attico-antral disease.

Radiological investigation

Radiology of the petrous pyramids and paranasal sinuses is advised for all patients with a chronically draining ear.

Radiological translucency of the paranasal sinuses excludes sinus infection as a cause of the chronicity of the ear condition. If there is mucosal swelling or opacity within a maxillary air sinus then treatment will be required.

Radiographic studies of the temporal bone can give valuable information about the anatomical and pathological features particularly when the right and left ears are compared and correlated with the clinical findings.

Conventional radiographic views of the petrous pyramid include:

(1) Schuller's lateral view to demonstrate the extent of mastoid pneumatization, the position of the sigmoid sinus and tegmen and also the epitympanic space.

(2) Chaussé's third projection, an oblique view to demonstrate the bony walls of the tympanic cavity, especially the lateral wall of the attic.

(3) Stenver's view of the petrous pyramid to show the petrous apex, the inner ear structures and also the mastoid tip.

In chronic suppurative ear disease of the benign or safe mucosal type, the mastoid may be well-pneumatized with normal cell outlines, the mastoid air cells may show clouding due to retained secretions and swollen mucosa, or there may be signs of new bone formation with progressive sclerosis, thickening of bony septa and obliteration of mastoid cells. If the middle ear infection is long-standing, having begun in early childhood, the mastoid may fail to pneumatize and appears sclerotic and acellular. Sequestra due to osteomyelitis may be seen on rare occasions radiographically.

Cholesteatoma associated with a small sclerosed mastoid may be demonstrated as a radiological bone defect with smooth margins of the attic and antrum, with erosion of the lateral attic wall, and sometimes with erosion or a fistula of the lateral semicircular canal. Lateral and frontal tomograms are more helpful than conventional views in giving detailed information about the extent of a cholesteatoma. Tomography is also especially desirable in patients with huge aural polyps that fill the auditory meatus and thereby preclude otoscopy.

MANAGEMENT OF TUBOTYMPANIC TYPE OF CHRONIC OTITIS MEDIA

The factors predisposing to chronicity of the infection must be identified and dealt with to make the ear dry and inactive. Then, ideally, all patients should have some form of tympanoplasty, to prevent re-infection by repairing the tympanic membrane and to restore hearing by reconstructing the defective ossicular chain.

Local aural toilet

Aural toilet is required in all cases of chronic otorrhoea and should be carried out meticulously, ideally at intervals determined by the presence and quantity of secretion. Painstaking suction clearance of debris and discharge by the otologist under the operating microscope at weekly or twice weekly intervals will often produce a dry ear within days or a few weeks.

Dry mopping with cotton-dressed probes by nursing staff, relatives or the patient himself is less satisfactory.

Syringing of ears with warm sterile Ringer's solution may be necessary to clear out thick purulent material, but may extend the area of mucosal infection, or precipitate an acute labyrinthitis in unsuspected erosion of the bony labyrinth by cholesteatoma.

Keeping water out of the ear

Constant re-infection by allowing water to enter the ear during bathing or washing is quite common and should be prevented by putting Vaselined® cotton wool into the meatus. Many patients seem never to have been instructed about the importance of this measure.

Topical medications

Topical medications include insufflations and ear drops, commonly applied after completion of aural toilet.

Powders

Insufflations of various antibiotic powders must be used sparingly because they tend to cake into hard masses obstructing drainage. Iodized boric acid powder is an old nostrum with the double advantage of dissolving in the presence of moisture at the same time as releasing nascent iodine which is bactericidal. The powder is blown through the perforation into the tympanum once or twice weekly after aural toilet. In most cases tympanic infection is brought rapidly under control with diminution of drainage and the attainment of a dry middle ear. The diameter of the perforation must be greater than 2·5 mm for this preparation to gain access to the middle ear. Sensitization to the powder is rare and is indicated by the appearance of a profuse serous otorrhoea within a matter of minutes of its application.

Ear drops

Thrice daily instillations of antibiotic-corticosteroid ear drops forced into the perforated tympanum by tragal massage are commonly used to reduce mucosal oedema and infection within the middle ear and Eustachian tube. Many ear drops in current use seem to be potentially hazardous because the antibiotic or solvent used as the carrier of the drug is ototoxic. The effects on the cochlear microphonics of guinea-pigs of various drugs and solvents at various concentrations instilled into the tympanum for periods varying from 1 to 3 days have been studied [2]. Gentamicin 0·3%, chloramphenicol sodium succinate ⩾5%, propylene glycol ⩾50% and 70% alcohol for one day all produced deafness. Neomycin, kanamycin and framycetin have all been shown to have ototoxic effects. Alcohol 70% applied to the round window niche for 10 minutes did not cause hearing loss.

Although the risks of ototoxicity seem to be slight, these antibiotic or antiseptic instillations must be used with care. They should not be used for longer than 7–10 days at a time because prolonged use might increase the risk of cochlear damage, might sensitize the patient's canal skin causing an intractable otitis externa, or might allow the growth of antibiotic resistant organisms.

Treatment of nasopharyngeal sepsis

The removal of infected tonsils and adenoids and the washout of pus-containing maxillary sinuses are often required in children. Adults with gross sinus disease and nasal polyposis or other obstructive nasal deformities may need septal and sinus surgery to restore nasal function before the ear can be satisfactorily treated.

Granulations and polyps

Granulations are red sessile protrusions usually situated on the promontory and which often pout through a central perforation. As mucosal infection diminishes, the granulations recede and may disappear.

A polyp in the external meatus may become large enough to obstruct drainage and prevent local treatment of the middle ear. In this circumstance it is better to remove it during a formal operation to explore the state of the mastoid, attic and middle ear, rather than blindly to attempt its avulsion from the ear canal. The presence of severe mixed deafness and vestibular symptoms on manipulating the polyp suggest that it is arising from carious bone over a labyrinthine fistula, or from the oval window region, and it must be removed with great care. Most polyps arise from carious bone of the promontory, ossicles, attic or mastoid antrum, and so their local removal via the meatus is often followed by recurrence because of failure to cure the underlying disease. Mastoidectomy is therefore required if the discharge persists and the mastoid lining is chronically infected.

Chronic mastoiditis

In chronic otitis media with central perforation the mastoid is often quite well pneumatized. If conservative measures fail to result in a dry ear the mastoid antrum and attic must be explored through a burr hole posterior to the suprameatal (Henle's) spine. If the mastoid lining is seen to be chronically infected with swollen mucosa, granulations and secretion, a cortical mastoidectomy is needed; this is necessary in about 12% of type I tympanoplasties in South Australia.

The posterior bony wall of the external meatus must be retained to preserve the natural shape of the meatus and to avoid the problems of a large exteriorized mastoid cavity. Chronic suppurative mastoiditis and otitis media forms the most important and widely accepted indication for the use of the closed technique of mastoidectomy with intact posterior canal wall. The supplementary creation of a posterior tympanotomy through the small triangular cleft of the chorda-facial angle into the mesotympanum is necessary when this recess is occupied by a tract of diseased air cells affected by mucosal granulation, osteitis or squamous epithelial ingrowth. Tube drainage via the lower end of the postauricular incision for 5 days allows evacuation of secretions and aeration of the mastoid, both necessary if a tympanoplasty completes the operation.

MANAGEMENT OF CHRONIC OTITIS MEDIA WITH EPIDERMOID CHOLESTEATOMA

Epidermoid cholesteatoma, cholesteatosis or keratoma of the middle ear cleft is a slowly progressive and destructive disease which, if untreated, will eventually impair hearing and may cause serious intracranial complications. The treatment of chronic otitis media with cholesteatoma is therefore surgical, to remove all the disease and render the ear 'safe'. Since the prospects of preservation or reconstruction of the middle ear hearing mechanism are most favourable when least damage of existing structures has occurred, it follows that early surgery in skilled hands is the most desirable form of conservative surgical management.

Non-surgical management

The non-surgical treatment of cholesteatoma can only be justified in those rare cases where the patient refuses to undergo surgery, or when the patient is a poor surgical risk. Repeated local cleansing of the 'perforation' and keratoma cavity with removal of epithelial debris and granulation by hooks, forceps and suction can reduce drainage and eliminate odour. Irrigation of the epitympanic space through a cannula is unwise if the perforation is small because infection can be introduced producing acute complications.

The only other exception to surgical treatment is when a known, limited, non-infected keratoma permits adequate local clearance from attic, tympanum or mastoid. Such patients can remain trouble-free, but need periodic otoscopic examination under magnification throughout their lifetime. For example:

(1) The small keratoma limited to the lateral attic area of a normal hearing ear may be easily and completely evacuated using suction, hooks and forceps. The lining wall of the attic retraction pocket should be fully visible and intact after this procedure.

(2) A large atrophic indrawn scar of an intact pars tensa may form a deep retraction pocket behind the handle of the malleus and accumulate within it an asymptomatic dry keratoma that is easily removed.

(3) A large encysted epidermoid cholesteatoma may erode the outer walls of the mastoid antrum and epitympanum to create a near-perfect atticoantrostomy from which the keratoma can be extracted, leaving a smooth and soundly epithelialized atticomastoid bowl with good access for routine inspection. The pars tensa can remain intact with a sealed-off mesotympanum. Hearing may be profoundly impaired in some cases with existing labyrinthine 'fistulae'. Cleaning of these ears should always be gentle, careful and under magnification.

Surgical management

The otologist should be aware of the problems of surgical treatment. Cholesteatoma often re-appears after its removal despite the most meticulous techniques of micro-surgery and regardless of the experience of the surgeon. Complete removal of the cholesteatoma matrix may be impossible if it insinuates itself into every nook and cranny of the middle ear cleft including the sinus tympani, the stapes footplate and crural arch, the round window niche, the hypotympanum and the Eustachian tube; or may be undesirable when the matrix covers a labyrinthine 'fistula' or is adherent to the round window membrane. Most adults with cholesteatoma have a small, acellular or poorly pneumatized mastoid process that aggravates the technical difficulties of certain 'closed' surgical techniques by imposing limitations of access on removal of disease. About half of children's mastoids operated upon for cholesteatoma are cellular and often extensively pneumatized. In these patients elimination of cholesteatosis is more difficult because of the infiltrative growth of matrix into bone, and consequently the incidence of recurrence is much higher than in adults. Rarely the keratoma may extend beyond the limits of the middle ear cleft to invade the labyrinth and petrous apex or the posterior and middle cranial fossae. Subtotal removal of the petrous pyramid may then be required to excise the disease. Recurrences of cholesteatoma can take several years to become evident, so an extended period of re-examination of all patients after surgery is necessary.

Opinions vary about the best method of surgical treatment of cholesteatoma: the choice is between the wide-access or 'open' approaches on the one hand, and the 'closed' techniques that retain the bony canal wall on the other [3–10].

The operation chosen should take into account the radiological anatomy of the ear, should allow the otologist to remove disease completely, should not make the patient worse than he was previously and should facilitate detection and surgical management of cholesteatoma recurrence.

Modern concepts of open approaches

In the radiologically small, acellular or sclerosed mastoid, the cholesteatoma is conveniently approached from its site of origin using a trans-canal route to expose the middle ear and remove the outer attic wall. The bone work is extended posteriorly as far as necessary to uncap the total extent of the disease. The keratoma with its matrix can then be removed usually in its entirety. This concept of completely 'uncapping' the disease of the small mastoid case has made it possible to preserve the bony canal wall in nearly 40% of the author's cholesteatoma cases because there was no mastoid extension of the disease.

There are three main types of open approach.

(1) *Intact canal wall and transcanal tympanoplasty*

A limited cholesteatoma confined to the mesotympanum can be removed after elevation of a posterior tympanomeatal skin flap and appropriate curettage of overhang or osteitis of the posterior tympanic ring. Repair of tympanic membrane and ossicular chain completes the procedure.

(2) *Atticotomy with intact posterior wall*

If a cholesteatoma is limited to the attic (i.e. there is no posterior extension beyond the aditus) it is usually unnecessary to take down the posterior bony canal wall unless there are exuberant granulations in the mastoid antrum. An extended atticotomy affords wide access for removal of all attic disease. The remains of the incus and the head of the malleus should usually be removed to ensure complete evacuation of the keratoma and its matrix. The defect in the attic can then be repaired by grafting, and the hearing restored by ossiculoplasty (using allograft incus). The tympanomeatal skin flap with an underlay of fascial graft is replaced as a single entity to restore the ear to a near-normal appearance (Figs. 11.1 and 11.2). Severe attic retraction pockets have not been observed after this technique. Slight dimpling of the attic membrane may be noted, but all patients develop a self-cleaning ear.

(3) *Attico-antrostomy*

The outer walls of the attic and antrum are removed together with the posterior bony canal wall as far medially as the Fallopian canal to permit the widest possible access for removal of keratoma, diseased mucosa, and bone from the

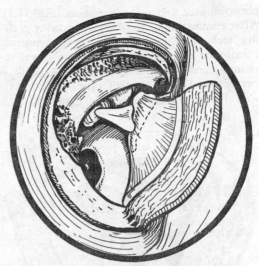

FIG. 11.1. Extended atticotomy: the outer attic wall has been drilled away completely to allow removal of the incus, the head of the malleus and the cholesteatoma sac. The crura of the stapes are absent in this case and an ossiculoplasty has been completed by transposing a remodelled allograft incus between the mobile stapes footplate and the malleus handle (malleoplatinopexy). In practice the tympanic membrane defect is repaired first by grafting before the ossiculoplasty is attempted.

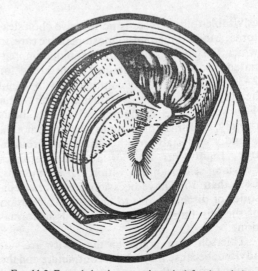

FIG. 11.2. Extended atticotomy: the attic defect is sealed by an underlay graft of temporalis fascia and the tympanomeatal skin flap is replaced to recreate a near-normal ear.

mastoid, attic and mesotympanum (Fig. 11.3). After elimination of the disease, underlay grafting techniques are used to repair tympanic membrane defects and seal off the mesotympanum, and an appropriate ossiculoplasty is performed (Fig. 11.4). Obliteration of deep mastoid recesses with connective tissue grafts is

Advantages of wide-access techniques

(1) In the small sclerosed mastoid, atticotomy or atticoantrostomy is a more efficient and adequate approach than the so-called 'closed' technique for removal of attic cholesteatosis. When the middle-fossa dura is exceptionally low-lying or if the sigmoid venous sinus is located

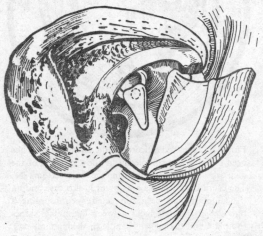

Fig. 11.3. Attico-antrostomy: the posterior bony canal wall has been removed as far medially as the vertical portion of the Fallopian canal. An allograft remodelled incus has been placed on the head of the normal stapes.

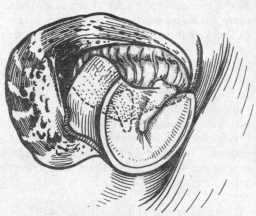

Fig. 11.4. Attico-antrostomy: an underlay graft of temporalis fascia has been used to seal the epitympanic area and the tympanomeatal skin flap has been replaced posteriorly to cover the small mastoid bowl. The interposed incus is in contact with the tympanic membrane immediately behind the malleus handle. The normal depth of the tympanum is retained, and hearing restored by this means.

advisable only if there is no invasive cholesteatoma. Modern methods of postoperative care, in which the cavity is filled with antibiotic-impregnated gelatin sponge retained undisturbed for 2–3 weeks, allow cavity contracture with sound healing and spontaneous epithelialization within 4–6 weeks. The mastoid bowl usually heals rapidly, is of small dimensions, shallow, smooth, soundly and stably epithelialized and trouble-free. Eighty per cent of attico-antrostomies become 'self-cleaning' within 12–18 months. Less than 10% have occasional and brief episodes of discharge due to temporary ulceration of the skin lining and granulation tissue formation.

Thiersch skin grafts to the cavity are not advised, because they inhibit contracture and the cavity remains the same size delaying the development of the important 'self-cleaning' capacity.

far forwards and overlies the antrum, transcanal attico-antrostomy is the only safe procedure available.

(2) The improved exposure of the attic and posterior recesses of the middle ear obtained by wide-access techniques facilitates removal of disease, and must reduce the chance of cholesteatoma recurrence.

(3) Detection of cholesteatoma recurrence is easier and earlier than in closed techniques. Epidermoid cysts developing from residual disease in the attic and mastoid can be removed usually as a minor out-patient procedure.

(4) Matrix can be retained undisturbed over a semicircular canal 'fistula' if circumstances necessitate this, e.g. an operation of the only hearing ear, or a large labyrinthine fistula with matrix adherent to the canal endosteum.

(5) This technique avoids the problem of retraction pockets in the presence of Eustachian tube malfunction.

Disadvantages of wide-access techniques

(1) If a large exteriorized mastoid cavity fails to heal by contracture and sound epithelialization there is sometimes a tendency (aggravated by climatic, social, or deficient dietary factors) for the lining epithelium to break down with ulceration and granulation, and to resist healing. Many patients fail to develop a self-cleaning mechanism and require periodic specialist attention for the remainder of their lives. A persistent problem requires obliteration of the cavity preferably after a period of 2–3 years when recurrence of cholesteatoma has been excluded by extended observation.

(2) Inadvertent entry of water into the ear should be avoided by the insertion of Vaseline®-impregnated cotton wool into the meatus as a precautionary measure before hair washing, showering or swimming.

(3) The labyrinth is relatively exposed and is unduly susceptible to thermal stimulation. Surfing and scuba diving must be forbidden.

(4) The functional disadvantages for hearing often attributed to atticotomy or atticoantrostomy are not proven.

Modern concepts of the closed technique

Jansen's method of a combined approach for tympanoplasty with mastoidectomy and retention of the bony posterior canal wall was adopted in the 1960s by many leading otologists. Of his several themes, two are important.

First, it is usually possible, even in the presence of mastoid and attic cholesteatoma, to preserve the whole length of the posterior bony canal wall, and outer attic wall, including the frame of the tympanic membrane, thus creating conditions for normal anatomical restoration of the ear with its benefits for hearing and the avoidance of an exteriorized mastoid cavity.

Secondly, it is possible, by the supplementary creation of a posterior hypotympanotomy in the triangular cleft of the chorda-facial angle (facial recess) between the sulcus of the tympanic membrane and chorda tympani nerve laterally, and the canal of the mastoid portion of the facial nerve medially, to expose the mesotympanum from a posterior viewpoint in order to remove disease in the facial recess and posterior tympanum, to ensure adequate drainage and

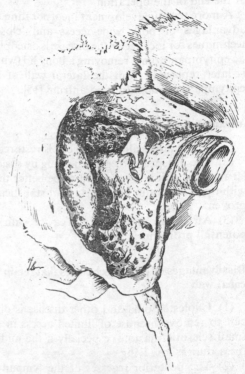

FIG. 11.5. Extended cortical mastoidectomy right ear: note preservation of the bony canal wall and the creation of a posterior tympanotomy in a well-pneumatized temporal bone.

aeration of the mastoid segment after operation and to provide a route for the insertion and correct positioning of any prosthesis used in ossiculoplasty after the tympanic membrane perforation has been grafted (Fig. 11.5).

Retention of the whole bony canal wall (to prevent later development of retraction pockets and 'recurrent' cholesteatoma) usually prevents adequate access to the anterior attic area and to the posterior tympanic sinus medial to the facial canal and pyramid despite posterior tympanotomy. The intact canal wall procedure has been modified by several surgeons to allow better exposure of the inaccessible areas of the posterior tympanum [11–14].

The posterior canal wall is divided by superior and inferior longitudinal osteotomies, and the bony segment with attached canal skin is mobilized anteriorly. This osteoplastic flap is replaced at the end of the operation.

A more recent development incorporating the advantages of both wide-access and 'closed' techniques for localized attic disease is osteoplastic epitympanotomy, removing a bony lid (which is later replaced) from the lateral wall of the epitympanum and aditus ad antrum [15].

Advantages of closed techniques

(1) An anatomically normal ear is restored.

(2) The prospects for good hearing by ossicular reconstruction are claimed to be better than with open techniques but this is not statistically proven.

(3) An exteriorized mastoid cavity with its potential problems is avoided.

Disadvantages of closed techniques that retain the canal wall

(1) Cholesteatoma and other disease is difficult to remove because of limited access in the small sclerotic mastoid, especially if the middle fossa dura is low lying.

(2) The posterior recesses of the tympanum (particularly the sinus tympani) are difficult to see if the canal wall is retained in its entirety.

(3) Damage to the facial nerve in an acellular bone is possible, although it is very rare in experienced hands.

(4) Recurrences of cholesteatoma in the attic and mastoid segments can progress unseen, shielded from view by the preserved bony canal wall. Detection of recurrences is difficult and delayed in closed techniques, unless a policy of deliberate mastoid re-exploration is adopted. The incidence of recurrence is seriously underestimated in most series of closed techniques.

(5) Late atrophy of a portion of the posterior canal wall with the development of a meatomastoid fistula has been reported in 16·7% of 156 cases of cholesteatoma treated by closed techniques [16]. This unexpected and often unsus-

pected complication is due either to thermal damage of bone and its blood supply during drilling and thinning down of the posterior canal wall necessitated by posterior tympanotomy or to osteoclasis associated with recurrence of cholesteatoma.

(6) There is a high incidence of residual cholesteatoma after closed techniques [17].

(7) A further mastoid re-exploration to exclude residual disease would seem necessary after all closed operations.

Indications for closed techniques in management of cholesteatosis

The compelling attraction of the closed techniques that retain the bony canal wall is the restoration of the ear to a desirably normal anatomical state. Their limitation is a failure to detect at an early stage the recurrences of residual cholesteatoma in the attic and mastoid. Given a high degree of technical skill, and the prior consent of the patient (or his guardian in the case of a minor) to allow a second mastoid operation to exclude residual disease 2–3 years later, closed techniques can always be attempted, particularly in those geographical regions where healing of the cavity after open techniques seems difficult to attain.

The low incidence of cavity problems after attico-antrostomy in patients with a small sclerosed mastoid has influenced the writer to reserve closed techniques of tympanoplasty in cholesteatoma entirely for the relatively rare case with the larger pneumatized mastoid.

Preservation or removal of cholesteatoma matrix

The preservation of matrix was debated in the era of the modified radical mastoidectomy. When the cholesteatoma was pea or bean-shaped with a smooth matrix free of any surface indentations, it was considered safe to leave the matrix *in situ* in the attic, aditus or antrum because it speeded up epithelialization of the cavity. Where the cholesteatoma matrix had an infiltrating tendency with an irregular surface it was considered more dangerous and demanded meticulous and complete removal [18].

Nowadays it is considered sound policy to

remove all vestiges of matrix from the middle ear cleft to avoid recurrence of cholesteatoma and to allow contracture of the cavity.

Removal of the matrix from the bony labyrinth is delayed to the last and dissection is carried out with great care under high magnification to avoid opening into the labyrinthine lumen if the matrix is adherent to the endosteum exposed in a 'fistula' or erosion of the bony labyrinthine wall. The eroded area should be covered immediately by bone dust and a fascial graft once the matrix has been removed. The risk of sensorineural impairment is not significantly different whether the matrix is retained over or carefully removed from a lateral canal 'fistula'. In the case of the rare cochlear 'fistula' even careful removal of matrix carries a high risk of cochlear deafness. Matrix over a cochlear 'fistula' should probably be retained and the disease exteriorized, especially if it is the patient's only hearing ear [19].

Recurrences of cholesteatoma after surgery

Classification
Reappearance of cholesteatoma after surgery may be iatrogenic, recurrent or residual according to the presumed mechanism of formation [20].

Iatrogenic cholesteatoma is a term reserved for the postoperative development of epidermoid cysts in ear canal, tympanic membrane or middle ear cleft of an ear previously free from cholesteatoma. Stratified squamous epithelium accidentally retained on malleus, tympanic membrane remnants or deep canal wall, and covered by a graft will form an epidermoid inclusion cyst. This is the 'graft' epidermoid that develops as a late iatrogenic complication of tympanoplasty. Such a mechanism is also possible in an ear treated surgically for cholesteatoma.

'Recurrent' cholesteatoma is seen almost exclusively as a complication of closed techniques that retain the posterior bony canal wall. After an otherwise successful operation, a retraction pocket (due to vacuum, adhesions or lack of support) develops in the intact tympanic membrane which collapses medially into the middle ear. This skin-lined pocket may then pass into the attic or into the chorda-facial recess, accumulating within it a mass of desquamated keratin that forms the bulk of a new keratoma. Recurrent cholesteatoma can also arise secondarily by migration of ear canal skin through a graft perforation into the middle ear.

Residual cholesteatoma refers to one which develops from residual fragments of living matrix inadvertently retained within the middle ear cleft at the original operation. Continued growth of the remnant forms a circumscribed slowly expanding cyst resembling a pearl.

Incidence of recurrent cholesteatoma
The incidence of reappearance of cholesteatoma is difficult to assess, and is likely to be underestimated for several reasons.

Patients may be unable or unwilling to attend for periodic review after surgery for many reasons such as forgetfulness, disinterest, expense, inconvenience, geographic problems, change of residence, infirmity, old age and death. The number of patients who attend for review falls off progressively so that information on recurrence rates is prejudiced.

After closed techniques, recurrences of cholesteatoma in the mastoid and attic are concealed from view, and so the incidence of recurrence will remain seriously underestimated unless every patient is submitted to re-exploration of the mastoid or to examination using a diagnostic telescope inserted via a post-aural incision.

After both open and closed techniques, recurrences in the middle ear remain undetected until the growing cyst makes contact with the tympanic membrane.

In 141 patients with cholesteatoma treated by wide-access techniques an average rate of emergence of residual cholesteatoma of 0·25% per month was noted during the first 5 years after which the discovery of residual disease almost ceased [21]. The cumulative incidence was 1·4% at 10 months, 14·9% at 5 years, and 17·0% at 8 years after operation.

Recurrence of residual cholesteatoma after closed techniques can be a problem of some magnitude [17]. Attic or mastoid cholesteatoma was encountered in 35% of patients when the mastoid was re-explored 1–2 years after an intact canal wall tympanoplasty and mastoidectomy. In patients with diffuse cholesteatosis of a pneumatized mastoid 56% later developed residual mastoid cholesteatoma.

Sites of predilection of cholesteatoma recurrence
After open techniques the cholesteatoma reappears at its original site and this finding lends support to the aetiological concept of the residual nature of the recurrence. There is no apparent predilection of cholesteatoma for recurrence at any one site. Involvement of the attic, mastoid and mesotympanum in recurrent epidermoid cysts is proportional to the involvement of these areas by the original cholesteatosis.

After closed techniques the attic seems to be disproportionally affected by recurrences presumably because of the difficulty of clearing matrix from this area, and also because of the additional mechanism of retraction pocket keratoma.

Factors influencing probability of recurrence
The chance of recurrence of cholesteatoma after removal depends on the age of the patient, the experience of the surgeon, and the surgical technique (open or closed).

The improved exposure for removal of disease afforded by wide-access approaches (extended atticotomy and attico-antrostomy) diminishes the probability of recurrence.

The chance of recurrence decreases with increasing experience of the surgeon, but this effect is less important.

The probability of recurrence depends primarily on the age of the patient and decreases with increasing age. Age has a very strong effect with an estimated probability of recurrence (author's data after open techniques) of 0·4 at 10 years, dropping dramatically to about 0·05 at 65 years. The explanation is that 40–50% of children with cholesteatosis have quite extensive mastoid pneumatization and the infiltrating nature of the matrix aggravates the difficulty of removal and enhances the possibility that some fragment of viable squamous epithelium is retained. Residual matrix in the child may have a greater potential

for growth and survival than similar remnants retained in the older patient.

Other variables such as sex and the pattern of involvement of middle ear cleft by cholesteatosis are not significant.

Growth rates of epidermoid cysts
The rate of growth is exponential but differs according to site [21]. In the attic, recurrent epidermoids tend to grow fairly rapidly, doubling in diameter about every 10 months. In the mastoid area, the growth rate appears to be slower, the cyst doubling in diameter every 25 months. The explanation of the differences in growth rates according to site is not known. Growth rates, however, may depend on:

(1) variations in growth potential of residual cellular remnants;

(2) vascular factors, including the haemodynamic changes accompanying infection; and

(3) availability of an adequate blood supply to the cyst matrix during its progressive enlargement.

Management of recurrent cholesteatoma

With open techniques, recurrences can be easily detected in the mastoid and attic as small epidermoid 'pearls' lying deep to the lining epithelium. These cysts can be removed readily at the time of consultation using sickle-knife and suction under the operating microscope.

Epidermoids within the middle ear are more difficult to detect early but eventually the cyst contacts the tympanic membrane, allowing a diagnosis to be made. Some of these residual cysts within the middle ear can be removed effectively by incising the tympanic membrane and the outer wall of the cyst to evacuate its contents by suction, thus marsupializing it. Other cases require a formal middle ear exploration, and a number turn up unexpectedly at a staged operation.

After closed techniques it is never possible, without surgical exploration, to detect residual or recurrent cholesteatoma in the mastoid or attic in the earlier stages. Formal mastoid re-exploration or some method of endoscopic inspection of the mastoid and attic by a small telescope, inserted via a retro-auricular stab incision, is therefore recommended for all patients who have had their cholesteatoma removed by closed methods of tympanoplasty which retain the posterior canal wall. Understandably, the patient is often reluctant to submit to a second exploratory operation 1–2 years later merely to exclude the possibility of recurrence of cholesteatoma, especially if he enjoys good hearing. For this reason many otologists do not restore hearing at the primary operation for cholesteatoma. The hearing deficit remains to be corrected later when the mastoid cavity and attic can be inspected. These considerations about a second operation apply especially to children to whom closed techniques have been applied and in whom the risk of recurrence is considerable. Small epidermoid cysts encountered in an uninfected ear at a second operation can usually be removed completely with the matrix intact. If there is any doubt about completeness of removal, or if the recurrence is extensive in an infected ear with osteitis, it is better to convert the closed case into an exteriorized attico-antrostomy by removal of the posterior canal wall and outer wall of the attic.

Timing of elective mastoid re-exploration in the closed case

The best time to re-open the mastoid electively should minimize the risk of missing the small early recurrence, and lessen the chance of allowing residual disease to destroy parts of anatomical and functional importance. Epidermoid cysts as small as 0·5 mm in diameter have been seen as late as 2 years after the first operation, but cysts larger than 5 mm have not been discovered earlier than 3 years in the non-infected case. It is therefore recommended that re-exploration of the mastoid and attic of the closed asymptomatic case be done no earlier than 2 years and not later than 3 years after the primary operation.

The development of discomfort, drainage, deterioration of hearing, meatomastoid fistula and obvious cholesteatoma in the operated ear are indications for early re-exploration. Such patients require experienced assessment and management for their successful outcome.

Tympanoplasty

Tympanoplasty is a term for those procedures which restore function to an ear that is damaged by chronic suppurative otitis media, previous surgery or congenital malformation. Tympanoplasty thus includes the careful eradication of disease from the middle ear and mastoid under magnification, the study of the integrity and mobility of the ossicular mechanism followed by the freeing of ossicular fixations, the bridging of defects in the sound conducting mechanism and the grafting of tympanic membrane perforations.

The principles on which functional success in tympanoplasty depends are: eradication of the disease; the provision of an intact and mobile tympanic membrane with vibratory characteristics resembling the normal so that it may transform sound pressure and protect the round window; the provision of an intact and mobile transmission system between the tympanic membrane and the oval window; and the restoration of a middle ear space aerated through the Eustachian tube.

The outcome of a tympanoplasty may depend on a variety of factors:

(1) The functional capacity of the Eustachian tube for aeration and clearance.

(2) The state of the middle ear mucosa, e.g. its secretory activity, the presence of adhesions or hypertrophy.

(3) Contractional forces of healing tissues after the mechanical system has been assembled.

(4) The mobility, mass, and viscoelasticity of the reconstructed tympanic membrane and transmitting system.

(5) The volume of the middle ear and mastoid pneumatic cell system.

(6) The sensorineural status of the diseased ear. This determines the best level of post-operative hearing after the conductive lesion has been surgically corrected. Reconstruction may be contra-indicated if the sensorineural reserve of the ear is extremely poor.

Although Wullstein's classification of tympanoplasty into five types (Table 11.1) was well recognized little or no attempt was made to reconstruct the ossicular chain in the 1950s and early 1960s. The operation was adapted to the

TABLE 11.1 Wullstein's classification of tympanoplasty

Type 1   Sound is conducted through a normal ossicular chain. A chronic tympanic membrane perforation is the sole abnormality and the middle ear is restored to normal by appropriate grafting techniques to close the defect.

Type 2   Sound is conducted through a deformed but functioning ossicular chain. The term now includes any reconstructive procedure which re-establishes the lever mechanism between the tympanic membrane and the oval window and maintains the normal lateral dimensions of the tympanum.

Type 3   The aim of the Type 3 is to establish a columella effect by bringing the tympanic membrane or graft into direct contact with the head of the normal stapes and with the medial attic wall. The mesotympanum is narrowed and there is a high risk of adhesions. The tympanic membrane acts as a sound pressure transformer through the intact stapes, and provides sound protection for the round window.

Type 4   Establishing sound protection of the round window with a graft may improve hearing where the stapes arch is destroyed, but the footplate remains mobile.

Type 5   If the stapes is fixed a fenestra into the lateral semicircular canal is required to improve hearing. An intact tympanic membrane forms a shallow middle ear cavity and provides sound protection for the round window without sound pressure transformation.

particular ossicular disorder when all diseased tissues had been cleared away. Since the mid 1960s further modifications of technique have been directed to improving the functional results by:

(1) Reliable grafting materials for the closure of defects of the tympanic membrane to achieve a mobile drumhead with vibratory characteristics resembling the normal.

(2) Avoidance of the Type 3, 4 and 5 tympanoplasties by using allograft ossicles to reconstruct the transmission mechanism and maintain a tympanum of normal lateral depth.

(3) Techniques that retain or restore the posterior bony canal wall of the auditory meatus thus avoiding the potential problems of the large exteriorized mastoid cavity.

(4) The restoration of Eustachian tubal function and the prevention of tympanic adhesions after operation.

Tissue transplantation in tympanoplasty

The repair of tympanic membrane defects by grafting with the patient's own tissues has been established since the early 1960s. Transposition of the patient's own incus or malleus to rebuild the sound-conducting mechanism within the middle ear was first reported in the 1950s [22].

One of the important advances of otological surgery in recent years has been the successful transplantation of middle ear ossicles and tympanic membranes from cadaver to patient in the surgical reconstruction of the middle ear [23–26, 29–31]. The following factors have been important.

(1) Technical limitations are no longer an obstacle due to the many excellent training programmes now established in most advanced countries.

(2) Cadaver material is plentiful and highly suited for otological procedures if obtained within 12–15 hours of death preferably from a 'disease-free' donor.

(3) Timing of operation. The operation need not coincide with the availability of fresh transplant material. Otological transplants, whether allograft or xenograft, are non-viable tissues stored in suitable preservative ready for instant use.

(4) Rejection phenomena. The most important advantage to the otologist of the use of preserved non-vital tissue is that the immunological phenomena of rejection (seen with a vital allograft and xenograft) seem to be inhibited, and neither the matching of tissues of donor and recipient nor immunosuppression are required. The host-versus-graft reaction is prevented by the denaturation of the graft proteins that apparently results from fixation in formaldehyde or storage in preservative (Cialit).

In other words the non-vital, denatured tissues used for transplantation in otology are immunologically inert.

It has been shown [27] that non-vital denatured allografts and xenografts demonstrate less local reaction after transplantation in experimental animals than do vital autografts.

Indications for allografts and xenografts in tympanoplasty

The chief reason for using allograft (or xenograft) materials in tympanoplasty is to allow a better reconstruction of the conducting mechanism and hence better hearing. Whereas ossicular allografts continue to fulfil an increasingly accepted and useful role as ossicular replacements in tympanoplasty the tympanic membrane allograft remains the subject of debate because of its generally lower 'take-rate' compared with autogenous temporalis fascia [28].

Marquet [29] has reported success rates of greater than 95% with allograft tympanic membranes fixed in 4% buffered formaldehyde (pH 5·6) and preserved in an aqueous solution of 1 in 5000 Cialit.

The advantages of the allograft tympanic membrane for the repair of total or subtotal perforations are their correct size and retained conical shape, their physiological stiffness giving better vibrational characteristics and improved functional results, and their capacity to inhibit the formation of middle ear adhesions; furthermore they allow an ideal method of implanting a malleus in preparation for later reconstruction of the ossicular chain.

It is also possible, after using formaldehyde fixation of the temporal bone, to dissect out a complete tympanic membrane with malleus and articulating ossicular chain [29]. This monobloc tympano-ossicular graft with its natural joints, ligaments and tendons can be used for cases in which there has been radical removal of diseased tissue from the middle ear and mastoid, provided the bony posterior canal wall has been retained or reconstructed. The correct positioning of the monobloc tympano-ossicular graft is critical because any minor displacement inevitably leads to bony ankylosis at the point of contact of the malleus-incus with the host's attic wall. For this reason many otologists continue to by-pass the attic in middle ear reconstruction by creating direct ossicular connections between malleus-tympanic membrane and stapes-oval window.

Allograft material may be hard to get and the preparation of the allograft tympanic membrane can be time-consuming so that allografts should not be used indiscriminately, but should be restricted to certain well-defined situations.

The allograft tympanic membrane with attached malleus handle is best reserved for total or subtotal loss of the tympanic membrane in association with total absence of the malleus and incus (as after radical mastoidectomy), absence or severe shortening of the malleus handle, or a malleus handle involved in cholesteatoma matrix necessitating complete removal of the ossicle.

The allograft tympanic membrane is rarely indicated for patients with a healthy and functioning malleus because repair of subtotal defects of the tympanic membrane using a temporalis fascial graft gives satisfactory results.

The allograft incus (and malleus or stapes) is useful in ossicular reconstruction when the patient's own incus is absent, or is so severely necrosed that the remnant of the ossicle is inadequate for reconstruction. It is also useful when the patient's incus is so involved in active disease (osteitis or cholesteatoma matrix) that it is necessary to remove and discard it. Ossicles involved by cholesteatoma nearly always show an advanced degree of osteitis, and tiny deposits of squamous epithelium that are only visible on histological examination, thus avoiding recognition with the operating microscope. Therefore, if ossicles are involved by cholesteatoma they should never be used as autografts for middle ear reconstruction.

Fate of allografts

In animals, preserved non-vital allograft bone chips and ossicles are invaded by host vascular tissue, and new bone is formed subperiosteally at the surface, and perivascularly in the interior. The new bone originates from the perivascular tissue of the host and is induced by the non-vital bone graft. Remodelling of the intercellular substance of the bone transplant can be demonstrated by the techniques of tetracycline labelling and fluorescent microscopy, or by autoradiography after administration of tritiated amino acids. In comparison with bone chips, ossicular allografts retain their shape better and are thus more useful for reconstructive surgery [30].

In man, transplanted allograft ossicles undergo similar changes, but more slowly: even after 3–6 years new bone formation is incomplete. The implanted ossicle is tolerated well, is covered by mucous membrane, and retains its form unaltered over many years.

The allograft tympanic membrane acts as an inert framework over which migrates a sheath of vascularized living connective tissue and epithelium [31].

Myringoplasty

The aim of myringoplasty is to restore an intact and mobile tympanic membrane having vibratory characteristics resembling the normal.

Graft materials

Despite the unique situation of the tympanic membrane in the depth of the auditory meatus with its special conditions of blood supply and aeration, perforations can now be repaired successfully in a high percentage of cases by grafts of various origin, autograft, denatured allograft and xenograft; meatal skin, fascia, periosteum, perichondrium, vein, dura or heart valve [32].

The majority of tympanic membrane repairs today are with mesodermal grafts of autogenous fascia or perichondrium, both of which are readily available and have excellent prospects of survival because of their low metabolic requirements and their resistance to infection. Less commonly, in special circumstances, denatured allograft tympanic membrane or dura are used.

Application of full-thickness skin as an onlay graft in the 1950s and early 1960s from sites such as the postaural region, arm, leg or abdomen was discontinued when the drawbacks of this material became apparent: graft cholesteatomas arising from hair follicles, the presence of sweat and sebaceous glands leading to adenohyperplasia, the failure of development of a migratory capacity and excessive desquamation of epithelial debris necessitating frequent aural toilet, and the occasional appearance of eczematous changes in the transplanted skin with thickening, oedema and a raw granulating surface.

Skin from the external meatus, however, has proved to be a reliable graft because it maintains its self-cleaning capacity, it does not contain hairs or glandular elements and being free of elastic fibres it does not shrink or curl up and

allows trimming of the graft to the desired size and shape. The graft has a thin and smooth periosteal layer on its undersurface and is applied as an onlay to the bed prepared for it on the denuded remains of the lamina propria of the tympanic membrane. Covering all mesodermal grafts by a meatal skin graft adapted to the margin of the defect in order to hasten epithelialization is strongly advocated [32].

Autogenous temporalis fascia has achieved almost universal popularity since the early 1960s as the best material for grafting perforations of the tympanic membrane. Not only is it readily available in the desired amount of 1 or 2 cm² by an endaural or postaural incision, but it also takes successfully (in competent hands) in over 95% of repairs of subtotal perforations whether the graft is living, dried or pressed. Graft failures are usually partial in that the residual defect is smaller than before and is amenable to revision. It is used as an onlay or inlay graft, as an interleaf, or as a plug.

Transplants of non-vital cadaver ear drums fixed in buffered formaldehyde (pH 5·6) and preserved in an aqueous solution of Cialit (1 in 5000) have been used in tympanic membrane reconstruction [33, 34].

The place of allograft tympanic membrane in myringoplasty remains debatable, and its use is only rarely indicated in patients with an intact and functioning malleus handle. The allograft drumhead with attached malleus is useful for patients with total loss of the tympanic membrane in addition to absence or defect of the malleus handle. The chance of success in transplantation of cadaver tympanic membranes is increased by attention to factors that improve the resistance of the graft (fixation in buffered formaldehyde, selection of a sclerotic drum), that allow adequate surgical exposure, that facilitate positioning of the graft (retaining a cuff of meatal periosteum attached to the annulus) and that speed up epithelialization (covering the allograft with an autogenous meatal skin graft).

Allograft dura is a very strong mesodermal graft usefully used in the closure of perforations where the site of the perforation (over the Eustachian tube) or the nature of the causative injury (welding spark burn) renders the usual temporalis fascial graft liable to breakdown.

Role of the graft

Mesodermal grafts serve as a supporting framework for the regeneration of the new tympanic membrane. The success of grafting is related to the blood supply available to the graft from the periphery and to the rate of epithelial migration over both medial and lateral surfaces of the graft. The rate of vascularization and epithelialization of the graft surfaces is accelerated by preserving the maximum of healthy marginal epithelium with its blood supply and by implanting the graft material between the mucosal and squamous epithelial layers of the recipient's tympanic membrane remnants. The most critical stage for allograft necrosis seems to be about 6 days after operation [31].

Myringoplasty in the wet ear

In the early 1960s grafting of perforations of tympanic membrane was attempted only if the ear had been dry for a period of 6 months but this may not always be possible to obtain without surgery. More than half of Smyth's patients came to operation with frank purulent otorrhoea [35]. Increasing experience of tympanoplasty has shown that whether the ear is wet or dry makes little difference to the outcome provided that operation is postponed during an acute infection.

Age limits for grafting

Grafts can be successfully applied to the perforated tympanic membrane of patients of all ages. Since the presence of the perforation in the tympanic membrane is often an important factor in the chronicity of tubotympanic disease, tympanoplasty in early childhood can be justified, and often gives gratifying results provided that social factors are not adverse. Tympanoplasty exerts a healing effect upon the middle ear mucosa in that the secretory activity of the epithelium diminishes and there is almost certainly a reduced liability to the later development of tympanosclerosis and ossicular fixation.

Complications of grafting

(1) Blunting or obliteration of the anterior tympanomeatal angle by fibrous tissue;

(2) excessive fibrous thickening of the grafted membrane;

(3) failure of the reconstructed tympanic membrane to retain an attachment along the whole length of the malleus handle with consequent lateralization of the grafted area;

(4) the formation of retraction pockets due to intratympanic adhesions, vacuum or lack of support;

(5) persistent perforation due to graft necrosis or technical failure; and

(6) the late appearance of epidermoid inclusion cysts – superficial or deep – from remnants of stratified squamous epithelium inadvertently retained on the malleus, tympanic membrane remnants or deep canal wall and covered by the graft.

Incidence of complications

The incidence of complications from grafting is greatest with onlay techniques, and least with underlay or interleaf techniques.

Graft acceptance is very high with both onlay and interleaf techniques. The risk of residual perforation is greater with inlay techniques for subtotal defects unless special care is taken to ensure adhesion of the graft to the peripheral remnant of the tympanic membrane particularly anteriorly.

Lateralization of graft from the malleus handle and blunting or obliteration of the sharp anterior and inferior tympanomeatal angle is exceptional with underlay or interleaf techniques, but is quite common (about 20%) with onlay techniques (Fig 11.6). The risk of epidermoid inclusion cysts of the deep variety is greater with onlay techniques than with underlay methods. These cysts gradually enlarge and eventually bulge the tympanic membrane outwards into the auditory meatus. Inclusion epidermoids after interleaf methods are usually superficial.

Ossiculoplasty

The middle ear is an impedance matching device by which the molecular vibrations of air are transmitted to the perilymph of the cochlea through the tympanic membrane and ossicular chain. The functional significance of the three-bone mammalian ear compared with the one- or two-bone columella of birds and reptiles is unknown but the columella-like prosthesis frequently used in middle ear reconstruction is as efficient a procedure for clinical purposes as the more complicated tympano-ossicular systems.

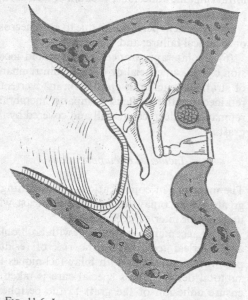

Fig. 11.6. Lateralization of the graft from the malleus handle and blunting of the inferior tympanomeatal angle after onlay grafting methods. (By courtesy of Professor Dietrich Plester.)

The reconstruction of the absent, damaged or fixed ossicular chain to restore transmission of vibrations from the tympanic membrane to the stapes footplate is known as ossiculoplasty.

Basic situations for ossiculoplasty

There are five basic situations in middle-ear reconstruction.

(1) *The ossicular chain is functioning normally, but the tympanic membrane is defective.* Closure of the perforation restores the sound pressure transformer to normal (Type 1 tympanoplasty).

(2) *The incus is partially or totally defective, but*

the stapes is normal. Here a connection is established between the head of the stapes and the malleus handle or tympanic membrane. These procedures are respectively named malleo-stapediopexy and myringo-stapediopexy.

(3) *The stapes footplate is mobile but the crura are absent.* Connections are made between stapes footplate and malleus, tympanic membrane or incus depending on the circumstances. These procedures are respectively called malleoplatinopexy, myringoplatinopexy or incudoplatinopexy.

(4) *The stapes footplate is fixed.* If it is not possible to mobilize the footplate of the stapes stapedectomy or footplate fenestration is required at a second stage when the tympanic membrane and middle ear are healed. The mobile malleus handle or long process of the incus is used to connect the prosthesis to the tissue graft sealing the oval window after stapedectomy. These procedures are known as malleovestibulopexy or incudovestibulopexy respectively.

(5) *The whole ossicular system is absent.* Either a monobloc tympano-ossicular implant can be used or an allograft tympanic membrane with the malleus handle and columella interposition as a one- or two-stage procedure.

Anatomical and functional considerations in ossiculoplasty

Reconstruction of the tympanic membrane precedes any attempt to reconstitute the ossicular chain because it is easier to position the elements of the new ossicular chain precisely once the tympanic membrane graft is in place and stabilized, and in certain situations such as gross mucosal damage, stapes fixation and uncertainty about removal of all cholesteatoma matrix, the ossicular replacement is postponed until the tympanic membrane is intact and the condition of the middle ear is favourable.

The perpendicular axis from the stapes footplate passes outwards through the posterior tympanic ring. Columellar ossicular implants of bone thus tend to fix to the posterior wall of the tympanum at the bony annulus unless the posterosuperior portion of the tympanic ring is removed by a curette to allow proper centring of the prosthesis.

The distance between the head of the stapes and the undersurface of the tympanic membrane is normally about 3 mm. Any prosthesis used to span the gap between the tympanic membrane and the head of the stapes must have this length if it is to be effective. The lateral dimension of the body of the incus is only 2 mm, so that methods of incus interposition that apply the lateral surface of the body of incus to the stapes head may not allow good transmission.

The placement of an incus prosthesis between the tympanic membrane and the head of the stapes or between the tympanic membrane and the footplate gives support for the tympanic membrane in that area (behind the malleus handle) most prone to retraction pocket formation.

The line connecting the stapes footplate with the umbo of the malleus handle passes close to the promontory. Fixation of a malleus-footplate columella to the walls of the oval window niche can occur, especially if this is narrow.

The columellar system is unable to compensate against sudden changes in barometric pressure if there is tubal malfunction. Accordingly, there can be a risk of protrusion of a columella through the tympanic membrane, or a subluxation of stapes into the vestibule with fistula formation and sensorineural hearing loss.

The columella may slip from its proper position because of the mechanical forces of healing or because of sustained negative middle ear pressure.

In contrast to the columella, the tympano-ossicular implant used with combined approach tympanotomy is said to retain the advantages of elasticity to compensate for abnormal static pressure imbalances.

Implant materials

Many materials have been used to replace the ossicular chain:

Autografts: remodelled auditory ossicles, bone from the mastoid cortex, tragal and septal cartilage.

Allografts: cadaver ossicles and septal cartilage, complete tympano-ossicular transplants.

Wire and plastics: stainless steel and tantalum wire, polyethylene, teflon, silicone rubber and Plasti-Pore® struts.

Apart from the complete allograft tympano-ossicular complex, all other materials are used as a columella directly from malleus-tympanic membrane to stapes-oval window. The columellar implant must avoid touching the walls of the middle ear if later fixation is to be avoided. The columella should be stable in position if later displacements are to be prevented, and this can usually only be achieved if the prosthesis is placed securely in contact with the medial aspect of the malleus handle or in contact with the tympanic membrane immediately posterior to the malleus handle. Development of adhesions can limit the function of the system, so that many otologists place implants of silicone rubber sheeting within the middle ear to prevent this happening after ossiculoplasty.

A few further comments about various materials would seem necessary.

Autogenous ossicles if carious or covered by cholesteatoma matrix must be discarded and should never be used for ossiculoplasty.

Preserved allograft ossicles, especially the incus, continue to play an increasingly useful role in middle ear reconstruction and are highly recommended. They may be remodelled by drilling to suit individual requirements. They are well tolerated and show little alteration to their shape, volume or quality over many years (Fig. 11.7).

Mastoid cortex bone, shaped as an incus or strut, can undergo serious changes in its surface form and volume within 2 years of its transposition, and is therefore not recommended.

Preserved allograft cartilage is not entirely suitable for reconstruction because it may soften and buckle, and it has a high incidence of later necrosis, especially in the presence of an active middle ear inflammation. Many otologists find it necessary to insert stainless steel wire into nasal septal cartilage to give it rigidity.

Wire of stainless steel or tantalum may be used to create an attachment between the malleus handle and the neck of the stapes (malleo-stapediopexy) or between the malleus and stapes footplate (malleo-platinopexy) particularly when the oval window niche is rather narrow, or when the facial canal overhangs the oval window niche.

Wire, however, is technically more difficult to use than an allograft incus interposition.

Plastic struts of various types tend to slip or to extrude through the tympanic membrane. A new porous high-density plastic material (Plasti-Pore®) has been developed in an attempt to avoid these problems in the short and long term.

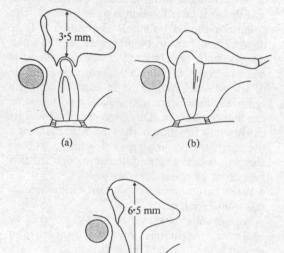

FIG. 11.7. Practical methods of ossiculoplasty with an allograft incus. (a) Myringo-stapediopexy. (b) Malleo-platinopexy. (c) Myringo-platinopexy.

Problems of tympanoplasty

Eustachian tube occlusion

Failure to demonstrate patency of the Eustachian tube before operation should direct the surgeon's attention to the anterior part of the mesotympanum because some cases of tubal blockage are easily remedied by removal of mucosal polyps, a cholesteatoma sac or a membranous diaphragm from the tubal orifice.

Permanent stricture or occlusion of the osseous part of the auditory tube is fortunately uncommon because it precludes a successful outcome.

Tubal malfunction, due to oedema of the tubal lining, often improves after tympanoplasty. It is desirable to explain, and stress the importance of, adequate middle ear ventilation to the patient before operation, and to teach him how to do the Valsalva manoeuvre. Even children under the age of 10 years can learn how to inflate their own tubes. Valsalva's manoeuvre is required only for those patients whose mucosa has been extensively damaged by the disease or by the operation and in whom the risk of postoperative adhesions is increased.

Several procedures have been advocated for tubal stenosis which can be demonstrated radiographically by radio-opaque dyes.

1. *Dilatation of the tube by the passage of bougies;* this is rarely successful.

2. *Insertion of silicone rubber or polyethylene tubing* down the auditory tube for a period of several weeks. This is worth a trial especially when the occlusion is at the protympanum.

3. *Middle fossa Eustachian tuboplasty.* A surgical procedure necessitating middle fossa craniotomy and elevation of the temporal lobe of the brain for reconstruction of the osseous portion of the Eustachian tube when it is obstructed by bone or fibrous tissue has been described and reported as restoring tubal function in six patients [36].

4. *Tympanomaxillary shunt.* The creation of a permanent communication between the middle ear and the maxillary air sinus by means of silicone rubber tube of 1·2 mm internal diameter has been reported as successful in four patients [37].

Middle ear fibrosis and chronic adhesive process

The presence of a non-aerated middle ear cleft due to collapse and adhesion of the atrophic tympanic membrane to the medial wall of the tympanum, or to the filling of the middle ear cavity with fibrous tissue are conditions which many otologists would prefer to leave alone and manage by prescribing a suitable hearing aid for the patient when this seems necessary.

In some of these patients the anterior part of the middle ear is still ventilated through a patent Eustachian tube. Careful exploration of the ear to elevate the collapsed atrophic tympanic membrane, to create a plane of cleavage to the aerated protympanum, to allow insertion of a stiff cadaver tympanic membrane with suitable implants of silicone rubber on the promontory can then make re-aeration of the middle ear possible. Ossiculoplasty is delayed for 8–12 months until the ear seems stable.

Sensorineural deafness

Sensorineural hearing loss is measured before operation by BC threshold audiometry and is a predictor of the best level of hearing that can be attained by any patient after surgical correction of the conductive mechanism of the middle ear. If the cochlear reserve is poor ossiculoplasty is not justifiable.

Sensorineural deafness occurring unexpectedly after uncomplicated myringoplasty may be due to the inadvertent pooling of antiseptics within the middle ear cavity and round window niche during the surgical preparation of the ear. All antiseptics are potentially ototoxic, and combinations of detergents with alcohol greatly increase the risk of toxic effects. Solutions of Hibitane and Savlon, and the tinctures of Metaphen and Zephiran are especially dangerous [38].

Sensorineural deafness can occur during tympanoplasty from inadvertent trauma to the intact ossicular chain by a cutting burr, from subluxation of the stapes footplate during ossiculoplasty, from exposure of the labyrinthine lumen during removal of cholesteatoma matrix, or from elective stapedectomy when the risk may be as high as 10%. Connective tissue grafts must be applied immediately to seal any fistula or the open oval window. A protective fascial graft over the mobile stapes footplate is recommended before placing an ossicular columella.

Results of tympanoplasty

Some of the many factors that can influence the result of a tympanoplasty operation have been mentioned already. Reliable long-term statistics of large series of tympanoplasties that have been carefully analysed at various times after operation to determine their mean audiometric bone–air gaps and variances and to relate these to the many variables such as

(1) the pathological condition for which surgery was indicated;

(2) the type of reconstructive procedure used; and

(3) time-lapse after operation;

and on which the outcome of the operation may depend are not readily available. This is possibly because of the near-Herculean effort required to mount such a survey, because the number of patients available for follow-up decreases with the passing of time, and because the great number of variables in tympanoplasty that can affect the outcome of operation makes interpretation of results difficult without multivariate statistical analysis.

Stapedectomy for otosclerosis, in skilled hands, gives stable long-term results, because the middle ear cleft is not infected. Stapedectomy therefore establishes a base line of early and long-term results from which to assess tympanoplasty.

A dry ear and successful grafting of defects of the tympanic membrane can now be achieved for over 95% of patients. The problem of long-term recurrence of cholesteatoma remains. If tubal function is adequate, if the middle ear mucosa is of good quality and heals without adhesions, and if the sensorineural reserve is satisfactory, hearing gains after tympanoplasty can be anticipated in nine out of ten patients with a Type 1 defect, and in six to eight patients out of ten where the ossicular chain requires a reconstruction (Type 2). In the classical Type 3 reconstruction, six or seven patients out of ten achieve initial good results provided the anatomical conditions are such as to allow the stapes head to tent the graft lateral to the facial canal. In these cases it is necessary to lower the posterior canal wall severely to achieve this. The narrow middle ear, however, is prone to develop adhesive process if any further attacks of middle ear inflammation occur.

The most frequent cause of unsuccessful tympanoplasty is now partial or complete closure of the Eustachian tube, but this is encountered in only a small percentage of patients.

References

[1] Tos M. (1974) Tubal function and tympanoplasty. *The Journal of Laryngology and Otology* **88,** 1113.

[2] MORIZONO T., JOHNSTONE B. M. & NG P. (1974) Ototoxicity of topical antibiotics. *Journal of the Oto-Laryngological Society of Australia* 3, 666.

[3] JANSEN C. (1963) Cartilage-tympanoplasty. *Laryngoscope* 73, 1288.

[4] JANSEN C. (1968) The combined approach for tympanoplasty. *The Journal of Laryngology and Otology* 82, 779.

[5] JAKO G. J. (1966) The posterior bony ear canal wall and the antrum threshold angle in conservative middle-ear surgery. *Laryngoscope* 76, 1260.

[6] MARQUET J. (1971) Human middle ear transplants. *The Journal of Laryngology and Otology* 85, 523.

[7] PORTMANN M. (1968) Open or closed technique in surgery of the middle ear. *The Annals of Otology, Rhinology and Laryngology* 77, 927.

[8] SHEEHY J. L. & PATTERSON M. E. (1967) Intact canal wall tympanoplasty with mastoidectomy. *Laryngoscope* 77, 1502.

[9] SMYTH G. L. D. (1962) A preliminary report of a technique in tympanoplasty designed to eliminate the cavity problem. *The Journal of Laryngology and Otology* 76, 460.

[10] SMYTH G. D. L., ENGLAND R. M., GIBSON R. & KERR A. G. (1967) Posterior tympanotomy: its importance in combined approach tympanoplasty. *The Journal of Laryngology and Otology* 81, 69.

[11] SCHNEE I. M. (1963) Tympanoplasty: A modification in technique. *Archives of Otolaryngology* 77, 87.

[12] LAPIDOT A. & BRANDOW E. C. (1966) A method for preserving the posterior canal wall and bridge in the surgery for cholesteatoma. *Acta Oto-Laryngologica* 62, 88.

[13] GUILFORD F. R. (1971) *Clinical Otology*, eds. Paparella M. M., Hoffmann A. & Huff J. S., Chap. 13, p. 128. Saint Louis: C. V. Mosby Co.

[14] RICHARDS S. & KILBY D. (1971) Mastoidectomy using an osteoplastic flap. *The Journal of Laryngology and Otology* 85, 1007.

[15] WULLSTEIN S. R. (1974) Osteoplastic epitympanotomy. *The Annals of Otology, Rhinology and Laryngology* 83, 663.

[16] WEINBERG J. & SADÉ J. (1971) Post-operative cholesteatoma recurrence through the posterior wall. *The Journal of Laryngology and Otology* 85, 1189.

[17] SHEEHY J. L. & CRABTREE J. A. (1973) Tympanoplasty: staging the operation. *Laryngoscope* 83, 1594.

[18] PLESTER D. (1961) Problems of tympanoplasty. *The Journal of Laryngology and Otology* 75, 879.

[19] GACEK R. R. (1974) The management of labyrinthine fistulae in chronic otitis media with cholesteatoma. *The Annals of Otology, Rhinology and Laryngology* 83, Supplement No. 10.

[20] SHEEHY J. L. (1970) The intact canal wall technique in management of aural cholesteatoma. *The Journal of Laryngology and Otology* 84, 1.

[21] GRISTWOOD R. E. & VENABLES W. N. (1976) Growth rate and recurrence of residual epidermoid cholesteatoma after tympanoplasty. *Clinical Otolaryngology* 1, 169.

[22] HALL A. & RYTZNER C. (1957) Stapedectomy and auto-transplantation of ossicles. *Acta Oto-Laryngologica* 47, 318.

[23] MARQUET J. (1966) Reconstructive micro-surgery of the eardrum by means of a tympanic membrane homograft. *Acta Oto-Laryngologica* 62, 459.

[24] HOUSE W. F., PATTERSON M. E. & LINTHICUM F. R. JR. (1966) Incus homografts in chronic ear surgery. *Archives of Otolaryngology* 84, 148.

[25] PULEC J. L. (1966) Homograft incus. Symposium on tympanoplasty. *Laryngoscope* 76, 1429.

[26] HILDYARD V. H. (1967) Transplant of incus homograft in the human. *Archives of Otolaryngology* 86, 294.

[27] HILDMANN H. & STEINBACH E. (1971) Experimental studies on closing of artificial eardrum perforations in rabbits. *The Journal of Laryngology and Otology* 85, 1173.

[28] SMYTH G. D. L., KERR A. G. & GOODEY R. J. (1971) Tympanic membrane homograft: further evaluation. *The Journal of Laryngology and Otology* 85, 891.

[29] MARQUET J. F. E. (1975) Homografts in middle ear surgery – ten years of experience. *Transactions of American Academy of Ophthalmology and Otolaryngology* 80, 30.

[30] HILDMANN H., STEINBACH E. & KOBURG E. (1974) The fate of bone transplants in the middle ear. *The Journal of Laryngology and Otology* 88, 531.

[31] MARQUET J., SCHEPENS P. & KUIJPERS W. (1973) Experiences with tympanic transplants. *Archives of Otolaryngology* 97, 57.

[32] PLESTER D. (1971) In *Clinical Otology*, eds. Paparella M. M., Hohmann A. & Huff J. S., Chap. 12, p. 120. St. Louis: C. V. Mosby Co.

[33] PERKINS R. (1970) Homograft tympanic membrane with suture sling. *Laryngoscope* 80, 1100.

[34] MARQUET J. (1973) Homografts in surgery of the ear. In *Otorhinolaryngology, Proceedings of the X World Congress, Venice, 1973.*, Arslan M. & Ricci V., p. 245.

[35] SMYTH G. D. L., KERR A. G. & GOODEY R. J. (1971) Current thoughts on combined approach tympanoplasty. Part I. Indications and pre-operative assessment. *The Journal of Laryngology and Otology* 85, 205.

[36] GLASSOCK M. E. & HOUSE W. F. (1970) Middle fossa Eustachian tuboplasty. *Otolaryngologic Clinics of North America,* 3, 111.

[37] DRETTNER B. & EKVALL L. (1970) Chronic obstruction of the Eustachian tube treated with a tympano-maxillary shunt. *Acta Otolaryngologica* 263, 29.

[38] MORIZONO T., JOHNSTONE B. M. & HADJAR E. (1973) The ototoxicity of antiseptics. *Journal of the Oto-Laryngological Society of Australia* 3, 550.

CHAPTER 12

Intracranial Complications of Ear Disease

MENINGITIS

Of all tissues of the body the central nervous system offers the least resistance to infection. Micro-organisms which are feebly pathogenic if they gain access to the brain may cause intracranial infection with fatal consequences.

Pathology

With the advent of antibiotics the mortality rate of bacterial meningitis has dropped sharply. It is unfortunate, however, that inappropriate therapy and diagnostic delay have not totally eliminated both a significant mortality and severe morbidity. Also, widespread use of antibiotics makes the identification of the responsible organism impossible in many patients with purulent meningitis. Virtually any pathogen gaining access to the central nervous system may cause meningitis. However, for practical clinical purposes there are two broad categories.

(1) Infants and young children – mostly *H. influenza, N. meningiditis,* and unknown in equal proportions with a low incidence of pneumococci.

(2) Older children and adults – highest incidence in these age groups of meningococci, pneumococci, *Streptococcus pyogenes* and a smaller but definite involvement of *Staphylococcus pyogenes.*

Infection of the meninges normally comes from the blood-stream. This is the usual sequence in meningococcal and some cases of pneumococcal meningitis. Local sources of infection cause a significant number of cases mostly from the middle ear, mastoid, paranasal air sinuses, from scalp and facial lesions and from intracranial trauma. Pneumococci and streptococci are organisms usually found in these instances.

Clinical features

The classical features of an acute illness are headache, photophobia, altered states of consciousness, nuchal rigidity and constitutional upset and need not be further elaborated here. Diagnosis is confirmed by lumbar puncture. It is important to carry out a comprehensive analysis of the cerebrospinal fluid so obtained. Every effort should be made to identify the infecting organism whether by spinal fluid or blood culture or from any local source of infection.

An accurate analysis of the cellular pattern present and an evaluation of the protein and sugar levels together with bacteriological findings should clarify any differential diagnosis such as aseptic meningeal reactions, meningism, etc.

Treatment

The principles of therapy of meningitis are well established, including general support, specific antibiotics and the eradication of any local source of infection. Whether regular intrathecal antibiotics should be used is a matter of contention. We would recommend this in the more severely ill.

Finally, the possible long-term sequelae must be kept in mind, in particular cranial nerve palsies such as deafness, facial palsies, etc. For these patients very little can be done but the other major complication, hydrocephalus, can be arrested by an appropriate ventricular bypass procedure with a valve-regulated shunt.

BRAIN ABSCESS AND SUBDURAL EMPYEMA

Macewen in 1893 [1] claimed that if an uncomplicated abscess of the brain is diagnosed at a relatively early stage recovery ought to be the rule. Few would agree with this view today. Ever since the turn of the century surgeons have been trying to equal his results – one death out of fifteen cases. Despite the advent of antibiotics and very considerable advances in diagnostic and surgical techniques the mortality associated with brain abscess and subdural empyema remains unacceptably high. Reports of mortality vary from 40% to 60% [2–4] for suprasellar abscesses. Posterior fossa abscesses fare equally badly with mortality figures of around 55% in some series plus a significant morbidity in survivors. Late referral and delay in instituting radical therapy account for a high proportion of deaths. The most important factor influencing survival is the relief of raised intracranial pressure by surgical means while the patient is neurologically alert [6].

Pathology

Since the introduction of antibiotics there has been a steady diminution in the number of brain abscesses due to ear disease and a rise in the proportion due to pulmonary infection with haematogenous spread. In spite of this, however, one series [8] showed that although otogenic causes are low the temporal lobe continues to be a favourite site for abscess formation. Since these are usually of otogenic origin, the reasons for the discrepancy must be a matter of speculation. Nevertheless the ear is the commonest source of a cerebellar abscess and the paranasal sinuses of a subdural empyema [5, 7]. In over 80% of otitic abscesses the ear disease is chronic, however, in many an acute exacerbation of the ear disease occurs at or about the time intracranial complications occur. It is twice as common for ear disease to infect the temporal lobe as the cerebellum. 'Haematogenous' brain abscesses are due to endocarditis and pyaemia from foci of suppuration anywhere in the body; a small proportion complicate cyanotic heart disease particularly with right to left shunts giving rise to so-called paradoxical emboli.

A great diversity of micro-organisms have been found in brain abscesses, *Staphylococcus aureus* and a diversity of streptococci being the most common. The pus often contains more than one organism or may even be sterile. The sensitivity of the organism is of primary importance in planning a rational antibiotic policy.

Infection penetrates the skull by two routes:

(1) via naturally-occurring portals such as the olfactory foraminae, the labyrinth, the internal auditory meatus and the vestibular aqueduct, via suture lines or via fracture lines.

(2) after the development of an area of localized osteomyelitis by spread through veins penetrating the dura.

The dura offers considerable resistance to the spread of infection, but penetration probably takes place along small vessels which traverse its thickness. If the wall of a venous sinus is involved thrombosis may ensue. Purulent exudate may then form on the inner surface of the infected dura giving rise to a subdural empyema. The exact manner whereby the brain is infected from a source in the middle ear is speculative, occasionally the brain is adherent to an area of infected dura in which case the abscess then involves the pia-arachnoid and the cerebral cortex. But the usual cerebral abscess develops in subcortical white matter. Initially an area of suppurative encephalitis develops with very considerable oedema, necrosis of the centre of infection and liquefaction. The so-called wall of the abscess is developed from fibroblasts derived from proliferating capillaries, and is of variable thickness, being thinnest in the deeper subcortical regions. This area of the cavity is the weakest and expansion tends to be towards the ventricles with possible subsequent catastrophic rupture. Multilocular lesions are common. Profound cerebral oedema is a major problem in all cerebral abscesses.

In the cerebellar otogenic abscess the abscess is attached to the dura superior, anterior and medial to the internal auditory meatus at the site of the venous connections between the inferior and superior petrosal sinuses [8].

The cause of a cerebral abscess to a very large degree determines the site of the lesion. The commonest abscess is of the frontal lobe arising from the infected sinuses, facial sepsis and facial injuries. Otogenic lesions are either temporal or cerebellar. Parietal abscesses are usually haematogenous.

Clinical features

Three groups of symptoms are usual, namely intracranial hypertension, focal signs and systemic upset.

Features of raised intracranial pressure dominate the picture and usually determine the outcome. Headache is the most frequent and significant initial complaint. It is suboccipital in cerebellar lesions but is not lateralizing in supratentorial lesions. Infection of the frontal sinus or ear very often gives rise to severe local pain, but the development of a brain abscess leads to a change in the distribution and nature of the pain which becomes more widespread and may alter with posture. Vomiting is a feature of cerebellar lesions. Confusion, lethargy and coma are due to increasing pressure and the development of internal brain shifts and herniae. These ominous features may present at a varying rate sometimes with startling rapidity. Papilloedema is inconstant and may be absent in the fulminating case.

The physical signs of transtentorial herniation may dominate the picture and conceal localizing signs. In particular, pupillary abnormalities and oculomotor palsies signify considerable urgency. Epilepsy is another common feature, but only focal attacks are of localizing value. A hemiparesis may be caused either by a posterior frontal abscess but may well be due to herniation. A contralateral quadrantic hemianopia is a feature of an otogenic temporal lobe abscess, and dysphasia is a valuable localizing sign, but the patient's condition may make it impossible to detect these two signs. Nystagmus with ataxia and defective conjugate eye movements are features of cerebellar lesions but again these findings may be difficult to elicit and evaluate in the very ill patient.

The degree of systemic upset is very variable: most patients are pyrexial with evidence of infection (increased sedimentation rate, leucocytosis, and increased polymorphonuclear cells in peripheral blood smears). The development of meningitis significantly increases these clinical features.

Special investigations

A number of diagnostic techniques have been evaluated in the literature [2, 9, 10]. Early and accurate diagnosis is a primary requirement because of the unpredictable behaviour of a patient with an abscess. A wide range of investigations are available but many are of neither diagnostic or localizing value, and since they usually increase the delay they should be avoided.

(1) *Plain radiographs* of the skull and chest are mandatory. In the skull views the presence of a calcified pineal may be very helpful in determining a midline shift. Mastoid and sinus views may help in establishing evidence of a primary source as may a chest radiograph.

(2) *Electroencephalography* (EEG) can give considerable help and serial observations in the doubtful case are useful. It has no localizing value in posterior fossa abscesses.

(3) *Radioisotope brain scanning* (Fig. 12.1) is of great value but suboccipital muscle can obscure the picture over the cerebellum. The technique is rapid without risk and so repeated scans may be carried out without morbidity.

(4) *Computerized transverse axial tomography* (EMI scan). This technique is of the greatest value in the localization and diagnosis of a space-occupying lesion [11]. It is non-invasive, has no morbidity and is rapid. With iodine enhancement its accuracy is increased (Fig. 12.2). This method is vastly superior to the EEG isotope scanning and it may be better than arteriography. Posterior fossa lesions are well demonstrated and the degree of internal herniation can also be assessed. Finally it can be used after operation to evaluate progress.

(5) *Arteriography* is the main investigation recommended at present – shifts, avascular areas and capillary blush are the features of an abscess, but its accuracy has been questioned [2] (Fig. 12.3).

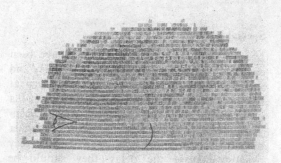

FIG. 12.1. Radioisotope brain scan with ^{99m}Tc. Lateral vein showing marked increase in uptake in frontal region.

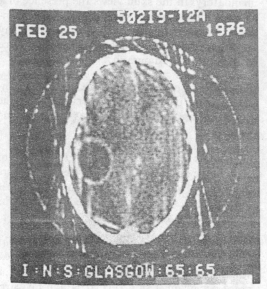

FIG. 12.2. Computerized axial tomogram showing clear temporal lobe abscess after iodine enhancement. (Courtesy of Dr. J. Stevens, Institute of Neural Sciences, Glasgow.)

(6) *Ventriculography* for many years was the mainstay of diagnosis and is recommended only as a last resort particularly in the diagnosis of a posterior fossa abscess. It has an undoubted morbidity and mortality.

(7) *A lumbar puncture* should not be performed because it is dangerous in this condition, it lacks localizing information and can be frankly misleading.

The sequence of investigations at present recommended therefore is: plain radiographs of skull and chest followed by an EMI scan with enhancement. If the latter is not available then do an EEG and a radioisotope scan.

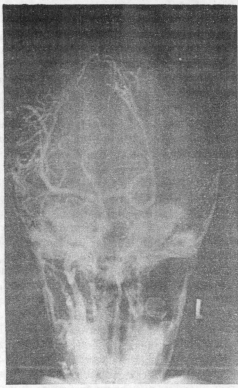

FIG. 12.3. Right carotid arteriogram showing substantial midline displacement of anterior cerebral artery, the appearances are those of a frontal mass.

All these investigations should be accomplished within a few hours of suspecting the diagnosis. Arteriography which may be quite superfluous at this stage should be done if in doubt.

Treatment

The brain abscess
Over many years several techniques have evolved for the treatment of brain abscess. Initially simple aspiration via a burrhole was used but in the 1930s excision of the lesion seemed to give better results. Whether these abscesses are best

treated by aspiration, drainage or excision has been a recurrent theme of many reports and no controlled approach has ever been adopted to resolve this controversy. In addition, advances in diagnostic therapeutic techniques make it impossible to compare different series [3, 4, 6, 8]. A complete excision via a craniotomy is more likely to be achieved if the abscess has a well-developed capsule, and this feature *per se* improves the survival rate. Where the abscess involves vital areas whose removal causes severe neurological deficit, aspiration and drainage are probably preferable. If the latter course of therapy is adopted progress can be followed with pyograms using microbarium suspension (Fig. 12.4). There is no evidence that intracavity antibiotics are of value but appropriate very substantial doses of broad spectrum antibiotics should be started as for a patient with meningitis while a definite diagnosis is being established and until bacteriological results are available. Penetration of the abscess by a wide variety of antibiotics is effective provided sufficiently high blood levels are present [12]. Anticonvulsants, steroids and cerebral dehydrating agents, e.g. mannitol, are adjuvant lines of treatment.

The primary focus

If the source of infection is known this must be treated appropriately, but brain abscess constitutes the immediate threat to life and must be accorded priority. Suppuration in the paranasal sinuses or in the ear should be eradicated as soon as the patient's condition allows it. A radical mastoidectomy has been recommended after the intracranial procedure under the same anaesthetic [13]. Bone should be resected to the point at which the abscess is attached to the dura if this is the case and is mandatory if extradural pus has been found. Drainage of the intracranial infection through a mastoidectomy is not recommended.

A final comment should be made on subdural abscess which is a very sinister complication of sinusitis. Symptoms may be sudden due to focal seizures or more insidious with headaches and depression of consciousness. A hemiparesis is the risk because pus in the subdural space has a profoundly paralysing effect on the underlying brain [14]. An acute subdural abscess is one of the

most imperative neurosurgical emergencies. The principles of diagnosis and therapy are the same as for intracerebral abscess but the urgency is very much greater [4, 7].

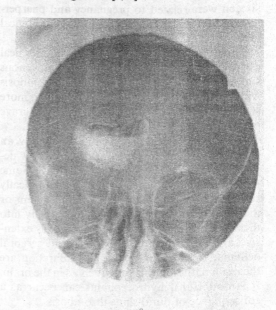

FIG. 12.4. Subfrontal abscess – pyogram after drainage and instillation of microbarium suspension.

CEREBRAL THROMBOPHLEBITIS AND DURAL SINUS THROMBOSIS

The clinical syndromes caused by thrombosis of the cerebral venous system vary as do all cerebrovascular diseases and are similarly dependent on the site, extent and speed of the obstructive process. The evolution of present day concepts of dural sinus thrombosis and thrombophlebitis has been extensively documented [15].

Pathology

The main aetiological factor in the development of dural sinus thrombosis is the presence of an adjacent septic focus, namely facial sepsis and cavernous sinus lesions, middle ear and mastoid infections and transverse sinus lesions. Sagittal sinus thrombosis is, however, more frequently idiopathic, but may be secondary to frontal osteomyelitis, sinusitis or compound skull fractures.

Krayenbuhl [16] reported seventy-three cases of which thirty were secondary to infection, sixteen were related to pregnancy and puerperium and fifteen had no demonstrable aetiological factor.

There are no valves or other anatomical obstructions between the intracranial venous sinuses and therefore a focal sinus thrombosis with few clinical signs may easily extend to more strategic areas with florid features and a grave prognosis.

If the pathological process is relatively slow an adequate collateral venous drainage may develop and limit the degree of brain damage. Some patients do not, however, have an anatomically sufficiently well-developed collateral system or the thrombotic process extends too rapidly into these channels. In these brain damage is extensive and frequently fatal. Widespread cerebral oedema, focal haemorrhage and infarction are the main pathological consequences in the brain. It is doubtful if hydrocephalus can occur as a consequence of dural sinus thrombosis.

Clinical features

There are three main clinical features with considerable overlap.

(1) *Raised intracranial pressure* due to cerebral oedema presenting with headache, drowsiness, vomiting and papilloedema.

(2) *Focal symptoms and signs* – usually heralded by generalized or focal epilepsy, and leading on to hemiparesis and dysphasia. This combination of epilepsy and paralysis is considered to be due to involvement of cortical veins.

(3) *Constitutional disturbance* – hyperpyrexia, tachycardia and leucocytosis. The degree of constitutional upset is very variable and in many instances the development of raised intracranial pressure confuses the interpretation of standard chart recordings.

The differential diagnosis of the above clinical features must include any infective intracranial process such as brain abscess. In addition one should eliminate the possibility of pregnancy, oral contraceptive medication, cerebral haemorrhage and encephalitis.

Special investigations

(1) *Lumbar puncture* – if a brain abscess can be excluded this procedure may have to be performed to exclude meningitis and cerebral bleeding. In severe cases of dural thrombosis xanthochromic cerebrospinal fluid may be present but an elevation of protein, pressure and cells is more usual.

(2) *The EEG* is consistently abnormal, indicating a graver prognosis in patients showing a florid abnormality early in the disease process.

(3) *Arteriography and dural sinus venography* are usually confirmatory of a major sinus obstruction but may be normal, or show a non-specific mid-line shift if focal cerebral oedema due to cortical thrombophlebitis is present.

(4) *The CAT scan* has not yet been evaluated as a diagnostic tool in these conditions.

Treatment

Five separate areas need consideration.

(1) *The raised intracranial pressure* should be vigorously treated with cerebral dehydrating agents, particularly intravenous mannitol. Surgical decompression by use of bitemporal craniotomies is debatable and probably of limited value. High dose steroids are frequently advocated but there is little real proof as to their value.

(2) *Antibiotic therapy* should be used probably in every instance even if a focal infective process has not been detected.

(3) *Epilepsy,* particularly status epilepticus, is the greatest hazard. Effective rapid control of seizures may be secured by the use of intravenous clonazepam and phenytoin. In a very small number of patients controlled ventilation may

help to gain complete remission of the status and improve the incracranial hypertension.

(4) *Anticoagulants* and low molecular weight dextran have been advocated [15, 16]. No cases of intracranial haemorrhage due to anticoagulant treatment have been described.

(5) *Surgery* has only a very restricted role and should be used only in the eradication of the primary focus if one is present and the very few patients requiring bitemporal decompression. A dural sinus thrombectomy is not recommended.

The prognosis of reported series is very variable; probably overall about 30% die and a small proportion of the survivors are disabled by a hemiparesis and epilepsy.

BENIGN INTRACRANIAL HYPERTENSION

Pathology

This condition involves the development of a pure syndrome of intracranial hypertension (i.e. headaches and papilloedema) and virtually no neurological deficits. It has been attributed to a variety of aetiologies but unfortunately some of the terminology used, particularly 'otitic hydrocephalus' has tended to obscure the essential nature of the condition. Ventricular enlargement does not occur; in fact the converse happens. The majority of cases are of unknown cause. In a few transverse sinus thrombosis may be a factor. There is a significant female preponderance with women between 20 and 40 years of age being most affected, but no proven endocrine factor has been described. Steroids are of proven value in the treatment yet in some children on steroids for other reasons the condition may develop.

Investigations

As a large number of space-occupying intracranial lesions present as raised intracranial pressure this condition can only be diagnosed safely by exclusion. Classically in the syndrome of benign intracranial hypertension skull X-rays,

EEG, isotope scan, CAT scan, angiography and ventriculography are all normal. Only the CSF pressure is raised without any other corresponding abnormality in fluid constituents.

Treatment

Treatment is directed at restoring intracranial pressure to normal and thereby protecting the retina from the effects of sustained papilloedema.

The vast majority of patients respond to the use of dehydration with frusemide, or a similar agent, and steroids. In a few, a bitemporal decompression may be needed, and some patients require ventricular-peritoneal shunts with standard valve systems as are used in congenital hydrocephalus. Progress of therapy can be assessed by repeated lumbar punctures, or by careful evaluation of blind spot areas [17].

References

[1] MACEWEN W. (1893) *Pyogenic Infective Diseases of the Brain and Spinal Cord.* Glasgow: Maclehose.
[2] GARFIELD J. (1969) Management of supra-tentorial intracranial abscess; a review of 200 cases. *British Medical Journal* 2, 7.
[3] JOOMA O. V., PENNYBACKER J. B. & TULTON G. K. (1951) Brain abscess, aspiration drainage or excision. *Journal of Neurology, Neurosurgery and Psychiatry* 14, 308.
[4] LE BEAU J., CREISSARD P., HARISPER L. & REDONDO A. (1973) Surgical treatment of brain abscess and subdural empyema. *Journal of Neurosurgery* 38, 198.
[5] SHAW M. D. M. & RUSSELL J. A. (1975) Cerebellar abscess. *Journal of Neurology, Neurosurgery & Psychiatry* 38, 429.
[6] CAREY M. E., CHOU S. N. & FRENCH L. A. (1972) Experience with brain abscesses. *Journal of Neurosurgery* 36, 1.
[7] KAUFMAN D. M., MILLER M. H. & STEIGBIGEL N. H. (1975) Subdural empyema: analysis of 17 recent cases and review of the literature. *Medicine* 54, 485.
[8] KRAYENBÜHL H. A. (1967) Abscesses of the brain. *Clinical Neurosurgery* 14, 25.
[9] SAMSON D. S. & CLARK K. (1973) A current review of brain abscess. *American Journal of Medicine* 54, 210.
[10] HASS R. & LAUBICHLER W. (1967) On the significance of EEG for the diagnosis of brain abscesses. *Acta neurochirurgica* 16, 79.
[11] AMBROSE J., GOODING M. R. & RICHARDSON A. E. (1975) An assessment of the accuracy of computerized transverse axial scanning (EMI Scanner) in the diagnosis of intracranial tumour. *Brain* 78, 569.

[12] BLACK P. J., GRAYBILL J. R. & CHARACHE P. (1973) Penetration of brain abscess by systemic antibiotics. *Journal of Neurosurgery* **38**, 705.

[13] WRIGHT J. L. W. & GRIMALDI P. M. (1973) Otogenic intracranial complications. *Journal of Laryngology and Otolaryngology* **87**, 1085.

[14] SCHILLER F., CAIRNS H. & RUSSELL D. S. (1948) The treatment of purulent patchy meningitis and subdural suppuration with special reference to penicillin. *Journal of Neurology, Neurosurgery and Psychiatry* **11**, 143.

[15] KALBAG R. M. & WOOLF A. L. (1967) *Cerebral Venous Thrombosis.* London: Oxford University Press.

[16] KRAYENBÜHL H. (1967) Cerebral venous and sinus thrombosis. *Clinical Neurosurgery* **14**, 1.

[17] JEFFERSON A. & CLARK J. (1976) Treatment of benign intracranial hypertension by dehydrating agents with particular reference to the measurement of blind spot areas as a means of recording improvement. *Journal of Neurology, Neurosurgery and Psychiatry* **39**, 627.

CHAPTER 13

Ear Infections

While infections of the external ear remain a constant problem in otolaryngological practice, infections of the middle ear have decreased as social and economic standards within the community have improved. The decrease in chronic middle ear diseases in most parts of the developed world has also cut down the incidence of bacterial complications within the inner ear. Viral infections at this site, however, have not diminished.

EXTERNAL EAR

Infections of the external ear and meatus are skin infections which lie within the province of the dermatologist. However, due to their anatomical relationship with the upper respiratory tract they commonly present to the otologist who is also better equipped to examine and treat the external meatus. But if the disease is obviously primarily dermatological with only secondary otologic involvement he should seek the help of the dermatologist, who may help in the management of intractable otitis externa.

The skin is composed of two major layers, the outer epidermis, which is a stratified epithelium with no blood vessels, and the underlying dermis with its fibrous network, rich capillary bed, nerve endings and the epidermal appendages (sweat glands, sebaceous glands and hair follicles). In the region of the pinna and external meatus, the subcutaneous tissue is sparse, leaving little room for inflammatory oedema, hence the association of severe pain with ear infections.

When the skin is involved by the acute inflammatory reaction, the vascular response is restricted to the dermis which becomes hyperaemic and oedematous. The cellular response is concentrated in the epidermis, and causes changes in its various layers producing vesiculation, wet desquamation, dry scaling and hyperkeratosis. In planning management of these conditions it is important to distinguish between the acute and chronic phases of inflammation. In the acute phase, the skin is red and oedematous, with a profuse exudate; pain is also prominent. The principles of treatment are systemic disinfection and local cleansing to remove the exudate and allow recovery of the epidermis. In the chronic phase the patient complains of irritation and the epidermis shows dry scaling, hyperkeratosis and occasional fissure. Local treatment is indicated in this phase – cleansing to remove debris and topical applications to eradicate infection and relieve irritation.

Perichondritis

Perichondritis may follow an infection of the closely applied skin, but it more generally follows trauma, infection in a subperiosteal haematoma or mastoid surgery in an infected ear, in which exposure of the cartilage allows entry of the bacteria, *Pseudomonas pyocyaneus* being the common pathogen. A similar appearance may occur with an allergic reaction to BIPP* packing.

The pinna is uniformly enlarged and inflamed with a shiny surface. Pain is severe and there is often considerable constitutional disturbance. Localized areas of fluctuation indicate subperichondrial abscess.

Treatment
During the acute phase the severe pain may require the use of powerful analgesics and local heat is often soothing. In the presence of hyperaemia, systemic antibiotics give high tissue levels

* Bismuth iodoform paraffin paste.

and treatment should be started with intramuscular penicillin unless a more appropriate antibiotic is indicated by bacteriological investigations. If treatment is prompt full resolution can be expected but if treatment is delayed or inadequate, the onset of the chronic inflammatory process necessitates prolonged treatment, and often the final result is poor due to cartilage necrosis. The appropriate antibiotics must then be continued to prevent spread of the infection. The main aims of the treatment are adequate drainage of the subperichondrial abscess and careful débridement of all necrotic cartilage, followed by frequent careful local dressings.

Otitis externa [1, 2]

Otitis externa can be classified into two main groups:
    (1) Localized otitis externa (furunculosis).
    (2) Diffuse otitis externa.

Furunculosis

Clinical features
This is the infection of one or more of the hair follicles in the cartilaginous meatus; the usual pathogen is the Staphylococcus. It may occur spontaneously but often follows diffuse otitis externa.

The acute inflammation causes oedema of the skin, which may cause painful meatal occlusion. The inflammation often extends over the mastoid process, obliterating the post-auricular sulcus, and may extend anteriorly into the parotid region. There is generally an associated acute lymphadenitis of the adjacent lymph nodes.

The patient often gives a history of previous otitis externa, but the first symptom is a pricking sensation in the ear. This rapidly proceeds to severe pain aggravated by movement of the pinna, and occasionally by opening the mouth. Examination of the ear shows the localized inflammation, and there is an associated conductive deafness if meatal stenosis is present.

Treatment
Pain is relieved by local heat and analgesics. Systemic antibiotics are always necessary due to

the soft tissue infection, and intramuscular penicillin is indicated. Only if the abscess points should it be drained by local incision; otherwise infection may be introduced into the subperichondrial plane. The oedema of the meatus, and hence severe pain, may be relieved by a gently inserted hygroscopic wick of glycerine. This wick should be changed daily and the meatus carefully cleaned of any exudate. With antibiotic therapy recovery is generally rapid, but care of the meatus must be maintained until it returns to normal (see below).

Diffuse otitis externa

There are many predisposing factors of diffuse otitis externa but all exert their action by interference with the normal physiological self-cleansing function of the external auditory meatus.

Skin throughout the body decontaminates itself by the migration of its superficial layers towards the surface in the process of desquamation. Such a mechanism in the deep meatus would soon result in a build-up of squamous debris. This is overcome by a modification of the migration process whereby the superficial layers pass laterally along the meatus as well as superficially to the surface [3]. The secretion of cerumen in the cartilaginous meatus no doubt aids this migration by acting as a 'moisturizing' agent preventing the completion of desquamation before the pinna is reached.

The predominant cause varies from centre to centre. In warmer climates the frequent contamination of the meatus with infected or chlorinated swimming pool water is the usual factor, and otomycosis is common. In temperate zones habitual self-cleaning appears to be the most common cause. It is a common belief that, 'wax is dirty' and the cleaning habit starts with the mother cleaning her baby's ear with the notorious cotton bud. The habit is ingrained by adult life and most patients will admit to regular intrameatal cleaning of their ears. Many of these patients have an obsessional habit of scratching their ears. The removal of the wax has several deleterious effects and initiates a vicious circle of recurrent infections (Fig. 13.1).

The primary effect of cerumen removal is the disturbance of normal desquamation, the epider-

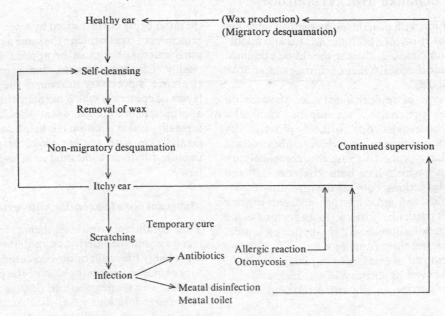

Fig. 13.1. The common pathogenesis and management of diffuse otitis externa

mal layer being shed within the meatus causing irritation, which induces further cleaning or scratching. Cleaning leads to epidermal trauma and in the absence of the protective cerumen infection soon results. The usual pathogens are the staphylococci or streptococci. The acute inflammatory response causes a low-grade otalgia and purulent otorrhoea, but as the infection is localized to the skin there is little constitutional upset. Antibiotics either topically or systemically achieve resolution of the infection, or at least relief of symptoms. If the meatus is full of squamous debris, the pathogen may persist and cause a rapid recrudescence of the infection. Alternatively the infection may resolve completely, but persistence of the self-cleaning habit soon causes a new infection.

As well as the direct spread of dermatosis, skin allergies can be caused by the topical application of ointments and cosmetics such as hair lacquer.

Clinical features
The patient generally presents to the otologist with a history of recurrent otitis externa, or 'itchy' ear. The bacterial flora is often different with mixed infections including Gram-negative organisms and fungi predominating. Examina-

tion of the ear shows an inflamed skin with a purulent exudate in the acute phase; movement of the pinna is often painful indicating involvement of the dermis. In the chronic stage the appearances are often minimal; there may be no discharge and the skin is dry and scaly, and in long-standing cases hypertrophy of the skin may cause meatal stenosis. The presence of fungi may be obvious by the presence of spores but more often the meatus is full of thick moist squamous debris, like blotting paper.

Treatment
The management of this condition has two aims: eradication of the infection, and care of the meatal skin until normal physiology is restored. Resolution of the infection and relief of the patient's symptoms are achieved by topical means, as the pathogen is generally confined to the avascular epidermis but severe cellulitis necessitates systemic disinfection. However, before the topical medication can be applied all exudate and squamous debris must be removed to allow access to the epidermis. This may be achieved by dry mopping, suction clearance or most effectively by gentle irrigation. This is not necessarily contra-indicated in the presence of a

perforation with otorrhoea, as such an infection will already involve both the meatus and middle ear. After cleaning, the ear should be examined to exclude the coexistence of chronic suppurative otitis media.

The type of topical agent used depends on personal preference, but topical antibiotics should be avoided due to the hypersensitivity reactions (neomycin and chloramphenicol are particularly prone to cause this complication). Vioform® which has both bacteriocidal and fungicidal actions, combined with a topical steroid for its anti-inflammatory and anti-pruritic effects is particularly useful. In an acute case, the topical medication should be applied on a wick. The wick has three functions:

(1) removal of exudate by capillary action;

(2) the close application of the drug; and

(3) a barrier to prevent scratching by the patient.

After the acute phase has passed, the medication should be continued as ear drops twice daily and repeated as necessary for relief of irritation. The follow-up depends on the severity of the condition and response to treatment, but in some cases daily supervision is necessary.

The patient must be advised regarding the cause of his complaint; in particular he must be instructed not to get water in his ears and to avoid cleaning or scratching them.

Recovery is generally rapid unless there is an underlying reactive cause. If a straightforward infection does not respond rapidly, bacteriological examination of the discharge should be done and a short course of the appropriate antibiotic given topically. Prolonged courses of antibiotics are unnecessary and predispose to otomycosis.

Following resolution, the patient must be continually supervised until the return of normal physiology is evident by the return of cerumen. Before discharge he must again be counselled regarding the cause and its avoidance.

Otomycosis

This condition is particularly common in tropical and subtropical climates but also follows prolonged local antibiotic therapy which eradicates the normal bacterial flora. The usual pathogenic fungi are *Candida albicans* and *Aspergillus niger*,

the latter being characterized by severe pain. The principles of treatment are the same as for diffuse otitis externa, but must be applied more thoroughly. Cleansing is vital, and gentle suction clearance is necessary to remove the superficial layers of epidermis which harbour the fungi. An appropriate antifungal agent should be used topically, and in addition it is helpful to paint the meatal skin with gentian violet or methiolate tincture for their additional antifungal properties.

Malignant otitis (necrotizing otitis externa) [4]

This condition, which is being increasingly recognized in the elderly and/or diabetic patient, is probably the result of the decreased inflammatory response seen in the skin of the patient due to small vessel atheromatous disease. The infection starts insidiously and is characterized by persistent pain and discharge; the pathogen is *Pseudomonas pyocyaneus* but recent unpublished work indicates that the primary causative organism is an anaerobic bacteria probably of the Bacteroides group. Ulceration or granulation are often seen in the floor of the meatus and the infection can spread to involve the adjacent soft tissues.

A facial palsy is a particularly poor prognostic sign. In the diabetic patient the infection increases insulin requirements and diabetic control becomes difficult. Management requires careful diabetic control, and careful surgical judgement. Chronic perichondritis and osteitis can occur and require wide local débridement under appropriate antibiotic therapy, preferably covering exposed bone with local flaps. In anaerobic infection metronidazole should be used.

Bullous myringitis [5]

This condition is often associated with influenza epidemics and in a few cases influenza A viruses have been isolated. The patient presents with severe otalgia and mild deafness. Examination shows haemorrhagic bullae in the skin of the tympanic membrane and deep meatus. They rupture rapidly releasing a sero-sanguinous fluid. The condition is often complicated by acute otitis media, and rarely meningo-encephalitis. Treatment is with analgesics and topical antiseptic drops to prevent secondary infection.

Herpes infection

Herpes simplex may involve the pinna, although more commonly it is found on the lips. It is preceded by a prickling sensation followed rapidly by vesicles on the skin. It tends to be recurrent and the frequency of recurrence can be reduced by the prompt application of idoxuridine ointment.

MIDDLE EAR

Acute otitis media [2, 6, 7]

Pathology and clinical features
Strictly speaking this term includes all inflammations of the *mucoperiosteal lining* of the middle ear, and includes the viral inflammation that occurs as part of the common cold. This diagnosis is often made by general practitioners in children with upper respiratory tract infections but most otologists prefer to restrict the term to bacterial infections. The usual pathogens are the Gram-positive cocci, but *Haemophilus influenzae* is often found. The inflammatory process involves the lining of the whole of the middle ear, but often some parts are more inflamed than others. It generally results from an ascending infection via the Eustachian tube, following an upper respiratory tract infection. Tubal dysfunction is the main predisposing factor, and those factors which affect this function are listed in Table 13.1. Tubal dysfunction is more common in children and hence otitis media is more often seen at this age.

The effects of the acute inflammation on anatomy and physiology explain the clinical presentation and natural history of the condition. The normal function of the middle ear as an impedance matching mechanism requires it to be filled with air at atmospheric pressure. However, oxygen is being continually absorbed from the middle ear spaces by the blood vessels in its mucosa. To correct this developing negative intratympanic pressure, the Eustachian tube is opened periodically to allow aeration and pressure equalization [8].

A disturbance in the normal aeration of the middle ear may cause a pathological sequence of events leading to acute suppurative otitis media. The progress towards this condition depends on the virulence of the pathogen and the host's resistance. It may be further modified by treatment, but it is useful to study the sequence of events in the untreated ear.

Inflammation of the middle ear mucosa has several effects. The profuse exudation and oedema interfere with ciliary action in the Eustachian tube, and a barrier to infection is lost. The

TABLE 13.1. Factors contributing to Eustachian tube dysfunction

Anatomical variation
1. Tube is shorter, wider and more horizontal in infant
2. Well-pneumatized mastoid provides large volume buffer [8]

Obstruction of lumen
1. Inflammatory oedema from adjacent infection, e.g. adenoiditis, sinusitis, (?) tonsillitis
2. Allergic oedema
3. Nasopharyngeal tumour
4. Post-adenoidectomy adhesions
5. Post-nasal packing

Physiological malfunction
1. Paralysis of tensor palati muscle
2. Cleft palate
   (a) Preoperatively, the cleft divides the common tensor palati aponeurosis
   (b) Postoperatively, hamulotomy removes the fulcrum around which tensor palati works

oedema reduces the lumen and also interferes with the opening of the tube. Hyperaemia of the mucosa increases oxygen absorption, and with decreased aeration rapid collapse of the middle ear occurs with retraction of the tympanic membrane and serous exudation. During this stage of *tubal occlusion* the patient is aware of a fullness in the ear, and examination shows a retracted tympanic membrane with a mild conductive deafness. This stage is commonly reached in viral upper respiratory tract infections, but resolution soon occurs with re-aeration of the middle ear. However, if bacterial superinfection occurs, the serous exudate rapidly becomes purulent and its continued production within the bony confines of the middle ear cleft results in bulging of the tympanic membrane. At the stage of *purulent exudation* the patient complains of severe throbbing pain, there is a constitutional upset with pyrexia and malaise, particularly in children, and the deafness becomes severe. The increase of pressure from the exudate causes avascular necrosis of the mucosa and tympanic membrane with rupture of the latter. At this point there is a general improvement in the patient's condition, and pain disappears; however, deafness persists and purulent otorrhoea occurs. With relief of the pressure on the mucosa the exudate dries up, the mucosa heals, and the perforation is closed by proliferation of its fibrous layer and by epithelial migration.

Treatment

The first general step in treatment is relief of pain. The otalgia of tubal occlusion can be overcome easily with simple analgesics such as aspirin or paracetamol, but the severe throbbing otalgia of purulent exudate often requires more powerful analgesics. In children a mild sedative is often beneficial for both the child and its parents. If general malaise and pyrexia are evident, bed rest should be advised.

The effectiveness of any specific treatment depends on its ability to resolve the underlying pathology; consequently the type of treatment depends on the particular stage reached in the natural history of the disease. During the stage of *tubal occlusion*, decongestion to open the Eustachian tube is indicated. Few studies have confirmed the value of these measures, but the use of vasoconstrictor nose drops and systemic antihistamines are thought to be beneficial. At this stage there is no evidence of bacterial infection so that the use of antibiotics is inappropriate. However, if careful follow-up is not possible to ensure resolution antibiotics may need to be used prophylactically. During the stage of *purulent exudation,* in addition to decongestant therapy, systemic disinfection is necessary. Based on experience, and probable susceptibility of the pathogen, penicillin is the drug of choice. It should be administered by intramuscular injection, as the disadvantage of an injection is far outweighed by the benefits obtained in rapid and complete resolution of the infection. A rapid response to intramuscular

penicillin may permit a change to oral medication, but this should be continued for at least 7 days. This must be emphasized to the patient who is liable to stop therapy when the pain stops, leading to inadequate treatment.

Since the advent of antibiotics the place of myringotomy has been disputed. Whilst otitis media treated adequately with antibiotics usually resolves, the recovery period is often prolonged with persistent Eustachian tube dysfunction if not actual secretory otitis media. In those countries where otitis media is dealt with primarily by the specialist, myringotomy is performed early giving more rapid recovery and a decreased incidence of complication. Most otologists perform myringotomy under general anaesthesia for severe pain, a bulging tympanic membrane and slow response to adequate treatment. Its early performance, by reducing pressure necrosis of the middle ear mucosa, causes less scarring and more rapid resolution.

Following rupture of the tympanic membrane in addition to antibiotics and decongestants drainage should be promoted via the meatus. This may be achieved by frequent dry mopping, suction or gentle irrigation to prevent secondary otitis externa. Topical antibiotics applied to the meatus are unlikely to reach the infected area, and are unnecessary.

Following treatment of acute otitis media careful follow-up is essential to exclude the onset of complications and to ensure complete resolution, as evidenced by a normal appearing tympanic membrane, aerated middle ear, and normal hearing.

The results of treatment vary from centre to centre, but with adequate treatment 80–90% of attacks of acute otitis media resolve completely. The usual causes of failure are the onset of chronic secretory otitis media or chronic suppurative otitis media.

Recurrent otitis media

The incidence of acute otitis media has a close relationship with socioeconomic factors, but in the developed nations probably 5–10% of all children suffer true otitis media in their first decade. Of these about 20% suffer a later attack, and if we exclude socioeconomic factors, the usual cause is persistent infection in the upper respiratory tract, although allergy is important according to some workers. Patients with recurrent otitis media must be examined carefully, including mastoid and sinus radiographs to exclude a focus of infection, which must be treated if found; otherwise simple adenoidectomy is often curative.

Tuberculous otitis media [6]

Tuberculous otitis media is rare and occurs secondary to pulmonary tuberculosis with infection usually via the Eustachian tube. It presents as a painless otitis media, and is characterized by extensive necrosis, both of the tympanic membrane which often has multiple perforation, and the mastoid with cold subperiosteal abscesses. The diagnosis is often made incidentally by bacteriological examination of the pus, or following diagnosis of pulmonary tuberculosis. Systemic antituberculous therapy is essential, and the local management is excision of necrotic tissue and drainage.

Complications of otitis media [2]

Complication occurs when the infection spreads beyond the mucoperiosteal lining of the middle ear. Several general factors influence the development of complications.

(1) The virulence of the organism, and its susceptability to therapy.

(2) The host's immune state and general resistence.

(3) The adequacy of treatment of the primary infection.

Antibiotics have reduced the incidence of complications in otitis media and have modified the symptoms of these complications. In the pre-antibiotic era, the onset of complication was heralded by sudden deterioration in the patient's general condition. Today, the development of a complication in the presence of inadequate antibiotic therapy is often insidious. The insidious onset, and relative rarity of these conditions means that they are often unrecognized until late. This is particularly true for complications of chronic otitis media. Complications of chronic otitis media usually require urgent mastoid exploration. Complications of acute otitis media are more susceptible to medical treatment, and a trial of antibiotics and drainage is justifiable. However, if rapid improvement does not occur drainage by cortical mastoidectomy should not be delayed.

The actual extension of infection beyond the mucoperiosteal lining generally occurs by one or more different pathological processes.

(1) Direct extension with bone erosion by osteitis or cholesteatoma.

(2) Direct extension along preformed pathways in the bone, e.g. labyrinth, congenital dehiscences, un-united sutures or old fractures.

(3) Retrograde venous thrombophlebitis.

Mastoiditis

Mastoiditis occurs when the infection spreads beyond the mucoperiosteal lining to involve the compact bone of the mastoid air cells. As well as the general factors already mentioned, it is also influenced by the anatomy of the aditus region [9]. If this is obstructed by mucosal oedema, the increasing pressure of purulent exudation in the mastoid segment cannot be relieved by rupture of the tympanic membrane. The resultant back pressure causes osteitis and bone necrosis, and with coalescence of the cells the infection tends to spread peripherally to break through the mastoid cortex causing a subperiosteal or an extradural abscess.

The classic form of acute mastoiditis is not commonly seen in the developed nations; due to the use of antibiotics, masked mastoiditis is more usual, but still uncommon.

Acute mastoiditis

In the untreated patient the progression from acute otitis media to acute mastoiditis is generally clinically obvious with a sudden dramatic deterioration in the general condition with an increased swinging pyrexia, tachycardia and severe malaise. It is particularly obvious when it occurs during the convalescent phase of acute otitis media.

The signs depend on the extent of the inflammation. The mastoid is tender, especially over the antrum, and has a variable degree of oedema from a slight palpable thickening to an obvious anteroinferior displacement of the pinna. A similar area of oedema over the posterosuperior meatal wall gives a sagging appearance to the deep meatus. Increased pain and deafness are present. In the presence of a perforation, the otorrhoea may increase, or decrease if the aditus is obstructed. Although the diagnosis is generally made clinically, mastoid radiographs may be helpful in showing clouding of the mastoid air cells. As the disease progresses the coalescence of cells may be detected on radiographs but this tends to be delayed. Serial radiographs are occasionally helpful in the less acute case.

Before antibiotics the treatment of acute mastoiditis was drainage by cortical mastoidectomy. With the advent of antibiotics it became possible to treat the condition medically, and antibiotic therapy became standard. However, it has become increasingly realized that although antibiotics can eradicate the infection, they do not always prevent the onset of chronic inflammation. This chronic inflammation eventually heals by fibrosis, but has a deleterious effect on the function of the middle ear, secretory otitis media and adhesive otitis media commonly resulting. Consequently there is a tendency now among otologists to perform a cortical mastoidectomy. As the diagnosis is essentially a clinical one, a short trial of systemic antibiotics is justifiable, but a failure to improve rapidly tends to confirm the diagnosis of mastoiditis, and cortical mastoidectomy should not be delayed.

Masked mastoiditis

The underlying pathology is the same with osteitis and bone necrosis but the time scale is prolonged due to the use of antibiotics. The usual history is of a recent attack of otitis media treated with an inadequate course of antibiotics. The antibiotics presumably decrease but do not eradicate the infection, which continues in a low-grade form within the mastoid air cells causing osteitis. There is a recrudescence of the infection and the patient presents with recurrent otitis media. Careful questioning often shows that the child never completely recovered either in general health or locally in the ear. Mastoid radiographs are essential and show cloudy cells with some blurring of cell margins on the affected side compared with the normal.

The basic pathology is an acute or chronic inflammation and the correct treatment is cortical mastoidectomy under antibiotic cover. Mastoiditis, although usually a complication of acute otitis media, may occur after chronic suppurative otitis media. With the occurrence of an acute infection superimposed on the basic chronic inflammation the patient complains of mastoid pain, and a pulsatile otorrhoea is seen. Treatment is excision of all diseased tissue, to establish drainage. In the presence of cholesteatoma an open cavity must be made.

Petrositis

The petrous apex is pneumatized in about 30% of temporal bones, usually by a posterior track of cells from the antrum by way of the semicircular canals. Less commonly there is an anterior track arising from the hypotympanum and passing medially between the cochlea and the carotid canal. If mastoiditis occurs in such a bone, inflammation may involve the petrous apex, and irritate the adjacent abducent nerve and trigeminal ganglion. Gradenigo, in 1904, described the classic triad of symptoms that results: otitis media, lateral rectus palsy and pain in the trigeminal distribution.

Management is the same as for mastoiditis of which it is merely an extended form. If cortical mastoidectomy is performed the appropriate cell tracks must be explored and, if diseased, the cells must be opened to allow drainage of the petrous apex. The classic approaches to the petrous apex are now rarely required with the advent of antibiotics.

Subperiosteal abscess

With infection of the mastoid, erosion of bone may occur as a result of osteitis or cholesteatoma. If the cortex of the bone is breached a collection of pus may occur beneath the overlying periosteum giving a subperiosteal abscess or extradural abscess depending upon which cortex is breached.

The usual sites for the subperiosteal abscesses are as follows:

(1) Post-auricular via the lateral cortex;

(2) Zygomatic via the zygomatic cells;

(3) Within the substance of the sterno-mastoid muscle, via the mastoid tip (Von Bezold's abscess);

(4) In the digastric triangle via the mastoid tip (Citelli's abscess);

(5) In the parapharyngeal space via the petrous tip.

They are clinically obvious due to their fluctuant nature, and indicate extensive infection. Consequently, urgent mastoid exploration under antibiotic cover is indicated. If the abscesses are not in direct continuity with the mastoid separate drainage should be performed.

Extradural abscess

Due to its intracranial site the extradural abscess is not clinically obvious. In the acute ear its symptomatology is generally indistinct from that of the mastoiditis, but in the chronic ear it may present with low-grade headache unresponsive to treatment. Whenever a mastoid is explored for an infection the dural plates should be inspected to detect the presence of an extradural abscess, and if present it should be drained via the mastoid cavity.

Lateral sinus thrombophlebitis

The extension of the mastoid infection to give a perisinus abscess causes an underlying mural thrombus. If this becomes infected progressive thrombophlebitis may occur with extension both intra- and extracranially. The early symptoms are malaise and headache, but with progressive thrombophlebitis septic emboli may occur, giving the typical rigors and bouts of high fever typical of septicaemia. If the thrombophlebitis extends to involve the mastoid emissary vein, a localized tender oedematous area may be felt over the mastoid (Greisinger's sign). With inferior extension the internal jugular vein may feel tender and neck stiffness may be apparent. Thrombosis of the lateral sinus can usually be demonstrated by the Toby–Ayer test, in which pressure on the ipsilateral jugular vein fails to cause an increase in CSF pressure as measured by a lumbar puncture.

The treatment of this potentially serious condition is drainage, with progressive exploration of the sinus in both directions until the limits of thrombophlebitis are reached. Ligation of the jugular vein and anticoagulants are rarely required, unless there is rapidly progressing thrombophlebitis.

Facial palsy

In acute otitis media facial palsy probably results from pressure on the nerve via one of the congenital dehiscences of the Fallopian canal. Electrodiagnostic tests should be performed and in the absence of degeneration, treatment with antibiotics and myringotomy may be adequate. In the presence of degeneration, or if the acute infection does not resolve rapidly, cortical mastoidectomy should be performed. Formal facial nerve decompression should only be performed when degeneration is present.

Intracranial complications are considered in Chapter 12.

INNER EAR

Labyrinthitis

The membranous labyrinth is protected by the osseous labyrinth, and unless the bone is breached infection is rare. Although infection may enter via one of the windows or via the internal auditory meatus, the usual cause is erosion of the lateral semicircular canal. This occurs more commonly in chronic suppurative otitis media especially with cholesteatoma. Labyrinthitis may also occur as a complication of acute otitis media or may be due to viral infection. It is generally classified into four types.

Para-labyrinthitis

Erosion of the osseous labyrinth exposes the membranous labyrinth causing a *fistula*. There is no inflammation of the membranous labyrinth, so that spontaneous nystagmus is not present. However, due to its exposure, the membranous labyrinth is susceptible to exogenous stimulation, usually a pressure change but occasionally a loud noise (the Tullio phenomenon). The patient may complain of vertigo on pressing his tragus, but the fistula is usually demonstrated by the fistula test, where alternate positive and negative pressures are applied to the external auditory meatus. A positive pressure causes an ampullo-petal flow of endolymph, increased labyrinthine tonus, and nystagmus towards the affected ear. A negative pressure has the reverse effect. Actual nystagmus is not always produced and vertigo alone is generally sufficient to make the diagnosis.

The presence of a fistula indicates a breach of the inner ear defences, a potentially serious condition requiring urgent mastoid exploration. It is important to exteriorize the fistula, but the surgical removal of any overlying granulation or cholesteatoma matrix may result in serous or even suppurative labyrinthitis.

Serous labyrinthitis

With extension of the inflammatory process and involvement of the membranous labyrinth, direct labyrinthine stimulation occurs, probably by a direct effect on the nerve endings, but possibly by caloric effect secondary to the hyperaemia. The resultant increase in labyrinthine tonus, or *irritative lesion*, produces a spontaneous nystagmus to the affected side. The patient is very dizzy with nausea and vomiting. Typically he lies curled up in bed with the affected ear downward. (In this position looking up is in the direction of the slow phase and the nystagmus is decreased – Alexander's Law.) Any movement aggravates the vertigo, and on standing the patient falls to the unaffected side. A variable amount of cochlear deafness is present. The diagnosis is a clinical one, and caloric investigation is contra-indicated as it may spread the infection; audiometry gives a useful baseline.

Treatment is by antibiotics but as penicillin does not readily enter the labyrinthine fluids, ampicillin and sulphadiazine in high doses are preferred. Heavy sedation and bed rest are required. In the presence of chronic otitis media surgical exploration and exteriorization of the fistula are indicated as for para-labyrinthitis.

Resolution is indicated by recovery of hearing, but some residual labyrinthine imbalance often persists. With return of hearing, the diagnosis of serous labyrinthitis can be made. A complete loss of cochlear and labyrinthine function indicates that suppuration has occurred, and the diagnosis was purulent labyrinthitis.

Purulent labyrinthitis

This diagnosis is made retrospectively when there is a failure in recovery of cochlear and labyrinthine function following labyrinthitis. The initial clinical picture is identical to serous labyrinthitis, with an *irritative lesion*. With the onset of suppuration destruction of the end organ occurs with a *paretic lesion*, and reversal of the nystagmus to the unaffected ear. The severe vertigo persists.

Treatment is the same as for serous labyrinthitis, but if during mastoid exploration pus is seen to be arising from the bony labyrinth, it must be opened widely; this, however, is rarely required.

Viral labyrinthitis [6]

Sudden cochlear or vestibular failure in the young with the absence of middle ear infection is generally thought to be of viral origin (in the elderly, vascular causes are more common). The mumps virus is most commonly associated with sudden deafness, although other viruses, such as measles, have been proven causes of deafness. Fortunately the deafness is generally unilateral: there may be no associated parotitis in which case the diagnosis is made by rising serological titres. High doses of steroids given early are thought to be beneficial but there are no controlled studies.

Prenatal rubella is also a well known cause of deafness. It may follow a maternal infection in the first trimester; unfortunately the infection is often subclinical and missed by the mother. Diagnosis is made by a raised rubella titre in the deaf infant. Treatment is prophylactic with rubella vaccination of susceptible women; high doses of gamma globulin following exposure to infection in the first trimester are thought to be useful.

Herpes zoster oticus [10]

Viruses play an important part in most infections of the upper respiratory tract. In the inner ear the commonest viral conditions are viral labyrinthitis and herpes zoster oticus. Unfortunately to confirm virological diagnosis by either isolation or serological tests is difficult and may only be successful in about 50% of cases. Consequently most virus infections are diagnosed on clinical grounds only.

When the *herpes zoster* virus affects the skin of the meatus and occasionally the concha it is termed *herpes oticus*. It is typified by severe pain for several days before vesiculation, and this may persist as post-herpetic neuralgia. The underlying pathology is an acute inflammation of the sensory ganglia of the cutaneous nerve. The auriculotemporal branch of the trigeminal nerve is usually involved, but sensory branches from the glossopharyngeal and vagus nerves may also be involved. It is unlikely that a vestigial sensory branch of the facial nerve is involved causing a geniculate ganglionitis, and it seems that the Ramsey–Hunt syndrome is due to a multiple zoster infection of the motor and sensory roots of the facial and statoacoustic nerves respectively.

The management is essentially symptomatic, but with a degenerating facial palsy decompression either surgically or with high doses of steroid may be considered.

Syphilis [7, 11]

Although the middle ear cleft may be involved by a gummatous osteoperiostitis in tertiary syphilis, the usual aural manifestation is syphilic labyrinthitis. This generally occurs with congenital syphilis, but is also seen with neurosyphilis. The patient presents with a fluctuating deafness, and although bilateral, the loss is often asymmetrical. Episodic vertigo and tinnitus are also present, similar to Ménière's disease. A false-positive fistula sign may be present due to abnormal mobility of the stapes – Hennebert's sign. The diagnosis may be difficult as the screening blood tests may be negative, but examination of the cerebrospinal fluid is often positive, and there may be other stigmata of congenital syphilis. Treatment requires very intensive therapy: high doses of ampicillin combined with steroids improve hearing, but the success of treatment is difficult to assess due to the fluctuation of the symptoms.

References

[1] SENTURIA B. M. (1957) *Diseases of the External Ear*. Springfield, Illinois: Charles C. Thomas.

[2] MAWSON S. R. (1974) *Diseases of the Ear*. London: Edward Arnold Ltd.

[3] ALBERTI P. W. R. M. (1964) Epithelial migration on the tympanic membrane. *Journal of Laryngology and Otology* 78, 808.

[4] CHANDLER J. R. (1972) Pathogenesis and treatment of facial paralysis due to malignant otitis externa. *Annals of Otology, Rhinology and Laryngology* 81, 648.

[5] DAWES J. D. L. (1953) Myringitis bullosa haemorrhagica. *Journal of Laryngology and Otology* 67, 313.

[6] SCHUKNECHT H. F. (1974) *Pathology of the Ear*. Cambridge, Massachusetts: Harvard University Press.

[7] GLORIG A. & GERWIN K. S., eds. (1972) *Otitis Media*. Springfield, Illinois: Charles C. Thomas.

[8] FLISBERG K. (1970) The effect of vacuum on the tympanic cavity. *Otolaryngologic Clinics of North America* 3, 3.

[9] RICHARDSON G. S. (1963) Aditus block. *Annals of Otology, Rhinology and Laryngology* 72, 223.

[10] CRABTREE J. A. (1968) Herpes zoster oticus. *Laryngoscope* 78, 1853.

[11] KERR A. G. SMYTH G. D. L. & CINNAMOND J. J. (1973) Congenital syphilic deafness. *Journal of Laryngology and Otology* 87, 1.

CHAPTER 14

Tympanosclerosis

Tympanosclerosis is an abnormal condition of the middle ear in which whitish plaques of collagen are laid down beneath the lining mucosa of the tympanic cavity. Plaques occurring in the tympanic membrane, so-called chalk patches, have been recognized for over two centuries but the first comprehensive description of tympanosclerosis and its effects on the hearing was given by Von Tröltsch in 1869 [1]. The condition attracted little serious attention, possibly because of the lack of an effective remedy, until the introduction of the operating microscope. Thereafter a paper by Zöllner and Beck [2] describing in detail the magnified appearances of tympanosclerosis and suggesting possible methods of surgical treatment, stimulated fresh interest and led to an appreciation of the importance of the condition as a cause of conductive deafness.

PATHOLOGY

While the exact cause of tympanosclerosis is unknown, the location of the plaques in the middle fibrous layer of the tympanic membrane or between the mucosa and periosteum elsewhere in the middle ear, is strong evidence that tympanosclerosis is of mesodermal origin. There is also widespread acceptance of the belief that the condition is not a disease *per se* but an abnormal healing response to a previous episode or episodes of otitis media. The latter may precede the onset of tympanosclerosis by many years but clear cut evidence of the previous inflammatory incident frequently persists either in the form of a perforation or scar of the tympanic membrane: perforations are typically large in size and devoid of discharge, the absence of active infection or cholesteatoma giving support to the author's belief that tympanosclerosis is more frequently a sequel to acute rather than to chronic middle ear inflammation. The precise cause of the excessive collagen deposition remains unexplained but it seems probable that in certain circumstances a collagen stimulating factor is released in the course of an otitis media and tympanosclerosis results. Such a reaction appears to depend on local conditions and there is no apparent association between tympanosclerosis and the systemic connective tissue disorders nor is there any known relationship to keloid. Tympanosclerosis does not appear to be the result of any specific viral or bacterial infection.

Histological changes

Soft tissue
Under the operating microscope two distinct types of tympanosclerotic plaques can be recognized:

(1) a softer form, creamy in colour, with a rubbery or cartilaginous texture: this type when removed separates off in onion layers;

(2) an extremely dense, hard, white form often firmly adherent to the surrounding bone.

Light microscopy shows the plaques to be covered by a rather flattened epithelium and typically to consist of masses of birefringent collagenous material almost totally devoid of cells and blood vessels. In some areas the collagen is arranged in bundles many of which show an irregular fibrillar structure whilst in other areas the fibrillar character is lost and the collagen assumes an amorphous hyaline appearance: deposits of calcium are common and areas of new bone formation may be encountered.

Electronmicroscopy shows masses of collagen fibres exhibiting the characteristic periodicity of around 640 nm. The following additional features have also been observed [3]:

(1) Marked proliferation of collagen fibres in the extracellular space, and electron-dense materials within or close to collagen bundles suggesting degeneration of collagen fibres with early calcium deposition.

(2) Degeneration of cytoplasm with fusion to the cell membrane to form an amorphous granular opaque mass.

(3) Electron dense masses within the matrix of mitochondria of the fibrocyte-like cells, in the membrane bound fragment, in the 'autophaged lysosomes' or in the collagen fibres indicating destruction of the fibrocyte-like cell.

(4) Shrinkage and increased density of nuclear chromatin.

The author has been able to confirm many of the above findings and has in addition observed bundles of mast cell granules and fat-like globules in the tympanosclerotic plaques.

Infra red spectrophotometer studies of the molecular structure of tympanosclerotic tissue typically show a broad absorption band centred at 1000 cm^{-1}, which is a region of phosphate compound absorption frequencies. Absorption bands indicating carbonate groups appear at approximately 1410 cm^{-1} and 1450 cm^{-1} while additional evidence of the presence of these groups may be visible at approximately 1520 cm^{-1} and 870 cm^{-1}. The presence of calcium can be confirmed by atomic absorption or scanning electronmicroscopy analysis. The foregoing observations indicate that the tympanosclerotic compound has all the characteristics of carbonate apatite.

Adjacent bone
Ossicles surrounded by tympanosclerotic tissue frequently appear demineralized and porous when viewed under the operating microscope. Histological sections show areas of bone absorption with replacement by tympanosclerotic tissue: severe bone destruction may result in ossicular discontinuity.

Harris [4] felt that the bone destruction was a direct result of the tympanosclerotic process, and recognized two types of tympanosclerosis – a non-invasive superficial form (sclerosing mucositis) in which the adjacent mucosa and periosteum remain intact and a deeper invasive type (osteoclastic mucoperiostitis) in which there is progressive bone destruction. However, there is considerable doubt regarding the existence of the latter type, since, in some cases at least, it appears to have been mistaken for coexisting cholesteatoma.

In general, tympanosclerosis is inactive, resembling the terminal scar of a burnt out inflammatory process which doubtless took place many years previously. The bone destruction so often observed in tympanosclerotic ears is probably a sequel to the preceding otitis media rather than to the tympanosclerotic process itself. Nevertheless a low-grade active destructive process may occasionally be observed in cases of tympanosclerosis of relatively recent origin, while in long-standing cases of an advanced nature devitalization and bone resorption may occur in those areas of the ossicular chain with a precarious blood supply, e.g. long process of the incus, due to strangulation by the surrounding sheath of dense avascular tympanosclerotic tissue.

Sites of involvement

Tympanosclerosis is encountered in cases with both intact and perforated tympanic membranes. The condition may thus be classified into 'closed' and 'open' forms [5]. The open form is more common if the tympanic cavity and mastoid are involved.

Tympanic membrane
'Chalk patches' in the tympanic membrane invariably occur in the stratum fibrosum of the pars tensa, varying in size from small clinically insignificant deposits to very large plaques occupying the entire surface area of the tympanic membrane. In many cases these chalk patches are the only evidence of tympanosclerosis.

Middle ear and mastoid
Plaques within the tympanic cavity and mastoid may occur with or without associated deposits in the drumhead and in both open and closed forms of tympanosclerosis. The deposits at times are enormous and may virtually obliterate the tympanic air space. The distribution of plaques throughout the tympanum follows a characteristic pattern. The oval window niche together

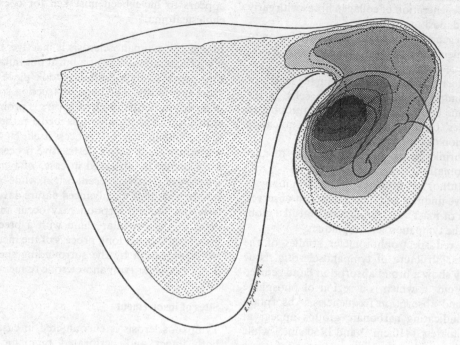

FIG. 14.1. Distribution of tympanosclerotic plaques in middle ear and mastoid (incidence indicated by shadow density).

with the stapes and stapedial tendon, the long process of the incus, the horizontal portion of the Fallopian canal, the 'sub-Fallopian groove' and the adjacent part of the promontory are the commonest sites. Deposits are also common in the attic but occur much less frequently in the hypotympanum and mastoid: plaques occluding the round window niche or the mouth of the Eustachian tube are comparatively rare.

EFFECT ON FUNCTION

The effect of tympanosclerosis on middle ear function depends on the site and extent of the collagenous deposits. In mild cases there is often no noticeable or measurable alteration; in others a severe conductive deafness occurs due to one or more of the following:

(1) reduced mobility of the tympanic membrane or ossicular chain;

(2) loss of continuity of the tympanic membrane or ossicular chain;

(3) reduction of the tympanic air space.

Reduced mobility

Tympanic membrane
The mobility of the tympanic membrane may be impaired by:

(1) massive plaque formation involving a large area of the tympanic membrane surface;

(2) adherence of a large plaque to the tympanic ring, to the handle of the malleus or to both;

(3) a massive tympanic membrane deposit resting against the promontory.

The most typical situation encountered in practice is that of a huge plaque involving the whole anterior portion of the tympanic membrane attached to the annulus anteriorly and to the handle of the malleus posteriorly: such a plaque not only affects the mobility of the tympanic membrane but immobilizes the malleus at the same time.

Ossicular chain

Stiffness of the ossicular chain results from the splinting effect of the tympanosclerotic envelope which can be likened to a layer of cement around the ossicles. As the oval window niche is the commonest site of tympanosclerosis it is not surprising that the stapes is the ossicle most frequently affected, stiffness occurring in approximately one-third of patients [6]. Upper ossicular fixation is also common since the narrow attic spaces are readily occluded by tympanosclerotic deposits: the liability to severe epitympanic fixation is increased if the deposits are calcified or ossified. Tympanosclerosis constitutes an important cause of the 'fixed malleus syndrome'.

Loss of continuity

Discontinuity is frequently encountered in tympanosclerotic ears although it is not necessarily the direct result of the tympanosclerotic process. Both the tympanic membrane and ossicular chain may be affected.

Tympanic membrane

Perforations of the tympanic membrane are encountered in roughly two-thirds of ears affected by tympanosclerosis [6]. They invariably occur in the pars tensa, are generally large and may cause significant conductive deafness. Active suppuration and cholesteatoma are rare.

Ossicular chain

Erosion of the long process of incus causing discontinuity of the incudostapedial joint is by far the most common ossicular defect. Destruction of the stapedial arch and the handle of the malleus are also relatively common but gross ossicular erosion is rare.

Reduction of tympanic air space

Massive deposits of tympanosclerosis may reduce or at times almost entirely obliterate the tympanic cavity and thereby impair sound transmission by altering its physical characteristics.

DIAGNOSIS

Accurate diagnosis is extremely important since the surgical treatment of tympanosclerosis is usually much more complicated than other types of conductive deafness. Thus tympanosclerosis, unsuspected before operation and manifesting itself for the first time at tympanotomy, may confront the otologist with a surgical problem far more difficult than anticipated and with a much poorer prognosis than he may have conveyed to the patient prior to operation.

Tympanosclerosis should always be suspected in patients with conductive deafness if:

(1) 'chalk patches' are visible in either tympanic membrane;

(2) the tympanic membrane shows evidence of scarring;

(3) there is no family history of deafness;

(4) there is a history of past otitis media followed by a non-progressive conductive deafness; and

(5) the mastoid is radiologically acellular.

Otoscopy. Tympanosclerosis occurring as chalk patches in the tympanic membrane seldom presents a diagnostic problem since the appearances are quite typical. The diagnosis of the intratympanic condition is more difficult except in cases of open tympanosclerosis where plaques are visible through the perforation: even these may be confused with cholesteatoma and careful examination under the operating microscope is often necessary to reach a diagnosis. Occasionally both conditions coexist but less often than might be expected, considering the fact that a longstanding perforation leaves the middle ear constantly open to infection and epithelial invasion.

Audiometry. Closed tympanosclerosis is liable to be confused with otosclerosis and other conditions which cause conductive deafness in the presence of an intact tympanic membrane. In such cases full audiological investigation is essential to assess the exact state of the middle ear. Tuning fork tests, pure tone and speech audiometry and tympanometry are of great help in detecting impaired mobility of the tympanic membrane, ossicular stiffness or discontinuity, inadequate function of the Eustachian tube or coexisting sensorineural hearing loss.

TREATMENT

Surgical management

In general, treatment is directed towards the relief of deafness and plaques not interfering with sound conduction are as a rule left alone. The three basic principles of surgical treatment are as follows:

(1) Restoration of mobility to stiffened or fixed structures.

(2) Repair of defects in the sound transmitting structures.

(3) Circumvention of severely affected areas by creation of a bypass.

The techniques employed differ little from those used in other forms of middle ear disease.

Tympanosclerosis of the tympanic membrane

Plaque removal

Plaques should be removed if they interfere with sound transmission, preserving the overlying epithelial layer of the tympanic membrane. The plaque is approached either by way of an existing perforation or by employing a stapes approach if the tympanic membrane is intact. An angled elevator of the Marquet type is then insinuated between the plaque and the outer layer of the tympanic membrane employing ×16 magnification. The plaque is separated by careful dissection and as it is freed it is displaced inwards thus detaching it not only from the remnant of the tympanic membrane but also from adjacent structures such as the handle of malleus and annulus. When all attachments are freed the plaque is removed leaving the outer layer of the tympanic membrane intact.

Myringoplasty

In suitable cases of open tympanosclerosis graft-

ing of the perforation should be carried out employing any of the standard myringoplasty techniques. Plaques are removed if necessary during the course of the operation. Excision of plaques by the technique described automatically denudes the inner surface of the tympanic membrane of its mucosal lining thus creating an ideal bed for an underlay type of graft. However, it may not always be advisable to remove plaques adjacent to a perforation if it is thought that there is a considerable risk of enlarging the defect due either to epithelial retraction or to tearing of a very thin remnant of the tympanic membrane in the neighbourhood of the plaque: grafts take surprisingly well even when placed on avascular plaques. The success rate of myringoplasty is likely to match closely that achieved in non-tympanosclerotic tympanic membranes.

Tympanosclerosis of the ossicular chain

In mild cases of tympanosclerosis removal of plaques with restoration of ossicular mobility is the operation of choice since plaques do not normally recur and there is a reasonable prospect of permanent hearing improvement. In more severe cases the loss of mucosa inherent in this technique is likely to cause excessive postoperative fibrosis leading in the long-term to hearing regression. Some form of tympanoplastic procedure is therefore preferable depending on the extent and site of the pathological process.

Stapes fixation

Severe involvement of the stapes area is best treated by stapedectomy but the pathology in tympanosclerosis differs from that in otosclerosis so that the technique may need to be modified and the results are not comparable. The following problems may arise:

(1) Footplate fixation is nearly always caused by a covering layer of collagen of variable thickness binding the surface of the footplate to the adjacent bone: annular ligament invasion by tympanosclerosis is unusual but may be encountered from time to time. In most cases removal of the surface layer of collagen immediately frees the stapes, and a floating footplate may result unless the otologist is aware of the danger and takes appropriate precautions.

(2) The viability of the long process of the incus is frequently impaired in tympanosclerosis and the attachment of a prosthesis may cause further devitalization. Late conductive deafness may result from incus necrosis.

(3) The incidence of post-stapedectomy sensorineural deafness in tympanosclerosis may be greater than in otosclerosis. Whether this is due to increased cochlear fragility directly related to the tympanosclerotic process or to sensitization of the cochlea by previous ear surgery is not known: the incidence of second stage stapedectomies is certainly much higher in tympanosclerosis and this may be the critical factor. Irrespective of the cause the possibility of cochlear fragility should be recognized.

(4) Attic tympanosclerosis may coexist with stapedial disease and must be carefully excluded before stapedectomy especially if a prosthesis is used. Epitympanic ossicular fixation unrecognized at operation or developing at a later date may create problems at a subsequent operation since the existing prosthetic mechanism must be dismantled or removed prior to undertaking further surgery in the attic to protect the cochlea from transmitted vibrations.

Attic fixation

At operation it is essential to inspect the attic in selected cases to exclude tympanosclerosis there. Exposure may be achieved in several ways, by permeatal atticotomy, by an attic inspection window or by a mastoid approach with or without posterior tympanotomy, the appropriate method being selected according to each individual situation. The last named procedure requires a more extensive operation than the other methods but it affords an opportunity to exclude unsuspected cholesteatoma in the mastoid.

As a rule, attic tympanosclerosis results in reduced mobility or total fixation of the malleus and incus: in these cases the stapes, even on careful inspection, may also seem fixed: doubt as to its mobility can readily be resolved by disarticulating the incudostapedial joint and testing the stapes independently.

Mobilization
Mobilization of the ossicular chain by removal of plaques from the attic is seldom successful and is generally considered inadvisable because of the high risk of ossicular refixation.

Attic bypass
(1) *In attic fixation with an intact and mobile stapes*, the fixed structures in the attic should be bypassed. The incus and head of malleus are removed and an ossiculoplasty is carried out by interposing one or other of the removed ossicles, suitably modified if necessary, between the handle of the malleus and the head of the stapes. This technique is also applicable to cases of ossicular discontinuity caused by erosion of the long process of incus. A type III tympanoplasty might be considered as a possible alternative, the transposed ossicle being placed between the head of the stapes and the tympanic membrane.

(2) *In attic fixation with the stapes superstructure missing and the footplate mobile*. After removal of the incus and the head of the malleus, the patient's own incus, or a homograft incus or malleus, is inserted between the handle of the malleus and the footplate of the stapes.

(3) *In attic fixation with the stapes intact but fixed*, if the tympanosclerosis fixing the stapes is not too extensive and the superstructure is intact, it may be possible to restore mobility of the stapes by removal of the plaques in the oval window area and then carry out an appropriate ossiculoplastic procedure.

In more severe cases stapedectomy is required in addition to an attic bypass, the hearing mechanism being restored by a malleus handle – oval window prosthesis using either a Sheehy wire or a teflon piston. The results of this procedure are somewhat unpredictable, but good long-term hearing improvement occurs in a reasonable proportion of cases.

An alternative procedure is fenestration of the horizontal semicircular canal.

(4) *In attic fixation with stapes fixation and gross tympanic membrane involvement* the best treatment is fenestration of the horizontal semicircular canal provided the tympanic membrane is intact. Removal of plaques involving the tympanic membrane, with the associated risk of cre-

ating a perforation, is unnecessary. The mobility of the tympanic membrane, so essential in tympanoplasty, is not vital to success in the fenestration operation because this depends primarily on the creation of a 'phase difference' between the oval and round windows. The obvious disadvantages of an open mastoid cavity and the inability to close the airbone gap completely in this operation are offset by the avoidance of several operations which are often necessary if tympanoplastic techniques are employed: furthermore the prospects of completely closing the airbone gap by tympanoplastic methods in advanced tympanosclerosis are in any case poor. A possible single stage alternative to fenestration is excision of the affected structures and replacement by a monoblock transplant of tympanic membrane and ossicles. This procedure must be regarded as the operation of choice if, in addition to the extensive pathological changes already indicated, the tympanic membrane is also perforated. The short-term results of these operations are encouraging but the ultimate fate of middle ear homografts is not yet certain and it may be some years before this technique can be fully evaluated.

Non-surgical management

The results of surgery in tympanosclerosis are less successful than those achieved in other forms of middle ear pathology and for this reason consideration may have to be given to alternative methods of management.

The fitting of a suitable ear-level hearing aid is indicated in cases where the chances of hearing improvement by operation are uncertain or where surgery carries an undue risk of sensorineural loss. Patients who do not wish surgical interference and those in whom surgery has failed may also derive help from a suitable hearing aid provided cochlear function is not seriously impaired.

References

[1] TRÖLTSCH A. VON (1869) *Lehrbuch der Ohrenheilkunde.* Leipzig.
[2] ZOLLNER F. & BECK C. (1955) Die paukensklerose. *Zeitschrift für Laryngologie, Rhinologie, Otologie und ihre Grenzgebiete* 34, 137.
[3] WON CHANG I. (1969) Tympanosclerosis. *Acta oto-laryngologica* 68, 62.
[4] HARRIS I. (1961) Tympanosclerosis – a revived clinicopathologic entity. *Laryngoscope* 71, 1488.
[5] GIBB A. G. (1971) Tympanosclerosis. *Acta oto-rhinolaryngologica Belgica* 25, 956.
[6] GIBB A. G. (1976) Tympanosclerosis. *Proceedings Royal Society of Medicine* 69, 155.

CHAPTER 15

Otosclerosis

Otosclerosis is a disorder of bone which is entirely confined to the human race; its cause is unknown. It occurs only in the otic capsule, where it begins in the middle layer, i.e. the endochondral layer. If it spreads to the region of the oval window and impedes the mobility of the footplate of the stapes a conductive type of hearing loss results. There is also strong evidence that it can produce a sensorineural hearing impairment by involvement of the cochlea.

PATHOGENESIS

Incidence

The important temporal bone studies undertaken by Guild [1] and since confirmed by others indicate that about 10% of the population has otosclerotic foci somewhere in the otic capsule and that about 1% has stapedial fixation. Even in children under the age of 5 years, autopsy material showed foci in about 0·5% of cases at some site.

A clinical diagnosis in the living patient is made rather less often; only between three and five per thousand of the adult Caucasian population have clinical conductive deafness due to stapedial otosclerosis [2]. Although various studies on the sex incidence of histological otosclerosis have failed to show any significant difference between males and females, in the experience of most otologists more women present for treatment than men. In the mongoloid and negroid races histological and clinical otosclerosis are much less frequent than in Caucasians; the disease is reported to be common in southern India.

Other statistical studies indicate that although otosclerosis is most common bilaterally it is unilateral in between 11% and 15% of patients. There is a positive family history in rather more than half of patients, whilst the likelihood of a sibling being affected amounts to approximately 10% [3].

Aetiology

Despite extensive studies by such respected investigators as Politzer, Siebenmann, Whitmark, Mayer, Weber and Nager, the essential cause remains unknown. The various factors which have been recognized are summarized by Schuknecht [4] under three main headings, viz. constitutional, local and general factors, as follows:

Constitutional factors

Constitutional factors in otosclerosis have long been recognized by otologists; very detailed studies led to the conclusion that inheritance was most probably by 'monohybrid autosomal dominant inheritance with a penetration of the pathological gene of between 25% and 40%' [5]. Subsequent chromosomal studies have nevertheless failed to identify with absolute certainty any specific chromosomal abnormality. The mode of inheritance has been further examined by Morrison [6] who regarded the evidence in favour of an autosomal dominant inheritance as conclusive. For simple genetic counselling he states that if two otosclerotic parents have children then about half the children will develop the clinical condition, and if an otosclerotic marries a non-otosclerotic about a quarter of their offspring will become deaf. He emphasizes that the degree of manifestation of the disorder varies tremendously from family to family and can be anywhere between 10% and 100%. Other genetic studies have failed to demonstrate any linkage between otosclerosis and such factors as blood groups, although its curious relationship with the generalized skeletal disorder of osteogenesis imperfecta has long been recognized.

Local factors

Of the possible local factors concerned in the aetiology, interest has centred upon the cartilaginous rests which are often found in the middle layer of the otic capsule. These areas of residual cartilage appear to be the usual sites of origin of otosclerosis and the most constant is found in the area known as the fissula antefenestram just anterior to the oval window (Figs. 15.1 and 15.2). It is suggested that certain factors activate these cartilaginous rests and that their subsequent replacement by abnormal bone is an attempt at a healing mechanism. It has also been suggested that the erect attitude assumed by man produces abnormal mechanical stresses in the base of the skull and that otosclerosis represents a healing process. Indeed, microfractures are a frequent finding in human temporal bone studies. It is difficult to understand, however, how significant mechanical stresses could be produced actually within the stapes footplate, one of the sites at which otosclerosis can begin.

General factors

That general factors probably play a significant role is suggested by the influence of pregnancy in either initiating or increasing the deafness of otosclerosis. Deafness which is clinically and histologically identical with that found in many patients with osteogenesis imperfecta also suggests a generalized disorder, possibly in the nature of mesenchymal hypoplasia. Ogilvie and Hall [7] supported this idea and expressed the view that otosclerosis was essentially a localized

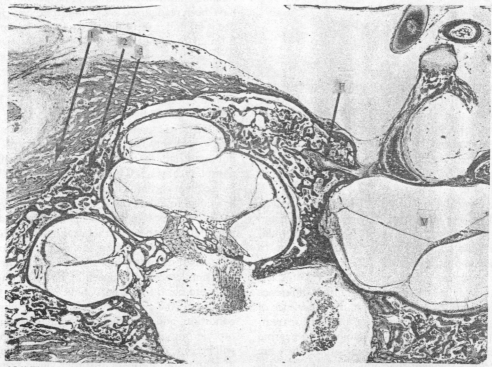

FIG. 15.1. The otic capsule in the fetus at 25 weeks, its three layers are clearly shown. (1) The outer periosteal layer. (2) The middle endochondral layer in which fibrocartilaginous rests tend to persist. (3) The endosteal layer. Note also the fissula antefenestram at (F) around which cartilaginous rests have a particular tendency to occur. The fissula postfenestram is a somewhat similar structure lying posterior to the oval window although less constantly present. The vestibule is indicated at (V).

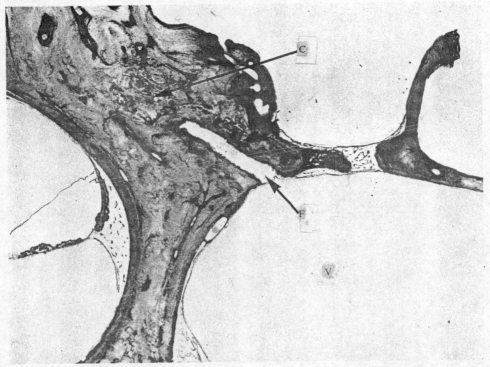

FIG. 15.2. The fissula ante fenestram (F) in the adult; cartilaginous rests are arrowed at (C); (V) indicates vestibule.

manifestation of osteogenesis imperfecta but it is difficult to understand why the disease should be so often localized to the otic capsule.

The disease has never been found in animals nor produced artificially in animals although otosclerotic bone has been grown *in vitro* successfully in a number of laboratories. The cultured bone retains all the original changes including continued osteoclasis, presumably due to an abnormal enzyme system persisting in the tissue culture. Further experiments suggest that the resorptive stage of otosclerosis is caused mainly by lysosomal hydrolases and electronmicroscopy has shown that certain cells containing numerous lysosomes (from which destructive enzymes are released) are present in the areas of bone resorption [8]. It is possible that the cells containing these lysosymes are indeed altered osteocytes. Osteolytic resorption is more usually recognized as a function of osteoclasts which exert their activity through the use of hydrolytic enzymes, such as acid phosphatase. Whatever the significance of these studies, further studies of bone

metabolism at cellular, enzymal and biochemical levels are clearly necessary.

Histopathology

Four stages are recognizable by light microscopy [9].

(1) Osteoclastic destruction of mature endochondral bone occurs and is sometimes referred to as the 'active phase' of otosclerosis, though the process is really one of otospongiosis rather than sclerosis. Resorption spaces containing a very cellular fibrous stroma are developed.

(2) Mucopolysaccharide and osteoid deposition occur in the resorption spaces with the production of highly cellular immature basophilic bone. The term 'blue mantles' is sometimes applied to these areas of abnormal newly formed basophilic bone deposited in the resorption spaces (Fig. 15.3).

(3) There is a continuing process of bony resorption and new bone formation with eventually the production of a more mature lamellar, eosinophilic type of bone.

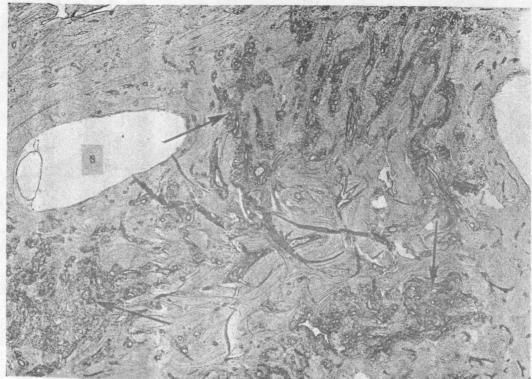

FIG. 15.3. Blue mantles of newly formed abnormal bone: three of the larger mantles are arrowed. (S) illustrates the semicircular canal. (By courtesy of Professor H. F. Schuknecht.)

(4) There is the formation of highly mineralized bone which because of the irregular pattern of resorption and new bone formation takes on a mosaic-like appearance. Even in the later healed stage of otosclerosis the matured lamellar bone is still very thick and cellular compared to the normal.

Finally, it must be emphasized that events are not necessarily as orderly as this description suggests. Otosclerotic foci may become quiescent or reactivated at any time, and it is by no means unusual for one particular focus to contain areas of different stages of activity.

As previously indicated, the commonest site for otosclerosis is in the region of the oval window. Indeed, 85% of otosclerotic foci are said to be found in this area. Temporal bone studies show that the other sites of predilection in descending order of frequency are the round window niche, focal areas of the otic capsule, the anterior wall of the internal meatus and the stapes footplate. Otosclerosis confined to the footplate is found in between 5% and 12% of various histological series. On extremely rare occasions an otosclerotic focus has been described in the incus or the head of malleus, though at such sites its presence is very difficult to explain. It has been known since the days of lateral canal fenestration that 7% of material obtained at operation from the lateral semicircular canal shows otosclerotic bone histologically.

As the otosclerotic bone replaces the normal an actual remodelling occurs without invasion of the adjacent spaces of the labyrinth even rarely in the grossest disease. Otosclerosis can even occur in the modiolus and in the osseous spiral lamina of the cochlea without invading adjacent spaces.

The surgeon will be most familiar with the appearances in the oval window area. At this

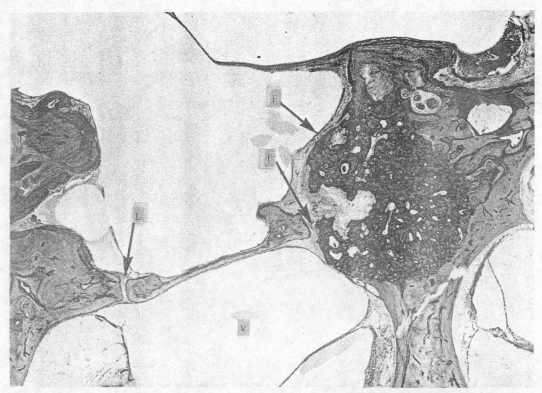

FIG. 15.4. A focus of 'nonclinical' otosclerosis is indicated at (F). The intact annular ligament is indicated at (LL), the vestibule is seen at (V). (By courtesy of Professor H. F. Schuknecht.)

point the focus in the anterior margin of the window occasionally may grow under the footplate and subluxate it laterally. More often the footplate becomes involved and fixed to a varying degree. In advanced diseases the footplate and oval window become completely obliterated.

For operative purposes the following clinical classification is useful (Figs. 15.4 to 15.7):

Stage 1 – less than half the footplate is involved;

Stage 2 – whole footplate involved but not grossly thickened;

Stage 3 – whole footplate is thick but its margin can still be recognized;

Stage 4 – the margins of the footplate are unrecognizable.

Obliterative disease of this type is common in Australia where it is perhaps the result of fluoride deficiency [10].

Otosclerosis confined to the round window niche is less frequently observed at operation;

experimental studies have demonstrated that hearing is not affected until the round window niche is totally obstructed.

The clinical significance of otosclerotic foci adjacent to the cochlea and the internal meatus are of great interest in relation to sensorineural deafness in otosclerosis and will be discussed in a later section.

Pathophysiology

Various analyses indicate that in about 70% of patients the disease begins between the ages of 11 and 30 years. If the onset of conductive deafness occurs after the age of 45 the possibility of Paget's disease (osteitis deformans) should be seriously considered as an alternative diagnosis. Characteristically the severity of the conductive deafness reaches its maximum in the third decade of life and any further deterioration in hearing is likely to be due to sensorineural degeneration.

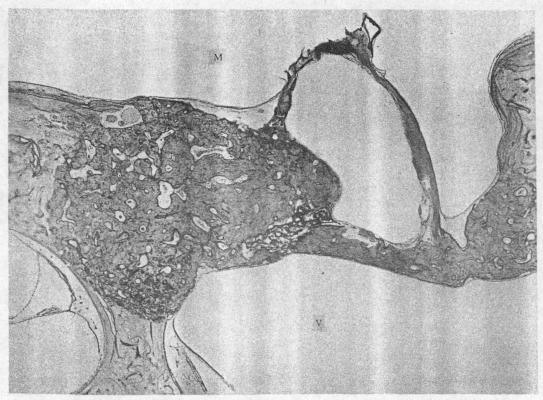

FIG. 15.5. Stapedial otosclerosis. A large focus fixes the stapes footplate anteriorly, the footplate itself is also involved and in addition there is ankylosis present posteriorly. (M) indicates the middle ear, (V) indicates the vestibule. (By courtesy of Professor H. F. Schuknecht.)

Generally, the severity of the conductive deafness corresponds to the extent of the footplate involvement, although exceptions do occur. The air–bone gap from fibrous fixation of the footplate is usually less than 30 dB; firm anterior ankylosis creates a conductive deficit of about 40 dB; and when the complete circumference of the oval window is involved a conductive loss may occur greater than 40 dB. A gap greater than 50 dB is very unusual even in cases of oval window obliteration, since at such high intensities sound transmission can occur directly through fixed ossicles. An air–bone gap greater than 50 dB is more probably due to ossicular discontinuity rather than ossicular fixation [11].

Sensorineural deafness in otosclerosis

The incidence as well as the cause of sensori-neural deafness in otosclerosis is still undecided. The majority of surgeons have the clinical impression that an undue proportion of their patients with stapedial otosclerosis also have some sensorineural loss. Various authors quote between 5% and 25% of patients over the age of 40 as showing some involvement audiometrically, but statistical surveys indicate that up to the age of 60 the occurrence of sensorineural deafness is the same in otosclerotic patients as in the general population and only over the age of 60 do otosclerotics show any increased susceptibility to sensorineural deafness [12].

The histological changes which affect the cochlea are clearly defined. Areas of atrophy of the spiral ligament and stria vascularis tend to occur where the otospongiotic foci impinge upon the endosteum, which is usually in the lateral wall of the various turns of the cochlea. However,

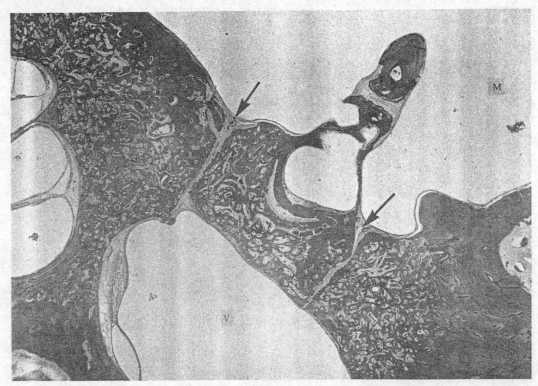

FIG. 15.6. Obliterative otosclerosis with extensive involvement of the promontory. The remains of the annular ligament are arrowed. (M) indicates the middle ear and (V) indicates the vestibule. (By courtesy of Professor H. F. Schuknecht.)

they bear no spatial relationship to the type of cochlear hearing loss present and the bone conduction curve is nearly always of a descending type. Moreover, the hair cell and neurone populations are frequently relatively normal until a very advanced stage of the disease is reached (Figs. 15.8 and 15.9).

Very gross atrophy of the spiral ligament can predispose occasionally to spontaneous rupture of the basilar membrane in which case a profound sensorineural deafness is present. Histological studies indicate that it is only very rarely that otosclerotic foci encroach upon the spaces of the cochlea or on the internal meatus with consequent physical effects which could result in possible impairment of sensorineural function.

The various histological changes such as spiral ligament and strial atrophy are interesting, but do not in any way explain why a sensorineural deficit should occur. Such impairment therefore has been theoretically attributed to toxic pro-

ducts arising from tissue degradation in the foci of disease around the cochlea or to biochemical disturbances, or to disturbances caused by venous shunts from the abnormal bone. More recently enzymal causes have been suggested. The nature of this enzyme and the manner by which it reaches the interior of the cochlea and its mode of action remain obscure. It is suggested that the enzyme is associated with the active, i.e. the absorptive spongiotic stage of the disorder; if maturation of such foci by fluoride therapy can be promoted then the sensorineural hearing loss can be arrested.

Valvassori [15] has shown by polytomography that patches of bony absorption occur around the cochlea in patients with mixed deafness due to otosclerosis. Both he and Shambaugh have taken the concept of cochlear involvement a stage further and have put forward evidence that sensorineural deafness can occur without stapedial fixation. As it appears to occur in the active,

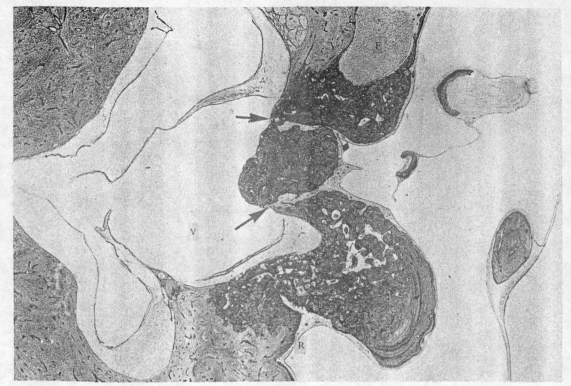

FIG. 15.7. Vertical section illustrating extensive obliterative otosclerosis. The margins of the oval window are arrowed. The round window niche is seen at (R), and the facial nerve at (F). The vestibule is indicated at (V). (By courtesy of Prof. H. F. Schuknecht.)

i.e. resorptive, stage of the disease, they prefer the term 'pure cochlear otospongiosis' rather than otosclerosis. It is suggested that the diagnosis of pure sensorineural deafness due to a pure cochlear otospongiosis may be suspected in patients who show one or the other of the following features:

(1) A family history of conductive deafness due to otosclerosis.

(2) Stapedial otosclerosis in the opposite ear with or without cochlear involvement.

(3) A flamingo flush in one or both ears.

(4) Areas of bone erosion around the cochlea on polytomography.

(5) Audiometric evidence of a flat or mid-frequency sensorineural loss.

(6) Sensorineural deafness of unknown cause starting insidiously in early or middle adult life.

The concept of pure cochlear otosclerosis has been strongly opposed by Schuknecht [16] on

histopathological grounds. Of 910 temporal bones studied by him 92 specimens showed clinical otosclerosis, i.e. stapes fixation. Another thirty-two specimens showed histological evidence of otosclerosis without stapes fixation and of this second group only in three specimens was cochlear otosclerosis present, i.e. histological otosclerosis which had replaced some part of the endosteal layer of the cochlea. In one of the patients with cochlear otosclerosis similar atrophic changes were present in the opposite temporal bone which contained no evidence of otosclerosis. In the other pair of temporal bones obtained from a patient with a mild hearing loss and histological evidence of cochlear otosclerosis, atrophic changes present in the cochlea were identical with those observed in ageing individuals without otosclerosis. He was forced to the conclusion that 'sensorineural hearing loss occurring in pure form without a conductive

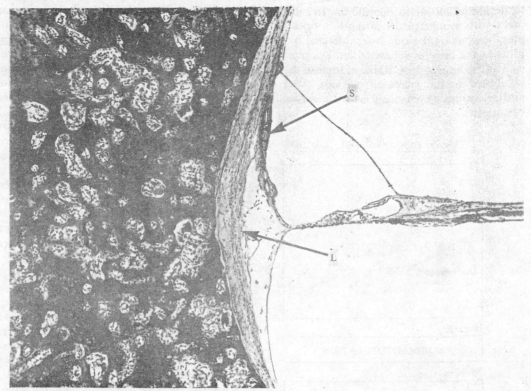

Fig. 15.8. Extensive otosclerotic invasion around the cochlea. Note the atrophic changes in the adjacent spiral ligament (L). Stria vascularis is indicated at (S). The organ of Corti was normal. This patient's audiogram and cochleogram are shown in Fig. 15.9. (By courtesy of Professor H. F. Schuknecht.)

deafness cannot be attributed to otosclerosis, because when the otosclerotic lesion is sufficiently severe to cause atrophy of the supporting, sensory and neural structures within the cochlea it invariably also fixes the stapes.'

Discussions have been summarized by Hoople [17] and by Shambaugh [14]. Further reference should be made to the important work of Friedmann [18] for further discussion on this question and for detailed comment on the pathology of many other aspects of both stapedial and cochlear otosclerosis.

CLINICAL FEATURES

Symptoms

Hearing loss is the cardinal symptom; it is generally bilateral and of gradual onset. The patient often states that she can hear better in the pre-

sence of background noise, a phenomenon known as *paracusis Willisii*. The explanation perhaps lies in the fact that normal people when speaking against a noisy background automatically raise their voices with consequent benefit to the patient with stapes fixation.

Tinnitus is present to some degree in a high proportion of patients and can be a troublesome symptom in about 25% of them; occasionally it is the presenting symptom. Often it is part of a sensorineural degeneration (whether caused by the otosclerosis or whether due to concomitant disease or presbyacusis), but occasionally it is seen in patients with a normal or near normal sensorineural reserve. In these patients it may well be due to the abnormal degree of vascularity of the otosclerotic bone. Tinnitus in otosclerosis can sometimes be helped by a successful stapedectomy. This symptom is also useful in helping to decide which ear to operate on. In bilateral cases with symmetrical hearing loss operation may be done on the side worse affected by tinnitus in the hope of relieving that symptom as well as the hearing loss. Relief of tinnitus can be attributed to the increased masking effect of ambient noise which occurs after a successful operation.

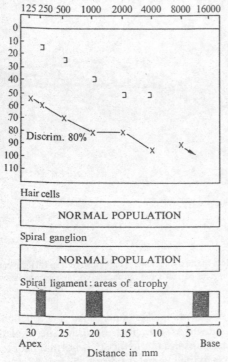

FIG. 15.9. Audiogram and cochleogram of patient shown in previous figure, the hair cell and spiral ganglion populations were normal. The areas of spiral ligament atrophy have no spatial relationship to the bone conduction loss. There is no anatomical explanation for the sensorineural deficit. (By courtesy of Professor H. F. Schuknecht.)

Giddiness is a symptom which is particularly difficult to evaluate in patients with otosclerosis though as already mentioned it has been recognized since the days of fenestration that otosclerosis can affect the bony capsule of the vestibular labyrinth just as it affects the cochlea. It is also known that occasionally an endolymphatic hydrops can occur, especially in advanced cochlear

otosclerosis. A variety of vestibular symptoms are described in otosclerosis, the most common of which is a true benign positional paroxysmal vertigo. Schuknecht [19] states that otosclerotic patients often exhibit vestibular disturbance, and various objective disturbances such as caloric hypoexcitability can be found in 57% of patients according to Virolainen [20]. Elevated thresholds for angular acceleration and deceleration, directional preponderance and positional nystagmus were also present in a high proportion of patients studied by him. If vertigo is a symptom of any great significance then true coexistent Menière's disease is to be seriously considered. Both otosclerosis and Menière's disease are common disorders and inevitably at times will occur in the same patient as has been demonstrated from temporal bone studies [21].

Examination

Characteristically the tympanic membranes are normal in otosclerosis, but thickening or scarring of the membrane may occasionally be present due to previous healed coincidental disease. The flamingo flush, originally described by Schwartze, may be caused by vascular bone on the promontory or by prominent blood vessels running over the promontory. In the former case, especially if seen in young patients, it is said to be associated with very active and rapidly advancing disease and a poor prognosis with or without stapedectomy.

Tuning fork tests indicate a conductive hearing loss and must never be omitted. The same applies to the use of the noise box whether the case be a unilateral or a bilateral one, if the surgeon wishes to avoid the error of failing to identify a false-negative Rinne and subsequently operating upon a dead ear. The Bing and the Gelle tuning fork tests may be useful in diagnosing stapes fixation. Testing of the level of hearing loss against a conversational and a whispered voice gives some indication of the level of the hearing loss and of the severity of any discrimination loss. It is again wise to confirm the findings by using the noise box before proceeding to audiometry which likewise must be done with correct masking.

The otosclerotic patient often has a typically

soft voice. though in time this may become harsh and badly modulated if a sensorineural deafness supervenes.

Audiometry

High quality audiometric testing with proper masking is essential. The minimum audiometric requirements are pure tone air and bone testing, as well as the speech reception threshold and the discrimination score. Useful though accurate bone conduction audiometry is, it must always be remembered that it is not always a precise measurement of the true sensorineural reserve. It is for this reason that not infrequently after a successful stapedectomy the difference between the pre-operative air and bone conduction thresholds, the 'air–bone gap', can be more than closed. It is also necessary to remember that the bone conduction output of most clinical audiometers is only about 60 dB with the result that occasionally very deaf patients are seen, with the diagnosis of otosclerosis, in whom no bone conduction threshold can be established on audiometry, but who nevertheless can be benefited by stapedectomy.

The most common type of pure tone audiogram seen in stapedial otosclerosis shows an air–bone gap and a hearing loss which is greatest in the lower frequencies. Later when the patient develops sensorineural loss for any reason the pattern will change to give a falling type of bone conduction curve in some patients. Reference must be made to the possible disadvantage from loss of speech discrimination which can occur if a stapedectomy is carried out on a patient with a large air–bone gap for the lower frequencies, a small gap for the upper frequencies and a descending type of bone conduction curve.

The Carhart notch is seen in about one-third of patients, most commonly at 2000 Hz. This phenomenon is not satisfactorily explained, although its reversibility in some patients after a successful stapedectomy favours a mechanical origin, possibly arising from the interference with the normal cochlear hydrodynamics by an immobile oval window. If reversal does not occur the surgeon must conclude that some actual cochlear degeneration is present. The interesting questions of cochlear degeneration and 'pure'

cochlear otosclerosis have been discussed in an earlier paragraph.

Differential diagnosis

Stapedial otosclerosis must be differentiated from other types of conductive hearing loss which may be associated with a normal or near normal tympanic membrane. In those patients in whom a detailed history and examination of the tympanic membrane using the microscope do not enable a diagnosis to be made, impedance audiometry and stapedial reflex testing may be of help; but in certain patients the true state of affairs may only be discovered at tympanotomy. The diagnosis of pure cochlear otosclerosis has been discussed previously.

Congenital stapes fixation, though fairly rare, is the commonest congenital ossicular lesion to be differentiated. It is to be suspected if a conductive hearing loss is discovered which there is good reason to think may have been present since birth, especially in the presence of a normal bone conduction audiogram and a fairly flat air conduction threshold at about 60 dB. *Congenital fixation of the head of malleus* is rare and only likely to be diagnosed at tympanotomy. *Adhesive otitis* and *tympanosclerosis* can both affect any part of the ossicular chain and although the great majority of patients have a previous history of otitis and show an abnormal tympanic membrane the occasional patient does not. Tympanosclerosis and adhesions are so common that they sometimes coexist with stapedial otosclerosis. Indeed, an essential step in stapedectomy is to ensure that the malleus and incus are not impeded in their normal movement by such coexistent lesions.

Ossicular discontinuity or dislocation must be considered as an alternative to fixation. Ossicular discontinuity of congenital origin is rare; as is necrosis of the long process of the incus arising from previous acute otitis media or irradiation. Dislocation of the incus may be caused by a previous head injury or simple mastoidectomy and the clue may be given in the history. A fracture-dislocation of the stapes is rarer and occurs only in severe head injuries. The otologist seldom sees such patients until very late by which time a severe degree of irreversible cochlear damage is also present which makes hearing improvement after tympanotomy unlikely.

Generalized bone diseases causing hearing loss are of great interest but seldom produce difficulty in differential diagnosis. The most important is *osteogenesis imperfecta*: a high proportion of patients who survive into adult life develop a deafness which is clinically and histologically identical with otosclerosis. The hearing loss develops as the tendency towards fractures decreases; the management of the deafness is identical with that of otosclerosis. Stapedectomy in the early active stage of the disease is best avoided because of the very vascular nature of the bone. In those patients demonstrating the features of osteogenesis imperfecta with otosclerosis-like deafness and with blue sclerotics the eponym 'van der Hoeve–de Kleyn syndrome' is applied. *Osteitis deformans* or Paget's disease, as previously indicated, is to be suspected in older patients developing symptoms suggestive of otosclerosis. Clinical suspicion is increased by the enlarged head and tortuosity of the terminal branches of the superficial temporal artery. The diagnosis is confirmed by a radiograph of the skull and by the high serum alkaline phosphatase. Stapedectomy in Paget's disease is of very limited value because of the high incidence of sensorineural impairment as well as the diffuse nature of the changes affecting the ossicular chain. Any improvement after stapedectomy is generally only temporary.

TREATMENT

Although surgery is the mainstay of treatment, a hearing aid and rehabilitative training may be preferable for some patients and there may be certain patients for whom administration of sodium fluoride can be considered.

Surgical treatment

Fenestration of the lateral canal now has a very minor place in the surgery of otosclerosis, but may merit consideration in patients with either an abnormal facial nerve or a persistent stapedial artery crossing the footplate, or those in whom

stapedectomy for obliterative otosclerosis has been followed by reclosure. A hearing aid may be considered preferable to a fenestration cavity even for these few patients, and the functional result is likely to be superior. Mobilization of the stapes likewise has almost entirely been superseded by stapedectomy, although it may on rare occasions still be considered for those patients with a small anterior focus of mature otosclerosis causing a minor degree of fixation.

Stapedectomy has become the operation of choice since Shea [22] and Schuknecht and his colleagues [23] published their techniques and results. Many modifications of stapedectomy have been introduced since the early 1960s and almost as many abandoned since then. It is not the policy of this book to describe surgical techniques, but briefly it may be said that the footplate may be partially or totally removed depending upon the pathology (the current tendency is to create a small opening in the middle third of the footplate). Some surgeons in suitable cases prefer to retain the crura when possible rather than insert a foreign material to replace the suprastructure. But whatever technique is used and whatever kind of prosthesis is inserted, the operation is one of the most predictable in the entire field of surgery, provided that it is carried out by a skilled surgeon on properly selected patients. The necessary skill can only be acquired by prolonged practise in the temporal bone laboratory, combined with assisting at many stapedectomy operations being done by someone already skilled. The operation can be relatively straightforward, or can be extremely difficult even in experienced hands. But generally the results as well as the failures and complications are directly related to the surgeon's skill and experience. For a detailed account of the operation and of other aspects of stapedectomy, reference should be made to the monograph by Schuknecht [4] based upon 6200 operations. For the latest changes in fashion reference should be made to the current literature.

Selection of patients for stapedectomy

To some extent selection depends upon skill, experience and the results of the surgeon concerned. One rule, however, is inviolate: the patient with a dead ear on the opposite side is not for operation, though she may be considered for stapedectomy if the time eventually arrives when she is no longer able to use any hearing aid effectively. This is seldom.

In younger patients the disease is generally in a more active stage so that a higher incidence of oval window reclosure is to be expected. Operation, therefore, should seldom be done under the age of 25 years. The upper age limit of stapedectomy is more difficult to define. The disease is usually less active in older patients so if the sensorineural reserve is adequate and if the patient is fit enough for local or general anaesthesia a good hearing improvement is to be expected. Even a minor degree of vestibular damage, however, may be associated with impaired vestibular compensation so caution may need to be exercised on these grounds especially if an operation is being considered on the second side. It should also be remembered that the membranous labyrinth in elderly patients often shows atrophic changes which may be greater if foci of cochlear otosclerosis have produced areas of spiral ligament atrophy.

The level of the sensorineural reserve is a basic consideration when contemplating stapedectomy. Two points arise from this:

(1) The bone conduction audiogram is not always an exact measure of the sensorineural reserve so a proportion of patients get 'overclosure' of the air–bone gap and a correspondingly gratifying result;

(2) Sometimes in the presence of a poor or very poor sensorineural reserve with impaired speech discrimination, operation may nevertheless be worthwhile either to enable the patient to use a hearing aid or to enable her to use one more effectively, even though it is realized that the patient may not be able to discard her hearing aid completely.

The clinical decision is even more complex if the patient has normal or near normal hearing on the better side. Opinion is divided concerning such patients: some otologists think that the surgical risk and results do not justify operation in such patients but many such patients do suffer a substantial degree of disability, inconvenience and social embarrassment and are grateful for any hearing improvement, even though the operated ear is still not as good as the normal one. The essential point is that the patient must be fully forewarned and must fully understand what benefits she may or may not expect. To a great extent this is a personal decision by the patient, even more than in the 'routine' case with a bilateral hearing loss.

Further criteria for operability consist of a negative Rinne test at least at 512 c.p.s., and an air–bone gap of at least 20 dB for the speech frequencies. The side selected for operation will be the worse side. The surgeon must always beware of the patient with the falling bone conduction curve, as previously mentioned. What may initially appear to be a satisfactory result in terms of air–bone closure on pure tone testing can in fact be a disadvantage to the patient in that what was formerly a fairly flat air conduction curve (well helped by a hearing aid) becomes a falling curve with further impairment of speech discrimination consequent upon the disproportionate improvement in the relatively unimportant low frequency carrier components of speech and greater consequent difficulty in using a hearing aid.

'Second side' stapedectomy calls for the greatest possible care in selection of patients. The patient with two ears functioning at an adequate level has only approximately a 10 dB advantage in a free field situation, although the inconveniences and embarrassments of one-sidedness have been referred to above. It has also been emphasized that vestibular compensation on the second side is often more difficult – sometimes very difficult – consequent upon unsuspected vestibular damage on the first side. Smyth and his colleagues [24] have emphasized the importance of adequate vestibular testing of patients for second side operations as well as the high incidence of vestibular abnormality after stapedectomy and the importance of avoiding an operation on the second side if there is any residual abnormality found in the first. The criteria for operating on the second ear depend to a great extent on the surgeon concerned. The following points are important:

(1) A certain time interval must have elapsed since the operation on the first side.

(2) A good hearing result must have been obtained with no impairment demonstrable on

either bone conduction audiometry or in speech discrimination testing. The patient must have had no unusual degree of post-operative vertigo and have normal vestibular responses.

(3) The operation should have been easy and atraumatic.

(4) It should preferably have been done by the same surgeon who has all details of any operative and post-operative problems – of which there should have been none.

The time interval varies between individual otologists: some of the best respected American surgeons will operate on a patient's second ear as early as 6–12 months if the first side was satisfactory. Many European surgeons are unwilling to operate until at least 2 or 3 years have elapsed and some will not operate at all on a patient's second side. A 'dead' ear can occur 8 or even 10 years after stapedectomy from the development of perilymph fistula (it can also occur, of course, with or without otosclerosis and with or without stapedectomy and from various unrelated causes). The author has now seen two patients, both with bilateral dead ears after stapedectomy in whom the time interval between operations was somewhat short.

Counselling of the patient for stapedectomy

It is essential that the patient should know exactly what she may and may not expect, especially if the disease is unilateral and the sensorineural reserve is impaired. The patient can be told that the likelihood of air–bone closure is approximately 90% and that partial air–bone closure will be obtained in a further 8%. The patient must also realize that hearing impairment can result from the operation and that this occasionally is severe and of sensorineural type. An incidence of 1 or 2% should generally be quoted for a primary operation. This may be more or less depending upon the surgeon and on the technical difficulty of the particular operation consequent upon anatomical factors or oval window obliteration. It must be emphasized that the incidence of sensorineural deafness is substantially greater (and the degree of success is less) in the case of revision operations.

Patients are usually interested not only in the short-term hearing gain, but also in how permanent any gain is likely to be. Recurrence of conductive deafness, for example, due to adhesions, or necrosis of the incus, or displacement of the prosthesis, or reclosure of the oval window can occur in a fairly small percentage of patients, the frequency varying substantially in reported series. More significant perhaps is the slowly progressive impairment of cochlear function that is sometimes seen. It is not always easy to determine whether this is due to a later effect of surgery, due to a late reaction to the graft or prosthesis, or whether it is due to effects of the otosclerotic process itself, or even to presbyacusis. Two studies have shown that approximately 12% of patients had sustained a loss between 11 and 25 dB for the speech frequencies at 6 years [25, 26]. Other reports of major series followed over an equal or longer period demonstrate no such deterioration.

The incidence of sudden severe sensorineural deafness occurring a long time after operation is even more difficult to define. The risk is small but always present. In a substantial proportion of patients this is probably due to the development of a perilymph fistula, a condition which may be preceded by a fluctuating level of hearing which demands immediate investigation and urgent exploration (see page 204).

The patient must be warned that slight dizziness in the first day or two is not unusual, and can generally be assured that any prolonged or severe unsteadiness or vertigo is not normally expected. Evidence of impaired vestibular function has been found in as many as 30% of patients during electronystagmography in the early months after operation though most patients become asymptomatic with the passage of time [24, 27, 28].

Excessive noise exposure after operation may cause some anxiety, but there is no evidence that stapedectomy predisposes to acoustic trauma. The temporary effect of industrial noise after stapedectomy is the same as in the normal patient [29].

After operation most European surgeons will insist upon the patient not flying for at least 1 or 2 months but in countries such as the United States where patients have often travelled a great distance for operation the surgeon will be asked how soon they can fly home again. American otologists who have been long experienced in stapedectomy will allow homeward flight 2 or 3 days after operation, though Shea [30] will permit it the day after operation if a living tissue seal has been used at the oval window.

Patients who have had a stapedectomy even months or years previously may be considered to be at some additional risk in view of the pressure changes involved, but the risks are apparently very small and probably negligible. In this respect a living tissue graft is perhaps safer than a piston prosthesis. It is probably unnecessarily cautious to advise patients never to fly as passengers, although perilymph fistula has been reported after flying in pressurised aircraft or even motoring in the mountains.

Contra-indications to stapedectomy

There are few contra-indications and to some extent these will be obvious from what has already been said in respect of age, impairment of the sensorineural reserve and other factors, such as general health. Active external otitis or a recent otitis media are clear contra-indications and both conditions must be fully healed and have remained healed before operation can be contemplated. A clean, dry central perforation of the tympanic membrane must be securely repaired by a preliminary operation if coexistent stapedial otosclerosis is suspected.

Vertigo of any significant severity is to be regarded as due to coexistent Menière's disease and most otologists will rightly regard this as an absolute contra-indication to stapedectomy. However, others state that they may consider operation if the condition has been in remission for at least 12 months, though in view of the frequent adhesions seen histologically in Menière's disease between footplate and saccule this seems somewhat risky.

Stapedectomy is contra-indicated in patients whose work demands frequent or major changes in barometric pressure or in whom a minor degree of vestibular decompensation could represent a major disability. Such occupations include professional pilots, divers, ballet dancers, professional athletes and those working at heights and in similar hazardous occupations. Caution should also be exercised in operating on the highly-trained ear of the professional musi-

cian especially if there is some preceding cochlear degeneration present. Distortion and recruitment may become manifest with the improvement in the hearing for air-conducted sound, even though the patient was formerly unaware of such problems.

Finally, it is again emphasized that the presence of a non-functioning ear on the opposite side is an absolute contra-indication to stapedectomy, except perhaps if and when the stage is finally reached at which the patient can no longer utilize any kind of hearing aid satisfactorily. It should also be emphasized that if tympanotomy shows that the round window is occluded, operation should be abandoned: attempts to re-open the round window almost invariably produce a profound sensorineural deafness.

Revision stapes operations

Revision stapes operations give the best results when the initial procedure has been a mobilization. In respect of stapedectomy itself it is again emphasized that the first operation should preferably be the last one because revision operations carry an increased risk of post-operative sensorineural hearing loss, are less likely to give an improvement than a primary procedure, and generally give a lesser amount of improvement.

Revision may be necessary for the relief of recurrent conductive deafness due to adhesions affecting any part of the reconstructed conducting mechanism, from necrosis of the incus, from displacement of the prosthesis or from reclosure of the oval window. The latter is unlikely to occur except in cases of oval window obliteration or active disease in young patients.

Urgent re-exploration must be carried out in those patients suspected of having either the early complication of reparative granuloma, or the later complication of perilymph fistula.

For the techniques and results of revision stapes surgery reference should again be made to Schuknecht [31].

Fenestration to stapedectomy

Stapedectomy in the previously fenestrated ear may be considered for certain patients in whom the fenestrated ear is the poorer one and in whom there is substantial residual ear–bone gap.

The following criteria must be satisfied:

(1) the sensorineural reserve is adequate;

(2) the fenestration cavity has been clean, dry and stable for at least several months;

(3) the malleus is mobile and in a satisfactory anatomical relationship to the oval window;

(4) the tympanic membrane is normally situated, without any medial displacement caused by loss of the posterosuperior segment of the tympanic annulus.

The operation is one which demands a high degree of surgical skill but which in good hands can produce a satisfactory level of hearing gain. The prosthesis should preferably be of fat/wire type [32].

Complications of stapedectomy

Most of the possible complications of stapedectomy will be self-evident from what has been written in previous paragraphs. The various complications can arbitrarily be classified as operative, early post-operative and late. For the various operative problems and complications which may be encountered reference should be made to texts dealing with operative surgery.

Facial palsy, *taste disturbance*, *perforations of the tympanic membrane*, *vertigo* and *infections* may occur as early post-operative problems, but only *reparative granuloma* should require any special comment. The exact cause is unknown, though it is said to occur in about 1% of stapedectomies. This complication can occur with both tissue graft and piston techniques. Contamination of the implant with foreign particles, trauma or crushing of tissue grafts, and excessive work within the margins of the oval window, the use of gelfoam, and surgical trauma in any form are probable aetiological factors. The development of such a granuloma probably accounts for the majority of cases of early sensorineural hearing loss. Reparative granuloma must be recognized promptly if a profound sensorineural loss is to be prevented. If 1 week after operation the flap and tympanic membrane appear red and boggy and there is a failure of hearing improvement the possibility of a granuloma filling the middle ear is to be borne in mind and urgent reopening of the middle ear should be considered. Typically, the granuloma fills much of the mesotympanum and completely obscures the region of the incus and oval window. Management consists of completely evacuating the granuloma, carefully removing the prosthesis and any extension of the granuloma into the oval window followed by the insertion of a different kind of prosthesis. Delay in treatment invites the development of a profound sensorineural deafness.

Of the late complications *suppurative labyrinthitis* and *meningitis* have been described due to perforation of the oval window graft by a sharp strut, but should not occur with modern stapedectomy techniques. *Recurrence of a conductive deafness* occasionally occurs and in the majority of patients is due to a *prosthesis problem. Delayed sensorineural deafness* can occur as late as 10 years after operation and in a high proportion of patients is due to the development of *perilymph fistula*. This complication should be suspected if a drop in hearing occurs which is of sensorineural type. The speech discrimination score may be disproportionately affected. Partial recovery of function may occur, only to be followed some time later by a more severe recurrence with less recovery until eventually a profound deafness is present. Giddiness is not necessarily a very prominent symptom and is sometimes quite insignificant. Perilymph fistula can occur with any kind of prosthesis, but probably has the least incidence if a living tissue graft has been used and the maximum incidence if gelfoam has been used. This complication is more common when the footplate has been removed completely or if the prosthesis is eccentrically placed. Urgent re-exploration is called for, but may not necessarily preserve the residual hearing. The leak is not always easy to identify, expecially if flimsy adhesions tend to obscure the oval window area. It is probably best not to remove the prosthesis, but simply to reinforce the region of the fistula by a fresh tissue graft supplemented by blood clot and a mucosal flap from the promontory.

Non-surgical treatment

Hearing aids

Not all patients are suitable for operation because of such factors as general health, small air–bone gap or poor sensorineural reserve. Not all patients who would benefit from operation will opt for surgical treatment. In every case it is the surgeon's duty to remember that stapedectomy is purely an elective procedure and to point out to his patient the relative advantages and disadvantages of a hearing aid. The misguided over-enthusiastic surgeon who pressurizes or unduly influences a patient towards operation will sooner or later regret the day.

For most patients a carefully selected hearing aid will give all the hearing advantages that a stapedectomy can offer with none of the risks or complications of surgery, infrequent though these may be in experienced hands. Moreover, modern aids are cosmetically unobtrusive and very reliable. It must also be remembered that any kind of conductive deafness is very easily compensated by means of an aid, especially conductive deafness due to otosclerosis, and that an aid can also help overcome any associated sensorineural impairment, something which surgery cannot do.

Although some very suitable patients will totally reject surgical help, there are by the same token many patients who although more suitable for a hearing aid are totally opposed to the idea and will opt for an inferior surgical result. The choice must essentially be that of the patient after all the facts have been clarified and in borderline cases a trial period with a hearing aid should be insisted upon.

In the very deaf otosclerotic patient with a poor sensorineural reserve, a hearing aid and stapedectomy together may provide the best means of successful rehabilitation. Moreover, the extremely deaf patient with little or even no bone-conduction thresholds recordable with a conventional clinical audiometer, but in whom otosclerosis is suspected either from the family history or from previous knowledge of the patient, may be enabled to use a hearing aid successfully after replacement of his fixed stapes.

As in all very deaf patients from whatever cause the fitting of an aid (or aids) should be combined with appropriate auditory retraining, lip-reading and other rehabilitative measures if necessary.

Medical treatment

As already indicated, considerable differences of opinion surround the question of sensorineural loss in otosclerosis. The question of medical treatment by the administration of sodium fluoride in order to cause maturation of the diseased bone and to arrest the development or progress of associated sensorineural deafness is even more controversial.

Fluoride treatment is based on the theory that foci of active disease, i.e. otospongiotic bone around the cochlea, release a product which is damaging to cochlear function and thereby produces a sensorineural deafness. The supporters of medical treatment argue that such damage will cease if the spongiotic foci can be altered into a mature otosclerotic bone.

The relationship of sodium fluoride to the prevention of dental decay is now generally accepted as is the fact that it exerts its benefit during the growth and development of the young tooth. There is good experimental evidence to indicate that fluorides have similar profound effects on young bone. Studies with labelled strontium in baby rats show that sodium fluoride promotes skeletal calcification and maturation. It also promotes the calcification of callus after experimental fractures. Likewise, skeletal decalcification initiated by steroids experimentally can be counteracted by sodium fluoride. In the human patient Valvassori [33] claims to be able to monitor the otospongiosis-otosclerosis process by polytomography and to show healing and calcification in patients receiving fluoride treatment.

Although the exact role of fluoride medication is still to be determined, Shambaugh [34] has put forward a strong case for its use in selected patients who have been diagnosed as having sensorineural deafness associated with cochlear otospongiosis with or without stapedial fixation. In presenting his preliminary results he concludes that fluoride medication is the 'only known method that gives promise for promoting recalcification and inactivation of an actively enlarging spongey otosporotic type of otosclerotic lesion'.

Sodium fluoride is a gastric irritant and must therefore be given in enteric-coated capsules. The drug is toxic, overdosage is dangerous and optimum dosage has still to be determined. It is probably in the range of 40 mg or possibly more daily in divided doses with meals. The duration of treatment is not defined, but normally should last at least 12 months and depends on poly-tomographic control to decide when the otospongiotic foci have become recalcified into mature bone. Skeletal fluorosis can occur if treatment is too prolonged. Because of its effect on the fetal skeleton medication is clearly contra-indicated in pregnancy and in patients with impaired renal function because of the risk of fluoride retention and consequent generalized skeletal effects. If fluoride medication fails it is suggested that 'Calcinar' (a synthetic calcitonin) can be used instead in the hope of promoting maturation of the otospongiotic foci.

References

[1] GUILD S. R. (1944) Histologic otosclerosis. *Annals of Otology, Rhinology and Laryngology* 53, 246.

[2] MORRISON A. W. (1971) Otosclerosis. In *Diseases of Ear, Nose and Throat*, eds. Ballantyne J. & Groves J., 3rd edn., Vol. 2, p. 358. London: Butterworth and Co. Ltd.

[3] LARSSON A. (1960) Otosclerosis: a genetic and clinical study. *Acta Otolaryngologica Supplement No. 154.*

[4] SCHUKNECHT H. F. (1971) *Stapedectomy*, p. 3. Boston: Little, Brown and Company.

[5] LARSSON A. (1960) Otosclerosis: a genetic and clinical study. *Acta Otolaryngologica Supplement No. 154.*

[6] MORRISON A. W. (1971) Otosclerosis. In *Diseases of Ear, Nose and Throat*, eds. Ballantyne J. & Groves J., 3rd edn., Vol. 2, p. 359 *et seq.* London: Butterworth and Co. Ltd.

[7] OGILVIE R. F. & HALL I. S. (1953) Observations on the pathology of otosclerosis. *Journal of Laryngology and Otology* 67, 497.

[8] CHEVANCE L. G., BRETLAU P., JØRGENSEN M. B. & CAUSSE J. (1970) Otosclerosis: an electron microscopic and cytochemical study. *Acta Otolaryngologica Supplement No. 272.*

[9] NAGER G. T. (1969) Histopathology of otosclerosis. *Archives of Otolaryngology* 89, 341.

[10] GRISTWOOD R. E. & VENABLES W. N. (1975) Otosclerotic obliteration of the oval window niche. *Journal of Laryngology and Otology* 89, 1185.

[11] SCHUKNECHT H. F. (1971) *Stapedectomy*, p. 40 *et seq.* Boston: Little, Brown and Company.

[12] GLORIG A. & GALLO R. (1962) Otosclerosis, ed. Schuknecht H. F., Chap. 4, *Henry Ford Hospital International Symposium*, p. 63. Boston: Little, Brown and Company.

[13] SHAMBAUGH G. E. JR. (1967) *Surgery of the Ear*, Chap. 18, p. 489. Philadelphia and London: W. B. Saunders and Company.

[14] SHAMBAUGH G. E. JR. (1976) Panel discussion on cochlear otospongiosis at *Fifth International Workshop, Chicago* – to be published.

[15] VALVASSORI G. E. (1976) Proceedings of the *Fifth International Workshop, Chicago* – to be published.

[16] SCHUKNECHT H. F. & KIRCHNER J. C. (1974) Cochlear otosclerosis: fact or fantasy. *Laryngoscope* 84, 766.

[17] HOOPLE G. D. (1966) Summation on discussion of sensorineural deafness in otosclerosis. *Annals of Otology, Rhinology and Laryngology* 75, 584.

[18] FRIEDMANN I. (1974) *Pathology of the Ear*, Chap. 5, p. 245. Oxford: Blackwell Scientific Publications.

[19] SCHUKNECHT H. F. (1974) in *Pathology of the Ear, Disorders of Growth, Metabolism and Aging.* p. 352. Cambridge, Mass.: Harvard University Press.

[20] VIROLAINEN E. (1972) Vestibular disturbances in clinical otosclerosis. *Acta Otolaryngologica Supplement No. 306.*

[21] BLACK F. O., SANDO I., HILDYARD V. H. & HEMENWAY W. G. (1969) Bilateral multiple otosclerotic foci and endolymphatic hydrops. *Annals of Otology, Rhinology and Laryngology* 78, 1062.

[22] SHEA J. J. (1958) Fenestration of the oval window. *Annals of Otology, Rhinology and Laryngology* 67, 932.

[23] SCHUKNECHT H. F., MCGEE T. M. & COLMAN B. H. (1960) Stapedectomy. *Annals of Otology, Rhinology and Laryngology* 69, 597.

[24] SMYTH G. D. L., KERR A. G. & SINGH K. P. (1975) Second ear stapedectomy – a continued controversy. *Journal of Laryngology and Otology* 89, 1047.

[25] MCGEE T. M. (1969) Fat-and-wire stapedectomy surgery. *Archives of Otolaryngology* 89, 423.

[26] HOUSE H. P. & GREENFIELD E. C. (1969) Five-year study of wire loop-absorbable gelatin sponge technique. *Archives of Otolaryngology* 89, 420.

[27] STROUD M. H. (1963) Permanent vestibular dysfunction in surgery for otosclerosis. *Laryngoscope* 73, 474.

[28] SPECTOR M. (1973) Electronystagmography after stapedectomy. *Annals of Otology, Rhinology and Laryngology* 82, 374.

[29] FERRIS K. (1967) A further study on the temporary effect of industrial noise on the hearing of stapedectomized ears at 4000 c.p.s. *Journal of Laryngology and Otology* 81, 613.

[30] SHEA J. J., JR. (1976) Panel discussion at the *Fifth International Workshop, Chicago* – to be published.

[31] SCHUKNECHT H. F. (1971) *Stapedectomy*, p. 109. Boston: Little, Brown and Company.

[32] SCHUKNECHT H. F. (1971) *Stapedectomy*, p. 103. Boston: Little, Brown and Company.

[33] VALVASSORI G. E. (1976) Paper presented to the *Fifth International Workshop, Chicago* – to be published.

[34] SHAMBAUGH G. E. JR. (1966) Therapy of cochlear otosclerosis. *Annals of Otology, Rhinology and Laryngology* 75, 579.

CHAPTER 16

Epistaxis

VASCULAR ANATOMY

For approximately 100 years it has been customary to divide the blood supply to the nose into that part arising from the external carotid artery and that from the internal carotid artery. The classical description of the blood supply of the nose was given by Zuckerkandl [1]. It is often said that Zuckerkandl stated that the blood supply to the nasal cavity is derived from branches of both the internal and external carotid arteries. He did not – he stated that the nasal cavity is supplied by the anterior nasal artery, the sphenopalatine artery and both ethmoidal arteries, but that the sphenopalatine artery is much more important, the other two branches only supplying collaterals. On entering the nasal cavity the sphenopalatine artery breaks up into three branches [2]: the inferior turbinate, the middle turbinate and the naso-palatine artery. These vessels and their chief branches run in the periosteum of the nasal mucoperiosteum. The inferior turbinate artery supplies the inferior turbinate and part of the common and inferior middle meatus. It has a main trunk which leaves the sphenopalatine artery and runs downwards and forwards to the posterior tip of the inferior turbinate where it divides into three terminal branches: the antral artery, and the medial and lateral terminal branches. The middle turbinate artery has a main trunk which leaves the sphenopalatine artery and runs along the lateral surface of the turbinate to the lower border of the bone where it enters a bony canal at the junction of the middle and posterior thirds of the turbinate and breaks up into three terminal branches which supply the anterior part of the turbinate and possibly a fourth branch, which supplies the bulla (Fig. 16.1).

The nasopalatine artery leaves the sphenopalatine foramen and passes along the antero-inferior border of the sphenoid to the septum. Before it leaves the lateral wall the superior turbinate branch is given off and a small artery to the sphenoid ostium. The superior turbinate artery gives off a branch which passes above the superior turbinate and anastomoses with the posterior and anterior ethmoid terminals in this area. The superior turbinate artery continues along the turbinate near its attachment supplying the posterior ethmoid cells and terminating in an anastamosis with the anterior ethmoid branches in the region of the anterior tip. The nasopalatine has two main branches: superior and inferior. The superior branch lies on the perpendicular plate; the lower just above the maxillary crest. The latter breaks into two further branches, one of which passes through the incisive foramen.

The anteroinferior region of the nasal septum is richly supplied with blood vessels and has been called at various times Little's area and Kiesselbach's plexus. These articles appeared in 1879 and 1880 respectively [3]. Little, who gave the earlier description, states that 'the septum at this point is supplied with branches of the anterior ethmoidal artery which anastomose freely with branches of the sphenopalatine artery. The lower portion of the septum is supplied by a branch of the superior coronary, the artery of the septum.'

The middle turbinate is said to be a useful landmark, in that bleeding above this is from a branch of the internal carotid system and below it from the external carotid system [4], but dye studies [5] have cast doubt on this. There are two opposing heads of pressure derived from the internal and external carotid arteries and the site of their interface depends on the relative pressure within them. In most of the cases studied by Shaheen injection of dye into the internal carotid artery did not cause discoloration of the upper part of the nasal cavity. It thus appears that the ethmoidal arteries contribute little to the arterial vasculature of the nose, as pointed out by Zuckerkandl. This may be due either to the interface of pressure between the two arterial systems or to the presence of a large branch from the sphenopalatine artery to the superior turbinate in the

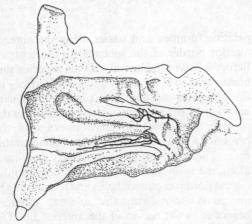

FIG. 16.1. The arterial supply of the lateral nasal wall, redrawn from Zuckerkandl [2].

equivalent area of the septum [2]. If arterial ligation is to be carried out this pressure interface must be borne in mind – ligation of the vessels on one side merely causes the vascular territory of the opposing vessel to increase and bleeding often continues. Furthermore, there is evidence to suggest that the anterior ethmoidal arteries are joined to one another by an anastomosis just anterior to the crista galli and this could account for persistent bleeding after ligature of one ethmoidal artery. Finally it should be noted that in about 15% of patients the anterior ethmoidal artery is absent on one side and in 2% on both sides [6].

Other vessels of less importance include the nasal branch of the descending palatine artery which leaves the canal just superior to the greater palatine foramen and supplies the floor of the nose, and the superior pharyngeal artery which supplies the choanal area.

SURGICAL PATHOLOGY

The cause of an epistaxis is not determined in about 30% of patients and the idiopathic group accounts for a further 55%. It can thus be seen that specific identifiable causes only account for 10–15% of all cases of epistaxis [7].

These causes will now be discussed in greater detail.

Hereditary haemorrhagic telangiectasia

This disease is also known as Rendu–Osler–Weber disease [8–10], but was first described in 1865 by Babington [11]. The gene of this hereditary disease is considered to be completely dominant and the defect may be passed from either parent to a child of either sex.

The presenting symptom in virtually all the patients is epistaxis. Telangiectases may occur on any mucous membrane or anywhere on the external surface of the body. The nasal mucosa is most commonly affected but lesions are frequently found in the tongue, palate, lips, buccal mucosa, pharynx and conjunctiva. The larynx, bronchi, stomach, colon, liver, bladder and brain have all been reported as sites for telangiectases. Isolated or multiple arterial venous fistulae may occur in the lung causing central cyanosis. On the skin the lesions occur on the face, the trunk, the arms, fingers, lips and nails, but bleeding rarely occurs from these sites because of the protective layer of squamous epithelium.

There are two basic vascular abnormalities: first, localized areas in the capillaries, where the walls have been reduced to the endothelial layers only, perhaps due to an inherited lack of elastic tissue, and secondly, visible dilatations of arterioles and capillaries leading to arteriovenous fistulae such as may be found in the lungs. Bleeding always occurs from the summit of the telangiectases and never extravasates into the surrounding tissue. It thus appears that the factors which determine whether the lesions bleed or not are to be found in the state of the overlying epithelium and not in the vessels themselves. It is this fact which has led to the forms of treatment which attempt to modify the overlying epithelium [12].

Infections

Epistaxis may occur in any infection due to the accompanying hyperaemia but certain infectious diseases have long been known to produce epistaxis including rheumatic fever, nasal diphtheria, smallpox, whooping cough, scarlet fever and typhoid fever, all of which are now fortunately uncommon. Local infection in the nose or sinuses secondary to a straightforward upper respiratory infection was found to be the cause of half the cases of epistaxis under the age of 15 in one series [13]. Epistaxis in children may also be due to the presence of an intranasal foreign body.

Epistaxis may occur from the edges of a chronic septal perforation of whatever cause due to separation of the crusts which form around the edge of the perforation, particularly if the cartilage is exposed.

Tumours

Benign tumours of the nose, sinuses and nasopharynx are uncommon and the only important benign tumour causing epistaxis is the juvenile angiofibroma. Haemangiopericytoma is a relatively rare tumour which has also been recorded as causing epistaxis.

Malignant tumours which are usually primary but may also be secondary are well known to cause a blood-stained nasal discharge, though not all do. Nasal symptoms are present in 34%, 55% and 91% respectively in tumours of the antrum, ethmoid and the nasal cavity. It can thus be seen that a nose bleed is not often an early symptom of carcinoma of the maxillary sinus [14].

Coagulation defects

These may be due to lung disease, liver disease or anticoagulants and appear to be responsible for about 5% of epistaxes. The most important diseases are leukaemia, haemophilia, von Willebrandt's disease, polycythaemia, macroglobulinaemia, myeloma and thrombocytopenia. The bleeding may also be due to administration of anticoagulants [7]. The spontaneous fibrinolytic activity of the plasma has also been measured in all patients with epistaxis and was found to be significantly higher in patients at the time of haemorrhage than after recovery some weeks later [15].

Idiopathic

The so-called idiopathic group includes about 85% of patients. These patients can be divided largely into those who bleed from the anteroinferior part of the septum (Little's area) in children, and those from the superior part of the nose in the elderly.

The exact pathology of bleeding from Little's area in children is not clearly known but it appears to be related to two factors: The hyperaemia and congestion of the upper respiratory tract which is notorious in children, and nose picking and repeated rubbing of an area where the mucosa is stretched over cartilage and bone. Other factors include the richness of the local anastamosis and possibly obstruction at the incisive foramen by anterior dislocation of the septum [16].

Much the commonest group of patients requiring hospital admission for a nose bleed are the so-called cardiovascular causes which form about half of the entire total. Although it is commonly thought that the cause in these patients is hypertension, careful studies [5, 15, 17] have shown that the blood pressure in these patients is no higher than in an age- and sex-matched controlled population. Shaheen has shown by histological studies that there is a loss of muscle in the tunica media which is replaced by collagen and the changes are most pronounced in persons suffering from epistaxis. This type of change resembles the arterial degeneration described in the cerebral arteries of patients dying from cerebral haemorrhage [18]. It therefore appears that whilst the hypertension may initiate the bleeding its persistence and severity are explained not by the elevated blood pressure but by the inability of the large vessels to contract.

Drugs and other toxic substances

Aspirin is a well-known cause of disorders of coagulation and was thought to be responsible in 5% of one series [19]. The significance of this is hard to assess since it has been shown that 33% of all patients attending hospital have recently been taking aspirin [20].

Inhaled toxins which can cause epistaxis include chrome, mercury and phosphorus.

CLINICAL FEATURES

Epistaxis is a common disease and it has been shown that approximately 10% of the normal population have suffered a significant nose bleed [17]. The disease may occur at any age but its maximum age incidence in adults is in the 60–69 age group in both sexes. It is more common in men than in women (6:4) and is subject to seasonal variation being half as common again in January as in June. The haemorrhage is often severe and the haemoglobin falls to 10 g/dl or less in approximately one-third of patients. The mortality rate is in the region of 1% due to cardiovascular disease or the progress of an underlying disorder such as liver failure [7]. Severe complications may also occur due to pulmonary oedema and reaction to transfusion; if radical treatment is needed such as arterial ligation this may also be attended by fairly severe complications.

MANAGEMENT

The management of epistaxis is traditionally divided into two phases: arrest of the haemorrhage and treatment of the underlying cause.

Arrest of haemorrhage

In general the bleeding may be stopped by one of two methods.

Local cautery

Chemical cautery, with silver nitrate in various percentages from 10–50% or trichloracetic acid, or electrocoagulation, require little further comment.

The silver nitrate may be used more elegantly in the form of a pre-packed silver nitrate stick (Wellcroft).

Packing of the nose

This may be done with gauze, preferably soaked in a mild antiseptic, and may need to be applied to one or both sides of the anterior part of the nasal cavity or to the post-nasal space.

Various methods of packing the nose with inflatable balloons have been used over the last 60 years beginning in 1917 [21]. Stevens described one of the best known: he states that the apparatus is very efficient and has produced no complications when used properly; in no case did he see a perforation except when the balloon was used after an SMR. He also measured the pressure in the balloon which amounted to 30 mmHg, which is well below the blood pressure so that ischaemic necrosis should not occur [22, 23]. A similar method for managing post-nasal epistaxis has been described using a Foley catheter. The procedure requires a Foley catheter (12 or 14) with a 30 ml balloon. The tip of the catheter distal to the balloon is removed to avoid trauma and irritation of the pharynx. The catheter is lubricated and passed along the floor of the affected nostril through the choana and into the nasopharynx. The balloon is then inflated with approximately 7 ml of water; the catheter is then drawn forward and a further 15 ml or so of water is added to fix the balloon in position. In order to provide the necessary powerful traction some means of anterior fixation is required and unless care is exercised this can lead to pressure necrosis of the ala of the nose. A sophisticated technique using a tripod traction mask to prevent this has been described in twelve patients with a satisfactory outcome [24].

A simpler method of occluding both the anterior and posterior choanae is provided by the Brighton balloon [26] (Fig. 16.2). The instrument is passed into one nostril and after the tip has reached the post-nasal wall, the fixed distal balloon is inflated with 8–12 ml of air. Tension is then applied to the shaft, thus occluding the posterior choana on that side. The mobile proximal balloon is moved up the shaft until it is within the nasal vestibule; it is then inflated thus anchoring the cuff to the shaft. By closing off the nasal cavity on that side, the haemorrhage is controlled.

Other inflatable balloons for occluding have been designed by Simpson, and by Mawson [26].

Arterial ligation

It is said that the first ligation of the common carotid artery for haemorrhage was carried out by Abernathy in 1795 [27]. The first ligation of this artery for epistaxis was reported in 1904 [28] in a patient with sarcoma of the maxilla. The operation was partially successful but it was later felt necessary to tie the other common carotid artery which resulted in the death of the patient.

The mortality rate of this procedure is high, in the region of 35%, and furthermore the almost uniform presence of a complete circle of Willis allows cross circulation and continuing haemorrhage.

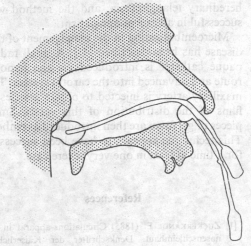

FIG. 16.2.

Ligation of the anterior ethmoidal artery is more successful and much less dangerous [29]. Ligation of the external carotid artery for postoperative nasal bleeding has been described [30] as has ligation of the internal maxillary artery [31]. In the latter procedure the maxillary sinus is opened from the oral cavity as in the Caldwell–Luc operation. Through a large opening in the posterior wall of the antrum the internal maxillary artery is separated by blunt dissection from the fatty tissue of the pterygo-palatine fossa and is then ligated using clips.

Treatment by drugs

Antifibrinolysins
Bacteria with fibrinolytic activity can be isolated from the nose of patients with epistaxis, and the fibrinolytic activity of patients with spontaneous activity is significantly higher than from the same patients some weeks later. The total fibrinolytic activity in the nasal mucosa is significantly higher

in patients with epistaxis while they are bleeding than a month later. In a double blind study to assess the effect of the anti-fibrinolytic drug tranexamic acid (cyklokapron) which is similar to the anti-fibrinolytic agent, aminocaproic acid (Epsikapron®) it was found that recurrent bleeding was significantly less in frequency and severity amongst the treated patients; furthermore, the hospital stay of the treated patients was reduced by 1·5 days compared with patients treated by placebo [15].

Vitamins
On occasion preparations containing vitamin C or vitamin K have been advised or prescribed. These vitamins have no part to play in the treatment of epistaxis except in the rare instance in which the patient is bleeding because of an actual deficiency of these vitamins.

Oestrogens
It has been suggested that spontaneous haemorrhage, including epistaxis, is a manifestation of a systemic disease due to a reduction of the circulating blood oestrogens and that this deficiency incited the formation of a tissue toxin which promoted vascular catabolism [32]. This is the rationale for treating patients with epistaxis by oestrogens; good results were claimed but the matter was not subjected to a trial. This view was encouraged by further work [33] in which a fibrinolytic enzyme was found in the circulating blood in women during menstruation, late toxaemia of pregnancy and prolonged labour, but not in non-menstruating women or uncomplicated pregnancy.

A properly controlled clinical trial of the effects of premarin and oestrogen [34] showed that oestrogens had no effect on the duration of the epistaxis and this method has not been heard of since.

Treatment of hereditary haemorrhagic telangiectasia

The following methods of treatment for epistaxis in this disease have been described [35].
(1) Electrocautery and various caustics.
(2) Partial resection of the nasal septum.
(3) Irradiation.

(4) Hormone therapy with oestrogens.
(5) Amputation of the nose.
(6) Septal dermoplasty.
(7) Microembolization.
(8) Cryosurgery.

Treatment of this disease with systemic oestrogens has been described [36] and it demonstrates that systemic oestrogens in guinea-pigs cause the ciliated columnar epithelium of the nose to undergo metaplasia to squamous epithelium. These experiments followed previous clinical observations [37], which suggested the use of oestrogenic hormones because of the apparent relationship between the recurrent epistaxis and the menstrual cycle. In one patient, the epistaxis occurred for a few days before the end of the secretory phase and disappeared shortly after the onset of menstruation. In animal experiments systemic oestrogens were used in an initial daily dose of 0·25 mg ethynyl oestradiol increasing by 0·5 mg per day at the end of 4 weeks if the epistaxis had not ceased. Twenty patients were treated successfully with this regime and biopsies from the nasal mucosa in many of these patients showed that squamous metaplasia had occurred [36].

The principle of squamous metaplasia was also employed by Saunders [38] who argued that although the telangiectases could occur anywhere in the nose, bleeding was usually from the anterior part of the septum because this is the part subjected to trauma, and if mucosa at this area was to be replaced with skin the latter tissue would prove much more resistant. In septal dermoplasty the septal mucosa is scraped off and a split thickness skin graft from the thigh or buttock is placed on the anterior third of both sides of the nasal septum. The graft extends from the dorsum to the floor of the nose and is carried far enough anteriorly to be sutured to the vestibular skin. This technique has proved to be successful in large numbers of patients with cessation of nose bleeding and return of the haemoglobin to normal values. Recurrence of the telangiectases within the skin graft has, however, been reported by others [39].

Cryosurgery has also been used in this disease [40]. In this report preliminary studies were first carried out on dogs with an experimentally produced severe epistaxis, which was controlled by

freezing at −20° C for 60 minutes; subsequent histological analysis showed that after 2 weeks the mucosa recovered completely and there was no destruction of the nasal cartilage. Cryotherapy was then tried on twenty-one patients with severe epistaxis. A Stevens nasal balloon was perfused with coolant at −20° C for 60 minutes and left in the nose to act as a tampon. The patients treated included nine patients with hereditary telangiectasia, and the method was successful in all except one patient.

Microembolization in the management of this disease has been described [41]. A small radiopaque catheter is introduced via the femoral route and advanced into the carotid system. The maxillary artery is injected to obtain a series of films of the distribution of this vessel. Small pieces of gel foam are then introduced as emboli. This technique appears to have been successful for a time at least in one very severe case.

References

[1] ZUCKERKANDL E. (1885) Circulations-apparat in der nasenschleimhaut. Denkschrifter der Kaiserlichen. Akademie der Wissenschafter Mathematisch-Naturwissenschaftliche Classe. Vol. 49, pp. 121–52.

[2] BURNHAM H. H. (1935) An anatomical investigation of blood vessels in the lateral nasal wall and their relation to turbinates and sinuses. *Journal of Laryngology and Otology* 50, 569.

[3] MCKENZIE D. (1914) Little's area of a locus Kieselbachii. *Journal of Laryngology and Otology* 29, 21.

[4] CAHN H. L. (1955) The control of epistaxis by arterial ligation. *Archives of Otolaryngology* 61, 641.

[5] SHAHEEN O. (1970) Studies of the nasal vasculature and the problems of arterial ligation for epistaxis. *Annals of the Royal College of Surgeons of England* 47, 30.

[6] SHAHEEN O. (1975) Arterial epistaxis. *Journal of Laryngology and Otology* 89, 17.

[7] JUSELIUS H. (1974) Epistaxis. *Journal of Laryngology and Otology* 88, 317.

[8] RENDU M. (1896) Epistaxis repetées chez sujet porteur de petits angiomes cutanes et muqueuex. *Bulletin et Memoires de la Sôcieté de Medicine des Hôpital de Paris* 13, 731.

[9] OSLER W. (1901) On a family form of recurring epistaxis with multiple telangiectases of the skin and mucous membranes. *Johns Hopkins Hospital Bulletin* 12, 333.

[10] WEBER F. P. (1907) A case of multiple hereditary developmental angiomata (telangiectases) of the skin and mucous membranes associated with recurring haemorrhages. *Lancet* 2, 160.

[11] BABINGTON B. G. (1865) Hereditary epistaxis. *Lancet* **2**, 362.

[12] HARRISON D. F. N. (1964) Familial haemorrhagic telangiectasia. *Quarterly Journal of Medicine, New Series* **33**, 25.

[13] EVANS J. (1962) The aetiology and treatment of epistaxis. *Journal of Laryngology and Otology* **76**, 185.

[14] LEDERMAN M. (1970) Tumours of the upper jaw. *Journal of Laryngology and Otology* **84**, 369.

[15] PETRUSON B. (1974) Epistaxis. *Acta Otolaryngologica* Supplement 317, 53.

[16] JONES R. M. (1971) Affections of the external nose and nasal cavities. In *Scott-Brown's Diseases of the Ear Nose and Throat,* eds. Groves J. & Ballantine J. C., p. 28, London: Butterworth.

[17] WEISS N. S. (1972) The relation of high blood pressure to headache and epistaxis and selected other symptoms. *New England Journal of Medicine* **287**, 631.

[18] RUSSELL D. S. (1954) The pathology of spontaneous intracranial haemorrhage. *Proceedings of the Royal Society of Medicine* **47**, 689.

[19] TUCKER W. N. (1963) Investigations and treatment of epistaxis. *New Zealand Medical Journal* **63**, 283.

[20] PARRY D. J. & WOOD P. H. N. (1967) The relationship between aspirin taking and gastro-duodenal haemorrhage. *Gut* **8**, 301.

[21] BECK A. L. (1917) An inflatable rubber ball for intranasal use. *American Journal of Surgery* **31**, 77.

[22] STEVENS R. W. (1936) Improved nasal packing. *Archives of Otolaryngology* **23**, 232.

[23] STEVENS R. W. (1951) Nasal packing. *Archives of Otolaryngology* **54**, 191.

[24] BELL M., HAWK M. & JAHAN A. (1874) New device for the management of post nasal epistaxis by balloon tamponade. *Archives of Otolaryngology* **99**, 372.

[25] WADSWORTH P. (1971) Method of controlling epistaxis. *British Medical Journal* **1**, 506.

[26] MAWSON S. (1956) Inflatable post nasal tampon. *Lancet* **1**, 486.

[27] HUNTER E. & GIBSON R. (1969) Arterial ligations for severe epistaxis. *Journal of Laryngology and Otology* **83**, 1099.

[28] BARTLETT W. & MCKITTRICK O. F. (1917) The stud_ secondary haemorrhage treated by ligation of the co. mon carotid artery. *Annals of Surgery* **65**, 715.

[29] GOODYEAR H. M. (1937) Nasal haemorrhage: Ligation of the anterior ethmoid artery. *The Laryngoscope* **47**, 97.

[30] BARRETT J. & ORR W. (1908) Two cases of epistaxis in which ligation of external carotid artery became necessary. *Intercolonial Medical Journal of Australasia* **13**, 314.

[31] SEIFFERT A. (1928) Unterbindung der Arteria maxillaris interna. *Zeitschrift Hals Nasen unt Ohrenkeilkunde* **22**, 323.

[32] JACOBSON P. (1954) Spontaneous haemorrhage. *Archives of Otolaryngology* **59**, 523.

[33] SMITH O. W. (1947) A menstrual toxin. *American Journal of Obstetrics and Gynecology* **54**, 204.

[34] GRANT J. H. (1961) Clinical evaluation of the use of premarin and the treatment of epistaxis. *Journal of Laryngology and Otology* **75**, 909.

[35] BRADBEER W. H. (1969) Treatment of hereditary telangiectasia. *Journal of Laryngology and Otology* **83**, 667.

[36] HARRISON D. F. N. (1964) Familial haemorrhagic telangiectasia. *Quarterly Journal of Medicine, New Series* **33**, 25.

[37] KOCH H. J., ESCHER G. C. & LOUIS J. S. (1952) Hormonal management of hereditary haemorrhagic telangiectasia. *Journal of the American Medical Association* **149**, 1376.

[38] SAUNDERS W. H. (1960) Permanent control of nose bleeds in patients with hereditary haemorrhagic telangiectasia. *Annals of Internal Medicine* **53**, 147.

[39] MCCABE W. P. & KELLY A. P. (1972) Management of epistaxis in Osler, Webber, Rondu Disease. *Plastic and Reconstructive Surgery* **50**, 114.

[40] BLUESTONE C. C. & SMITH H. C. (1967) Intranasal freezing for severe epistaxis. *Archives of Otolaryngology* **85**, 445.

[41] KENDALL B. E., JOYNER L. R. & GRANT H. (1977) Microembolisation in the management of epistaxis in hereditary haemorrhagic telangiectasia. *Clinical Otolaryngology* **2**, 249.

CHAPTER 17

Nose and Sinus Infections

RHINITIS

The common cold

The cold is the most common illness of man. The disease also has economic aspects because it is probably the most important cause of absenteeism from work.

Pathology

The common cold syndrome can be caused by a large number of agents but more than 90% are non-bacterial and are usually viral. The most important group are the rhinoviruses of which more than eighty different types have now been identified. Rhinoviruses contain RNA and are about 30 nm in diameter. They are inactivated at a pH3 which is the reason that they are not found in the intestinal tract. Other viruses include the myxovirus, the Coxsackie A and B viruses, ECHO viruses and the adenovirus [1].

The common cold occurs in all countries of the world. Although there is a widespread belief that exposure to cold is important this has never been convincingly demonstrated. The infection is transmitted by droplet infection; within 24 hours after infection the first changes in the epithelium of the nasal passages and pharynx begin: hyperaemia, oedema, and a leucocyte infiltration. After 2–5 days the ciliated columnar epithelium is desquamated followed by regeneration of new epithelium.

Oedema of the mucosa can close off the ostia of the nasal sinuses and the Eustachian tube, causing sinusitis and otological symptoms.

Clinical features

In the acute stage the illness is characterized by nasal obstruction, sneezing, and profuse watery secretion. There is a general feeling of malaise and a mild fever. The patient complains of a smarting feeling in the nose and nasopharynx. Rhinoscopy shows a swollen, fiery red mucosa covered with watery secretion.

In almost all cases this first viral stage is followed by bacterial infection of the damaged nasal mucosa. Secretion is then purulent. Normally this bacterial phase heals in several days with or without treatment. In 5–10 days unless complications occur the whole process is healed.

Taking into account the great frequency of the common cold, complications such as tubal catarrh, otitis media, and sinusitis are rare. In some cases the illness tends to descend into the lower respiratory tract causing laryngitis, tracheitis, bronchitis, and pneumonia. In patients with atopic rhinitis or bronchitis the course of the disease is more often chronic with a persisting purulent phase.

Treatment

There is no specific treatment known for viral rhinitis. Aspirin can be given as symptomatic treatment. It has never been convincingly demonstrated that high doses of vitamin C have a favourable effect on the course of the common cold [2].

Vasoconstrictor nose drops can relieve the troublesome nasal obstruction and may help to prevent complications. Nose drops containing sympathomimetic agents should always be prescribed in isotonic aqueous solution and never in an oily solution; the latter can cause lipid pneumonia if aspirated into the lower respiratory tract. In addition to their vasoconstrictor action the ciliary movement of the nasal mucosa may be paralysed preventing the normal drainage of secretions. This should be taken into account when prescribing nose drops. The second side effect of vasoconstrictor nose drops is the so-called rebound effect: after the desired constriction of the nasal mucosa a period of reactive vasodilatation and swelling occurs which encourages the patient to have recourse again to the nose drops. This may set up a vicious circle so that the patient uses more and more nose drops more and more often (*rhinitis medicamentosa.*) Nose drops should therefore only be prescribed for self-limiting diseases and then only for a period of at most 10 days.

In contrast to the viral phase of the common cold the bacterial phase is amenable to treatment. In the vast majority of patients this is not necessary since healing occurs spontaneously. Antibacterial treatment always needs to be given to 'at risk' patients with, e.g., recurrent sinusitis, nasal polypi, asthma, bronchitis; in that case a broad spectrum antibiotic active against the *Haemophilus influenzae* is to be preferred since this is the responsible organism in most instances. Antibiotics are also indicated in patients in which the bacterial rhinitis threatens to become or is already chronic.

In infants acute rhinitis is a serious and sometimes life-threatening disorder. The newborn is almost exclusively dependent on nasal respiration. Furthermore, a patent nasal airway is necessary for satisfactory breast or bottle feeding. As the result of the rhinitis a rise in temperature and convulsions can occur. Treatment consists of the administration of antibiotics as determined by culture, and care of the airway by regular suction of the nose and possibly by means of vasoconstrictor nose drops. The latter must be used very carefully and in low concentration since overdosage occurs very quickly. Overdosage can declare itself initially by motor excitement, and later by somnolence and even collapse. Naturally, prophylaxis is very important in infants; and therefore contact with patients with colds must be prevented.

In older children and adults a chronic rhinitis may proceed to hypertrophic or hyperplastic rhinitis, especially if there is an atopic rhinitis combined with chronic infection. In the long term irreversible changes then occur in the mucosa characterized by an increase of the mesenchymal elements of the nasal mucosa. The anterior end of the middle turbinate, and the inferior edge and the posterior end of the inferior

turbinate are particularly involved in this process. Chronic nasal obstruction then exists which no longer responds to nose drops satisfactorily. The diagnosis can be made simply from the rhinoscopic appearances; posterior rhinoscopy often shows an enormously swollen posterior end of the turbinate which resembles a raspberry in appearance and which can close the choana completely.

Management consists of the removal of the irreversibly altered epithelium and possibly a very conservative and preferably submucous turbinectomy. Naturally, the underlying condition (atopy, infection, or chronic sinusitis) must also be treated to prevent a recurrence.

Atrophic rhinitis (ozaena)

Pathology
Atrophic disease of the nose may cover a whole spectrum from mild atrophy of the mucosa to ozaena which renders the patient a social outcast. In the mild forms of atrophic rhinitis (*rhinitis sicca*) the complaint is usually of a crust formation in the nose; epistaxis also occurs. Anterior rhinoscopy shows a dry glazed nasal mucosa with crusting, especially in the anterior part of the nose. The cause of the disorder, as of ozaena, is not known.

With increasing severity of the disorder more nasal atrophy occurs: the nasal skeleton atrophies, the nasal passages become very wide, and histological examination of the nasal mucosa shows metaplasia of the ciliary epithelium to squamous epithelium, atrophy of the entire mucosa, and degeneration of the goblet cells and the glands. Anterior rhinoscopy shows a very wide nose, the turbinates are markedly atrophied and sometimes have even disappeared and there is crust formation but no foetor.

The term ozaena is used when the nasal atrophy is accompanied by a marked formation of crusts and foetor. There is a general impression that the disorder is now seen less often in Europe than several decades ago, possibly due to improved nutrition and hygiene. The aetiology of ozaena is not known. According to some authors the basic cause is chronic inflammation and according to others a chronic iron deficiency. Although *Klebsiella ozaenae* can be cultured from the nasal secretion of patients with ozaena it has never been demonstrated that this is the causal organism. It is well known that radical operations in which the nasal cavity is widened, such as turbinectomy, can cause ozaena.

Histological examination of the nasal epithelium in ozaena shows the same changes as in nasal atrophy but to a greater degree.

The disease can begin in early life but usually does so between the fourteenth and sixteenth year. Ozaena occurs three times more commonly in women than in men. There are clear differences in racial incidence so that ozaena is very rare in Negroes both in the USA and in Africa. There is also some evidence that hereditary factors may be important.

Clinical features

The principal complaint is of the intolerable smell emanating from the patient's nose. Since ozaena is almost always accompanied by anosmia the patient does not notice the smell himself but his attention is drawn to it by others. In serious cases the patient is forced to shun all social contact. Despite the wide nasal cavities patients often complain of nasal obstruction due to extensive formation of crusts, headache, and epistaxis. Anterior rhinoscopy shows the changes of nasal atrophy and the atrophic nasal mucosa is covered with yellowish-green or yellowish-brown crusts. Posterior rhinoscopy also usually shows crusts in the nasopharynx. The repulsive smell is typical and unmistakable.

Treatment

If little is known of the aetiology of ozaena even less is known of specific treatment. The source of the smell can be removed by keeping the nose free of crusts. This can often be achieved by nasal douches three times a day with an isotonic saline solution and instillation of drops of inert oil to loosen the crusts. The results of countless forms of medical treatment which are to be found in the literature such as hormones, vitamins, iron supplements, antibiotics, and so forth are at best doubtful.

If conservative treatment does not achieve the desired result, operation to narrow the nose may be successful. Submucous implants may be introduced into the nose, paying particular attention to the lateral wall and the posterior half of the nose. Plastic materials, bone, and cartilage can be used as implants.

Good results have been attained from a method in which the vestibule is completely closed off on one or both sides using skin flaps. The nasal mucosa returns to normal over the course of several months and the crust formation and foetor disappear. If the nose is reopened after a reasonable period, which is usually more than a year, healing may sometimes be permanent [3].

Occupational diseases of the nose

Damage may be caused to the nose by substances inhaled as a result of one's occupation. The inhaled substances may have a chemical, mechanical, or an allergic action. For a long time it has been known that workers in chromate factories may be affected by septal perforations. The perforations always occur in the cartilaginous septum 1–2 cm behind the columella and are seldom larger than 2 cm in diameter. The disorder often causes no symptoms. Soda, arsenic vapour, several salts, and inorganic acids can cause septal perforations by the action of their vapour or because they are deposited as fine powder on the nasal mucosa.

Atrophic rhinitis can also occur due to the influence of chemicals. Long continued inhalation of some substances can damage the olfactory epithelium causing anosmia and this has been described as being due to ammonia, formaldehyde, osmium trioxide, mercury, several inorganic acids, and chromium compounds amongst others.

Working in a dusty environment, e.g. near cement, coal metal, flour, and tobacco, can also cause septal perforation and in this case a mechanical factor is probably important.

Allergic occupational disorders are discussed in Chapter 18.

Finally it should be noted that carcinoma of the nose and sinuses occurs more frequently in those who work with nickel and chromium compounds, isopropyl alcohol, X-rays, and radioactive substances. Ethmoidal carcinoma occurs more frequently in workers in the wood and leather industries [4].

Specific infections of the nose

Syphilis

A primary chancre of the nasal mucosa is rare. It is usually found anteriorly on the septum or on the anterior end of the medial turbinate; it is almost always unilateral.

The nasal mucosa is swollen, there is a unilateral purulent rhinorrhea and sometimes oedema of the entire nose.

Marked swelling of the appropriate lymph nodes typically occurs. The equally rare primary chancre of the skin of the nose does not differ appreciably from that at other sites on the skin. The secondary stage of syphilis of the nose has few typical features: nasal obstruction, little secretion, and sometimes fissures of the vestibule of the nose. Lymphangitis and lymphadenitis almost always occur.

The tertiary stage of syphilis is the most important as far as the nose is concerned. The most common form of this disease is a diffuse infiltration involving all layers of the nose. The nose is swollen, blocked, and extremely painful; the local lymph nodes are usually not involved. In the long term, foetid sequestrae, necrosis, and rejection of part of the nose occur. In the healing phase synechiae, perforations of the septum, and marked cosmetic deformities occur. A rarer form of tertiary syphilis is the solitary gumma which if it occurs in the septum usually causes a perforation.

Congenital syphilis in the newborn is characterized by 'luetic sniffles': purulent rhinorrhoea, sometimes with crust formation and often accompanied by vestibulitis. The disease can be differentiated from other forms of rhinitis by the presence of lymphangitis and lymphadenitis. A later form occurs only about the tenth year of life and has many features in common with the diffuse infiltration of the nose in the third stage of acquired syphilis.

The diagnosis is confirmed by the presence of spirochaetes in the secretions and tissues and by positive serology. The treatment is carried out by the venereologist. Syphilis of the nose is nowadays extremely uncommon but since the frequency of venereal disease is increasing the possibility of this disease must always be borne in mind.

Tuberculosis

A primary tubercular focus in the nose is extremely uncommon and only occurs in children. The later stages of tuberculosis can have many forms, of which the most important is lupus vulgaris of the skin of the nose. This is a slowly progressive disease which leads to serious mutilation after some years in the absence of treatment. The characteristic of this disorder is that pressure with a glass spatula causes the so-called 'apple jelly' patches to appear. Acid-fast bacilli are not often demonstrated or cultured in this disorder so the diagnosis may be difficult. In this and in all other forms of nasal tuberculosis a careful search must always be made for a focus elsewhere in the body, especially, of course, in the lungs. In patients who have previously had lupus the development of lupus carcinoma must always be suspected; this disorder is always radio-resistant and metastasizes rapidly. There is probably a connection between the radiotherapy previously often used in lupus and the development of the carcinoma [5].

The nasal mucosa can also be affected by lupus vulgaris. A septal perforation eventually occurs, almost always of the cartilaginous septum.

In advanced stages of pulmonary tuberculosis, especially in patients in poor general condition, a rapidly progressive ulcerating tuberculous infection of the nasal mucosa can occur. In contrast to lupus vulgaris described above the secretions are in this case rich in tubercle bacilli.

Modern tuberculous therapy has made advanced nasal tuberculosis rare.

Rhinoscleroma

This disease is caused by *Klebsiella rhinoscleromatis* which has a certain relationship to *Streptococcus pneumoniae*. This disease is endemic in eastern Europe (Poland and Russia) but is an imported disease in western Europe. Rhinoscleroma is also encountered fairly often in North Africa, Indonesia, and South America. This disease is not very infectious, and its incubation period is unknown.

Initially the symptoms are those of chronic rhinitis, often with a clinical picture like that of ozaena. Later the nasal mucosa becomes thickened and in the third stage this thickening

...pands into very hard infiltrates which bleed easily and which cause nasal obstruction and later external deformity of the nose. Often the disease extends to the nasopharynx and sometimes to the base of the tongue and the epiglottis. Scar formation occurs after the disease has healed leading to stenosis of the nasal passages. The diagnosis in the early stages is difficult; Russell bodies and Mikulicz cells are typical but these are only encountered in large numbers in later stages. A history of having lived outside Europe is also very important. Long-term treatment with relatively high doses of antibiotics is indicated.

Leprosy

Leprosy is a skin disease caused by *Mycobacterium leprae,* which is an acid-fast bacillus showing marked similarities to the tubercle bacillus. The disease can extend to the nasal mucosa. In the first stage the clinical picture is similar to that of rhinoscleroma but later infiltrations (leproma) occur which ultimately ulcerate resulting in a foetid purulent rhinorrhoea. Later still the supporting tissues of the nose decay resulting in a septal perforation, usually of the cartilaginous septum, and broadening of the nasal skeleton.

Rhinosporidiosis

Rhinosporidiosis is a chronic granulomatous disease caused by the fungus *Rhinosporidium seeberi.* The disease is endemic in India and Ceylon but occurs sporadically throughout other parts of the world. The symptoms caused by nasal rhinosporidiosis are epistaxis, nasal obstruction, and purulent nasal discharge. Examination shows red polypoid, haemorrhagic tumours of the nose in which the rhinosporidium filled with spores can be demonstrated by histology. Treatment is usually confined to removal of the granulations.

Mucormycosis

The occurrence of the fungus mucor in the nose can lead to rhinocerebral phycomycosis. This is a severe, acute illness with fever and mental deterioration. Infarction in the nose and sinuses spreads to the orbit and the central nervous system. The condition occurs almost exclusively in diabetics and in patients in a poor general condition.

Examination shows a brownish-coloured nasal secretion, black crusts on the septum and the lateral wall of the nose with sometimes a septal perforation, proptosis, and in the later course of the disease, cranial nerve paralysis, saddle nose, and loss of vision. The diagnosis is made by histological examination of a biopsy in which the hyphae are found [6].

Early recognition of the disorder is important since the mortality is otherwise very high. Treatment consists of bringing the underlying disorder under control, especially diabetes, and intravenous administration of amphotericin B.

Other rare conditions

Chronic diphtheritic rhinitis is an inflammation of the nasal mucosa caused by *Corynebacterium diphtheriae.* A membrane forms in the nose which is difficult to remove and which causes bleeding. The diagnosis is confirmed by microscopic examination and culture. The treatment consists of immediate administration of antitoxin and penicillin.

Chronic glanders is caused by infection by *Actinobacillus mallei.* The disease is extremely uncommon and is caused by contact with horses; a severe rhinitis can be found amongst other symptoms.

The nose can furthermore be affected by fungi and yeasts such as *Coccidioides immitis,* and species of *Actinomyces, Blastomyces, Aspergillus, Candida, Histoplasma,* and *Sporotrichum.*

Nasal diseases which occur only in the tropics include nasopharyngeal *leishmaniasis* and *yaws.*

SINUSITIS

The nasal sinuses appear during development as pouches of the nasal epithelium and development of the sinus system continues after birth. The antrum achieves its greatest relative size about the seventh year, but the ethmoidal system only about the twelfth year. The frontal sinus is not present at birth; it remains rudimentary until the sixth year and then expands rapidly between the seventh and tenth year to its final size. The frontal sinus may be absent on one or both sides. The sphenoidal sinus only achieves its final size about the thirteenth year and sometimes much later [7].

Acute maxillary sinusitis

Pathology

This usually arises as a complication of viral rhinitis but it is possible that the disease begins as a viral sinusitis; the infection is always bacterial by the time the patient consults a specialist. The most frequently occurring micro-organisms are the *Haemophilus influenzae*, the pneumococcus, staphylococcus, and the streptococcus [8]. An acute bacterial sinusitis can also arise on the basis of atopy; a sinusitis of dental origin can be caused by extension of a periàpical inflammation or abscess. Swelling of the mucosa of the sinus occurs as a result of the infection and this can lead to closure of the ostium. The secretions can then no longer drain and a vicious circle is set up.

Clinical features

The symptoms of acute maxillary sinusitis can vary enormously. Often there is severe throbbing pain of the appropriate half of the face especially in the area of distribution of the infraorbital nerve. The pain is also often felt in the teeth especially during jerky movement such as riding in a bus or even whilst walking. Often pain above the eye is complained of in the absence of infection of the frontal sinus. Some patients only complain of a feeling of pressure in the cheek.

Examination usually shows a tenderness to palpation and pressure over the affected sinus. Anterior rhinoscopy shows a swollen nasal mucosa with pus in the middle meatus. The patient generally complains of malaise, but the temperature is usually elevated little or not at all. The affected sinus may transilluminate less well than the opposite side. Radiography shows complete opacity or a fluid level of the maxillary antrum, although the diagnostic significance should not be exaggerated [9]. The diagnosis is confirmed by antroscopy and antral lavage.

Treatment

Management of acute maxillary sinusitis in the less severe cases consists of the administration of broad spectrum antibiotics, possibly as dictated by sensitivity tests, and of nose drops to ensure good drainage. In patients with severe pain and pressure symptoms antral lavage is indicated since there is otherwise a considerable risk of complications. The lavage may be carried out via the natural ostium or by the inferior meatus. In children it is usually not possible to carry out lavage under local anaesthetic and in this case small drainage tubes can be introduced under general anaesthetic into the sinus which can thus be washed out several times daily whilst the child is in hospital. The lavage must be continued until the drainage is clear. Some authors feel that mucolytic agents given orally or locally shorten the course of the disease.

The patient with a persistently recurring acute maxillary sinusitis is a difficult problem. An intranasal antrostomy can then provide some improvement; although the sinusitis recurs there is now good drainage of the secretions and pain-free lavage is now possible. Any underlying allergy should be treated. Sometimes it is useful to advise these patients to take prophylactic antibiotics at the start of a cold. If an acute maxillary sinusitis does not heal completely then the picture becomes that of chronic maxillary sinusitis.

Chronic maxillary sinusitis

Clinical features

Symptoms here are usually very much less severe. The patients complain of pressure symptoms or of dull pain, and sometimes of neuralgias in the area of distribution of the infraorbital nerve. Usually the patient complains of nasal obstruction and a purulent nasal discharge. Chronic pharyngitis and laryngitis can be caused by the continual irritation due to the secretion and sometimes an irritative cough. The chronic sinusitis is sometimes accompanied by bronchitis (sinobronchitis, Mounier–Kuhn syndrome). Kartagener's syndrome (maxillary sinusitis, situs inversus, and bronchiectasis) [10] and mucoviscidosis may also underlie chronic sinusitis. The only symptom of maxillary sinusitis in children may be the so-called pseudo-appendicitis (Brenneman's syndrome) [11].

The diagnosis of sinusitis is made basically from the radiological appearances, possibly supported by antroscopy. Ultimately the sinusitis can lead to the formation of polyps which can grow out into the nasal cavity. It is not clear why polyps form quickly in some cases whereas in others they do not form even after years of purulent infection.

Treatment
Initially an attempt may be made to heal the chronic maxillary sinusitis by repeated lavage supported by antibiotics. A dental cause should naturally be treated. However, in many cases the antral mucosa is irreversibly damaged and recovery is not to be expected without operation. An intranasal antrostomy may suffice for a simple, chronic purulent inflammation; a radical operation must usually be carried out, however, particularly for a polypoid purulent inflammation. The aim of such an operation should be the following:

(1) the creation of a good drainage opening into the inferior meatus;

(2) removal of irreversibly diseased mucosa from the cavity; and

(3) to allow healthy mucosa to grow into the sinus.

The most commonly used radical operation on the antrum is the Caldwell–Luc operation.

In general a Caldwell–Luc operation should be avoided in children since damage to the roots of the remaining teeth is a real possibility.

The most important complications of this operation are damage to the nasolacrimal duct during the creation of the window in the inferior meatus, leading to epiphora, and neuralgia of the infraorbital nerve, usually caused by damage to the nerve by excess removal of the anterior wall of the maxillary sinus or by retractors during the operation. Fracture of the very thin posterior wall of the maxillary sinus can often extend to damage the maxillary nerve in the pterygopalatine fossa. Avulsion of the nerve must sometimes be carried out later for this neuralgia. An oroantral fistula can occur in the gingivolabial sulcus at the site of the incision and also in the alveolus after extraction of a carious tooth. In both cases

a closure with flaps is indicated after healing of the sinusitis.

Acute ethmoiditis

Since the ethmoidal labyrinth lies at the centre of the other accessory sinuses it is often involved in inflammation of the sinuses. From the anatomical point of view the ethmoidal labyrinth can be divided into an anterior part that drains into the middle meatus and a posterior part which drains into the superior meatus. This difference does not appear to be of any great clinical importance.

Clinical features
The symptoms of acute ethmoiditis are often non-specific. There is a feeling of pressure over the root of the nose and sometimes also in the temporal area, but true pain is usually absent. Since an acute ethmoiditis is usually accompanied by disease of one or more of the other sinuses the latter often determines the clinical picture. The diagnosis is made by plain radiographs, possibly supplemented by tomography.

Treatment
Acute ethmoiditis usually heals with conservative treatment. If there is a concomitant maxillary or frontal sinusitis, management of the latter is usually sufficient to heal the ethmoiditis. In children ethmoiditis combined with a maxillary sinusitis can have a very severe course, with high fever, oedema of the face and orbital cellulitis; nevertheless a drainage of the antrum appears often to be satisfactory in dealing with the acute symptoms. In some cases, however, external drainage of the ethmoidal labyrinth is required.

Chronic ethmoiditis

Clinical features
Chronic purulent ethmoiditis is very rare and is almost symptomless. The patient may complain of vague pressure sensations, nasal obstruction, and a purulent nasal discharge. The chronic hypertrophic form in which mucosal thickening occurs in the ethmoidal cells, occurs more frequently; the thickening continues to extend to finally appear as multiple polyps under the middle turbinate. One of the first symptoms is hypos-

mia which later proceeds to anosmia. Increasing nasal obstruction follows later.

Treatment

If chronic ethmoiditis, with or without polyp formation, does not react satisfactorily to conservative treatment surgery should be considered. The ethmoidal labyrinth can be approached in several different ways: via the nose, via the antrum, or by an external incision in the medial canthus. Surgery of the ethmoidal labyrinth is difficult and complications are not rare. The most important are:

(1) Damage to the dura caused by perforation of the anterior cranial fossa or of the cribriform plate. As a result of this a CFS rhinorrhoea or meningitis can occur. Damage to the cribriform plate also causes permanent anosmia. The defect must be closed intracranially; and

(2) The optic nerve can be damaged in external ethmoid operations via the lamina papyracea or in transnasal operations in which the dissection is carried too far laterally. Intraorbital bleeding can occur after the operation which can also lead to permanent blindness if it is not dealt with rapidly. The lacrimal apparatus or the ocular muscles, especially the trochlear muscle, can also be damaged, leading to epiphora or diplopia.

Acute frontal sinusitis

Clinical features

Acute frontal sinusitis usually causes severe pain over the affected sinus; this is usually accompanied by headache, and there is pain on pressure or on tapping over the sinus. The periodicity of the pain is typical of this disease: it usually begins several hours after getting up and decreases again in the afternoon. It has already been pointed out that supraorbital pain is often a symptom of maxillary sinusitis.

Examination sometimes shows purulent secretions anteriorly in the middle meatus, but since the frontonasal duct is often closed this symptom may be absent. Forehead and upper eyelid oedema is commonly seen.

The diagnosis is confirmed by radiography which shows opacity or a fluid level of the sinus.

Treatment

In some cases the sinusitis can be treated conser-

vatively by regular constriction of the mu[...] and by the administration of antibiotics. Ho[...] ever, if the pain is very severe or there is marke[...] oedema over the sinus, drainage is indicated. Probing of the frontonasal duct should never be performed because a number of serious complications have been described. Trephining can be carried out through an incision in or inferior to the eyebrow and a small drainage tube inserted. Several days of repeated lavage with physiological saline or an antibiotic solution is usually sufficient to control the infection.

Chronic frontal sinusitis

Clinical features

Chronic frontal sinusitis usually causes few symptoms. Sometimes the patient complains of a feeling of pressure locally over the sinus and sometimes there is a neuralgia of the supraorbital nerve. Examination also shows few specific symptoms but oedema of the nasal mucosa and chronic rhinitis may be seen. Again the final diagnosis is made radiographically.

Treatment

If surgery is necessary there are numerous operations to choose from. All these techniques are intended either to provide reliable drainage or to obliterate the cavity of the sinus. Good results are now claimed with the osteoplastic flap operation in which the anterior wall of the frontal sinus is preserved [12].

Complications do not often occur after operations on the frontal sinuses and are in principle the same as those described for the ethmoid sinuses. If the symptoms of the sinusitis are not improved after the operation the cause may be that an isolated cell of the frontal sinus has been overlooked. It is always necessary therefore to carry out a final inspection of the sinus at operation with the guidance of radiographs.

Acute sphenoidal sinusitis

Symptoms of acute sphenoidal sinusitis are very variable. Often the patient complains of pain in the occipital area and sometimes over the vertex. There is also often pain behind the eyes and over the mastoid process. Patients usually complain post-nasal discharge. If the ostium of the sinus an be seen by anterior rhinoscopy, which is seldom, purulent secretions can be seen coming from it. Radiography again forms the mainstay of diagnosis.

The disease is almost always healed by conservative treatment.

Chronic sphenoidal sinusitis

The symptoms of chronic sphenoidal sinusitis are similar to those of the acute form but are less pronounced.

If conservative treatment is not successful a sphenoidectomy should be carried out in which an attempt must be made to remove the irreversibly altered mucosa and to provide good drainage.

Complications can occur after sphenoidectomy because of the close proximity of the sinus with several important structures: the anterior and middle cranial fossa, the pituitary, the optic chiasma, the cavernous sinus, the internal carotid artery, and the third, fourth, fifth, and sixth cranial nerves.

Complications of sinusitis

Although sinusitis occurs frequently complications are infrequent. Furthermore, since the introduction of antibiotics mortality has decreased significantly. However, complications can lead to serious disease and it is therefore very important to recognize and prevent them as rapidly as possible. Probably one of the most important causes of these complications is a too aggressive surgical approach in acute sinusitis. It has already been pointed out that acute sinusitis can usually be controlled with exclusively conservative treatment.

The complications can be divided into three main groups:
(1) disorders of bony structures;
(2) disorders of the orbit; and
(3) intracranial complications.

Disorders of bony structures
These usually arise from the frontal sinus, less often from the ethmoidal sinus, and rarely from the antrum and the sphenoidal sinus. A benign form is hyperplastic osteitis, in which diffuse thickening of the bone or osteosis arises. Rarifying osteitis is of more importance clinically because it can spread externally via the vascular channels causing microfistulae and finally a subperiosteal abscess. In very severe forms sequestrae can occur.

Osteomyelitis is a rare complication which can occur especially in the frontal bone. This disease can occasionally also be caused by trauma or by haematogenous spread from another site. It occurs particularly in children and young patients in whom the cancellous layer is relatively thicker. The osteomyelitis can extend from the frontal bone to the other bones of the skull. Initially the symptoms appear to be those of a severe acute frontal sinusitis; this complication must always be kept in mind if swelling of the soft tissues begins to extend beyond the area of the frontal sinus. Radiology is of little value in the early stages since some time must elapse before dissolution of the bone becomes visible on radiographs. Without treatment the osteomyelitis finally leads to serious intracranial complications.

There is no unanimity of opinion over treatment. In the early stages antibiotics may be used, but once radiological abnormalities appear a radical operation on the frontal sinus with removal of all necrotic bone must be carried out [13].

Osteomyelitis of the upper jaw is almost always of dental origin; if the disease arises from the maxillary sinus, a radical operation must be carried out with removal of irreversibly diseased bone. An unusual form of osteomyelitis of the upper jaw, usually of haematogenous origin, occasionally occurs in infants. In this case the treatment should be as conservative as possible to prevent damage to the tooth germs and even hemiatrophy of the face.

Disorders of the orbit
Complications of the orbit are almost always due to disease of the frontal and ethmoidal sinuses. These complications should come to mind if oedema of the eyelids occurs, although this can be due to an uncomplicated sinusitis. More important signs are chemosis of the conjunctiva and displacement of the bulb. The direction of displacement is usually away from the affected

sinus: in frontal sinusitis in an inferior direction, in ethmoidal sinusitis externally, and sometimes in maxillary sinusitis superiorly.

Disease of the posterior ethmoid cells and of the sphenoidal sinus can cause exophthalmos. The ocular movements may be interfered with and abnormalities of the optic fundus can occur.

Osteitis and periosteitis of the orbital walls can occur due to progress of inflammation of a sinus and this may proceed to a subperiosteal abscess. In such a case a radical operation must be carried out in which the abscess is drained into the sinus. An external approach is seldom indicated, but if an abscess of the eyelids occurs this should be drained externally.

An orbital abscess is a severe complication which may lead to blindness, sinus thrombosis, and meningitis.

In this case a radical operation must be carried out on the appropriate sinus combined with incisions in the orbital periosteum. In very severe cases an orbital exenteration may be indicated. High doses of antibiotics should of course be given in all these diseases as dictated by a culture and sensitivity test.

Previously it was thought that retrobulbar optic neuritis usually had a nasal cause but nowadays it is thought that this condition is more often associated with diseases such as multiple sclerosis, intoxications, generalized vascular disorders, and infections. The treatment of the sinuses is only indicated if there is clear evidence of sinusitis, especially of sphenoid origin.

Intracranial complications

Inflammation of the sinuses can cause serious intracranial complications: extradural and subdural abscesses, meningitis, cerebral abscess, and septic thrombosis of the venous sinuses (Chapter 12).

Miscellaneous disorders of the sinuses

Pseudocyst

Pseudocysts of the sinuses occur frequently and usually have no clinical significance. They are due to fluid retention in the lamina propria of the nasal mucosa and are thus covered with epithelium. Treatment is almost never indicated.

Retention cysts

Retention cysts are caused by closure of the duct of a gland; they are thus covered with epithelium. Treatment is seldom indicated since they usually burst spontaneously before they are big enough to cause symptoms.

Mucocoele

A mucocoele (called a pyocoele if the contents are infected) arises when drainage from a sinus is impeded. They usually occur in the frontal sinus or in an ethmoidal cell, but rarely in the other sinuses. Since the secretion produced by the mucosa cannot drain, the size of the mucocoele increases slowly, leading to erosion of the surrounding bone which can become paper thin. An unusual sensation (the 'ping-pong ball' phenomenon) is felt on palpation. Marked displacement of the orbital contents and exophthalmos can occur.

The treatment is surgical: the mucosa is removed and if the sinus is not obliterated good drainage to the nose must be provided. In ethmoidal mucocoeles the latter is usually sufficient.

Pneumatocoele

A pneumatocoele is an air-filled expansion which usually affects only the frontal sinus and rarely the other sinuses. An intracranial pneumatocoele can also arise via a dehiscence of the inner table. The cause is not clear.

Polyps

Polyps can arise in the sinuses due to chronic inflammation. This topic is discussed on pp. 236–238.

Sinusitis caseosa

Sinusitis caseosa is caused if inspissated pus and debris cannot escape via the natural ostium. A yellow, cheesy, friable mass is found in the sinus, especially the frontal sinus.

Cholesteatoma

Cholesteatoma of the sinuses, especially of the antrum and the frontal sinus is rare. Squamous epithelium may be found in the sinus as a result of trauma, metaplasia of the mucosa, or ingrowth from outside and this may continue to expand rather like a cholesteatoma of the middle ear. Radical operation is indicated.

Aerosinusitis

Aerosinusitis (barotrauma) is caused by rapidly occurring alterations in pressure such as during rapid descent in an aeroplane. Since the air pressure in aeroplanes nowadays is almost always maintained at a normal level this disorder occurs much less frequently. Barotrauma causes a severe stabbing pain without many other symptoms; occasionally a haematoma of the sinus may occur. As a prophylactic measure attempts may be made to keep the ostia of the sinuses as wide as possible with vasoconstrictors.

DERMATOSES OF THE EXTERNAL NOSE

Since both the exterior of the nose and the nasal vestibule are covered with skin almost all the dermatological diseases can occur at this site.

Vestibulitis

This disorder is characterized by the formation of crusts and excoriation of the skin of the vestibule. Fissures also occur on occasion. Usually these patients suffer from a chronic purulent nasal discharge due to chronic rhinitis or sinusitis and they often have poor general hygiene. The fissures frequently become chronic because the crusts are picked off before the fissure has healed.

The most important treatment is to cure the underlying rhinitis. Local treatment consists of the application of antibacterial ointment possibly with corticosteroids added.

Impetigo

Impetigo is a superficial infection of the skin caused by the staphylococcus, the streptococcus, or both. Erosions occur which are covered with a yellowish seropurulent crust and often extend peripherally. Impetigo is a self-limiting disease but its course can be considerably shortened by specific treatment. Strict hygiene, short nails and regular washing with germicidal soap are very important. In serious cases oral antibiotics may be given but local treatment is usually sufficient.

Nasal furuncle

This is a necrotizing inflammation of a hair follicle. The cause is almost always *Staphylococcus aureus*. Formerly the nasal furuncle was to be feared because of its complications but these seldom occur because of modern antibiotics.

The symptoms are a fever, marked swelling and the affected part of the nose shows redness, a glazed appearance, and often oedema. There is usually marked pain in the nose. In an uncomplicated case the abscess bursts into the lumen of the nose, externally or sometimes into the gingivolabial sulcus. In serious cases a thrombosis of the angular vein and the inferior ophthalmic vein can occur and this can lead to a thrombosis of the cavernous sinus. It must be assumed that this complication has occurred if the patient's general condition deteriorates, if there is a high swinging fever or rigor, and if cerebral symptoms such as vomiting and alterations of the level of consciousness are seen. Symptoms such as oedema of the eyelids or conjunctiva and papilloedema develop as a result of the decreased venous drainage. The inflammation can also extend to the meninges causing meningitis and septic emboli can occur from breakdown of the thrombus causing distant septic metastases in the lungs, joints, muscles, and skin.

The most important point of the treatment of a furuncle is not to carry out any mechanical interference because of the danger of bacteraemia. Antiseptic ointments can be used and antibiotics must be given as determined by culture and sensitivity tests.

Erysipelas

Erysipelas is an acute inflammation of the epidermis and the dermis caused by pyogenic streptococcus. The disease often begins in the vestibule or on the dorsum of the nose from which it spreads rapidly over the entire face. There is a sharply demarcated, painful, red infiltrated area that extends peripherally. There is often a marked oedema of the adjoining part of the face. The patient usually has a high fever, sometimes with rigors, headache, nausea, and vomiting. The disease is treated by high doses of penicillin.

Rhinophyma

This is a complication of acne rosacea which

most often occurs in old men. There is a hyperplasia of the sebaceous glands and of the connective tissue of the nose which can sometimes reach an enormous size. The disease can be treated very effectively by dermabrasion.

References

[1] JACKSON G. G. (1973) Viruses causing common respiratory infections in man. *J. Infect. Dis.* **127**, 328.

[2] SCHWARTZ A. R., YASUSI T., HORNICK R. B., SUKETAMI T. & GLECKMAN R. A. (1973) Evaluation of the efficacy of ascorbic acid in prophylaxis of induced rhinovirus 44 in man. *J. Infect. Dis.* **128**, 500.

[3] YOUNG A. (1971) Closure of the nostrils in atrophic rhinitis. *J. Laryngol. Rhinol.* **85**, 715.

[4] ACHESON E. D., COWDELL R. H. & RANG E. (1972) Adenocarcinoma of the nasal cavity and sinuses in England and Wales. *Brit. J. industr. med.* **29**, 21.

[5] GOTTRON H. A. (1951) Hauttuberkulose. In *die Tuberkulose*, Stuttgart: Thieme.

[6] LOWE J. T. & HUDSON W. R. (1975) Rhinocerebral phycomycosis and internal carotid artery thrombosis. *Arch. Otolaryngol.* **101**, 100.

[7] DAVIS V. (1914) *Development and Anatomy of the Nasal Accessory Sinuses in Man.* Philadelphia: Saunders.

[8] LYSTAD A., BERDAL P. & LUND-IVERSEN L. (1963) The bacterial flora of sinusitis with an in vitro study of the bacterial resistance to antibiotics. *Acta otolaryng. (Stockholm)*, Suppl. **188**, 390.

[9] ILLUM P., JEPPESEN F. & LANGENBACK E. (1972) X-ray examination and sinuscopy in maxillary sinus disease. *Acta ololaryng. (Stockholm)* **74**, 287.

[10] HOLMES L. B., BLENNERHASSET J. B. & AUSTEN K. F. (1968) A reappraisal of Kartagener's syndrome. *Am. J. med. sci.* **255**, 13.

[11] BRENNEMAN J. (1927) The abdominal pain of throat infections in children and appendicitis. *J. Amer. med. ass.* **89**, 2183.

[12] ALFORD B. R., GORMAN G. R. & MERSOL V. F. (1965) Osteoplastic surgery of the frontal sinus. *Laryngoscope* **75**, 1139.

[13] BORDLEY J. E. & BISCHOFBERGER W. (1967) Osteomyelitis of the frontal bone. *Laryngoscope*, **77**, 1234.

CHAPTER 18

Allergic and Vasomotor Rhinitis

ALLERGIC RHINITIS

Types of hypersensitivity reaction

Hypersensitivity reactions are currently divided into four general types, as suggested by Gell & Coombs [1].

Type I hypersensitivity is mediated by reaginic antibody, mainly or even exclusively of the IgE class (anaphylaxis and allergy). Most allergic disorders of the nose fall within this group.

Type II hypersensitivity reactions are produced by reactions of antibody with cell-bound antigen followed secondarily by complement fixation (clinical examples include acute post-streptococcal glomerulonephritis, chronic rejection of transplants, and some instances of drug allergy).

Type III reactions are effected by soluble antigen–antibody complex deposition at the reaction site (toxic complex reaction). Following the formation of a complex, complement fixation occurs, mediating many of the biologic consequences of Type III reactions (seen clinically in serum sickness, possibly in auto-immune disease, and the hyperacute form of renal allograft rejection).

Type IV reactions (delayed or cellular hypersensitivity) are caused by the reaction of specifically sensitized small lymphocytes with antigens. Typically, a 24–72 hour delay occurs in onset of the reaction after exposure of a sensitized individual to a specific antigen (seen clinically in contact dermatitis, bacterial hypersensitivity and probably also in transplantation reactions and tumour immunity).

As emphasized above, the Type I reaction is the most important in diseases of the ear, nose, and throat. Other terms for this group are immediate type hypersensitivity, reaginic hypersensitivity, or atopy. This type of allergy is characterized by a particular type of circulating antibody, reagins, or skin-sensitizing antibodies. The reagins circulate freely in the serum but also demonstrate a great affinity for certain cells, especially in the intestinal and respiratory tracts. They can be differentiated from most other antibodies by the fact that their biological activity is lost after heating to 56° C. Reagins do not pass the placenta. When cell bound reagin combines with antigen a reaction occurs within several minutes ('immediate type hypersensitivity'). This reaction is due to the fact that mediators such as histamine, slow reacting substance and kinins are freed by the antigen–antibody complex causing vasodilatation, increased vascular permeability, and smooth muscle contraction. As a result, urticaria, rhinitis, bronchospasm, etc., can occur depending on the site and the severity of the reaction.

Reaginic activity in humans is mainly determined by IgE, a special class of immunoglobulins with a molecular weight of approximately 200 000 and a sedimentation coefficient of 8S [2]. There are several ways of determining the amount of specific IgE in human serum, of which the radioallergosorbent test (RAST) is the best for routine diagnostic use [3]. This test is a modified antiglobulin reaction based on a radioimmunoassay of reaginic IgE antibodies present in the patient's serum. Good agreement has been found between the results of RAST and those of passive transfer (Prausnitz–Küstner), as well as with those of in vitro histamine release from sensitized leucocytes and from human lung [4]. There is also a very good agreement for the results of skin testing provided that good extracts, such as those from pollen, are used.

The atopic syndrome

Atopic rhinitis with which we are now principally

concerned is only one facet of a complex of diseases which can be summarized as the 'atopic syndrome'. This hereditary syndrome shows a moderate degree of penetration and a variable expression; its manifestations include atopic eczema, rhinitis, asthma, eosinophilia, and production of reagins against many different allergens.

Atopic eczema (neurodermatitis)

The earliest stage of this disease begins in the second or third month of life and extends into the second year. Often there is a moist eczema, mainly localized to the scalp and the face. Typical sites affected during the second stage of this disease are the flexor surfaces of the elbow and the knee, and the face. This phase of the eczema is drier in character. At all stages the eczema is characterized by violent itching. About a third of patients with atopic eczema later develop asthma or atopic rhinitis.

Atopic rhinitis and asthma

Atopic rhinitis and asthma are two aspects of a single disorder of the respiratory tract due to reactions between allergens and reagins fixed to the mucosal cells. Since the nose receives a large share of the inhaled allergens as a result of its filtering action, it can be expected that in slight exposure to an allergen and in a patient who is only mildly sensitive a rhinitis only will occur. However, if a greater quantity of allergen is inhaled or if the patient is more sensitive asthma occurs. Individual reactivity of the nose and bronchi to histamine determines whether rhinitis or asthma occurs; infection of the nose or the lung can also influence the clinical course of the disease. The size of the inhaled particles largely determines the fact that pollen atopy characteristically causes rhinitis whereas house dust atopy manifests itself as asthma. A grass pollen grain has an average diameter of 50 μm and thus lands on the nasal mucosa, whereas house dust particles are much smaller (5 μm) so that a relatively larger proportion passes into the bronchial tree. In severe exposure or marked individual sensitivity a patient with hay fever can suffer bronchial symptoms.

Eosinophilia

There is at the moment no agreement over the role of the eosinophil in atopy. The cell has phagocytic properties and moves by chemotaxis towards a high histamine concentration [5]. It is assumed that the eosinophils fulfil a function in detoxifying histamine.

Eosinophilia is often found in the peripheral blood of patients with atopy, but this eosinophilia depends on several factors. Exposure to the allergen is a stimulus for the increase of the number of eosinophils in the blood of an atopic person. Thus patients with hay fever often show an eosinophilia during the pollen season whilst the eosinophil count in the peripheral blood is normal for the rest of the year. The seasonal eosinophilia shows lower values in long standing disease and also after consistently carried out desensitization. A very marked increase in the number of eosinophils is usually found in atopic children in the stage when the skin reactions are still negative.

It must be emphasized that eosinophilia is of itself not evidence of the existence of an allergy; eosinophilia can occur in a large number of diseases, such as parasitic infestations, malignancy, periarteritis nodosa, adrenal insufficiency, etc. In all diseases in which histamine is released, including allergic phenomena, a local eosinophilia occurs.

Thus the nasal secretion of patients with hay fever shows a large number of eosinophils during the hay fever season, but outside the season the number of eosinophils in the nasal secretion is normal although an eosinophilia of the nasal mucosa can be caused by provocation with grass pollen.

Formation of reagins

The most characteristic property of the atopic patient is his ability to produce reagins against different allergens. A child is not born allergic and the development of reagins begins gradually. Without contact there can be no atopic allergy! The degree to which the reagins are formed depends on several factors. First, the degree of atopy is constitutionally determined; some patients have a great number of positive skin reactions to several allergens very early in life, whereas in others these develop gradually and at a later age. Secondly, boys develop atopy more easily than girls and thus do so earlier and to a greater degree. Thirdly, the degree of exposure is important. Usually sensitivity to human dander appears first, since this is the material with which one comes into contact intensively and continuously. Sensitivity to house dust usually occurs next. Sensitivity to pollen, exposure to which only occurs for part of the year, is less frequent and usually begins at a later age. Naturally the severity of the individual allergen is also important: the dander of cats is notorious for its strong antigenicity.

Priming

It has been shown experimentally that the longer a nasal mucosa is exposed to an allergen the less allergen is required to cause the same reaction. This phenomenon is called 'priming' [6]. If a patient with a proven pollen atopy is challenged outside the pollen season with concentrations of pollen which are the same as those found on a day with a high pollen count, rhinitis does not occur. But if the same patient is challenged for an hour a day on several consecutive days, he will develop symptoms after about 3 days. Furthermore, if he is challenged daily, less pollen is required on each succeeding day to produce comparable episodes of rhinitis, and after several weeks of such exposure the amount of pollen needed to produce rhinitis is only one-fiftieth of the dose which caused a reaction on the first day of challenge.

This priming is a reversible process, that is, the sensitivity begins to decrease if challenges are stopped for a few days, and more pollen is then needed to produce symptoms. Priming is a local effect. If one nostril is primed the other nostril remains resistant to challenge. It has been shown that allergic rhinitis can be produced by a small dose of pollen in the primed nostril. At the same time there are no symptoms from the other nostril even after challenge with fifty times more pollen.

Priming is immunologically non-specific, i.e. a nostril primed with one antigen becomes more reactive to any other antigen to which the patient is allergic. Thus, the symptoms of a patient with a grass pollen atopy during the hay fever season are made worse by contact with another allergen to which he is only slightly sensitive and which would not cause symptoms outside the hay fever season; in other words, if his nasal mucosa has not been primed.

ATOPIC RHINITIS

Clinical features

A special allergy survey sheet is used in many clinics for taking history; whilst such a form has many advantages, it cannot replace a history taken by an experienced physician. The following points should be noted in the history of every patient:

(1) Chief complaint and history of the present illness.
(2) Previous allergic history:
    atopic eczema
    contact dermatitis
    rhinitis
    eye symptoms
    asthma and bronchitis
    allergy to insect stings
    food allergy.
(3) Family history.
(4) Results of previous allergic treatment:
    desensitization
    antihistamines
    steroids
    sodium cromoglycate
    antibiotics
    other treatment.
(5) When symptoms occur:
    time of year (seasonal variations)
    time of the week (weekend or weekdays)
    time of day (day or night)
    improvement during holidays.
(6) Where symptoms occur:
    at home, at work or at school
    indoors or outdoors
    special hobbies.
(7) What the patient thinks makes him worse:
    contact with dust or with animals
    specific occupations
    tobacco smoke, chemical agents.
(8) When the patient is free of symptoms.
(9) Description of the patient's home:
    damp or dry

city or rural

any moulds noticed

carpets, furniture, mattress, pillow, blankets.

(10) Influence of stress, menses, food, alcohol.

(11) Any further information.

Although atopic rhinitis can be caused by several different allergens, the clinical picture does not depend on the type that causes the reaction because the same mediators are released whatever the allergen. The most characteristic symptoms of atopic rhinitis are sneezing,watery rhinorrhoea, itching of the nose, and nasal obstruction. The symptoms occur within 5–15 minutes of exposure to the allergen and sneezing occurs in spasms of 10–20 at a time, which can exhaust the patient. The watery rhinorrhoea is usually very profuse; large numbers of handkerchiefs are used; a vestibulitis and excoriation of the upper lip are often caused as a result of the secretion. A very common complaint is the annoying itching in the nose, and nasal obstruction which is usually of moderate severity. Marked nasal obstruction without secretions, sneezing, and itching is seldom due to an uncomplicated atopy. Swelling of the ostia of the nasal sinuses can cause obstruction leading to sinusitis. Swelling of the mucosa of the Eustachian tube can cause tubal catarrh resulting in deafness.

The patients often complain of itching in the ears which is probably referred in origin. Eye symptoms (itching and epiphora) and itching of the palate and the throat are also common complaints. Depending on the type of allergen, the degree of exposure and the sensitivity of the patient, bronchial symptoms can also occur, varying from a constricted feeling in the chest and a dry cough, to serious asthma. Finally it must be pointed out that psychological factors are as important in atopic rhinitis as they are in asthma. Stress in the form of difficulties at school, work or home can exert an unfavourable influence on atopic rhinitis.

A number of typical stigmata occur, particularly in atopic children: facial grimaces and frequent nose rubbing (the 'allergic salute'), a transverse nasal crease due to the constant rubbing of the nose, and a bluish-black discoloration under the lower eye lid ('allergic shiners'). Various degrees of malocclusion may develop because of the constant mouth-breathing.

Examination of the nose in allergic patients often shows a typical boggy greyish-pink mucosa, particularly of the inferior turbinates, which may practically occlude the nasal passage. Atopic patients usually show a hyper-reactivity of the nasal mucosa to non-specific stimuli so that dust particles, tobacco smoke and irritant gases can make the symptoms considerably worse. Often examination of the nose with a nasal speculum precipitates a violent bout of sneezing, and swimming in an indoor pool with a high chlorine content often causes a worsening of the symptoms in atopic children. Finally, an atopic nasal mucosa is more susceptible to bacterial infection. An infective complication must be suspected if the nasal secretion is purulent (in uncomplicated atopic rhinitis it is always watery), if the nasal mucosa is markedly hyperaemic and if many polymorphonuclear neutrophils are found in a specimen of the nasal secretions.

Laboratory investigation

Eosinophil count. No abnormalities are found in a complete blood count in an uncomplicated atopic rhinitis, apart possibly from an eosinophilia of between 3 and 7%. It is again emphasized that an eosinophilia in the peripheral blood is not evidence of an allergy but also occurs in many other diseases; on the other hand, an eosinophilia in the peripheral blood can be absent in atopic rhinitis. The ESR is normal in uncomplicated atopy.

Cytology. Cytological examination of the nasal mucus is very important. The most convenient method of obtaining a sample of nasal mucus is to use a cotton wool pledget to wipe the surface of the inferior or middle turbinate lightly. Children are asked to blow their nose on to a piece of plastic film. Wright's or Hansel's stain may be used. In uncomplicated atopy an increased number of eosinophils may be found, at least in patients who have recently been in contact with the responsible allergen. An increased number of mast cells is often found, and in infection an increased number of neutrophils and bacteria; sometimes CCP cells with viral inclusions can be demonstrated with special stains. It has already been pointed out that the macroscopic appearance of nasal secretions provides important information.

Nasal biopsy. Further information can be obtained by histological examination of a nasal biopsy.

The biopsy can be obtained easily under local anaesthesia from the lateral or the middle part of the inferior turbinate with a small biting cup forceps. After appropriate staining, fairly typical changes are seen in atopic rhinitis: eosinophils, destruction of the basement membrane, and debris which appears to be the remains of the nuclei of the eosinophils.

In some patients a marked increase in the number of mast cells will be noticed. In the presence of infection there will be a polymorphonuclear infiltrate.

RAST test. The RAST test can provide important information in patients with dermographia as a result of which it is not possible to assess the skin reactions. Now that this test is available it is no longer necessary to carry out a Prausnitz–Küstner test in such patients; this test takes a long time and carries the risk of transmitting serum hepatitis.

Radiographs. Finally, it is often desirable to take radiographs of the nasal sinuses to exclude disease of the sinuses.

Skin tests

The purpose of skin tests is to assess if the patient is producing reagins and, if so, against which allergens and to what extent. Three types of skin tests are used in clinical practice: the scratch test, the prick test and the intracutaneous test. An immediate wheal and erythema characteristic of atopic sensitization are produced in all.

In the scratch test the antigen is applied to a superficial scratch which penetrates the outer cornified layer of the skin. The prick test is performed by pricking the skin with a needle through a drop of the antigen solution. The disadvantage of both tests is that they are rather

insensitive; since concentrated antigen solutions must be used there is also the risk of severe constitutional reaction.

In the intracutaneous test a small amount of antigen (0·02 ml) is injected into the superficial layers of the skin. The extracts used are 100–1000 times diluted compared to those used in the scratch and prick tests. The reactions are made on the back, or on the volar surface of the forearm; the arm has the advantage that a tourniquet can be applied if an anaphylactic reaction occurs so that further spread of the antigen through the body can be temporarily prevented. On the other hand, the back offers more space for a large number of skin tests which must naturally be placed at a reasonable distance (5 cm) apart since they can mutually influence each other. One-millilitre tuberculin syringes with 26 gauge needles are used; disposable syringes and needles are to be be preferred since glass syringes can be contaminated by previously used antigens. The tests are read after 20 minutes and are scored from 0 to 4 depending on the size of wheal and flare and the presence of pseudopod formation of the wheal.

The different factors which can influence the skin test must be taken into account. Antihistamines and sympathicomimetic amines can suppress the skin reactions so that the patient should not use these drugs for 2 days before the examination. Corticosteroids have no appreciable influence on skin reactions. The quality of the test allergen used is very important; very dilute allergens can rapidly lose their antigenicity. The reactions are often more strongly positive on warm days, when dermographia also occurs more often. In very nervous patients the reactions are sometimes incorrectly negative; if the history is positive the tests should be repeated on another occasion. The reactions are more difficult to interpret on sunburned skin, on which they are usually weaker than normal.

A control should always be carried out using the solution in which the test allergen is dissolved. A positive reaction indicates either an allergy to one of the constituents of the solution or dermographia. In the latter case, a Prausnitz–Küstner reaction, or preferably RAST, should be used.

It is advisable to carry out a skin reaction with a dilute histamine solution at the same time. This gives an impression of the ability of the skin to react to liberated mediators. Which allergens to use depends to a certain degree on the history and where the patient lives. A standard series can be maintained consisting of: a control, histamine solution, house dust, human dander, mixed grass pollens, mixed tree pollens, mixed weed pollens, mixed moulds, and mixed animal danders.

If necessary, further differentiation can be made by a second investigation, possibly with other less frequently occurring allergens added. The patient must remain under observation for at least half an hour after the skin test because constitutional reactions occasionally occur which can sometimes be serious. These anaphylactic reactions are characterized by urticaria, Quincke's oedema, restlessness, anxiety and, in serious cases, by bronchial constriction, hypotension, and even shock. If such a reaction occurs a tourniquet should be applied as quickly as possible to the arm to which the skin test has been applied and antihistamine given intravenously, in the other arm. In serious reactions adrenaline must also be given subcutaneously.

Provocation tests

Although the allergen can almost always be identified from the history and skin reactions, more detailed information can sometimes be obtained from provocation tests. The simplest of these is an ophthalmic test in which a little dried pollen or a watery extract of an allergen is introduced into the conjunctival sac; redness is then looked for 20 minutes later. The test gives little more information than the skin tests.

Further information can be obtained from nasal provocation; the nasal patency is measured by a rhinomanometer after which a drop of antigen is introduced on the nasal mucosa without touching the latter, to avoid causing non-specific stimulation; alternatively antigen is insufflated into the nose. After 20 minutes the nasal patency is measured again. The disadvantages are that the test is tedious to perform and that no more than one allergen at a time can be tested.

The different allergens
House dust
House dust is the most frequently occurring allergen which causes symptoms in western Europe. It consists of a mixture of fibres, moulds, human and animal danders, bacteria, and food remnants. It was discovered about 1920 that house dust had antigenic properties; it also appears that samples of house dust from all parts of the world have the same antigenic properties but in different degrees. Dust from old houses on damp ground especially appear to contain large quantities of antigen [7].

A mite, the *Dermatophagoides*, has been shown to be the responsible allergen [8]. The strength of extracts of different samples of house dust appear to be proportional to the number of mites in the specimen. In all patients with positive skin reactions to a house dust extract, the reactions to an extract of house dust mite also appear positive, whereas in a control group without atopy for house dust positive reactions to mite extract are never found. The house dust mite has been shown to produce the allergen in house dust.

The house dust mite can be cultured in a climate chamber, the optimal conditions for reproduction and growth being a temperature of 25° C and a relative humidity of 80%. This explains why samples of house dust taken in the late summer and early autumn have a higher antigenicity than those taken at other seasons and also why house dust taken from damp houses is more strongly antigenic than that from dry ones. It also explains why patients with house dust allergy have most symptoms in the autumn and why atopic asthma and atopic rhinitis usually improve during a stay in a dry moutainous area.

Grass pollen
Atopy to pollen occurs frequently and is usually an atopy to the pollen of grass. Cross-antigenicity occurs between the pollens of different grasses and it is therefore not necessary to differentiate between them in respect to hay fever. Grass pollinates in southern England from the middle of May to the middle of July with a peak in the last week of June and the first week of July, and at this time pollen can be found in the air. In more northerly regions pollination occurs later. The pollen count is highest on dry windy days and in country areas, and in these circumstances patients with hay fever have the most symptoms.

In a small proportion of patients with hay fever, tree pollens are the responsible antigens. There is no cross-reactivity between different sorts of tree pollen, and different trees which pollinate at different times may cause symptoms in the same patient. Almost all trees pollinate earlier than grasses. It is therefore important to correlate the patient's complaints with the daily pollen counts which are available in most countries. Hazel, willow, plane, and silver birch are the most troublesome; allergy to the pollen of conifers may occur but is rare. Allergy to birch pollen is quite common, particularly in the Scandinavian countries. Birches pollinate in early May and finish well before the grass pollen season begins. Hay fever caused by weeds and cultured flowers is rare, but in the USA allergy to a common weed, the ragweed (Ambrosia), is common and troublesome. The pollen from this weed is found in the atmosphere in the late summer.

Human dander

It is remarkable that man can become allergic to skin scales from the species. Skin reactions to human dander are usually the first to occur and are present in most patients with allergy. Despite this the antigen has a limited clinical importance. Allergy to human dander can occur in hairdressers and chiropodists in whom exposure to this antigen is an occupational hazard. This allergy can be the cause of a severe allergic rhinitis.

Animal danders

The skin scales of animals can be very potent allergens; it is the skin scales themselves and not the hairs which contain the antigen. Allergies have been described against all the mammals with which man comes into frequent contact. The more intensive the contact the greater the chance of sensitization: allergies to horses and cats occur often. Similar allergies can also arise indirectly so that members of the family of the patient who regularly rides horses can develop an allergic rhinitis to the skin scales brought into the house on clothing. This emphasizes again why a careful history is so important.

Moulds

It is probable that the spores of moulds can also cause rhinitis; large numbers of these spores are found in the air, especially in July, August, and September. The most important are the *fungi imperfecti* (*Cladosporium* and *Alternaria*). There is at the moment no general agreement about the role played by moulds [9].

Occupational allergies

Allergies occur in many occupations; it is not practicable to discuss all these and a few examples must suffice. An allergy can occur in pharmacists to Radix ipecacuanha, Folia sennae, lycopodium powder and Radix saponariae. Lycopodium powder is also used in the rubber, metal, and cosmetic industries. In woodworkers, allergies can occur to certain tropical types of wood: abachi, limba, and teak. Castor oil bean can also cause a severe rhinitis and asthma.

In laboratories working with insects atopy can occur especially for the larger species, such as the grasshopper, the Colorado beetle and the cockroach.

Treatment

In every exacerbation of atopic rhinitis the importance of the following factors should be assessed, in addition to the atopy: infection, non-specific stimuli, and stress. In infection, which often complicates atopy, treatment with antibiotics must begin according to the culture and sensitivity tests. The patient must be protected from irritant gases such as those that occur in industries; swimming in strongly chlorinated baths must be avoided. The role played by stress is often difficult to assess, but if it is proven then the appropriate measures must be taken. Sufficient rest and a well-balanced diet are also important factors.

The main steps in treatment are as follows.

Elimination

The most obvious and most effective procedure is elimination of contact with the causative allergen. In some cases this is fairly simple: a pet can be disposed of or a plant whose pollen is causing symptoms can be removed from the house. Sometimes it may be necessary for the patient to seek alternative employment, particularly if bronchial symptoms occur in addition to rhinitis. It is obvious that in advising such intervention it must have been shown irrefutably that the suspected allergen actually is the cause of the complaints, if possible by a provocation test. Often it is not possible to eliminate the allergen completely but it is certainly possible to reduce contact with it. Thus a patient with hay fever can try to arrange his holiday so that he spends the period of the worst symptoms in surroundings low in pollen (by the sea or in the mountains). Partial elimination is very important, particularly in house dust allergy. The patient should preferably live in a dry, centrally heated house. The surroundings must be kept as free from dust as possible by regular use of a vacuum cleaner. The bedroom is particularly important since the average adult spends a third of his day there and children much more. The mattress and pillow must be made of foam rubber and the blankets must be beaten frequently. Old kapok mattresses and quilts must not be used.

Often these measures suffice to get rid of the complaints or to reduce them to an acceptable minimum.

Desensitization

Several investigators have shown that desensitization, if it is indicated and properly carried out, can have a favourable effect on the symptoms of atopy [10, 11]. There is no general agreement about the mode of action of desensitization, but possibly the following factors, amongst others, are important:

(1) The so-called blocking antibodies of the IgE type may be stimulated by desensitization. It is said that these blocking antibodies prevent the allergen from reaching the mast cell. There is probably some connection between the titre of the blocking antibodies and the clinical effect of the desensitization.

(2) The titre of specific IgE antibodies in serum rises at the beginning of desensitization but falls after long continued treatment.

(3) The basophil cells show a considerably lesser tendency to degranulation after desensitization; thus fewer mediators are released as a result of the antigen–antibody reaction.

A course of desensitization imposes a prolonged burden on the patient and one should therefore assess whether the required aim cannot be achieved by other methods such as elimination or medical treatment. Further, one must be convinced that desensitization is actually being carried out with the allergen which is responsible for the symptoms; one should treat the patient and not the skin test. Finally, a course of desensitization is not indicated if the patient is not completely motivated and if the other factors which have also been responsible for originating the rhinitis such as infection, non-specific stimuli and stress are not also treated.

The best results from desensitization are undoubtedly achieved in grass pollen allergies; this method often succeeds in rendering the patient free of symptoms during the hay fever season or at least reduces his symptoms so that he is made comfortable with a minimum of medication. Good results are also achieved in house dust allergies; if desensitization is carried out, control of the environment should not be neglected. Desensitization to animal dander is only seldom indicated; in the first place it is almost always possible to keep the responsible allergen out of the patient's surroundings, and, furthermore, animal dander is usually a very powerful antigen so that there is an increased danger of serious generalized reaction.

There are three methods of desensitization: coseasonal, pre-seasonal and perennial, of which the last is undoubtedly the best. Desensitization should be carried out with gradually increasing doses. Only well-standardized extracts must be used. The patient must be observed for 20 to 30 minutes after each injection so that any possible anaphylactic reactions can be treated. At the present time treatment with a watery extract is preferred.

There are differences of opinion as to the effect of treatment with bacterial vaccines. Although several authors have claimed clinical improvement, no double blind trials have been carried out that show irrefutably that treatment provides better results than a placebo.

Sympathicomimetics

Oral sympathicomimetics have a favourable effect on the symptoms of atopic rhinitis and since they have a mild stimulating effect they can profitably be combined with antihistamines. Nasal drops containing sympathicomimetics should not be prescribed since these can lead in the long run to a rhinitis medicamentosa because of their rebound effect. They should only be used for a short time for the treatment of complications such as sinusitis.

Sodium cromoglycate

Sodium cromoglycate inhibits the release of histamine and SRS-A from sensitized human lungs *in vitro* thus acting after the antigen meets the reagin but before release of the chemical mediators. Consequently the drug allows antigen–antibody reaction to proceed in a less harmful way, possibly by the mechanism of membrane stabilization. It has been shown by several investigators that the drug is effective in atopic rhinitis [12]. As sodium cromoglycate is very poorly absorbed from the gastrointestinal tract it is given by insufflation into the nose. It is one of the few known drugs with no major side-effects.

Antihistamines

Antihistamines antagonize the histamine released in the atopic reaction and can counteract the histamine hyper-reactivity of the airways. All of them have a number of side-effects such as drowsiness and an atropine-like effect which can differ markedly between different patients. The type of antihistamine and its dosage must therefore be individually determined, often by trial and error, to achieve the best effect with the fewest side-effects.

Corticosteroids

Corticosteroids have a very beneficial effect both in atopic and non-atopic non-infective rhinitis. Their anti-inflammatory properties are probably responsible for this effect.

Since systemic corticosteroids have important side-effects, especially if they are given for a long time, they are seldom indicated in atopic rhinitis. In a serious exacerbation of an atopic rhinitis, e.g. during the middle of the pollen season, a short course of corticosteroids can certainly be considered, particularly in a relatively low and gradually decreasing dose beginning with 10–20 mg of prednisone a day. Intranasal beclomethasone diproprionate is probably an important advance. Several double blind trials have shown that it offers a marked benefit without the risk of

systemic side-effects [13]. Occasionally the use of beclomethasone may cause slight epistaxis or candidiasis which resolves rapidly after withdrawal of the drug.

VASOMOTOR RHINITIS

Besides true allergic rhinitis the rhinologist is often confronted with patients who have real nasal symptoms which are difficult to ascribe to any specific diagnosis. These nasal symptoms present in two different forms:

(1) chronic nasal obstruction without much nasal discharge; and

(2) attacks of sneezing, rhinorrhoea and lacrimation.

These symptoms have usually been classified as vasomotor rhinitis, but the term rhinitis is incorrect since there is no inflammation in these patients and it would be better to use the term vasomotor rhinopathy. The term vasomotor indicates that the symptoms can be explained by the instability of the autonomic system.

The nasal mucosa receives its autonomic innervation from the pterygopalatine ganglion, which is positioned in the pterygopalatine fossa. This ganglion contains three types of neural elements: sensory, sympathetic, and parasympathetic. Branches of the maxillary nerve cross the pterygopalatine ganglion and run towards the structures of the middle third of the face they innervate. The autonomic supply of the nasal mucosa and the lacrimal gland is provided by the vidian nerve (according to official anatomical nomenclature: nerve of the pterygoid canal). This nerve is formed by two components: sympathetic fibres coming from the superior cervical ganglion, via the carotid plexus and the deep petrosal nerve; and parasympathetic fibres, coming from the geniculate ganglion via the greater petrosal nerve.

The latter fibres form synapses in the pterygopalatine ganglion [14]. From the pterygopalatine ganglion the pterygopalatine nerve runs to the nose; this nerve supplies the main portion of the innervation of the nose. It appears that in the walls of the nasal vessels both noradrenaline- and acetylcholinesterase-containing fibres are present. Also the venous sinuses present a dense network of both types of fibres. However, in the nasal glands, both serous and mucous, only acetylcholinesterase-containing fibres can be demonstrated. It can be concluded that the vasomotor fibres are both sympathetic and parasympathetic, while the secretomotor fibres are parasympathetic [15].

On the basis of this distinction one can surmise that the chronic obstruction syndrome is caused by hypofunction of the sympathetic system, while the rhinorrhoea syndrome is caused by hyperfunction of the parasympathetic system.

The chronic nasal obstruction syndrome

Apart from disturbances of the autonomic system, chronic nasal obstruction can also be caused by misuse of nosedrops containing sympathomimetic agents (rhinitis medicamentosa). It is often difficult to break the patient's psychological dependence on nosedrops and it is often necessary to prescribe a sedative at night; phenergan is very satisfactory for this since it not only has a sedative action but is also an antihistamine with an atropine-like effect. During the day the patient can be given a combined preparation of a less sedative antihistamine and an oral decongestant containing pseudoephedrine, phenylephrine, or phenylpropanolamine. The patient may also be instructed to put drops in one side of the nose only; when the rhinitis medicamentosa is cured after 4–6 weeks the drops are then discontinued on the other side.

A cause of nasal obstruction which is often not appreciated is the use of certain drugs, especially the hypotensive agents such as the rauwolfia alkaloids and methyldopa. A different form of treatment may then be tried in consultation with the physician. Other drugs which can cause nasal obstruction are the ergot alkaloids which are used in migraine, cholinesterase blockers, and chlorpromazine.

Hormonal influences can also cause nasal obstruction which can occur at puberty and during menstruation. Possibly 'honeymoon rhinitis' also falls under this heading. A severe and troublesome rhinitis can occur during pregnancy and is difficult to manage because drugs should not be given at this time. Oral contraceptives can also cause nasal obstruction.

As in asthma, psychological influences can also aggravate or even cause vasomotor rhinitis. The rhinologist fairly regularly sees patients who complain about nasal obstruction for which there is no objective evidence. Often it is sufficient to explain to the patient that one side of the nose may become obstructed alternately as a result of the nasal cycle and that this is a normal physiological event. Sometimes the symptom of nasal obstruction appears to be an unconscious pretext for consulting the doctor about a supposedly misshapen nose.

The most reliable method of objective assessment of nasal obstruction is provided by rhinomanometry. Several different methods of this have been described but in principle these all depend on measuring the degree of fall in pressure which occurs in the nose with a specific airflow or, conversely, on measuring the airflow at a pre-determined differential pressure.

In anterior rhinomanometry the pressure difference between the nasopharynx and the ambient pressure is recorded. One nostril is used to measure the pressure. Since there is no flow in this nasal meatus, the pressure at the nostril is equal to the pressure in the nasopharynx. Simultaneously, the flow at the other nostril is measured. A drawback of this method is that due to the introduction of nasal obturators, distortions of the nasal valve area are practically unavoidable [16]. This problem can be obviated by using a facial mask. In posterior rhinomanometry the pressure difference between the oropharynx and the ambient pressure is recorded [17]. This probably is the most reliable test of nasal resistance, but its clinical significance is limited by the fact that about 40% of patients are unable to perform this.

The forms of nasal obstruction which are caused by dysregulation of the autonomic nervous system can be treated in the first instance by prescription of sympathomimetic drugs such as ephedrine or its derivatives. These can cause palpitations, gastric disturbances and nervousness and are therefore not well tolerated by all patients. It has already been emphasized that vasoconstrictor nosedrops should not be given for long-standing nasal symptoms.

Antihistamines are sometimes of benefit, a fact which may be explained by their atropine-like effect, but an objection is their sedative effect. In severe cases the turbinates may be cauterized and good results can also be achieved by submucosal diathermy of the turbinates or submucous turbinectomy. This last procedure must be carried out with care since excessive widening can cause crust formation and even atrophic rhinitis.

The rhinorrhoea syndrome

The other clinical picture with which autonomic dysregulation may present is with bouts of sneezing, excessive watery rhinorrhoea, and watering of the eyes. In this case nasal obstruction is often less conspicuous. These symptoms occur more commonly in women than in men. The attacks begin in the mornings immediately after getting out of bed and can last for several hours or even all day. Between the attacks the patient is usually entirely symptom free. The attacks can be so serious that the patient becomes entirely incapable of work.

A number of these patients can be treated successfully with disodium-cromoglycate, although its mode of action in the rhinorrhoea syndrome is still unexplained. Antihistamines, possibly combined with sympathomimetics, are also often successful. Almost all patients with this form of vasomotor rhinitis respond very favourably to corticosteroids but in view of the known complications of this treatment it should seldom be used over a long period. It is possible that a beclomethasone nasal spray will be successful in this respect.

In very resistant cases division of the vidian nerve may be considered. Although the vidian nerve contains both post-ganglionic sympathetic fibres and pre-ganglionic parasympathetic fibres, it is assumed that the parasympathetic influence predominates [18]. Division of the vidian nerve therefore results in a relative parasympathectomy.

If the indications are correct (i.e. there is no allergy and the patient suffers from a type of vasomotor rhinitis that is characterized by excessive sneezing and rhinorrhoea) it appears that the symptoms are relieved immediately after the op-

eration in almost all patients [19]; unfortunately after 9–12 months about half of these patients suffer a recurrence. It has been shown experimentally in rats that after transection of the supplying nerves an initial disappearance of the autonomic nerve endings in the nasal mucosa takes place, but that between 2 and 12 months post-operatively reinnervation can be demonstrated [20].

Unilateral watery rhinorrhoea, especially if this occurs after trauma, can be due to a CSF leak. The diagnosis can be confirmed by determining the glucose content of the secretions and by introducing radioactive iodine or fluorescine in the CSF and assessing if this material appears in the nose.

Episodic unilateral rhinorrhoea can occur in cluster headache and in the unusual syndrome of gustatory rhinorrhoea after parotidectomy.

NASAL POLYPS

Pathology

The aetiology of nasal polyps is not completely clear.

The vast number of theories include: the polyp is an adenoma [21], a soft fibroma [22], a myxomatous degeneration of the mucosa [23], a consequence of necrosing ethmoiditis [24], a result of effusion and vascular congestion [25] or of cystic dilatation of glandular ducts and acini [26]. All these theories at present only have historical significance. In 1933 Kern and Schenck [27] put forward the theory that nasal polyps were a consequence of allergy; however, it has been shown more recently in a large series of patients with nasal polyps that only in 28% was an atopy present and that most probably chronic infection was the causative factor. On the other hand, nasal polyps occur more commonly and at a younger age in atopic rather than in non-atopic people [28].

A recent pathogenetic theory holds that polyps develop as a consequence of rupture of the epithelium as a result of tissue pressure from an oedematous and infiltrated nasal mucosa. The infiltrated and oedematous lamina propria prolapses caudally in the form of granulation tissue;

the vascular stalk is established and at the same time epithelization of the prolapsed tissue takes place from the edges of the ruptured epithelium. At this stage a small polyp has formed. Mucous glands then grow from the epithelium into the depths of it. At the same time the volume of the polyp increases, probably due to gravity and the haemodynamic conditions of congestion of the venous discharge through the thin stalk. Through passive growth of the polyp the characteristic, very long, tubular ducts arise and this explains the much lower density of glands than observed in the normal nasal mucosa. With increasing age of the polyp, fibrosing and round-cell infiltration of the stroma increase, the glands degenerate and become cystic [29].

At the sites of the polyps that are exposed to the current of air metaplasia may take place, so that the columnar pseudo-stratified epithelium changes into stratified epithelium. Malignant degeneration of nasal polyps does not occur, but nasal polyps can arise secondary to malignant disease in the nose. A unilateral polypus, especially if accompanied by a blood stained purulent discharge, should be treated with suspicion. The tissue removed at polypectomy should always be submitted to histologic examination.

Polyps usually form in the middle meatus, particularly near the ostia of the sinuses, and sometimes in the roof of the nose; it is not clear why they are never seen on the septum, in the lower meatus or in the lower respiratory tract. Nasal polyps are frequently accompanied by bronchial asthma and, as such, are an expression of a disorder of the entire respiratory tract which must be treated as one unit. Often nasal polyps are harbingers of asthma, which develops later.

In a number of patients with nasal polyposis, particularly if combined with non-atopic bronchial asthma, intolerance for aspirin, with often a crossed intolerance to indomethacine pyrazones and coal tar dyes, is encountered. Ingestion of these substances can lead to severe and even fatal dyspnoea and respiratory arrest; they should therefore be used with great care in these patients. The pathogenesis of this syndrome is not quite clear, but there is evidence that it is related to the inhibitory action these compounds exert on the biosynthesis of prostaglandins [30].

Nasal polyps occur rarely during childhood. If nasal polyps are found in a child it must be suspected to be the first symptom of mucoviscidosis. This syndrome consists of

(1) pancreatic insufficiency,
(2) chronic bronchopneumonia and obstructive emphysema,
(3) high chloride content in the sweat,
(4) positive family history.

In approximately 90% of patients a chronic maxillary sinusitis is found [31]. One out of every 10–20 children with mucoviscidosis is suffering from nasal polyposis. The polyps can be present at a very young age, even in the second year of life. In about 15% of the patients with mucoviscidosis an allergy is demonstrable. If this combination is present then nasal polyps are found in one out of every three patients. Therefore, in all children with nasal polyposis, mucoviscidosis should be excluded by means of a sweat test and, possibly, jejunal biopsy [32].

Nasal polyps also occur in the rare Kartagener's syndrome of bronchiectasis, situs inversus and chronic sinusitis. They have also been described in children with Peutz–Jeghers' syndrome of pigmented spots on the skin, especially around the mouth and polyposis of the gastrointestinal tract.

A specific type of polypus is the antro-choanal polyp which occurs especially in the second and third decades of life but can also occur in children. The polyp is solitary arising from the maxillary antrum (most frequently from the lateral wall) and passes via the ostium and the nasal cavity into the nasopharynx. A few cases have been described in which a polyp arose from the sphenoidal sinus or from the posterior ethmoidal cells. Histologically, the polyp does not differ from other nasal polyps. The choanal polyp can reach an enormous size and has a marked tendency to recur so a Caldwell–Luc operation is usually necessary to eradicate it.

Treatment

The problem in management of nasal polyps is the tendency to recurrence after removal. The polypectomy can be carried out either under local or general anaesthesia. If the nasal polyps are the result of a chronic maxillary sinusitis a Caldwell–Luc operation should be carried out at the same time. If there have been multiple recurrences an ethmoidectomy may be indicated.

Vasoconstrictor nose drops are almost always contra-indicated in the medical treatment of the polyps. If the nasal polyps are due to atopy this should be treated in the usual manner. Purulent infections of the nasal mucosa should be treated with antibiotics. This is even more important than usual since every patient with polyps is a potential sufferer from asthma. Corticosteroids have an extremely powerful effect but it is not usually justifiable to prescribe oral corticosteroids over a period of years for this chronic disorder. It is probable that sprays containing beclomethasone, which have been shown to be useful in bronchial asthma, will also prove useful in nasal polyps. However, good results are not expected from insufflation with cromoglycate which often has such a good effect in atopic rhinitis.

References

[1] GELL P. G. H. & COOMBS R. R. A. (1963) *Clinical Aspects of Immunology*, Oxford: Blackwell.

[2] ISHIZAKA K., ISHIZAKA T. & HORNBROOK M. M. (1966) Physicochemical properties of human reaginic antibody IV. Presence of a unique immunoglobulin as a carrier of reaginic activity. *J. Immunol.* **97**, 75.

[3] AAS K. (1974) The radioallergosorbent test (RAST): diagnostic and clinical significance. *Ann. All.* **33**, 251.

[4] FOUCARD T., AAS K. & JOHANSSON S. G. O. (1972) Concentration of IgE antibodies, PK-titres and chopped lung titres in sera with hypersensitivity to cod. *J. Allerg. Clin. Immunol.* **1**, 157.

[5] KAY A. B., STECHSCHULTE D. J. & AUSTEN K. F. (1971) An eosinophilic leukocyte chemotactic factor of anaphylaxis. *J. Exper. Med.* **133**, 602.

[6] CONNELL J. T. (1969) Quantitative intranasal pollen challenges. III. The priming effect in allergic rhinitis. *J. All.* **43**, 33.

[7] VAREKAMP H., SPIEKSMA F. TH. M., LEUPEN M. J. & LYKLEMA A. W. (1966) House dust mites in their relation to dampness of houses and the allergen content of house dust. *Proc. 5th Interasma Congress*, Pressa Trajectina, Utrecht.

[8] VOORHORST R., SPIEKSMA F. TH. M., VAREKAMP H., LEUPEN M. J. & LYKLEMA A. W. (1967) The house-dust mite (*Dermatophagoides pteronyssinus*) and the allergen it produces. Identity with the house-dust allergen. *J. All.* **39**, 325.

[9] PEPYS J. (1969) *Hypersensitivity Diseases of the Lungs due to Fungi and Organic Dusts*. Basel: S. Karger.

[10] JOHNSTONE D. E. & DUTTON A. (1968) The value of hyposensitization therapy for bronchial asthma in children—a 14-year study. *Pediatrics* **42**, 793.

[11] LOWELL F. C. & FRANKLIN W. (1965) A double-blind study of the effectiveness and specificity of injection therapy in ragweed hay fever. *New Engl. J. Med.* **273**, 675.

[12] GIRARD J. P. & BERTRAND J. (1975) Study of 2% solution of sodium cromoglycate in perennial rhinitis assessed by subjective and objective parameters. *Clin. All.* **5**, 301.

[13] HOFFBRAND B. I. & HARRIS D. M. (Eds.) (1975) Beclomethasone dipropionate aerosols. International Symposium. *Postgrad. Med. J.* **51**, Suppl. 4.

[14] WENTGES R. T. R. (1975) Surgical anatomy of the pterygopalatine fossa. *J. Laryngol. Otol.* **89**, 35.

[15] CAUNA N., CAUNA D. & HINDERER K. H. (1972) Innervation of human nasal glands. *J. Neurocytol.* **1**, 48.

[16] KORTEKANGAS A. E. (1971) Clinical application of rhinomanometry. *Rhinology* **9**, 144.

[17] INGELSTEDT S., JONSON B. & RUNDCRANTZ H. (1969) A clinical method for determination of nasal airway resistance. *Acta Oto-Laryng. (Stockh.)* **68**, 189.

[18] JACKSON R. T. & ROOKER D. W. (1971) Stimulation and section of the vidian nerve in relation to autonomic control of the nasal vasculature. *Laryngoscope* **81**, 565.

[19] GOLDING-WOOD P. H. (1973) Vidian neurectomy: Its results and complications. *Laryngoscope* **83**, 1673.

[20] GROTE J. J. (1974) The autonomic innervation of the nasal mucosa. *Thesis*, Nijmegen.

[21] BILLROTH T. (1855) *Über den Bau der Schleimpolypen*. Berlin: Reimer.

[22] HOPMANN C. M. (1855) Über Nasenpolypen. *Monatsschrift für Ohrenheilkunde und Laryngo-Rhinologie* **19**, 161.

[23] MACKENZIE M. (1884) *A Manual of Diseases of the Throat and Nose*. New York: Wood.

[24] WENTGES R. TH. R. (1972) Edward Woakes, the history of an eponym. *Journal of Laryngology and Otology* **86**, 501.

[25] HAJEK M. (1896) Über die pathologischen Veränderungen der Siebbeinknochen im Gefolge der entzündlichen Scheimhauthypertrophie und der Nasenpolypen. *Archiv für Laryngologie und Rhinologie* **4**, 277.

[26] YONGE E. S. (1907) The determining causes of nasal polyps. *British Medical Journal* **ii**, 964.

[27] KERN R. A. & SCHENCK H. P. (1933) Allergy, a constant factor in the etiology of so-called mucous nasal polyps. *Journal of Allergy* **4**, 485.

[28] WENTGES R. TH. R. (1973) Nasal polyps and atopy. In *The Atopy Syndrome and Organ-Challenge Procedures*. Zeist.

[29] TOS M. & MOGENSEN CHR. (1977) Pathogenesis of nasal polyps. *Rhinology* **15**, 87.

[30] VANE J. R. (1976) The mode of action of aspirin and similar compounds. *J. Allergy Clin. Immunol.* **58**, 691.

[31] SHWACHMAN H., KULCZYCKI L. L., MUELLER H. L. & FLAKE C. G. (1962) Nasal polyposis in patients with cystic fibrosis. *Pediatrics* **30**, 389.

[32] METRE T. E. VAN, COOKE R. E., GIBSON L. E. & WINKENWERDER W. L. (1960) Evidence of allergy in patients with cystic fibrosis of the pancreas. *Journal of Allergy* **31**, 141.

CHAPTER 19

Cosmetic Facial Surgery

Patients may seek cosmetic facial surgery for two reasons. First, they may consider their face to be ugly or deformed and wish to have it improved by surgery and, secondly, they may reject the outward appearances of ageing and hope that surgery will arrest or reverse this process. Rhinoplasty, otoplasty and mentoplasty are performed generally to improve deformities while face lift, blepharoplasty and chemabrasion improve the ageing face. While these operations have traditionally been the preserve of the plastic surgeon they should now form part of the surgical repertoire of the otolaryngologist.

RHINOPLASTY

Surgical anatomy

The osseous nasal pyramid

The paired nasal bones and parts of the frontal processes of the maxillae form the main part of the osseous nasal pyramid. At the nasal radix the nasal bones are supported by the nasal spine of frontal bone which provides a shelf-like support, so adding strength to the nasal bridge.

The upper lateral cartilages and quadrangular septum

The paired upper lateral cartilages are somewhat triangular in shape and are attached to the nasal bones and frontal processes of maxillae which override them for a few millimetres. In their upper part they meet in the midline and are also continuous on their under surfaces with the quadrangular septal cartilage. The two upper lateral cartilages and the septal cartilage make up the upper part of the cartilaginous vault and are

developed from the same mass of cartilage. The inferior free edge of the upper lateral cartilage tends to project into the nasal vestibule for a few millimetres, so forming the limen nasi which is clearly visible on anterior rhinoscopy. They are attached to the overlying alar cartilages by connective tissue, and it is in this region that the intercartilaginous incision is made. Towards the midline the lower edge of the cartilage is separated from the septal cartilage by a well-defined cleft and this ingenious design provides the necessary mobility to form a valve-like device with the septum, so enabling the nose to vary the resistance to airflow. It is generally conceded that about 80% of the nasal resistance in the Caucasian nose is dependent upon the liminal valve.

Lower lateral cartilages (alar cartilages)

The paired alar cartilages which form the lower part of the cartilaginous vault have a lateral and medial crus which make an angle with one another and are joined at the dome. The domes are joined together in the midline by the interdomal ligament which gives important support to the nasal tip. Each lateral crus overlaps the lower part of the upper lateral cartilage and is firmly attached to the pyriform opening by dense connective tissue in which there are often sesamoid cartilages. This fibro-sesamoid complex is also an important aid in the support of the nasal tip. The medial crura of each alar cartilage meet in the midline below the domes and form the columella which in turn is attached to the caudal edge of the cartilaginous septum by the membranous septum. The feet of the medial crura are attached to the inferior portion of the cartilaginous septum and provide support to the nasal tip. The area in the supratip above the domes of the alar cartilages is known as the weak triangle of Converse. The anterior septal angle of the quadrangular cartilage tends to project between the diverging lower edges of the upper lateral cartilages and is sometimes visible in subjects with thin nasal skin (Fig. 19.1a and b).

Types of nasal deformity

Deviation

The deviated nose is caused by an unreduced fracture of the nasal bones, displacement of the quadrangular cartilage or displacement of both bone and cartilage. If injury occurs in childhood the deformity tends to become accentuated as the nose grows.

Hump

The nasal hump may be purely bony, purely cartilaginous or may consist of both bony and cartilaginous elements. The cause may be familial, racial or post-traumatic; the mechanism of the latter is usually a subperiosteal haematoma which ossifies. The nose appears sharp from the front and long and drooping from the side.

Saddle

The saddle nose may be due to an unreduced fracture of a backward displaced nasal pyramid or destruction of the septum with backward displacement of the upper lateral cartilages. Injury may produce a haematoma and subsequent loss of cartilage or the deformity may be due to removal of excessive septal cartilage as was performed in the once popular radical septal operations.

Tip deformities

Deformities of the lower cartilaginous vault or 'tip' are many and varied and are often confusing to the beginner in rhinoplasty. The tip may be:

(1) *Too long:* The tip is lower than the nasolabial angle giving the appearance of a hooked nose (Fig. 19.2a)

(2) *Too short:* If the tip is too short it projects upwards and while this might be acceptable in a woman who is just over 5 feet tall it is generally

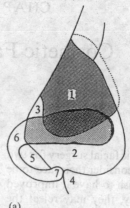

(a)

1. Upper lateral cartilage
   Note the under running of the nasal bones and frontal process of maxilla by the upper lateral cartilage

2. Septal cartilage

3. Cleft

4. Nasal spine of maxilla

5. Membranous septum

6. Medial crus of alar cartilage

7. Alar foot in close relation to septal cartilage

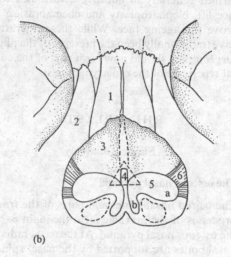

(b)

1. Nasal bone

2. Frontal process of maxilla

3. Upper lateral cartilage

4. Septal angle

5. Lower lateral cartilage
   (a) Lateral crus (b) Medial crus

6. Fibro-sesamoid complex

△ Weak triangle of Converse

FIG. 19.1. Illustrating the important parts of nasal anatomy.

unacceptable because both nares are visible and the upper lip looks too long (Fig. 19.2b).

(3) *Too high:* If the distance from the nasolabial junction to the end of the tip is too long then the tip will project. This may be part of a nose that is too big in its bony and cartilaginous components but if it exists on its own the nose in profile has the appearance of a ski jump (Fig. 19.2c).

(4) *Too low:* If the distance from the nasolabial junction to the end of the tip is too short then the nose will have a convex shape in profile. The tip appears too low in a patient with a cartilaginous hump which may be racial or due to the postoperative complication of 'polly beak' (Fig. 19.2d).

(5) *Too broad:* A broad tip is almost always accompanied by thick greasy skin which in itself forms most of the excess tissue. The deformity may however be due to abnormally large lateral crura of the lower lateral cartilages.

(6) *Too narrow:* A tip that is too narrow is usually caused by an operation in which the excision of the alar cartilages has been too enthusiastic.

Angle deformities

(1) *Nasolabial angle:* In the male this should ideally be 90° and in the female 105°. If this angle is too obtuse it is usually due to a tip that is too short. The more usual deformity is an excessive acuteness of the angle. While this may be apparent due to a too-long tip it may be real after an SMR in which the maxillary spine has been removed allowing the soft tissue to recess into the space created.

(2) *Nasofrontal angle:* The nose should meet the forehead at an angle of 30°. While the procerus muscle can contribute to blunting this angle the deformity is usually bony in origin.

Alar deformities

The alae should meet the face at a perpendicular line dropped from the medial canthus. If it is inside this line they are too narrow and the nostrils will be constricted and the tip too high. If they lie outside this line they are too broad. This is the negro nose but it can also occur in a saddle nose or one with a too-short tip. The nostrils appear round instead of pear shaped.

Columellar deformities

The columella usually projects about 3–4 mm lower than the lower alar edge when viewed from the side. If it projects more than this it is a hanging columella and if less, it is retracted. The columella also may be deviated to one side by a dislocated septum.

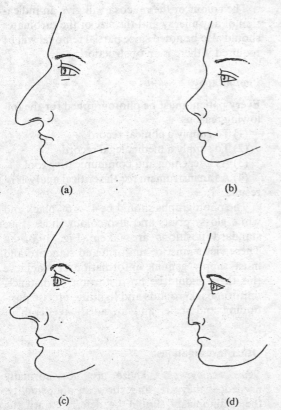

(a)   (b)

(c)   (d)

FIG. 19.2 Illustrating tip deformities: (a) too long; (b) too short; (c) too high; (d) too low.

Investigation

History

Patients want a rhinoplasty for one of three reasons and this must be established at an early stage. They want to be able to breathe better, or they want an obvious deformity corrected or they want to look beautiful. It is also important to establish whether the patient came of her own accord or because of the wishes of a relative. If the patient comes on her own find out what precipitated the visit – a divorce, a job failure, or another such emotional trauma which will require assessment prior to operating. If there is a breathing problem then the usual questions of allergy, sinusitis, discharge, etc. must be assessed.

The type of nose that the patient wants or requires must be pre-judged according to the sex, height, age, build, and race of the patient. A small girl needs a short nose, a tall girl a longer nose, a broad-faced patient will look worse with a narrow tip and an older woman would not suit a retroussé nose. It is not advisable to change a nose in a non-Caucasian patient to one which would not be ethnically appropriate.

The psychology of patients requesting a rhinoplasty has been studied mostly in North America where the demands and requirements of patients are different from those in Europe. In both continents however the following could be considered to be psychological danger signs:

(1) A history of multiple cosmetic operations.

(2) Exaggeration of minor defects.

(3) Expectation that rhinoplasty will make them beautiful.

Care should also be taken in treating young males or menopausal females.

Examination

Whilst examining the nose with a good light one decides about the type of deformity, noting at the same time the size of the face, the slope of the forehead and the proportion of the chin to the face. The deformity of the bony and upper cartilaginous vaults are then examined both from in front and each profile. By running a finger gently down the nasal dorsum irregularities can be detected and recorded. The texture of the skin is examined for it must be remembered that thick skin tends to minimize the effect of a reduction technique and, therefore, more dorsal septal cartilage is usually removed in these cases. Moreover, thin skin will tend to show any imperfection after surgery and, therefore, extra special care

must be made at the completion of surgery to ensure that all is well.

The lower nasal vault is then examined and some idea of the amount of intrinsic support can be determined by gently pressing down on the tip with the finger. As numerous types of variations exist in this region it is axiomatic that if the upper part of the nose is altered surgically then some form of tip plasty will be required to ensure that the nose retains harmony with the rest of the face.

Examination of the airways and particularly the septum is important because this will decide whether septal surgery needs to be added to the surgery of the bony and cartilaginous vault. If the septum is dislocated and causing an external deformity then a septoplasty is essential. If the obstruction takes the form of a small spur or minor convexity then it is preferable to perform a limited SMR especially if much alteration is required in the dorsum and tip.

The colour of the mucosa will give an indication of any allergy and the size of the turbinates should also be noted since partial removal will be required if there is an obstruction.

Photography

Every patient must be photographed for the following reasons:

(1) To supply a clinical record.

(2) To supply a medicolegal record.

(3) As a teaching and communicative tool.

(4) As an instrument for the critical analysis of results.

The photographs should be 4″ × 6″ black and white glossy prints and also colour slides. Five standard positions are taken (Fig. 19.3a–e). These views must be uniform and standard and must supply genuine information. To achieve this there should be no distortion of distance, uniform backgrounds and lighting, precise positioning and scale, and an adequate depth of focus.

Other investigations

Sinus radiographs. These are not normally needed; if they are, and show an abnormality, then rhinoplasty should be deferred until the infection has been treated.

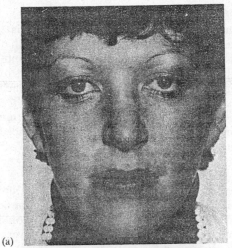

(a)

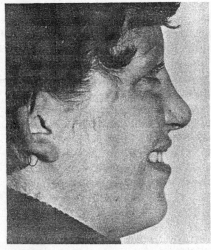

(d)

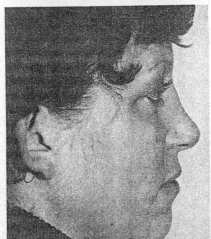

(b)

FIG. 19.3 Before a rhinoplasty is performed, the following photographs should be taken in black- and-white prints and colour transparencies: (a) full face; (b) right lateral smiling; (c) right lateral; (d) left lateral; (e) head back to show the base of the nose.

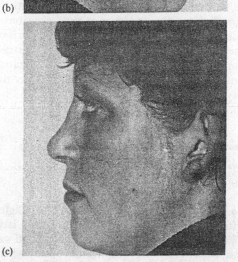

(c)

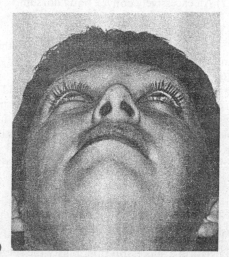

(e)

Rhinomanometry. There is no more indication for this in the rhinoplasty patient than in any other patient with nasal disease.

Psychiatric assessment. Assessing a patient prior to a rhinoplasty is a very specialized task and there are few such specialists in Europe. The authors feel that if they think they need a psychiatric examination of a patient requesting rhinoplasty then it might be better not to perform the procedure.

Errors in diagnosis and selection

The two most obvious errors are poor patient selection and incomplete evaluation of the deformity. A patient dissatisfied with a rhinoplasty will tend to keep visiting the surgeon with requests for a revision. Unless there is something obvious and easy to correct such as a bony spicule or an uneven hump such request should be resisted. Surgeons who perform rhinoplasty will also see patients who have had such rejections from their original surgeon; they should again resist the temptation to revise the procedure because they will almost certainly be visited with the sins of the first surgeon.

The types of noses that a beginner should avoid operating on are:

(1) Excessively large noses.
(2) An excessively convex bony dorsum.
(3) A shallow nasofrontal angle.
(4) Excessive tip projection.
(5) A wide bulbous tip with excessively thick skin.
(6) Ethnic noses.

Finally the rhinoplasty 'step ladder' should be borne in mind. Noses are categorized as follows – beautiful, normal, deformed, and horrible. Surgery can only move a nose up this ladder by one step and both the patient and the beginner in rhinoplasty should be aware of this.

Treatment

Basic surgical concepts

To perform a successful rhinoplasty the surgeon must master many different techniques and it is the successful selection of the most appropriate of these techniques to suit the individual case that gives a good result. The basic principle of rhinoplasty is to create mobility or to remove parts of the nasal skeleton, thus creating spaces on which the skin can redrape.

The most confusing part of the literature relates to the multitude of techniques described to alter the tip. Basically one can only do six things to the tip – lengthen, shorten, raise, lower, broaden, or narrow.

Scar tissue takes up to 18 months to mature and so a final assessment of the result cannot be made in under a year. The young surgeon should learn to think in terms of tissue dynamics over a long period.

Detailed description of all types of rhinoplasty is beyond the scope of this volume. An outline of the three major problems will be given.

Straightening the deviated nose

If the bony vault is deviated then medial and lateral osteotomies are performed. The bones should be over-corrected because scar tissue tends to shift them back to their original position. It is difficult to get the nasal bones to remain in a good position if they were badly displaced and injections of steroids do not seem to help.

If there is an external deviation of the cartilaginous vault a septoplasty is required to replace the septum in the midline. If this is done at the same time as the osteotomies then excision of tissue should be kept to a minimum. If there is no external deviation of the septum but an obstruction to the airway then serious consideration should be given to doing a partial SMR since this may disturb the nasal attachments less and not compromise the results of the osteotomies.

Reduction rhinoplasty

The following areas can be reduced in size or angle and thereby fall under this heading.

Nasofrontal angle: A straight nasofrontal angle is difficult to correct. Removal of procerus is ineffective because the area is eventually filled with scar tissue. The same complication occurs when a wedge of bone is chiselled out.

Bony hump: When this is removed, either by saw or chisel, the dorsum of the nose is left broadened and medial and lateral osteotomies are required to narrow this. Occasionally a bony hump may be due to a subperiosteal haematoma and this can be repaired by removal of the scar tissue or by rasping if there is ossification.

Cartilaginous hump: This is formed by both the upper lateral cartilages and the quandrangular cartilage. Removal must, therefore, include parts of both these cartilages.

Bony cartilaginous humps: A combination of the above two techniques is used.

Nasolabial angle: If this is obtuse the maxillary spine may be partially removed to allow the base of the columella to retract but it often causes the upper lip to appear too long.

Tip: If the tip is too high then it may be lowered by removing fragments of the medial crura of the alar cartilages. The problem however is not so often to deliberately lower the tip but to stop the tip falling too far due to natural scarring. If this happens then it accentuates the cartilaginous vault, giving the appearance of a 'polly beak'.

A tip that is too broad can be narrowed by removing a portion of the lateral crura of the alar cartilages. This is usually combined with the removal of a V-shaped wedge from the dome to allow the lateral and medial crura to form a more acute angle (Fig. 19.4). If the tip is too long then the basic manoeuvre to shorten it is to remove a V-shaped portion of the caudal end of the quad-rilateral cartilage based dorsally. Also by removing the cephalic ends of the lateral crura space is created for the tip to rotate into, thus shortening the nose (Fig. 19.5).

Ala: If the ala lies outside a perpendicular line drawn down from the medial canthus it is too broad. It can be narrowed by removing a full thickness wedge from its base and resuturing the defect (Fig. 19.6).

Augmentation rhinoplasty

Naso frontal angle: This is a very difficult defect to improve. Attempts can be made by cutting the procerus and allowing it to retract by detaching

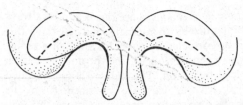

FIG. 19.4. To shorten the tip a portion of the cephalic part of the lateral crura of the lower lateral cartilages is excised. To narrow the tip a V-shaped portion is removed between the lateral and medial crura.

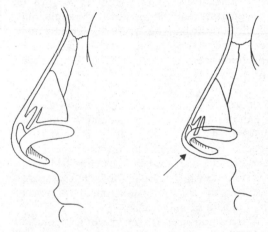

FIG. 19.5. In shortening the tip a V-shaped portion of the caudal end of the septum is removed to allow the lower lateral cartilages to move in a cephalic direction.

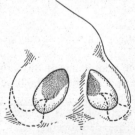

FIG. 19.6. To narrow the ala a wedge is removed as shown and the ala is stitched back on to the face.

the hump and pushing it up or by inserting a free graft via an eyebrow incision.

Bony saddle: This rarely exists on its own, usually being accompanied by a cartilaginous saddle.

Cartilaginous saddle: Since this is almost always accompanied by an internal septal deformity this must be corrected by either an SMR or a septoplasty depending on whether or not there is an external deviation. The saddle should be filled with pieces of cartilage obtained from the patient's own septum or cartilage stored in cialet obtained from other patients.

Cartilage is best obtained from the end of the eighth rib at the costal margin or from the lower border of the seventh costal cartilage. These sites are preferred because it is possible to obtain a big enough graft that will not warp. The tunnel into which the cartilaginous graft is inserted should be as small as possible and haemostasis should be absolute, because cartilage tends to resorb on contact with blood.

Bony-cartilaginous saddle: Discussion on the repair of this defect centres around whether bone or cartilage is the better graft. Bone partially absorbs but is replaced by fibrous tissue. It may also become displaced from its bony bed on the nasal bones which should also be infractured. It also runs the risk of not adhering to the underlying bone and being mobile.

Cartilaginous grafts, on the other hand, are liable to absorption if in contact with blood and are not sufficient to fill large defects.

There is no place for artificial grafts such as silicones or Silastic except in children on a short-term basis, since these are inevitably rejected in the long term.

Nasolabial angle: This defect may be apparent if the tip is too long or it may be real if the maxillary spine has been removed in an SMR operation. In this case the space between the base of the columella and the maxillary spine area is filled with a cartilage graft which is inserted as multiple small pieces threaded together.

Tip: If the tip is too short then the primary problem is lack of soft tissue and this is difficult to replace. A dorsal graft may push the tip down and cause a visible tenseness in the end of the nose.

A tip that is too low can be heightened by adding a small piece of cartilage as a 'button'. It can also be heightened by dividing the medial

from the lateral crura and resuturing the medial crura together. While this gives a pleasing profile it makes the tip look notched from the front.

A narrow tip is difficult to broaden but attempts can be made by moving the alae outwards and allowing sufficient relaxation of soft tissue by lowering the tip.

MENTOPLASTY

For the purposes of facial harmony there must be a satisfactory relationship between the length of the nose and the size and shape of the chin and forehead. A well-proportioned nose cannot appear aesthetically correct without a properly proportioned chin. If, for example, the chin is small then the nose may appear unduly prominent; and if at the same time the forehead is sloped with an abnormally wide nasofrontal angle, the nose will also appear unduly prominent.

Types of deformity

A chin may be too prominent (prognathic) or too small (micrognathic). Each of these deformities can be either real or apparent; the former situation exists if maxillary growth has been altered by a cleft palate or if the middle and upper thirds of the face, or the nose, are excessively large. Each deformity may or may not be accompanied by abnormal dental occlusion. There are three broad classes of occlusion:

Class I: 'Normal' maxillo-mandibular relationship.

Class II: The upper teeth are relatively anterior to the lower teeth; this is the situation which may exist in micrognathia.

Class III: The lower teeth are relatively anterior to the upper teeth; this is the usual accompanying dental feature in prognathism.

Investigation

History

The reason for the patient's request must be established. The pyschiatric complications which sometimes exist among patients seeking a rhinoplasty are uncommon in those wanting a mentoplasty. An ugly jaw, especially with malocclusion, is somehow more noticeable than a nasal deformity. These patients may also have speaking or eating difficulties.

Examination

Apart from noting whether the jaw is prognathic or micrognathic the single most important finding is to establish whether or not there is a Class II or III malocclusion. If either of these is present then the patient should be referred to an oral surgeon because any correction of the position of the jaw will have to be accompanied not only by dental fixation but also by reshaping of some of the occlusal surfaces. It is also important to assess the position of the lips. Competent lip posture occurs when the lips meet without strain when the mandible is in the rest position. When the lips are unable to form an adequate seal without strain then lip posture is incompetent. The latter situation often exists in malocclusion.

Decide also whether the mandibular problem is real or apparent.

Photographic analysis

Normally two right lateral photographs are taken as well as a full-face view. One of the lateral photographs is taken with the patient smiling because considerable accentuation of the mental soft tissue may take place when the mentalis muscle contracts and this might contra-indicate an augmentation mentoplasty. On the second photograph the position of the chin is assessed by drawing a line perpendicular to the Frankfurt plane so that it is tangential to the lower lip. The point of the chin should touch this line (Fig. 19.7).

Cephalometric evaluation

Cephalometric radiology allows comparable pre- and post-operative views of both the hard and soft facial tissue. It is essential if malocclusion exists but is not necessary if no dental work needs to be done.

Treatment

Mentoplasty may be done either to augment or to reduce the size of the chin. The operation falls into two other main categories:

(1) Major surgery requiring osteotomy or bone graft; and

(2) Minor camouflaging techniques such as onlays or implants.

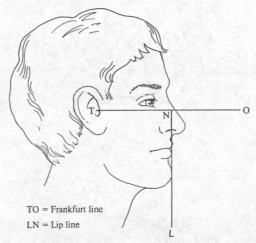

TO = Frankfurt line
LN = Lip line

FIG. 19.7. On a right lateral photograph a perpendicular line (LN) is dropped from the Frankfurt line (TO) to study the chin-lip relationship.

Augmentation mentoplasty without malocclusion

If the augmentation required is not great then an implant can be used. The best ones available at the moment are preformed Silastic implants with or without a backing of Dacron. There is some indication that resorption of the mandibular bone takes place under the implant but this tends to be self limiting and is unrelated to whether the implant is placed extra- or sub-periostially.

If a greater degree of augmentation is required then a horizontal osteotomy is performed from an intra-oral route. The mandible is divided horizontally below the alveolar canal, moved forwards and wired to the upper portion (Fig. 19.8).

Augmentation mentoplasty with malocclusion

This requires osteotomies in the vertical ramus,

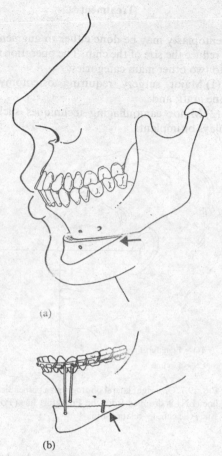

(a)

(b)

FIG. 19.8. Augmentation mentoplasty. In a simple augmentation the mandible is divided horizontally below the alveolar canal and moved forward.

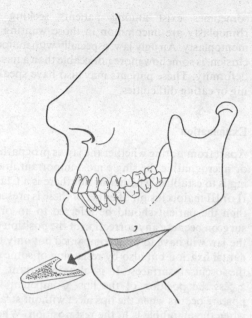

FIG. 19.9. Reduction mentoplasty. To reduce the height of the mandible a wedge of bone is excised and the remaining portions are wired as in Fig. 19.8.

Reduction mentoplasty with malocclusion

The most useful operation is to split the mandible vertically through the vertical ramus posterior to the lingula and neurovascular bundle. The horizontal portion is then moved posteriorly and the segments are immobilized by intermaxillary fixation.

OTOPLASTY

Deformities of the pinna are mainly congenital but may result from trauma or disease. The most common of the congenital deformities are prominent ears, but other defects occur and include asymmetry of the pinnae, cup ears, microtia or macrotia, and abnormalities of the lobules.

At the age of 5 years the child's ear is 95% developed. However, during the next few years the growth of the face catches up and so tends to make the defect less noticeable. This fact, together with the degree of prominence of the ears and the feelings of self-consciousness from teasing at school, must be considered before surgery is advised (Fig. 19.10).

resetting of the teeth in occlusion and intermaxillary fixation.

Reduction mentoplasty without malocclusion

This problem is usually related to an excessive height of the mandible and in order to reduce this height a wedge is removed below the alveolar canal and the lower segment is wired to the upper part (Fig. 19.9).

Removing the lower edge of the mandible in an effort to reduce size is unrewarding since the soft tissue scarring ultimately recreates the deformity.

length and width are 6·5 cm and 3·5 cm respectively, the width being measured from the tragus to Darwin's tubercle.

In general the ear projects from the cranium at an angle of 30° to the median saggital plane. The cephaloconchal angle (i.e. between the skull and the concha) is usually about 90°. The scaphoconchal angle tends to be more variable. In the normal ear it is usually about 90° but may be as much as 120° (Fig. 19.11).

Types of deformity

The two main types are prominent ears (bat ears) and cupped ears. They may be unilateral or bilateral and are often associated with either a relative or absolute macrotia.

There are two deformities of the cartilaginous pinna which lead to undue prominence of the ears and quite frequently the deformities coexist.

Poor definition of the antihelical fold and its superior crus leads to widening of the scaphoconchal angle and an abnormally *prominent ear*. The posterior part of the concha may be overdeveloped, resulting in a deeper than normal conchal concavity and, as this results in the antihelical fold being moved further laterally than usual from the head, the auricle becomes unduly

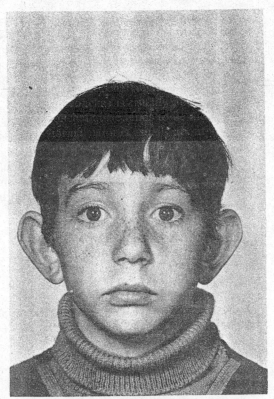

FIG. 19.10. Bat ears showing the prominence caused by an unfolding of the antihelical crease.

Surgical anatomy

The pinna consists of a single piece of yellow fibro-cartilage enclosed by a clearly identifiable perichondrium which supplies nutrition. A haematoma developing beneath the perichondrium jeopardizes the blood supply to the cartilage which then degenerates.

The cartilaginous framework is thrown into complicated curves and depressions; the posteromedial aspect, however, is relatively smooth and convex whilst the antero-lateral aspect is irregular and generally concave. The lobule is the only part of the pinna which has no underlying cartilaginous support. Its size varies considerably but as a general rule is not longer than 2 cm as measured from the anti-tragus to its free edge.

The skin on the anterolateral surface is firmly adherent to the perichondrium whilst that on the posteromedial side is relatively lax. The average

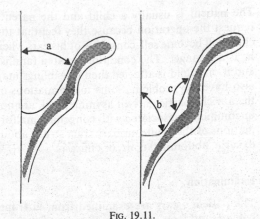

FIG. 19.11.

Horizontal section of ear to show

(a) Cephalo-auricular angle

(b) Cephalo-conchal angle

(c) Scapho-conchal angle

prominent. Any defect leading to a cephalo-auricular angle greater than 30° tends to result in a prominent ear and may be classified as such.

Two factors may modify the defect:

(1) Hair style. Most young girls wear their hair long, covering the ear deformity, and it is when there is a desire for a change of hair style that the problem of prominent ears has to be considered. Moreover, in recent years men's hairstyles have enabled the prominent ears to be similarly camouflaged.

(2) Head growth. As previously mentioned, as the child's head grows it tends to make prominent ears less noticeable and hence minor degrees of deformity may not require surgery.

The cupped ear is characterized by a hooded appearance of the pinna due to the upper helix being folded downwards over the antihelix.

The hooded defect is caused by both a shortened crus helix and short helical rim. There are often other coexisting deformities associated with cupping. In particular the antihelix is often underdeveloped and there is frequently some degree of microtia.

Investigation

History

The patient is usually a child and the parents request the operation because they feel that the child will become self-conscious of his ears when he is a teenager. The condition is often familial and if one child is affected then his siblings may also have the problem. Some malformations of the auricle, particularly if asymmetrical, are not uncommonly associated with congenital malformations of the genito-urinary tract so ask about dysuria, abdominal colic, or enuresis.

Examination

The patient's ears are examined from in front, behind, and from each side. The size of the ears are compared with each other and the projection from the head, i.e. the cephalo-auricular angle, is noted. A few degrees of difference is frequently found in normal individuals and is of little significance. It is useful to remember that the long

axis of the normal ear is parallel to the nasal bridge line and that its perpendicular height is roughly the same as the mid face area, i.e. from the glabella to the subnasale. The ears are then folded backwards to form a more normal projection with the head when the poorly formed or nonexistent superior crus and antihelix will immediately show up. Whilst performing this manoeuvre an idea of the thickness and resistance of the cartilage can be obtained. By the age of 9 or 10 years the cartilage becomes more adult in texture and in these cases cartilage incisions and excision are more frequently needed to obtain a satisfactory cosmetic result.

Photography

Four views are normally taken:
(1) Full face.
(2) From behind.
Both of these are taken with the hair lifted out of the way so all the angles are clearly seen.
(3) Right lateral.
(4) Left lateral.

Other investigations

If congenital urogenital anomalies are suspected an intravenous pyelogram should be performed.

Treatment

If otoplasty is indicated it is best performed at about 5 years of age, either just before or after the child commences school.

Prominent (bat) ears

There are a large number of different techniques to repair bat ears, all of which have their protagonists, but in general the operation has two main goals:

(1) To produce a well-defined superior crus and antihelical fold, i.e. to narrow the scaphoconchal angle. This may be produced, particularly in young children with easily mouldable cartilage, by sutures only (Mustardé) or by cartilage cutting and rolling procedures (McEvitt, Converse, Becker, Rubin).

(2) To reduce the amount of conchal projection. At surgery the site and amount of conchal cartilage to be excised is estimated, so setting the auricle nearer the head.

Cupped ears

In mild cases a V–Y plasty is performed on the crus helix to lengthen it, so allowing the rest of the pinna to unfurl (Grabb). A procedure similar to that for prominent ears may be necessary to form a proper antihelical fold. In more severe cases the auricle is straightened out by performing a series of radial incisions in the auricular cartilage.

BLEPHAROPLASTY

The earliest noticeable features of ageing appear in the periorbital region and, as we live in an age-conscious society, the demand for blepharoplasty continues to increase.

A patient who needs a face-lift operation will almost certainly require a blepharoplasty for the best cosmetic result but the converse is not true and blepharoplasty may antedate a face-lift operation by some 5 to 10 years. Moreover, some female patients develop prominent lid bags at an early age, probably as a result of an hereditary trait and can be helped by blepharoplasty when aged 30–35 years.

Surgical anatomy

There are usually two fat pockets in the upper lid – a small medial and a rather larger lateral pocket. The fat in the former compartment is white, less vascular, and has larger globules than that of the lateral compartment. The palpebral portion of the lachrymal gland lies in the lateral part of the upper lid and may become prominent in some patients in whom ptosis of the gland has developed.

There are usually three fat pockets described in the lower lid. However, the medial and intermediate are not uncommonly continuous and form a single large pocket, which is separated from the smaller lateral one by a fibrous band which runs obliquely from the lateral orbital margin to the posterior lachrymal crest (Fig. 19.12).

Types of deformity

(1) *Blepharochalasis*
This is defined as wrinkling and relaxation of the eyelid skin.

(2) *Formation of periorbital fat pads*
These changes occur in both upper and lower lids but, as yet, there is no clear consensus about their causation. The fatty bulges probably arise from accumulation of periorbital fat together with thinning of the septum orbitale, the orbicularis oculi muscle and the eyelid skin rather than true herniation of fat from the orbit. Fat tends to collect in certain definite anatomical sites in the lids and these are described as lid pockets.

Investigation

History

The patient must be asked about his or her reasons for requesting cosmetic surgery and the

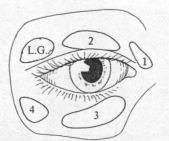

1. Medial upper lid pocket

2. Lateral upper lid pocket

3. Medial lower lid pocket

4. Lateral lower lid pocket

L.G.   Lacrimal gland

FIG. 19.12. Showing the usual fat pockets in the upper and lower lids.

surgeon must obtain some idea of the patient's insight and expectations from such an operation. The same psychological contra-indications as for rhinoplasty apply as they do in any facial cosmetic operation.

Examination of periorbital areas

The site and degree of wrinkling and the amount of fatty bag formation is judged and recorded. A careful assessment of the skin is made because the thin, atrophic skin usually found in older patients tears easily and must be handled with care, whilst the thicker skin occurring in younger patients contracts more after surgery and remains swollen for longer periods. When deep wrinkles are noticed they must be pointed out to the patient, as it is unlikely that these can be completely eliminated by blepharoplasty. Moreover, malar fatty bags are almost impossible to eradicate.

Examination of eyes

It is essential that an ophthalmological examination be made in all cases. Fundoscopy, examination of the fields of vision and tonometry should all be completed prior to operation.

Keratitis sicca, recurrent dendritic ulcers, recurrent allergic blepharitis, and lagophthalmos are contra-indications to surgery. Chronic glaucoma however is not an absolute contra-indication to blepharoplasty.

General medical examination

The patient is carefully examined to exclude any general medical condition which may produce swelling in the lids. Oedema from nephrosis, liver disease, and early hypothyroidism must be excluded, as well as swelling related to the menstrual cycle.

Blood dyscrasias and conditions which tend to produce easy bruising and uncontrolled bleeding must be excluded by a routine screening profile including a full blood count, prothrombin time, bleeding time, and prothromboplastin time. The presence of an undiagnosed bleeding problem will lead to disastrous complications – namely

massive haematomata in the lids and possibly intraocular bleeding and even blindness.

Photography

Four views are usually taken:
(1) Full face.
(2) Close up of both eyes, the field being limited to the area between the tip of the nose and the hairline.
(3) Close up lateral view of each eye to demonstrate periorbital swelling.

Treatment

Operations are designed to remove the redundant skin and fatty bags and bulges from both upper and lower lids. A brow lift to elevate the eyebrow may be indicated in the older patient. Absolute haemostasis is essential in all eyelid surgery.

Standard upper lid blepharoplasty

An ellipse of skin is removed from the upper lid with a 'dart' extending into the lateral canthus (Fig. 19.13). Although more skin can be removed here than in the case of the lower lid, care must be taken otherwise lagophthalmos may develop post-operatively. The fat bags are removed by making short incisions in the orbicularis oculi in the region of the medial and lateral pockets. The skin incision is closed with a continuous subcuticular suture to avoid production of skin tunnels

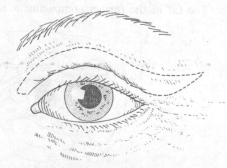

FIG. 19.13. Standard area of excision in upper lid blepharoplasty.

which may result from rapid epithelialization around interrupted sutures:

Standard lower lid blepharoplasty

This is the operation of choice for the older patient who exhibits wrinkling of the periorbital skin as well as fatty bulges and pads. The skin incision is made 2–3 mm from the ciliary margin and extended for a few millimetres into the lateral 'crow's foot' (Fig. 19.14). The skin is dissected from the underlying orbicularis oculi and

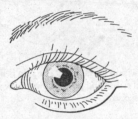

Fig. 19.14. Incision for lower lid blepharoplasty lies 2–3 mm from the ciliary margin and extends laterally in a suitable skin crease.

the fat pads are removed by incisions through the orbicularis oculi and septum orbitale. The skin is then redraped over the lid and slight tension made on the flap in an upward and lateral direction. The redundant skin is removed, care being taken to avoid too much tension in the lower lid which may lead to ectropion and epiphora.

Skin-muscle flap technique for lower lid blepharoplasty

This is the method of choice in the younger patient in whom the fat bags are present but with little or no wrinkling of the skin. The skin and muscle are freed from the underlying septum orbitale and the fat pads removed by clamping and fulguration of the pedicle, as in the standard blepharoplasty technique.

FACE LIFT (RHYTIDECTOMY)

The operation for removal of facial wrinkles has been performed for the past 70 years. In the last decade, however, it has achieved not only an enormous rise in popularity due to the fact that it represents a physical rejection of the ageing process but also the operation itself has lost much of its mystique.

Types of deformity

The skin owes its tensile property to its dermal collagen fibres which lie at right angles to the direction of the underlying muscle fibres and thus to the stretch force. While the formation of natural wrinkles of the skin is related to skin tension, some are due to anchorage of the underlying muscles of facial expression to the integument. Most of these latter creases are congenital and indicate the attachment of the skin to the tela subcutanea by connective tissue strands which extend from the epidermis through the dermis to the superficial aponeurosis.

As skin becomes older its capacity to stretch decreases, probably because the elastic fibre meshwork and collagen fibres are in a less active state of metabolism.

Age is the most constant factor in the production of wrinkles but familial and racial factors are also important. The process is accelerated in fair-skinned blondes and red-haired people. Dark-skinned people can be deceptive about their age and it is perhaps for this reason that fair-skinned people spend so many hours trying to darken their skins in the sun. While a sun tan undoubtedly makes one look better the effect of actinic rays on the skin is to overstretch the collagen fibres and accelerate the process of wrinkle formation.

The next commonest factor is weight reduction which in the older person leaves the skin lax and redundant. Hormonal factors such as hysterectomy and the menopause, and also cardiac and renal disease, have an effect on the ageing process.

Investigation

History

The patient is usually a woman but an increasing number of men are now requesting face lifts. The reason for seeking the operation is that the patient has noted the loss of skin elasticity herself and by pulling it back has given herself some idea of what the result of a face lift would be.

Examination

The first thing to establish is whether the patient needs a face lift, a blepharoplasty, or both. If she is primarily concerned about an ageing face then the best improvement may be achieved with a blepharoplasty. Conversely, if a face lift is performed without a blepharoplasty (if this was indicated) then the patient may not be satisfied with the final result.

It is also important to be able to tell the patient what can and what cannot be improved with the operation. The most dramatic effects are seen around the jaw line and the malar bones, especially if these are high. A face lift will not markedly improve deep nasolabial creases, excess skin and fat in the submental area, deep horizontal forehead creases or fine circumoral wrinkles.

Photography

The standard views are full face, right and left laterals, and a three-quarters view with the patient smiling.

Treatment

The face lift operation is now quite standardized and a description of its technique can be found in other texts. There is now general agreement that there is little place for anything other than a full face lift. Procedures such as a brow lift and the reduction of a double chin are best done as separate procedures after the full face lift (Fig. 19.15). If a blepharoplasty is required this can be performed at the same time but, if possible, it is better if the two procedures are done separately.

It is not possible to predict with any accuracy when a secondary face lift operation will be required. Older patients who have their first face lift in their fifties or sixties will require secondary surgery sooner than the patient in her forties. There is evidence to suggest that repeated facial operations involving repeated undermining and closure under tension results in a change in the dermal collagen.

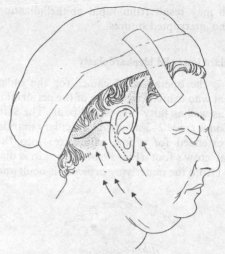

FIG. 19.15. Incision for face lift. The skin is undercut to the nasolabial crease and pulled upwards as shown, the excess being excised.

After the operation the face is swollen with some discoloration but this usually settles after 10–14 days.

CHEMABRASION

Fine wrinkles around the mouth and eyes unaccompanied by sagging of facial skin can be improved by chemabrasion. The basic agent for this is phenol which causes keratolysis and coagulation by disruption of the sulphur bridges of keratoprotein. Penetration and absorption is modified by the addition of soap. Croton oil is an additional irritant and speeds the destruction of the epidermal layer. The action of the mixture is prolonged by the application of a vapour barrier in the form of waterproof adhesive tape.

The solution should be freshly mixed for each patient in the following proportions:

Phenol 88%	3 ml
Croton oil	3 drops
Cetavlon soap	8 drops
Distilled water	2 ml

This is applied to the wrinkles by a cotton bud and small strips of adhesive tape are then applied and left for 48 hours.

Further Reading

ANDERSON J. R. (1976) Symposium: The supra-tip in rhinoplasty: a dilemma. III. Supra-tip soft-tissue rounding after rhinoplasty: causes, prevention and treatment. *Laryngoscope* **86**, 53.

BECKER O. J. (1952) Correction of the protruding deformed ear. *British Journal of Plastic Surgery*, **5**, 187.

BECKER O. J. (1956) General principles of corrective nasal plastic operation. *Transactions of the American Academy of Ophthalmology* **60**, 522.

BECKER O. J. (1968) *Principles of Otolaryngologic Plastic Surgery*. Chicago: Year Book Medical Publishers.

BROWN J. M. & McDOWELL F. (1965) *Plastic Surgery of the Nose*. Springfield, Illinois: Thomas.

CONLEY J. & DICKINSON J. T. (1972) *Plastic and Reconstructive Surgery of Face and Neck*, Vol. 1. Stuttgart: Georg Thieme Verlag.

CONVERSE J. M. (1950) Restoration of facial contour by bone grafts introduced through oral cavity. *Plastic and Reconstructive Surgery* **6**, 295.

CONVERSE J. M., NIGRO A., WILSON F. A. & JOHNSON N. E. (1955) Technique for surgical correction of lop ears. *Plastic and Reconstructive Surgery* **15**, 411.

CONVERSE J. M. & WOOD-SMITH D. (1963) Technical details in the surgical correction of the lop ear deformity. *Plastic and Reconstructive Surgery* **31**, 118.

CONVERSE J. M. & WOOD-SMITH D. (1964) Horizontal osteotomy of the mandible. *Plastic and Reconstructive Surgery* **34**, 464.

DENECKE H. J. & MEYER R. (1967) *Plastic Surgery of Head and Neck*, Vol. 1. Berlin: Springer Verlag.

FARRIOR R. T. (1971) Esthetic blepharoplasty. *Laryngoscope* **81**, 848.

FOMAN S. & BELL J. (1970) *Rhinoplasty: New Concepts*. Springfield, Illinois: Thomas.

GIBSON T. & DAVIS W. B. (1957) The distortion of autogenous cartilage grafts: its cause and prevention. *British Journal of Plastic Surgery* **10**, 257.

JANEKE J. B. & WRIGHT W. K. (1971) Studies on the support of the nasal tip. *Archives of Otolaryngology* **93**, 458.

LEWIS J. R. JR. (1973) *Atlas of Aesthetic Plastic Surgery*. Boston: Little, Brown.

MALINIAC J. W. (1938) Reconstruction of deformed chin in its relationship to rhinoplasty: dermal graft – procedure of choice. *American Journal of Surgery* **40**, 583.

MASTERS F. W. & LEWIS J. R. JR. (1973) *Symposium on Esthetic Surgery of Nose, Ears and Chin*. St Louis: Mosby.

McEVITT W. C. (1947) Problem of protruding ear. *Plastic and Reconstructive Surgery* **2**, 481.

MUSTARDE J. C. (1963) The correction of prominent ears using simple mattress sutures. *British Journal of Plastic Surgery* **16**, 170.

PAFF C. H. (1973) *Anatomy of Head and Neck*. Philadelphia: Saunders.

REECE T. D. & WOOD-SMITH D. (1973) *Cosmetic Face Surgery*. Philadelphia: Saunders.

REIDY J. P. (1960) Skin muscle flap. *British Journal of Plastic Surgery* **13**, 256.

RETHI A. (1934) Raccourcissement du nez trop long. *Revue de chirurgie plastique* **2**, 85.

RUBIN L. R., BROMBERG B. E., WALDEN R. H. & ADAMS A. (1962) An anatomic approach to the obtrusive ear. *Plastic and Reconstructive Surgery* **29**, 360.

RUTLEDGE L. J. (1963) Surgical anatomy of the nose. *Eye, Ear, Nose and Throat Monthly* **42**, 28.

SERCER A. (1958) Dekortikacija nosa. *Chirurgia maxillofacialis et plastica* **1**, 3, 149.

WRIGHT M. R. & WRIGHT W. K. (1975) A psychological study of patients undergoing cosmetic surgery. *Archives of Otolaryngology* **101**, 145.

CHAPTER 20

Facial Trauma

FACIAL FRACTURES

The commonest cause of bodily injury in the civilized world is a vehicular accident and 80% of these injuries are sustained in the head and neck regions.

General principles of management

Facial skeletal injuries may be divided into two main groups, each requiring a different approach and expertise with regard to management. Superiorly, the injury may involve both the orbital cavities and the cranium; inferiorly, the tooth-bearing structures may be disrupted. These maxillofacial fractures require a team approach whose composition varies according to the site of the injury. Obviously, it is also very important to rule out any serious injuries below the neck.

After the airway has been cleared and safeguarded and once bleeding has been brought under control, and blood volume is being maintained, a thorough assessment of the injuries must be made. This should include soft tissue injuries, any obvious fractures, and any missing teeth. It is prudent to suspect a neck injury in any trauma to the head. Therefore, in the conscious patient, the neck should be examined, particularly for undue pain or tenderness. Greater care should be exercised in a comatose patient. It might be most important to obtain a radiograph of the neck before moving the patient, to exclude a cervical skeletal injury. After the neck is considered to be safe, further assessment of skeletal injuries is then made by radiography.

The standard views that are usually requested in such cases include the following projections: Waters, Caldwell, basal and lateral. For certain fractures and in specific instances, additional views are requested and these will be mentioned under the appropriate headings.

In mid-third facial fractures, if bleeding is profuse and difficult to control, consideration may have to be given to emergency reduction of the fragments because torn vessels may be kept open by the distracted bony fragments.

Cerebrospinal rhinorrhoea should not be a cause for immediate alarm, although the diagnosis needs to be made as soon as possible. When mixed with blood, the simplest test for the presence of CSF is to let some of the fluid drop onto a dry, dark cloth. The halo sign is an indication of an admixture of cerebrospinal fluid. Most traumatic cerebrospinal fluid leaks will stop spontaneously after reduction of the fractures.

Fractures of the zygoma

Fractures of the zygoma may be divided into two groups: (1) fracture of the body of the zygoma (or fracture of the malar) and (2) fracture of the zygomatic arch.

Fractures of the zygomatic body

Pathology

These fractures may be sustained in a car accident, from fist fights, and occasionally in contact sports. Classically, and most commonly, this fracture involves the zygomatic arch, the fronto-zygomatic suture line and the infraorbital rim; hence, this is often erroneously referred to as the 'tripod' fracture. The actual fracture line is much more extensive and must be appreciated in order to obtain proper reduction.

From the frontozygomatic suture line the fracture extends along the inner aspect of the lateral wall of the orbit to the inferior oblique fissure. From here, the fracture advances forward and medially towards the infraorbital canal of the maxillary bone. The fracture may either enter the infraorbital foramen or skirt it, usually laterally. From the rim the fracture descends along the face of the maxilla toward the maxillary buttress – the lower portion of the zygomatic process of the maxillary bone. Consequently, a sharp ridge may be palpable within the buccal sulcus. The fracture then ascends superiorly along the posterior portion of this process to traverse the infratemporal fossa until it joins the fracture along the frontozygomatic suture line. There is also a fracture across the zygomatic arch. Thus, this fracture involves not only the body of the zygoma but also a portion of the maxillary bone and, therefore, includes the maxillary sinus as well. Moreover, the fracture along the arch may involve the temporal process of the zygoma, thus technically involving three bones.

Occasionally there may be more than one fracture involving the body of the zygoma and, more rarely, the upper extent of the fracture may be below the frontozygomatic suture line. On rare occasions, the malar eminence may be comminuted.

Clinical features

The usual displacement of a fractured body of zygoma is medially, inferiorly and posteriorly (Fig. 20.1). Thus, there is a step-off, or an angulation, at the infraorbital rim; separation, or some displacement, at the frontozygomatic suture line; disruption of the convexity of the arch of zygoma; and a step-off in the maxillary buccal sulcus at the buttress of the maxilla. Since the fracture traverses the floor of the orbit (Fig. 20.2), there may be ocular symptoms and signs, such as diplopia, conjunctival ecchymosis, lowering of the lateral canthus, entropion with a lowered level of the pupil, and there may be disruption in the vertical movement of the globe. Since the infraorbital canal is often involved

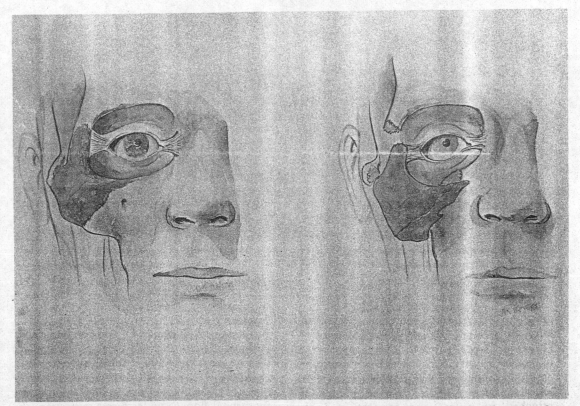

FIG. 20.1. Typical displacement of fractured body of zygoma – downward, medially and backward. Hence, depression of malar eminence and lowered lateral canthus.

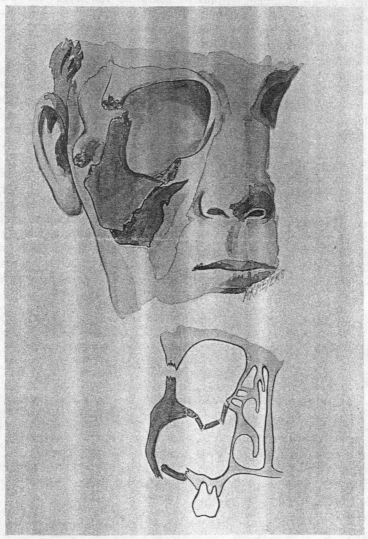

FIG. 20.2. In a fracture-dislocation of the zygomatic body there is concomitant fracture of the orbital floor and of the zygomatic process of the maxilla.

there may be hypoaesthesia or anaesthesia of the infraorbital nerve. There is no malocclusion. However, there is often trismus because of impingement of the displaced bone against the coronoid process of the mandible, because the anterior fibres of the masseter muscle are attached to a fractured segment, and also because of haematoma and oedema along the infratemporal portion of the zygoma (Fig. 20.3).

Treatment

The treatment of choice, in most instances, is to perform interosseous wiring along the infraorbital rim and the frontozygomatic suture and to explore the orbit in cases of preoperative evidence of entrapment of periorbital tissues. While the orbital floor is under direct inspection, the antrum should be packed with iodoform gauze which is left for 2 weeks.

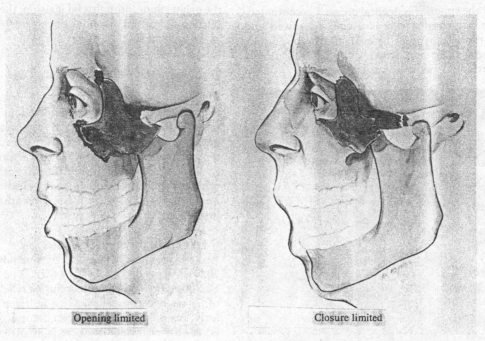

Opening limited

Closure limited

FIG. 20.3. Common type of trismus resulting from fracture of zygomatic body (left). Occasional impaction of fragment of zygomatic arch behind open coronoid process, shown on right.

Fracture of the zygomatic arch

Clinical features

This fracture invariably results from contact sports or from fist fights. The usual presenting sign is that of depression of the arch, and trismus. The latter may be due to actual impingement of the fragments, in addition to the factors enumerated above. Very rarely, the mandible may be caught in the open position, a fragment impinging behind the coronoid process. As a result the patient has difficulty in closing his teeth (Fig. 20.3). The radiographic projection that best demonstrates this fracture is the underexposed basal view (Fig. 20.4).

Treatment

Although numerous techniques have been described for reduction of this fracture, perhaps the most acceptable technique with the most predictable results is that described by Gillies. This consists of approaching the arch through a temporal fossa incision. Occasionally, if the fragments are unstable after reduction, the elevation plane may

need to be temporarily packed to maintain proper contour of the arch.

Fractures of the maxilla

Blow-out fracture of the orbit

Pathology

By definition this implies an isolated fracture of the maxillary component of the orbital floor, with an intact orbital rim. It is usually induced by sudden, blunt trauma which is not very severe. The orbital contents are forced into a cavity of decreased capacity and the weakest of its walls gives way into the sinus cavity.

Clinical features

Invariably there is immediate diplopia and this may be accompanied by epistaxis due to tearing of the mucoperiosteum of the maxillary sinus (Fig. 20.5). The patient usually presents with periorbital and conjunctival ecchymosis and, occasionally, there may be subcutaneous emphysema. There is apparent ptosis of the upper lid and the superior palpebral crease is accentuated. The palpebral fissure is usually narrowed and enophthalmos may be evident. The pupil may appear to be at a lower level. There is usually interference with upward gaze and, to a lesser

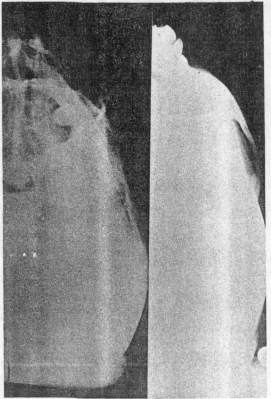

FIG. 20.4. Composite radiographic base views of skull. Left, routine normal exposure; right, underexposed view to show arch.

extent, with downward gaze as well. The infraorbital rim is always intact. Often there is accompanying hypoaesthesia or anaesthesia of the infraorbital nerve. In addition to radiographic evidence, the diagnosis is usually confirmed by a positive forced duction test performed on the inferior rectus muscle (Fig. 20.6).

Treatment
When indicated, the fracture may be reduced through a Caldwell–Luc antrostomy and the fragments held in place with iodoform gauze packing, or with a Foley catheter, for 2 weeks (Fig. 20.7). The alternate method is to approach the orbital floor through a lid incision; the gap in the floor is bridged by a bone or cartilage graft or by an implant (Fig. 20.8).

Transverse fractures of the maxilla

Pathology and clinical features
Fractures of the maxilla may involve the alveolar process, the frontal process (in fractures of the nose), or the tuberosity. However, the common type of injury in a car accident is a transverse fracture of the maxilla. This is commonly referred to as the *Le Fort fracture,* which may or may not be symmetric. Such fractures are divided into three categories:

> Le Fort I, floating palate;
> Le Fort II, pyramidal fracture; and
> Le Fort III, craniofacial dysjunction (Fig. 20.9).

Each fracture involves the occlusive relationship of the teeth, because the maxilla is driven posteriorly, causing an open bite deformity (Fig. 20.10). In each fracture there is involvement of the nasal septum.

In the lower and midfacial horizontal fractures, the fracture lines pass through the maxillary antra and in the Le Fort II fracture the orbital floor is often involved. In the high fracture, the most proximal line of fracture passes through the lateral and medial orbital walls, through the base of the nose, and through the zygomatic arches. It should be understood that a Le Fort II fracture often has elements in it of the Le Fort I, and the Le Fort III is often accompanied by fractures in the lower strata of the maxilla as well. The higher the level of the uppermost fracture line, the more force was required to induce the trauma and, consequently, the more serious the overall condition of the patient.

Treatment
The specific initial management of these injuries is to place the patient in intermaxillary traction by means of arch bars and elastic bands. Usually, reduction of the malocclusion will be effected within 24–48 hours. If this has not taken place, disimpaction of the maxillary segment may be very difficult. Sometimes this may be accomplished only through open reduction by exposure of the fracture lines.

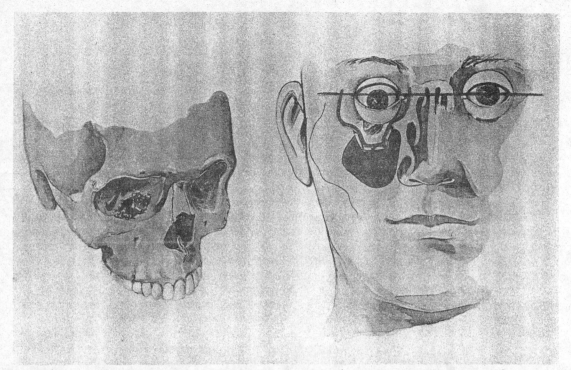

FIG. 20.5. Blow-out fracture right orbit. Note trap-door nature of fragments, displacement of periorbital tissue into antrum and lowered level of pupil.

The Le Fort I fracture usually only requires intermaxillary fixation and suspension from the zygomatic arches (Fig. 20.11). If a buccal sulcus laceration be present over the fracture site it may be prudent to insert interosseous wire ligatures at the pyriform aperture.

Le Fort II and III fractures may require

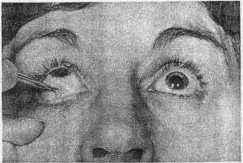

FIG. 20.6. Forced duction test being performed on inferior rectus muscle.

antrostomies and packing of the antra in addition to wiring at the infra-orbital margins. The Le Fort III also requires ligation at the fronto-zygomatic suture lines. Suspension of the Le Fort I and II fractures is to be established from the zygomatic arches and Le Fort III from the zygomatic processes of the frontal bones.

In all of the Le Fort fractures the nasal septum requires reduction and splinting. Since there is often a concomitant fracture of the nasal pyramid in Le Fort II and III injuries, this should be reduced at the same time.

Where a Le Fort fracture is accompanied by a fracture of the mandible, the mandibular fracture should be reduced first in order to obtain a base onto which to articulate the maxillary dental arch.

In some of these fractures there may be comminution of the infraorbital rim and of the orbital floor. In such circumstances the fragments should be wired and stabilized by antral packing and the orbital floor should be grafted with thin

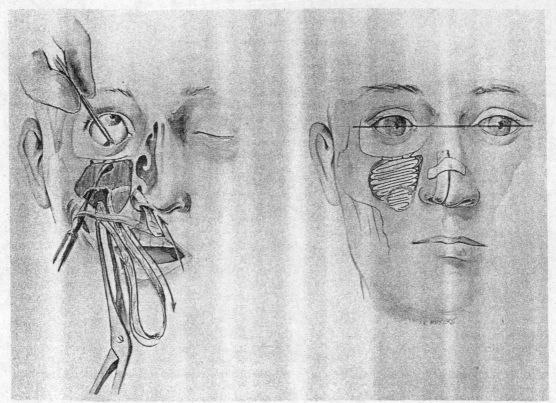

FIG. 20.7. Reduction of blow-out fracture via Caldwell–Luc antrostomy. Packing brought out through antromeatal fenestra. Forced duction test repeated at conclusion of procedure.

bone obtained either from the nasal septum or from a bone bank.

Fractures of the mandible

Fractures of the mandible are the most easily diagnosed of all the facial fractures since they always lead to some degree of dysfunction. Because multiple fractures of the mandible are common, it is important to look for a second or a third fracture, particularly on the opposite side. Correct diagnosis requires correct radiographic projections and it is helpful if the standard lateral oblique views are supplemented by a panoramic radiograph of the entire mandible (Fig. 20.12).

Clinical features
The diagnosis of a mandibular fracture is made on the basis of a history of external trauma, although pathologic fractures also occur. Invariably, there is malocclusion of the teeth and the normal functions of speech, chewing, and swallowing are disturbed. There may be obvious external disfigurement as well as ecchymosis and/or laceration of the overlying mucosa. Crepitation may also be noted, especially in multiple fractures.

Treatment
Since fractures of the body of the mandible are compound, early reduction lowers the risk of infection. Furthermore, early definitive treatment greatly facilitates reduction by the closed method. If a tooth with a devitalized pulp is in the line of fracture, it is best to extract it to prevent infection. In the presence of infection, intermaxillary fixation will aid in the control of the disease by preventing further devitalization of tissues that may be caused by mobility of the fragments.

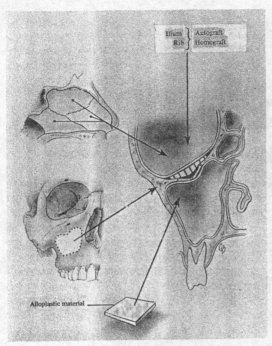

FIG. 20.8. Sources of graft or implant material.

Closed reduction. All mandibular fractures with a sufficient complement of suitable teeth should be given a trial of closed reduction, even if open reduction is contemplated. The method of choice is the application of arch bars to both upper and lower teeth and reduction of the malocclusion is attempted with intermaxillary elastic bands. If distraction is present at a fracture site, the arch bars may be applied in corresponding segments. Reduction of the malocclusion with elastic traction is usually achieved in 48 hours. The rubber bands may be left on for the period of immobilization, or they may be replaced by steel wire ligatures. If the fragments are impacted they may have to be reduced by manipulation before the application of the arch bars.

Open reduction. Open reduction of mandibular fractures may be indicated in the presence of (1) multiple fractures that cannot be reduced by intermaxillary traction alone; (2) unstable fragments; (3) fractures of the body with unfavourable obliquities (Fig. 20.13); (4) some fractures of the edentulous mandible; (5) telescoped, bilateral

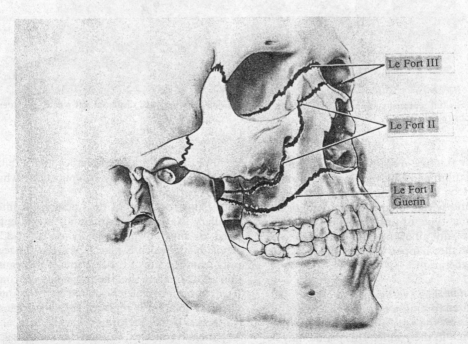

FIG. 20.9. Classification of transverse fractures of the maxilla. Le Fort I and Guerin are synonymous.

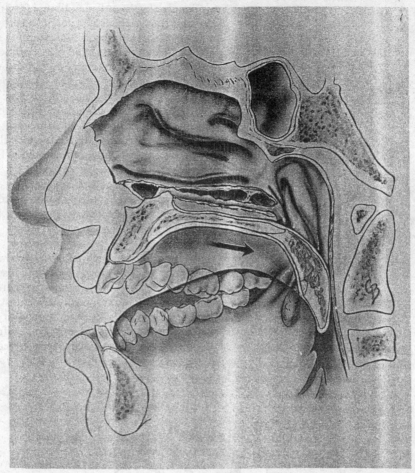

FIG. 20.10. Sagittal representation of Le Fort fracture. Note open-bite deformity and displaced soft palate, the latter tending to obstruct the airway.

subcondylar fracture-dislocations; (6) failure of closed reduction; and (7) overlying lacerations.

It cannot be stressed too strongly that open reduction and wiring of the jaws automatically require some type of intermaxillary fixation. Furthermore, not all of the fragments need to be wired, unless they happen to be readily accessible through a laceration.

Immobilization. The average period of immobilization required for union is from 4 to 6 weeks but this depends on the age of the patient, less time being required in the young. This period may be modified by other factors, such as the site and extent of the fracture, the accuracy and stability of the reduction, and any complications which may have arisen.

In testing for union of the fracture, the intermaxillary fixation is released and the patient is asked to bite down gradually on a wooden tongue blade which is placed between the teeth away from the site of the fracture. If this causes pain at the fracture site, the fragments are considered to be incompletely united and the intermaxillary fixation is replaced for an additional 1–2 weeks. If the fracture appears to be healed, the patient is restricted to a soft diet for a week or two and is instructed to exercise the mandible in

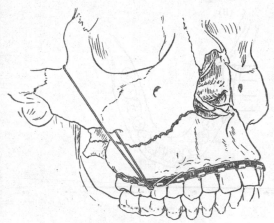

FIG. 20.11. Le Fort I fracture, showing suspension (ligature) from zygomatic arch to dental arch bar.

order to loosen the muscles and ligaments involved. The chewing of gum on both sides of the mouth should be encouraged for a time.

Fracture of the edentulous mandible

Although relatively infrequent, fractures of the edentulous mandible present special problems in management. Apart from the special technical considerations involved, these fractures occur in the older age group and the accompanying decrease of blood supply and atrophy of the bone may lead to delay in healing and to non-union of the fragments.

The patient's artificial dentures are invaluable in the management of fractures of the mandible. If the dentures are broken during the injury, they should be repaired because they will be of great assistance in the treatment even if some pieces of the denture are missing. An old discarded denture may be just as useful.

Without a denture it is rather difficult to determine the correct anatomic relationship between the maxilla and the fractured mandible. However, it is more important to restore symmetry of the mandibular outline than to correct minor discrepancies of the bite, since the latter may always be remedied later by altering the denture or by making a new one. When no denture is available, an intra-oral splint should be made by

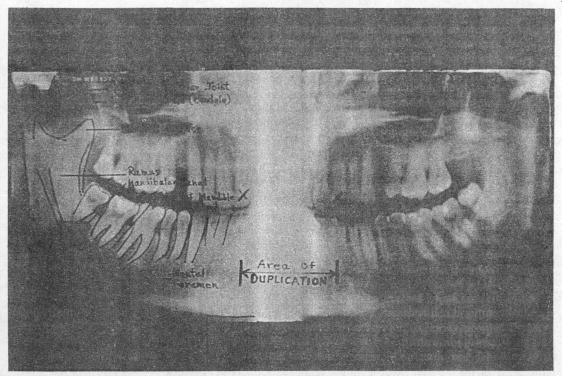

FIG. 20.12. Panoramic radiograph of mandible.

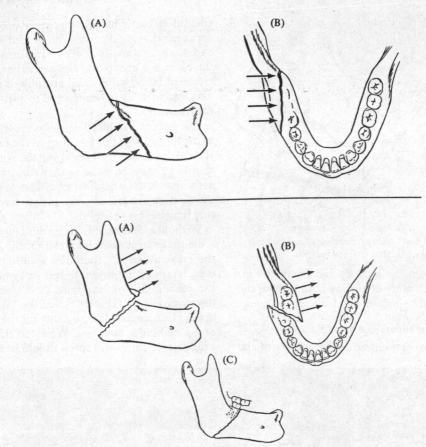

FIG. 20.13. Fracture obliquities of mandible. *Upper* shows favourable obliquities (minimal or no displacement); *lower* shows unfavourable obliquities (displacement due to distraction). C shows an unfavourable obliquity, negated by presence of an articulating tooth in the proximal fragment. Arrows show direction of muscle pull.

a competent and experienced prosthodontist. Fractures of the body behind the denture-bearing area, and of the mandibular angle, may require open reduction and wiring in addition to intra-oral splinting.

Fractures of the neck of the mandible

In children below puberty, open reduction and wiring should not be contemplated. There is a very important growth centre in the condyle and surgical intervention may lead to its atrophy with underdevelopment of that side of the mandible. If the condyle is not disturbed it usually becomes remodeled in the glenoid fossa within 3 years.

Therefore, it is necessary only to immobilize the fracture by intermaxillary fixation for approximately 10 to 14 days, depending on the age of the child.

Bilateral fracture-dislocations of the condylar processes of the mandible in adults, with telescoping or overriding of the fragments, must be corrected by open reduction to maintain the vertical height of the mandible. This is especially true in edentulous patients. If such fractures are not treated the mandibular rami telescopes superiorly and anteriorly and the mandible comes to rest against the maxillary tuberosities. If the patient's general condition does not permit a bilateral open reduction it may be satisfactory to wire one side only, provided that the principles of intermaxillary fixation are maintained.

Fractures in children

Usually fractures of the facial bones in children are not badly misplaced. Fractures of the mandible are most often of the greenstick variety. Vigorous treatment is neither indicated nor necessary and should be avoided since it may interfere with growth centres. Generally, the approach should be conservative.

However, when the fractures are severe, with marked displacement, they should be treated as in adults. When orthodontic appliances are in place they may be readily used for reduction and intermaxillary fixation. Because deciduous teeth are peg-shaped and will not hold arch bars or eyelet ligatures securely, immobilization by a cap splint is more desirable. Such a splint is cemented to the teeth or is circumferentially wired to the mandible, depending on the degree of injury. However, this procedure requires the services of a competent prosthodontist who is experienced in this type of management. It is also advisable to have the child's orthodontist involved in the management of such fractures.

Nasofrontal injuries

Septal haematoma and abscess

Pathology
A septal haematoma may arise after trauma to the nose, but in rare cases also spontaneously. A collection of blood occurs between the septal cartilage and the mucoperichondrium, usually on both sides of the nose. Since the septal cartilage does not possess a blood supply and is entirely dependent on the perichondrium for its metabolism, it may undergo necrosis after 1 or 2 days if adequate treatment is not instituted. Furthermore, a septal haematoma almost always precedes a septal abscess. A septal haematoma should, therefore, be regarded as a surgical emergency because, if it is neglected, falling in of the cartilaginous pyramid nearly always results.

Treatment
A septal haematoma or abscess should be widely incised and evacuated immediately, after which the incision must be held open with a small rubber drain and the nose must be packed to hold the mucosa against the cartilage. It should be inspected daily until resolution. At the same time as the incision is made the cartilage should be inspected; if this appears already to have been destroyed then a graft of cartilage or bone should be implanted to prevent further collapse due to scar tissue contracture. The patient should be treated for at least a week with broad spectrum antibiotics.

Nasal fractures

Pathology
The commonest facial fracture is that of the nasal skeleton. Although the usual nasal fracture may appear 'simple' on external examination, such a fracture is always compound on the inner surface, its lining being a mucoperiosteum. In fact, it is most likely that any external trauma to the nose that induces an epistaxis has resulted in some break in its bony–cartilaginous structure, even if this is not detectable clinically.

Fractures of the nasal pyramid may be unilateral, bilateral or complex. The unilateral fracture may be a simple crack with little or no displacement (Fig. 20.14). The bilateral fractures are by far the commonest. They usually cause deviation of the entire nose (Fig. 20.15). Lateral blows may distort the nose into either a so-called 'C' or an 'S' deformity of the dorsal line. Frontal blows may cause comminution of the nasal framework and septum, producing a flattened configuration to the nose.

Complex fractures commonly result from powerful frontal blows which drive the nasal pyramid into the ethmoid labyrinth and forces of such severity are occasionally capable of fracturing the frontal bone as well. Resulting from forces of high magnitude, these fractures are often comminuted. Not only is the nasal pyramid shattered, but the stout nasal process of the frontal bone is broken as well. Thus, a disruption of the entire nasofrontoethmoidal complex may occur, with a marked depression of the nasion and frequent telecanthus (Fig. 20.16).

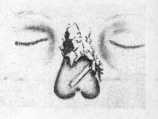

(a)

(a)

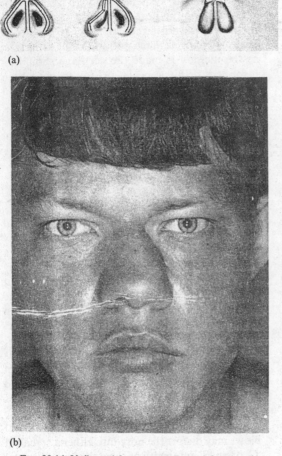

(b)

FIG. 20.14. Unilateral fracture. (a) Bony deformity. (b) external appearance.

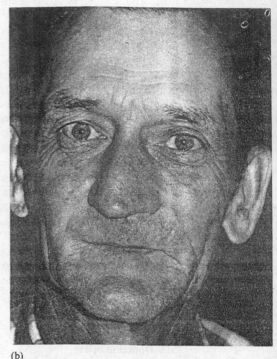

(b)

FIG. 20.15. Bilateral fracture from lateral blow. (a) Bony deformity. (b) External appearance.

The most serious nasal injury is the compound comminuted fracture with tissue loss. It is important to remember that a large laceration may create the illusion of missing tissue and that the avulsion of a portion of the nasal skin and/or underlying framework requires a major reconstruction.

Clinical features

A history of trauma to the midface accompanied by epistaxis, a noticeable deformity and nasal airway obstruction are the usual complaints. Although post-traumatic mucosal oedema may well result in nasal obstruction, this symptom suggests skeletal displacement, or a septal haematoma. Nasofrontoethmoidal complex fractures may produce symptoms of diplopia and epiphora.

The amount of swelling, ecchymosis and deformity seen on examination is usually directly proportional to the magnitude of the trauma. The fractured nose is commonly exquisitely tender. The absence of bony crepitus on palpation does not rule out a fracture, since the fragments may be impacted and because of swelling. The nasal swelling is commonly accompanied by

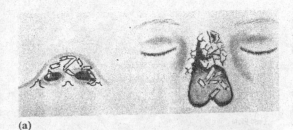

(a)

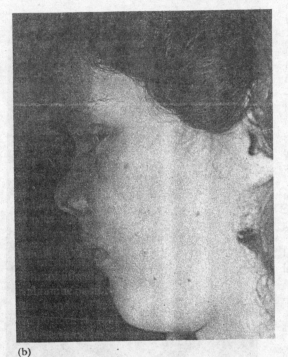

(b)

Fig. 20.16 Collapsed nasal dorsum from frontal blow.
(a) Bony deformity. (b) External appearance.

giving the nose a flattened, pushed-in appearance (Fig. 20.16).

The nasofrontoethmoidal complex fracture is characterized by marked deepening of the nasion, severe swelling, and telecanthus. There may be apparent telecanthus, an illusion created by the absence of the normal ridge lent by the dorsum of the nose between the eyes. Normally the eyes should be separated from one another by approximately the length of one eye (30–35 mm). In traumatic telecanthus, the medial canthal ligaments are displaced laterally, giving the appearance that the eyes are likewise displaced. If the fracture continues through the cribriform plate or fovea ethmoidalis, a CSF rhinorrhoea may complicate the fracture.

Nasal fracture accompanied by avulsion of tissue is fortunately rare. The nasal skeleton and overlying soft tissue may be ripped from the face but is usually pedicled and infrequently torn away completely. Vigorous epistaxis commonly accompanies these injuries.

The availability of a detailed pretraumatic photograph of the patient may be helpful in making an accurate assessment of the injury. Radiographic examination in these injuries is of limited diagnostic value as vascular markings and sites of previous fractures may confuse the physician. Radiographs, however, may be important medicolegally.

Treatment

Reduction and fixation should be done as soon after the injury as possible, because of the tendency of these fragments to become stabilized rapidly. Closed reduction may be readily performed under local anaesthesia.

The most effective instruments for reducing these fractures are the Asch forceps, the paired Walsham forceps, and a broad, flat, stout elevator such as the Ballenger's. With one of these instruments in the nose and the other hand palpating the bony pyramid, the fractured bones are manipulated into place. Two goals must be kept in mind as reduction proceeds. The septum must be straightened, thereby opening the airway, and the bony pyramid must be restored to its pretraumatic configuration. Both goals may be thwarted because of pre-existing deformity. For example, the fractured septum may be impossible to

periorbital swelling and ecchymosis, as well as occasional subscleral haemorrhage.

The direction of the traumatic force often determines the direction of the deformity. A lateral blow can create a unilateral fracture of the nasal pyramid producing a depression on the lateral side of the nose. A more forceful injury may cause a collapse and shortening of the side opposite the blow and elongation of the side on which the blow is received. This will produce a deviation of the dorsum of the nose to the shortened side. A frontal blow that crushes the nasal skeleton will cause collapse of the nasal pyramid reduce due to a previous fracture. An extremely conservative trimming of the septum may be done through a small mucoperichondrial tunnel so that the septum may be returned to a midline position. In no circumstances is a radical septoplasty or a rhinoplasty recommended in the early treatment of the trauma patient.

Maintenance of position is accomplished by the use of intranasal packing and the application of an external splint. Internal septal splints may be fashioned from Silastic-sheets. Half-inch ribbon gauze packing, impregnated with iodoform powder, is antiseptic and imparts a pleasant medicinal aroma. It can maintain the septum in the midline, provide tamponade against haemorrhage, and may approximate any mucosal lacerations. Enough packing should be inserted into each nasal cavity to prevent portions of the fractured nasal pyramid from collapsing into the nasal cavity. However, overpacking can produce widening of the pyramid, especially of comminuted fractures. Moulding of the nose with the fingers and repeated visual checks of the profile and frontal appearance must be done as packing proceeds.

When reduction of severe collapse of the nasal framework cannot be maintained by intranasal packing, support of the fragments can be accomplished by the use of hammock wires. Two parallel wires are passed through the bony nasal base, then are twisted to one another over lead plates (Fig. 20.17).

The pack is usually removed at 3–5 days. The position of the nose must be checked frequently and, if it tends to wander from the desired position, it should be replaced by firm digital pressure. If the deviation of the nose persists after a week or 10 days, the patient should apply firm digital counter pressure frequently to the bony pyramid to correct the deflection.

Most lacerations of the mucosa require no suturing. Synechiae or webs may be avoided by the insertion of a Silastic sheet on each side of the septum. In injuries compounded through the skin, a layered closure resulting in everted wound edges should be done.

Complications. Airway obstruction may result from septal deflection, a combination of septal and skeletal deformity, or scar tissue. A purely

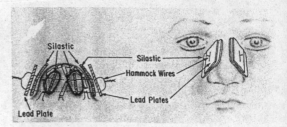

(a)

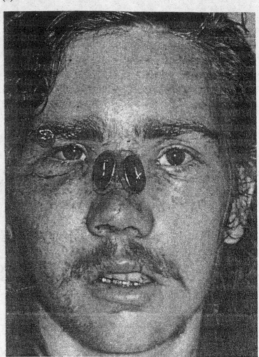

(b)

FIG. 20.17. Hammock wires are placed to support a collapsed nasal dorsum. (a) Two wires are passed through the skin of the lateral aspect of the nose near the nasofacial angle. They are passed through the bony fragments of one side, through the septum, the fragments of the opposite side and the nasal skin of that side. (b) The wires on each side are passed through a pad that may be cut from a sheet of Teflon felt or foam rubber and then through a lead plate and are twisted together.

septal deformity may be corrected early. Synechiae should be lysed when diagnosed, and the raw surfaces kept apart by a sheet of Silastic. A web may be removed by either incision and Silastic sheet interposition or by the use of Z-plasties.

Occasionally, a septal perforation or epiphora

may complicate more severe injuries. Septal perforations may present with periodic crusting and epistaxis, or the patient may complain of whistling sounds as he breathes.

External nasal deformities may require correction by means of rhinoplastic techniques, either to reposition the fragments in their proper positions or by building up depressions with grafting materials.

Presistent epiphora is a troublesome complication of nasofrontoethmoidal fractures and may require a dacryocystorhinostomy for relief.

Frontal bone fractures

Pathology
Severe trauma to the midface is occasionally accompanied by fracture of the frontal bone. The pyramidal-shaped frontal sinus is the pneumatized central portion of this bone. Fractures may involve the thick anterior wall, the relatively thin posterior wall, the nasofrontal duct, or any combination of the three. The fractures may be undisplaced or depressed, and simple or compound. Severe penetrating wounds may pass through both walls of the sinus, pierce the underlying dura, and macerate the frontal lobes of the brain.

Clinical features
The patient, often a victim of a motor vehicle accident, has usually sustained sufficiently severe trauma to render him unconscious. Once awake, pain, tenderness, and swelling are common presenting features. A depressed anterior wall fracture, if seen early, will appear as a visible indentation. As swelling increases, the defect becomes less apparent and, in the presence of substantial haematoma, may be very difficult to palpate (Fig. 20.18). Occasionally the diagnosis of a depressed fracture may be made erroneously if the edges of a subgaleal haematoma are palpated.

Epistaxis often results from tears in the mucosal lining of the frontal sinus. If the posterior wall is fractured and the dura lacerated a CSF rhinorrhoea is often present.

Through-and-through injuries have a fatal outcome at the scene of the accident in 70–80% of cases. The survivors present with an obvious

dehiscence in the central forehead from which blood, CSF and brain may ooze.

Radiographic examination includes the Caldwell, Waters, submentovertical, and lateral views. Fractures in the walls, and air-fluid levels in the sinus are usually seen in these projections. The hyperextended base view is often very useful in detecting fractures of the posterior wall but the most helpful radiograph is obtained by lateral tomography. Both anterior and posterior wall fractures may be clearly seen, and the

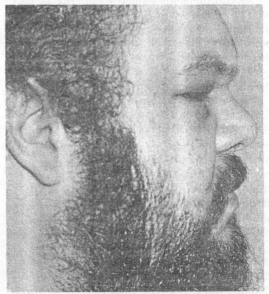

(a)

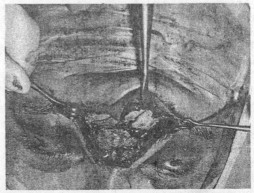

(b)

Fig. 20.18. (a) Anterior wall frontal sinus fracture with no apparent external deformity. (b) Same patient showing the comminuted depressed fracture.

degree of displacement usually can be accurately ascertained.

Treatment

Linear, undisplaced, anterior wall fractures probably require no surgical repair. Depressed fractures should be elevated in order to correct any cosmetic deformity but, more especially, to preclude the formation of a mucocoele that may ensue from the entrapment of mucosa. The approach can be made through either an overlying laceration or the standard 'butterfly' or coronal incisions. All mucosa within 6 or 8 mm of the fracture line should be excised and the bare bony margins cleaned with a cutting bur. Once the normal forehead contour has been restored by elevation of the fragments, holes are drilled in the bone and the fragments are secured with wire.

Some controversy exists over the management of the undisplaced posterior wall fracture. Sufficient reports in the literature and our own experience indicate that this fracture not only allows bacterial contamination of the intracranial cavity from the nasal cavities but may also set the stage for the future formation of a mucocoele. Because of this risk most posterior wall fractures should be treated by ablation with fat through an osteoplastic flap approach, or by frontal sinusectomy if the circumstances warrant it. Reconstruction of the contour will have to be considered at a later date. However, it is important that all dural rents be closed either by direct suture or by grafting with fascia.

Any damage to the frontonasal duct requires frontal sinus obliteration. The predisposition of this duct to closure by scarring, after even a relatively minor injury, makes eventual mucocoele development almost inevitable. Evidence of a fluid level that will not clear after 10–14 days following the injury, must force the decision to ablate the sinus.

Through-and-through injuries should be treated conjointly with the neurosurgeon. Any devitalized brain should be debrided and cerebral haemorrhage must be stopped. Dural tears are repaired by fascia lata patching or direct suturing. The posterior wall of the sinus is completely removed and all mucosa of the remaining sinus walls is excised with a bur. The frontonasal ducts are plugged with temporalis muscle, and

the anterior frontal sinus wall fragments that had been removed at the beginning of surgery, burred free of their mucosa and soaked in Betadine (povidone-iodine), are now wired into place. During the next 12–36 hours, the frontal lobes should fill in the defect and ablate the sinus (Fig. 20.19).

Complications

The early complications of these fractures are related to trauma to the cranial contents and the accessibility of bacteria secondary to lacerations of the dura. Frontonasal duct injuries create a closed cavity in the sinus. In the presence of chronic sinus disease, the contained fluid may become infected. Fractures of the sinus floor may entrap orbital contents causing limitation of gaze.

Undiagnosed depressed fractures of the anterior wall may not show an obvious deformity until the overlying haematoma resolves. The defect is very disfiguring and usually requires correction by means of an onlay graft.

The most serious late complication is the formation of a mucocoele, which may take many years. This strange entity, whose precise mechanism of formation has thus far eluded investigators, seems often to have its genesis in entrapped frontal sinus mucosa. Fractures involving the nasofrontal duct or the anterior or posterior tables, especially if there is displacement, have a high frequency of mucocoele development. The bone erosive qualities of the mucocoele with the potential for pyocoele development put the patient in continuous danger of meningitis, encephalitis or brain abscess, in addition to the accompanying external deformity and displacement of the orbital contents.

SOFT TISSUE INJURIES

Trauma to the face produces injuries of varying severity and complexity whose ultimate functional and cosmetic outcome depends on the skilful repair of the soft tissues. Wide, raised, or depressed scars are obvious on the face, whereas fine, flat scars are less conspicuous and are camouflaged by cosmetics.

The principles involved in the management of

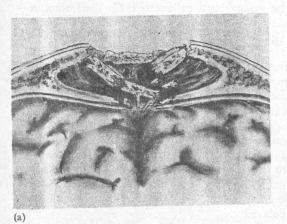

(a)

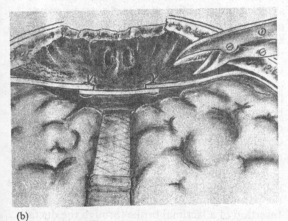

(b)

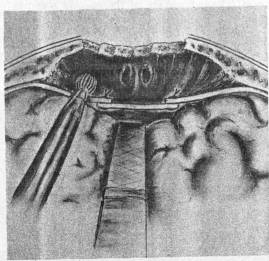

(c)

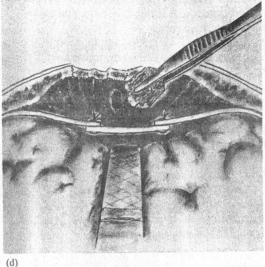

(d)

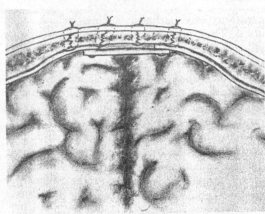

(e)

FIG. 20.19. (a) 'Through and through' fracture of the frontal sinus into the anterior cranial fossa. (b) Posterior frontal sinus wall is removed following debridement of devitalized brain and placement of dural graft to stop CSF leak. (c) Remaining frontal sinus cavity is burred free of mucosa. (d) Temporalis muscle plugs seal the frontonasal ducts. (e) Previously removed anterior wall fragments have been meticulously cleansed, divested of mucosa and soaked in povidone-iodine. They are now wired into place. The brain comes forward and obliterates the space.

facial wounds that should lead to minimal scarring are a knowledge of the anatomy of the area, performing a thorough examination of the wound and making a precise assessment of the injury, meticulous cleansing with conservative debridement, detailed approximation of the lacerated tissues in a layered fashion, and attentive postoperative care.

The direction of a laceration in relation to the facial crease lines invariably determines the prognosis of the subsequent scar. For many years Langer's lines [1] were thought to be the most favourable direction in which to make a surgical incision. In 1951 Kraissl [2] pointed out that in the face the most favourable scars are those that fall in the natural crease or wrinkle lines. When facial muscles contract they produce a series of parallel wrinkles that run across the long axis of the muscles and render expression to the face. These crease lines do not all coincide with Langer's lines and in some areas, as in the upper lip, run at right angles to them.

Pathology

Lacerations may be linear, slicing, stellate, or avulsed. They may be clean or contaminated, fresh or old. They may or may not involve injury to underlying viscera or skeletal elements.

Linear lacerations are usually made by a sharp object like a knife or broken glass. There is minimal contusion wide of the cut edge and the wound is usually relatively clean.

A slicing laceration may be linear as viewed in its course along the skin surface but, when closely inspected from its superficial epithelial surface to its deep dermal aspect, it is seen to be obliquely angled. The epidermis on the sliced side of the cut is thin, like a split thickness skin graft, and will tend to form a wide scar on healing.

Stellate wounds are usually the result of blunt trauma. These wounds have an exploded appearance with ragged and irregular margins. There is usually much contusion at the edges.

Avulsion lacerations involve injuries in which portions of skin, and even deeper layers, have been ripped out or blown away. These severe injuries may result from animal bites, motor vehicle accidents or gunshot wounds. It is important to remember, however, that in many extensive lacerations the gaping of the wound may give the illusion of tissue loss. This is especially true in those lacerations which lift up a flap of tissue.

The degree of contamination and the age of the wound must be assessed. *Contamination* in the sense that we use here implies gross soilage with substances such as gravel and soil. The depth of the wound must be explored for foreign material. Pieces of glass, gravel and organic material may be found and must be removed meticulously to prevent wound infection, or extrusion, with subsequent disfigurement. The *age of the wound* is important from the standpoint of bacterial invasion and timing of the surgical repair. Because of the rich blood supply to the face, most lacerations may be closed primarily up to 4 days following the injury. However, if it becomes infected, closure should be delayed.

Injuries to underlying structures must be assessed and remedied prior to closure whenever possible. However, in certain cases of a laceration overlying a fracture it is permissible to close the laceration over the fracture and delay the reduction and fixation until a time when the patient's sensorium may be clearer, facial swelling has diminished, or operating room time becomes available. Diplopia or malocclusion raises a strong suspicion of a facial fracture. Careful palpation in the depths of the wound may confirm this.

A flow of saliva from a wound that does not penetrate the oral cavity usually indicates that the parotid gland or Stensen's duct is lacerated. Insertion of a lacrimal probe through the ductal papilla helps to reveal the site of the ductal dehiscence. The cut surface of the parotid gland is distinctive, due to its slightly greyish colour and lobular appearance. In most instances saliva in the wound is due to a cut gland; the duct often escapes injury.

When the parotid is cut, or when a laceration is present in the vertical axis of the face, evidence of damage to the facial nerve must be searched for. Diagnosis of facial nerve severence is facilitated by familiarity with the extratemporal course of the nerve and its branches.

Treatment

General considerations

A patient presenting with facial lacerations often has multiple injuries and so his general condition should be assessed first and any respiratory embarrassment, or signs of shock, must be treated immediately. All debris should be quickly removed from the upper airway and any obvious bleeding controlled locally.

Tetanus prophylaxis should be instituted either by the administration of toxoid or human antitoxin.

In terms of gravity of injury, facial lacerations have a low priority. While the patient's other problems are being cared for, an antiseptic dressing should be placed in the wounds until definitive closure may be performed. This will keep the wound moist and help to prevent infection. Prophylactic antibiotics are not recommended routinely in clean, fresh lacerations.

Wound preparation

Initial assessment is usually done in the emergency room. Although uncomplicated facial lacerations may be treated adequately there, the same care should be administered as would prevail in the operating room. Thorough cleansing of the wound under either local or general anaesthesia is the first step in definitive treatment. Shaving of a beard or moustache is important for cleanliness and clear visibility. However, the eyebrow should never be shaved as it sometimes fails to regrow; it should merely be clipped with scissors. The area is scrubbed with a germicidal soap and flushed with copious amounts of sterile saline or half strength hydrogen peroxide until all foreign material is washed away. Any road tar must be meticulously removed with a brush, as any remaining vestige will invariably result in the formation of an unsightly tattoo. Occasionally, a shave excision of parts of the wound is necessary to remove this tar.

Conservatism is the rule in debridement and should be limited to devitalized tissue and tissue either stained by road tar or in which the dirt cannot be scrubbed out. Lacerations in which a bevelled cut has been made should have the thin portion excised and this edge countersunk into the opposing side to avoid the widened scar previously alluded to. It is unwise to excise the tips of jagged, irregularly shaped lacerations if they are viable; they should be treated as small flaps that fit into opposing small defects. When approximated, they impart an irregular configuration to the resulting scar which actually tends to camouflage it. This is based on the fact that a straight line scar, even when very thin, may easily be noticed by the observer because of the predictable nature of a straight line. On the other hand, the eye finds it difficult to follow an irregularly shaped scar due to its unpredictable course and the difficulty of picking up the changing pattern of the scar once it is lost in areas of obscurity.

Suture technique

There is nothing magical about the 'plastic surgical repair' of facial cuts. Over the years, this appellation has conjured up an undeserved mystique that has dissuaded many fine surgeons from repairing facial wounds. These lesions are easily amenable to treatment if a few basic principles are followed. The main rules to adhere to are:

(1) Take time to make careful stitches;
(2) Use delicate instruments and fine needles and sutures;
(3) Use a layered closure;
(4) Place the cutaneous sutures in such a way as to evert the edges; and
(5) Instruct the patient in meticulous postoperative care.

Delicate instruments and fine sutures complement accurate surgical technique. Needle holders designed by Webster, Castroviejo or Gillies are designed for the small needles. Small skin hooks and small tissue forceps hold the tissues atraumatically while the stitch is being taken. Iris scissors are ideal for trimming small bits of skin.

Skin edges on the face should be approximated with 6–0 non-absorbable suture material. The various polymers, such as nylon, polypropylene and dacron, are inert and, although they do not tie as readily as silk, are eminently suitable as skin suture. Four or more knots are necessary to prevent spontaneous untying of the suture. Subcutaneous sutures may be absorbable or nonabsorbable. Catgut, 4–0 or 5–0, is commonly used as are Dexon® and Vicryl®.

The oral mucosa is best sutured with 3–0 or 4–0 chromic catgut on a cutting needle. The mucosa of the nasal cavity is difficult to suture and so a micropoint needle should be used.

A layered closure involves placing sutures in each anatomic plane that has been incised. If a muscular or fascial layer has been violated, then it must be sutured, as must the dermal layer, the subcuticular layer and the epidermal layer. The subepithelial sutures should be placed so that the knot is buried in the depths of the wound. These sutures serve not only to accurately coapt each anatomic layer involved in the wound, but also to eliminate dead space where blood or tissue fluid may collect. They also assist in placing the skin edges in precise edge-to-edge contact.

Careful suturing entails taking an equal bite of tissue on both sides of the wound. This means that the suture must not only be the same distance from the wound edge but also at the same depth from the cutaneous surface on both sides of the laceration. Subcutaneous sutures should be placed approximately every 5 mm and they should hold the wound surfaces together so that the external skin sutures will serve merely to coapt the epithelial edges. The skin stitches should be placed about every 1·5–2·0 mm. They should be about this same distance from the wound edge and not tied too tightly.

The skin sutures must be placed so that the skin edges will be everted. This is because the scar will contract, causing some depression of the wound edge. Such a scar will cast a shadow, making it conspicuous. This eversion is produced by taking a wider bite of tissue in the depth of the needle's excursion than at the surface. When the suture is tied, this wider bite of the deeper tissue pushes the wound edges higher than the skin surface. Performing this manoeuvre is facilitated by the use of a skin hook which puts traction on the dermis towards the wound. The suture needle is then driven into the tissue with the angle of attack at 30–45 degrees to the epithelial surface. When the hook is relaxed it is apparent that the skin suture runs a course that is wider in the depths than at the surface. Care is taken to ensure that the suture is symmetrically placed on each side of the wound.

Missing tissue

Only rarely will one see actual tissue loss in a facial wound. When tissue is missing, however, and simple undermining of the skin locally will not effect adequate tension-free closure, then the raw surface should be covered by a flap or a graft.

Skin grafts may be partial thickness or full thickness. The partial-thickness grafts may be classified as thin (8/1000–12/1000 inch), medium (12/1000–18/1000), or thick (18/1000–28/1000). Full-thickness grafts include both the epidermis and dermis.

Partial-thickness grafts have the advantages of ready availability, and good take on the recipient site. The principal disadvantages are contracture and poor colour match. Because of this, the use of split-thickness grafts on the face following trauma is usually limited to those instances in which a tissue dressing is needed until a flap can be mobilized to reconstruct the defect. The thicker a split-thickness graft, the more closely will it resemble the qualities of a full-thickness graft.

Full-thickness grafts are superior to partial thickness grafts in colour and texture and undergo less contracture. The major disadvantage is their relatively inferior take rate. These grafts are frequently used instead of flaps when skin has been avulsed in such areas as the lip, nose, eyelid or eyebrow. Full-thickness grafts for use in the head and neck should be taken from an area that will provide a good colour match. The post-auricular and supraclavicular areas provide skin of excellent colour and texture for resurfacing facial skin loss.

Both partial and full thickness grafts should be kept in place with a tie-over bolster of cotton, gauze or sponge rubber to facilitate the establishment of circulation and prevent the formation of haematoma. Thorough excision of fat from the undersurface of a full-thickness graft is essential to ensure adequate contact between the dermis of the graft and the recipient surface. The bolster is removed at 10 days.

A much more satisfactory method of restoring avulsion defects is the use of regional flaps. The major disadvantage of flaps is the addition of incisions which will increase the amount of scarring. There are three basic types of flaps: advancement, rotation and transposition.

The simplest type of flap is the advancement flap. Two parallel incisions are made from each limit of the defect and the underlying tissue is elevated until gentle traction will approximate the flap edge to the edge of the defect. 'Dog ears' created at the base of the flap may be eliminated by the excision of Burow's triangles. If the defect is too large to be accommodated by a single advancement flap, two flaps may be used from opposing sides of the wound.

The rotation flap is one of the best methods of closing a triangular defect. A semicircular flap is cut, the diameter of which is roughly twice the width of the defect. This rule dictates a rather large flap and its geometry necessitates careful planning so that the incision does not fall across too many natural crease lines in obvious areas. A back cut may be made at the base of the flap opposite the defect to enhance closure. It must be remembered that such a cut narrows the flap's pedicle. This is an excellent flap in the scalp or for moving tissue from under the chin or from the neck on to the face.

The transposition flap involves the swinging of a flap from a donor area across healthy tissue into the defect. The donor site is closed primarily by generous undermining, or it is skin grafted. The donor site is usually selected in a relatively camouflaged area in the neck or in an area where primary closure will result in the suture line being in a natural crease line. Major defects resulting from a gun blast or other severe mechanical trauma may be restored by large transposition flaps from the forehead, nape of neck, or chest.

An ingenious application of the principle of the transposition flap is the Z-plasty. This is composed of two triangular flaps disposed around a common axis. This common central axis may be a scar, or small avulsion defect, a web or a contracture. When the flaps are transposed, the defect is obliterated, the web effaced or the contracture lengthened. The gain achieved by the transposition of the Z-plasty flaps is at the expense of tissue lateral to the original defect. The three limbs of the Z-plasty must be of equal length but the angle of the two outside limbs to the central axis need not be the same. The ideal angle is 60 degrees, and as the angles are made smaller the amount of lengthening achieved diminishes and the amount of blood supply to the flap tips is less. When the angles are increased, the amount of lengthening achieved increases but the ease of transposing the flaps is less. These extremes of angle range from 20 to 75 degrees in practice. It is always necessary to elevate around the base of each flap to facilitate transposition.

Post-operative care

Since absolute haemostasis must be secured prior to wound closure, no drains are usually needed. The only dressing used is a layer of antibiotic ointment over the suture line. Alternate sutures are removed on the fourth or fifth postoperative day and the remainder 1 or 2 days later. Once the sutures are removed, the skin is painted with tincture of benzoin and Steristrips® are placed across the wound edges for a period of several weeks. The strips are replaced every 48–72 hours. The purpose of this manoeuvre is to relieve any tension on the maturing scar in those lacerations that cross natural crease lines.

The patient should be advised that the final appearance of the scar should not be judged for about a year. The initial scar, until about 2–3 weeks, is usually narrow and pink but becomes somewhat wider and red over the ensuing 3–6 months, then gradually blanches at around 12–18 months. Scar revision should be delayed for 12 months or longer until the scar has matured.

Complications

The repair of facial lacerations has few complications and most of these are the direct result of poor technique.

The commonest early complication is *infection* but most of this is minor and easily treated by removal of a few sutures to release any entrapped pus, repeated cleansing, and the application of antibiotic ointment. Because of the rich vascular supply to the face these infections tend to stay localized and should clear easily with vigorous local therapy. Only occasionally is a systemic antibiotic indicated. One should not be lulled into a state of complacency, however, as disastrous progression can occur in neglected facial wounds. Recalcitrant infections should raise the suspicion of a foreign body in the depths of the wound.

Slough of the wound edges, or of small flaps involved in the repair, may occur as the result of infection, trauma or maceration of the skin. Poor blood supply to the area, in diabetic patients or in those with skin damaged by irradiation, may be the cause of major necrosis at the wound site. The slough should be treated by careful attention to the metabolic status of the patient, control of diabetes, or restoration of a depressed haemoglobin level and local therapy to control any existing infection. Any debridement should be avoided until a clean line of demarcation between dead and viable tissue ensues. Infection is usually easily controlled in these patients by the application of saline or acetic acid soaks. Once the sloughed area is debrided the granulating wound can be left to heal by secondary intention, if small, or it may be skin grafted or covered by a flap, if large.

Tattooing of the wound will occur if road tar or gunpowder is not adequately removed at the time of closure. This usually requires treatment by excision of the affected areas.

Hypertrophic scars may form, especially in the dark races. These may be controlled to some extent by the intralesional injection of a long-acting steroid preparation. Steroid injections and massage may soften hypertrophic scarring in many cases.

Keloids may also respond to steroid therapy but are uninfluenced by massage. This heaped up invasive process of continuing scar formation may be treated by irradiation with a 250 kV source or by intralesional suturing of radioactive iridium wire. Many radiotherapists are reluctant to use these modalities in keloid treatment because of their carcinogenic potential. Excision and early regular steroid injections are occasionally successful in ablating keloids.

References

[1] Goss M. G. (1975) *Gray's Anatomy*, 29th American Edition, pp. 1102–3. Philadelphia: Lea and Febiger.
[2] Kraissl C. J. (1951) The selection of appropriate lines for elective surgical incisions. *Plastic and Reconstructive Surgery* **8**, 1.

CHAPTER 21

Facial Pain

The recognition of the causes of facial pain, an essential precursor of treatment, demands an understanding of certain fundamental principles about pain generally.

PHYSIOLOGY OF PAIN

Perception of pain

Perception of pain depends on:

(1) The integrity of its underlying neural mechanisms, viz. pain receptors in organs and tissues, the peripheral and central nervous system conducting paths; and

(2) The 'sensorium', a neutral word to describe where and how the pain stimulus is received and translated into a sensation of 'pain'.

Intensity of pain

The intensity of pain depends upon:

(1) The strength of the stimulus causing it;

(2) The area stimulated, e.g. the cornea is more sensitive than the skin; and

(3) The sensitivity of the 'sensorium' which varies with each individual's 'threshold' for pain.

Reaction to pain

Reaction to pain is not necessarily related to the strength of the stimulus causing it. It varies with the psychical, physical and metabolic state of the victim and many other factors. Facial pain tends to produce stronger reactions than pain in more caudal areas of the body, partly because the face seems to be a more intimate part of one's personality and partly, no doubt, due to the denser innervation of the face and head.

The reference of pain

No matter where in its path a sensory nerve is stimulated – and this is true of cranial, spinal, or autonomic nerves – the patient most commonly experiences pain in the peripheral terminations of that nerve, though occasionally in a neighbouring nerve or nerves sharing the same central nervous (usually spinal) segment. It is this latter to which the term 'referred pain' properly applies, e.g. when irritation of the diaphragm, from liver or pleural lesions, causes pain in the shoulder area, because both receive their innervations from the third, fourth and fifth cervical segments.

Quality of pain

The work of Sir Thomas Lewis and his colleagues led to the classification of pain into two types – superficial and deep.

Superficial pain produced by a brief stimulus, e.g. pin-prick, cut, heat, cold, faradic current, etc. is felt as a sharp pain varying in intensity with the strength of the stimulus and the patient's threshold for pain, and it is accurately localized. If the stimulus, even intense cold, is prolonged, the result is a 'burning' sensation.

Deep pain has a dull, aching quality and is often accompanied by nausea and changes in pulse rate; its localization is imprecise and often vague.

The classification of pain into superficial and deep is not as explicit as Lewis believed, for all shades and combinations occur. For practical purposes it can be said that *superficial* pain arises from skin, buccal mucosa and periosteum, and *deep* pain from bone, joint, muscle, blood vessels and viscera; the latter is usually 'referred'. Pain arising from the air sinuses tends to be deep in quality though from the frontal, and maxillary sinuses it is localized to a great extent in relation to their sites; whereas from the ethmoidal and sphenoidal sinuses pain tends to be felt at the base of the nose and in the temporal regions.

'NEURALGIA'

'Neuralgia' is often used by the public as a synonym for pain but it should be confined to pain which is felt in the area of distribution of a sensory nerve – whether the noxious stimulus is applied to a nerve trunk, posterior spinal root(s) or ganglion (ganglia). On this basis two forms of neuralgia can be differentiated clinically:

(1) primary; and
(2) secondary or symptomatic.

Characteristics of primary neuralgia

Primary neuralgia, occurring usually in certain cranial nerves, is unassociated with any objective signs of impaired nerve conduction. It has a characteristic quality – paroxysmal, shock-like, lightning pains like the stab of a knife or a red-hot needle, which last only seconds, but with remissions between the spasms which may be so short as to be overlooked by the patient who will complain of the pain being continuous unless directly questioned. The pain is excruciatingly severe so that the face is distorted (some gargoyles are said to represent the pain in trigeminal neuralgia), the eyes fixed, speech arrested, and a look of profound apprehension tells of the dread of a return of the pain. In primary neuralgias there are 'trigger zones' – which when stimulated, e.g. by touching, brushing, or eating, precipitate a paroxysm of pain. These 'trigger zones' tend to be localized and since they are less likely to be stimulated during sleep, the nights are usually freer from pain than the days.

The cranial nerve in which primary neuralgia occurs most commonly is the trigeminal, but it occasionally appears in the glossopharyngeal, the facial (geniculate ganglion) and superior laryngeal. In all these nerves, ganglia are found in their first sensory pathway to the central nervous system and the frequency of neuralgia is related directly to the size of these ganglia. Very occasionally the 'tic'-like pain of a primary neuralgia may recur as the presenting sign of a pathological lesion, e.g. from compression of the Gasserian ganglion by a tumour, granuloma, or aneurysm in the middle or posterior cranial fossa, but as a rule this stage is short-lived, and signs of motor or sensory paralysis appear. In slowly progressive lesions though, e.g. multiple sclerosis, cranial hyperostosis, Paget's disease, etc., the primary neuralgia may persist for a longer period without signs of nerve dysfunction though the causative lesion is usually unmasked easily.

Many explanations have been advanced to explain the mechanisms of primary neuralgia. It has been suggested that it is analogous to epilepsy [1], namely a sudden, explosive, irregular discharge of energy from the ganglion cell, hence the value of anticonvulsive drugs, e.g. carbamazepine ('Tegretol') in trigeminal neuralgia.

Characteristics of secondary neuralgia

Secondary neuralgia is due to a gross pathological lesion directly involving the nerve (e.g. trauma, neoplasm), posterior root (e.g. tabes dorsalis) or ganglion (e.g. herpes zoster). Three features characterize symptomatic neuralgia.

(1) The pain is usually a mixture of superficial and deep; sometimes it is pricking and burning but usually it is boring and aching; it is often continuous, with frequent exacerbations and rare remissions;

(2) Associated with the pain are objective signs of interruption of continuity of the nerve, viz. anaesthesia, paresis, muscle wasting, diminished or absent reflexes, or trophic changes; and

(3) These objective signs tend to progress gradually and involve neighbouring structures.

PRIMARY NEURALGIAS

Trigeminal neuralgia

Clinical features

About 50% of patients are between the ages of 50 and 70, and it is rare under 40 years; it is somewhat commoner in women, and involves the right side of the face almost twice as often as the left. Most commonly the second and third divisions of the fifth nerve are involved but the pain can first appear in any of the three divisions and spread to the others. Bilateral disease is found rarely (about 1 in 25 cases) and is most commonly associated with chronic multiple sclerosis.

The quality of the pain and its distribution stamp the diagnosis, but the earlier mentioned caveat, viz. that rarely gross pathological lesions may present with 'tic'-like pain, should be remembered and compel continuing observation. At the onset of herpes there may be no rash but it appears within days almost invariably and especially in the ophthalmic branch of the fifth cranial nerve (Fig. 21.1).

Paroxysms of pain usually return in cycles and last for weeks or even months. These cycles tend to recur with greater frequency and severity; spontaneous recovery is rare.

Early recognition of trigeminal neuralgia will avoid much unnecessary suffering. Almost every patient will have had unnecessary dental extrac-

tions, sinus drainage, etc. Yet no oral or nasopharyngeal disease gives pain which accurately reproduces the pain of trigeminal neuralgia and this pain is never relieved permanently by dental or nasal treatment though a spontaneous remission may follow and be falsely interpreted on the basis of *post hoc ergo propter hoc*. In primary neuralgia local treatment to teeth, sinuses, etc., should be given only if that treatment would be justified in the absence of the primary neuralgia, i.e. only if intrinsic oral or nasal pathology calls for it. This is important since there is always a possibility that infection may lead to an ascending neuritis reaching the ganglion and rendering it more unstable.

Treatment

This applies to all the primary neuralgias. The most effective drugs are carbamazepine ('Tegretol'), and diphenylhydantoin. Both are anticonvulsants. Carbamazepine should be started with a dose of 200 mg daily and gradually increased to a maximum of 600–800 mg daily, in divided

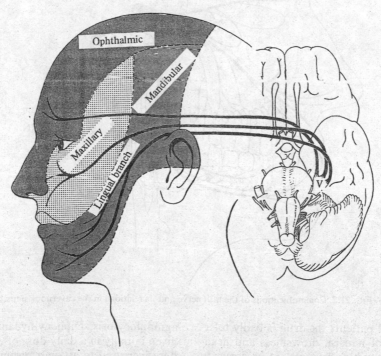

FIG. 21.1. Branches of fifth cranial (trigeminal) nerve.

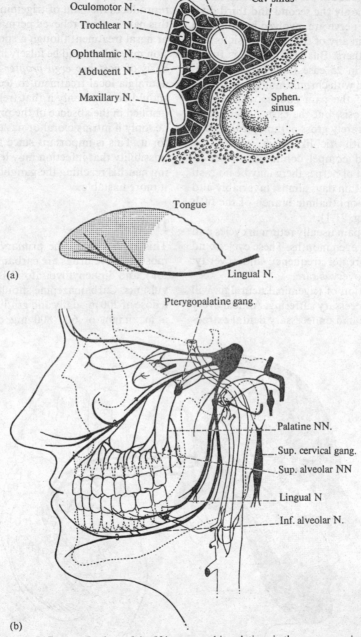

(a)

(b)

Fig. 21.2. Communications of the fifth nerve and its relations in the cavernous sinus.

doses. In some patients the drug is badly tolerated because of nausea, drowsiness and headache, and regular blood counts are necessary to detect the early signs of aplastic anaemia or agranulocytosis. Diphenylhydantoin should be given initially in a daily dose of 300 mg and the dose increased to attain a serum level of 12–18 mg per ml.

In both trigeminal and glossopharyngeal neuralgia 'trigger zones' in mouth and pharynx may prevent the patient taking food or drink and severe malnutrition can result. However, the paroxysms may recur with such frequency that the patient is driven to suicide. Thus if drug treatment fails to give relief there should be early resort to surgery – preferably pre-ganglionic root section (Fig. 21.2).

It is preferable not to delay surgery as soon as it is clear that medical treatment gives inadequate relief. Too often the patient has been rendered edentulous in an attempt to relieve the pain. After root section the jaw is anaesthetic, and so there is great difficulty in fitting a denture correctly in order to prevent ulceration from pressure. Also, where there are alveolar 'trigger zones' the patient fears to brush his teeth, with resulting dental disease often necessitating extractions with the resulting hazards mentioned earlier. Moreover, if the concept of an ascending neuritis be valid, delay in sensory root section may no longer be effective because the nerve cells in higher stations, e.g. brain stem, may have become more unstable. This last may indeed play a part in producing the virtually intolerable burning pain of 'anaesthesia dolorosa' which follows, very occasionally, sensory root section, and for which leucotomy may offer the only relief.

Other methods of destroying the Gasserian ganglion in whole or part by alcohol injection, freezing or heat coagulation are less effective than sensory root section.

It should be added that the only analgesics likely to relieve the pain of primary neuralgias, e.g. the opiates, are addictive though their use may nevertheless be justified in the aged.

Glossopharyngeal neuralgia [2]

Clinical features

This neuralgia is much rarer than trigeminal neuralgia and commonly overlooked.

Fig. 21.3 shows the distribution of the glossopharyngeal nerve. It carries sensations from part of the pharynx, the palatine tonsil, the posterior third of the tongue, the mucous membrane lining

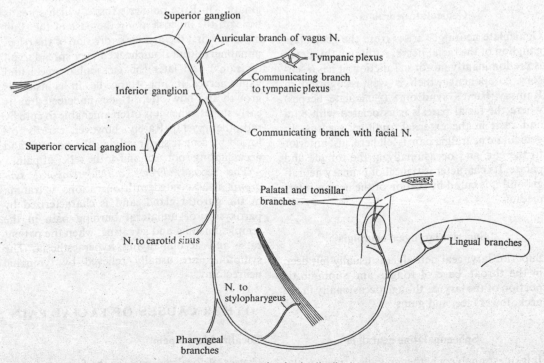

FIG. 21.3. The glossopharyngeal nerve showing its distribution and connections.

the tympanic cavity, Eustachian tube and mastoid air cells; and clinical evidence suggests also from the posterior wall of the external auditory meatus, part of the concha, a strip of the posteromedial surface of the auricle and the immediately adjacent mastoid region.

It is in this distribution that the pain is felt and its quality conforms to that of primary neuralgia. Paroxysms are 'triggered' by swallowing, chewing, talking, yawning, coughing, sneezing, stooping or syringing the ear. 'Trigger zones' are the tonsils, the pharyngeal wall, the base of the tongue, and the ear.

Treatment

Objective signs of dysfunction of the glossopharyngeal nerve are not easily detected and so section of the nerve leads to little disability. The intracranial approach for preganglionic root section may reveal a gross pathological lesion. The position of the ganglia on the nerve sometimes allows extracranial avulsion to be effective.

Geniculate neuralgia

Geniculate neuralgia arises from the geniculate ganglion of the facial nerve. Although this nerve is predominantly motor in function, it has a sensory component which is well recognized in Ramsay Hunt's syndrome (geniculate herpes) where the facial paresis is associated with pain and rash in the external auditory meatus. In geniculate neuralgia pain is felt here, just anterior to the ear, and occasionally in the tongue and palate. Its character is typical of primary neuralgia and it is cured by section of the nervus intermedius.

Superior laryngeal neuralgia

Superior laryngeal neuralgia is usually felt deep in the throat, base of tongue and supraglottic portion of the larynx, though occasionally in the neck, lower face, and gums.

Sphenopalatine neuralgia

It is questionable whether so-called sphenopalatine (or Slüder's) neuralgia is a true primary neuralgia. Its features resemble more closely the 'cluster' headaches of vascular origin.

Great auricular neuralgia (Fig. 21.4)

Very occasionally, tic-like pain is felt in the area of the angle of the mandible and arises in the posterior root ganglia of the second and third cervical nerves.

SECONDARY NEURALGIAS

Pain in the face may arise from any lesion which irritates its nerve supply at any level. Such lesions are conveniently divided into three groups:

(1) *Intracranial*, e.g. neoplasms, granulomata, reticuloses, aneurysms, syringobulbia, thrombosis of posterior inferior cerebellar artery.

(2) *Lesions of the bony cranial base*, e.g. fractures, carcinomatosis, osteitis deformans, cranial hyperostosis, petrous osteitis.

(3) *Extracranial*. These are too numerous to detail but there are two which justify references.

The first is a *nasopharyngeal carcinoma*, originating in Rosenmüller's fossa, which spreads beneath the mucosa along the base of the skull involving first the maxillary division of the trigeminal nerve (but if unchecked may spread to all divisions) and later the glossopharyngeal and vagus nerves. Its importance lies in its insidious growth and how often it goes undetected in its early stages, when it is often amenable to cure by radiotherapy [3]. Rarely, however, cure is followed by scar tissue involving the nerve(s) and necessitating root section for the relief of pain.

The second, *Frey's auriculotemporal syndrome*, is associated with operations or trauma to the parotid gland, and is characterized by paroxysms of unilateral burning pain in the temple, flushing and sweating, when the patient eats, and accompanying hyperaesthesia. The symptoms are usually relieved by tympanic neurectomy.

OTHER CAUSES OF FACIAL PAIN

Localized facial pain

Causes of localized pain in the face are legion. Amongst these are:

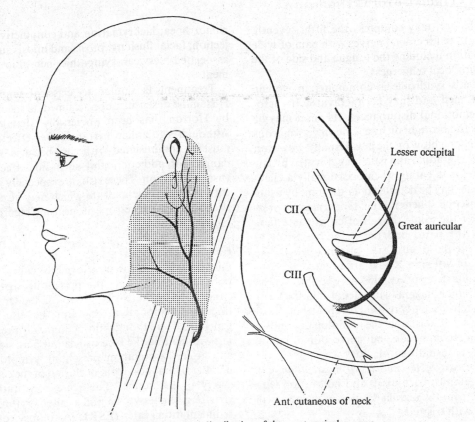

FIG. 21.4. Origins and distribution of the great auricular nerve.

(1) *Disease of paranasal sinuses*, especially infection or neoplasm. Infection of the maxillary sinus may involve the apices of adjacent teeth and present as dental pain: very rarely the infection may involve the maxillary nerve and present as maxillary neuralgia; similarly sphenoidal sinus infection may involve the nerve of the pterygoid canal (vidian nerve).

(2) *Diseases of teeth and jaws* are the commonest cause of facial pain. Examples are caries, periapical infection, lateral periodontal abscesses, pulp stones, osteomyelitis (actinomycosis is not to be overlooked), fractures, rarefying osteitis following tooth extraction, and neoplasms. Pain due to a diseased tooth may be referred to a normal tooth (*vide supra*) but the affected tooth can be indicated by the pain being aggravated by temperature extremes or percussion and eased by local anaesthesia (not, of course, a nerve block).

(3) *Disease of the ears*, especially otitis externa, may give preauricular pain.

(4) *Disease of the eyes*. Glaucoma, ocular muscle imbalance, etc., may present with frontal pain.

(5) *Disease of the temporomandibular joint* commonly gives rise to preauricular and temporal pain, in, for example, rheumatoid arthritis. But in *Costen's syndrome* pain arises in the absence of any evidence of gross pathology in the joint. This syndrome normally occurs in edentulous patients, over the age of 40, in which the joint is overstrained due to malocclusion, loss of molar support with over-closure of the jaws or to non-equilibrated dentures. Amongst the factors said to be responsible are compression of the chorda tympani and auriculotemporal nerves, and pressure on the Eustachian tube. It has been suggested that distortion of the thin tympanic plate, which ends in a free edge at the petrotym-

panic fissure, may compress the fifth, seventh, ninth and tenth cranial nerves with pain of wide distribution including the tongue and side of the nose with local tenderness.

Costen's syndrome is commoner in women than in men and may be aggravated by associated emotional disturbances. Its onset may be sudden and brought on by a wide yawn, vigorous chewing, or a blow on the jaw. Usually, however, its onset is gradual and pain is aggravated by jaw movements in eating when occasionally a clicking sound may be detected over the joint by using a stethoscope. There is often tenderness on pressure over the joint (though often pressure here relieves the pain) and the mandible tends to deviate to the painful side on opening. In the absence of arthritis, X-rays are negative.

Although temporary relief may be obtained by infiltration of the joint with a local anaesthetic or corticosteroids, early referral to a prosthodontist is necessary. Excision of the mandibular condyle has been recommended but correction of dental occlusion is usually satisfactory.

(6) *Disease of the muscles of mastication*, e.g. injury, tetanus, trichiniasis and infiltration with tumour from the maxillary sinus or parotid, will present with trismus.

Facial pain of vascular origin

There are two conditions to which special attention should be drawn:

(1) *Migrainous neuralgia,* which appears to be similar to, or identical with, Horton's neuralgia, histamine headache, and ciliary, petrosal or Slüder's (sphenopalatine) neuralgia (note the use of 'neuralgia' as synonymous with 'pain'); and

(2) *Giant-celled (temporal) arteritis.*

Migrainous neuralgia

Migrainous neuralgia, unlike classical hemicrania, is associated with a constant, boring or burning pain, usually starting in one eye or temple and radiating widely to the face, ear, and often the neck and shoulder. The pain usually reaches its peak within 30 minutes and recedes fairly quickly but tends to recur in 'clusters' especially at night, for a few weeks; it may then disappear for a time only to recur in many patients. Accompanying the pain may be

rhinorrhoea, lachrymation and conjunctival injection; facial flushing, ptosis and miosis suggest associated cervical sympathetic nerve involvement.

Treatment is similar to classical migraine. Histamine desensitization, claimed as successful by Horton, has been universally abandoned. Although ergotamine tartrate is often effective, it must be administered with care because of the dangers of addiction and such side-effects as vasoconstriction. These risks are especially grave with methysergide maleate which may also give rise to irreversible retroperitoneal and pleuropulmonary fibrosis.

Giant-celled arteritis

Giant-celled arteritis was formerly called temporal arteritis because the presenting sign was commonly in the easily observed, tender, and thickened temporal artery. But the disease is generalized and though most commonly presenting with pain in the face or head, it may start in any artery; a common presenting symptom is unilateral blindness from occlusion of the central artery of the retina. There are constitutional signs, e.g. slight pyrexia and a raised erythrocyte sedimentation rate (ESR). A biopsy of an affected artery reveals the characteristic giant-cell pathology and often relieves local pain. The disease tends to occur in the older age groups.

Early treatment with corticosteroids in large doses (up to 40 mg prednisolone daily) should be instituted and a careful watch kept on the ESR so that the dose can be regulated. Response to this treatment is rapid. Ergotamine preparations are contra-indicated; they can, by aggravating the vasoconstriction, cause severe necrosis.

Atypical facial neuralgia

In this group, psychogenic factors play the major part. The victims are usually, but not exclusively, women over 40, and very often menopausal. The pain which they describe in extravagant terms ('excruciating', 'appalling', 'crucifying') is never of the primary neuralgia or 'tic' type, but is usually constant, dull, and boring; it spreads to the whole face and often to the neck and shoulders and there are innumerable 'trigger zones'. The pain sometimes appears after alleged trauma, e.g. slight injury or dental treatment. Unlike a true 'tic', where the patient usually carries on with his or her job, the patient with 'atypical facial neuralgia' complains that it incapacitates her for business or domestic duties.

These patients are often depressed, obsessive and dependent personalities; they tend to lack psychological insight and are constantly seeking an organic cause for their pains and demanding surgical intervention. One patient consulted 24 dentists; each treatment was followed by a few days' relief before the return of pain. Another patient with dominantly right-sided facial pain had successively, over a period of 6 years, avulsion of the supraorbital nerve, alcohol injection of the trigeminal ganglion, section of the sensory root of the fifth cranial nerve (with resulting keratitis and eventually blindness of the eye), injection of the stellate ganglion, stripping of the internal carotid, removal of the stellate ganglion, removal of the presumed sensory cortex on the left side (with temporary aphasia), a right-sided leucotomy followed by a bilateral frontal leuco-

tomy – all alas! with only transient benefit. Sedative drugs, analgesics, antidepressants, monoamine oxidases may give temporary relief but the pain inevitably recurs or is substituted by other psychogenic disturbances. Reference to a psychiatrist, once an organic cause has been eliminated, should not be delayed.

Referred pain to the face and jaws

This is rare but can occur in myocardial ischaemia associated with coronary artery disease, in cervical spondylosis, and very rarely, from lesions of the oesophagus and cardiac end of the stomach.

References

[1] LORD COHEN OF BIRKENHEAD (1959) Facial neuralgias. British Dental Journal 2, 9.
[2] COHEN H. (1937) Glossopharyngeal neuralgia. Journal of Laryngology and Otology 52, 527.
[3] SIR TERENCE WARD (1975) Closing the gate to pain. Annals of the Royal College of Surgeons 57, 229.

CHAPTER 22

Neck Masses

CONGENITAL NECK LUMPS

Lymphangiomas

The best known lymphangioma of the head and neck is the cystic hygroma [1], which is rare, but is part of the lymphangiomatous tumours which include simple lymphangiomas and cavernous lymphangiomas. These can sometimes be combined with haemangiomatous elements to a greater or lesser extent.

Embryology

The lymph system arises from five primitive sacs (two jugular sacs, two posterior sciatic sacs and a single retroperitoneal sac) developed from the venous system [2, 3]. Endothelial buds from these extend centrifugally to form the peripheral lymphatic system.

There are two theories of origin of lymphangiomas. They either are sequestrations of lymphatic tissue derived from portions of the primitive sacs, which retain their rapid and proliferative growth potential and have no connection to the normal lymph system [4], or they arise from endothelial fibrillar membranes which sprout from the walls of the cyst, penetrate surrounding tissue, canalize and produce more cysts [5].

Pathology

Lymphogenous conditions have been classified into three groups [6].

(1) *Lymphangioma simplex*, composed of thin walled capillary-sized lymphatic channels.

(2) *Cavernous lymphangioma,* composed of dilated lymphatic spaces often with fibrous adventitia.

(3) *Cystic hygroma*, composed of cysts varying in size from a few millimetres to several centimetres in diameter.

All these can be regarded as one entity but site may play some part in the final version – the smaller lymphangiomas occur in the lips, tongue, cheek and where the tissue planes are tighter, whereas the cystic hygroma has more space to expand into the tissue planes of the neck. Simple lymphangiomas can occur anywhere in the mouth as pale soft fluctuant lesions and form one-third of all lymphangiomatous tumours. More common are cavernous lymphangiomas which form 40% of these lesions, mainly in the tongue. At the base of the tongue they must be differentiated from a lingual thyroid, a lingual carcinoma or an internal laryngocoele. They also occur on the lateral border. Some cheek lesions reach an enormous size and are very difficult to eradicate since total excision produces an unacceptable cosmetic defect.

A cavernous lymphangioma of the floor of the mouth can be part of a cystic hygroma or a ranula. Macrocheilia usually affects only the upper lip (Fig. 22.1).

Cystic hygroma forms 30% of the series and consists of large multinodular cystic masses which may communicate or be isolated [7]. The walls are thin and the contained fluid can be clearly seen. A hygroma occurs in the cervico-facial region spreading into the cheek, mouth, tongue, parotid and even the ear canal (Fig. 22.2).

Histologically the cyst is lined by a single layer of flattened endothelium, with fetal fat and cholesterol crystals [8]. They are rare tumours forming 0·5% of large series of neck lumps [9–11]. There is no sex or side predominance. Two out of three are noted at birth, and nine out of ten before the end of the second year.

Thirty-five per cent of lymphangiomas of all

types occur in the cheek, tongue and floor of the mouth, 25% in the neck and 15% in the axilla.

Clinical features

Most of these tumours manifest themselves at birth or shortly afterwards. Lymphangiomas in

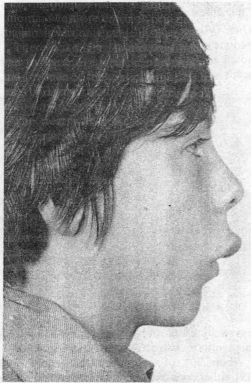

FIG. 22.1. Lymphangioma of the upper lip causes a rocheilia which is best managed by a lip shave, incision of lymphangioma and vermilion advancement.

the mouth can first appear in adult life as can recurrences of cystic hygromas after surgery in infancy. Recurrences usually occur on the periphery of the facial area where the main mass originally presented such as the ear, parotid or posterior triangle.

While size alone is the prominent first symptom and sign, if the cyst is big enough it can cause stridor. In very large cysts a lateral displacement of the trachea and even mediastinal widening may be seen on the radiograph.

Sudden increase in size by spontaneous haemorrhage may be fatal. Brachial plexus compres-

sion with pain and hyperaesthesia may also occur [12].

Treatment

Cystic hygroma should be excised. Other treatments described have been: aspiration, incision and drainage, injection of sclerosants and radiotherapy.

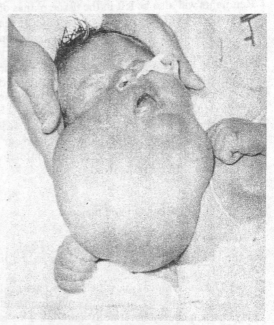

FIG. 22.2. A cystic hygroma in a neonate affecting the cheek, mouth, tongue, neck and external ear.

Incision and drainage should only be done for infection, which is rare. Injection with sclerosants should be avoided because of the proximity to major vessels and nerves; it also thickens the walls and tissue planes and makes surgery much more difficult.

Young patients should not be irradiated because of the dangers of retarded bone and tissue growth, thyroid malignancy and cosmetic deformities. Surgery should only be delayed in the premature infant; delay in otherwise healthy infants only leads to continuing morbidity and increased mortality. It has been suggested that complete regression occurs in 15% [13] but other authors claim never to have seen this [14].

No operation should be done without a preoperative chest radiograph to rule out mediastinal involvement. Damage to the facial, hypoglossal and accessory nerves should be avoided. It is difficult to get a good cosmetic result in huge cysts because of the tissue displacement and the large amount of skin that must be removed.

Intra-oral lymphangiomas should be removed from an external approach since they are almost certainly much more extensive than expected. Remnants will also be left in the tissue planes of the tongue. Lymphangiomas of the base of the tongue can often be dealt with by coagulation diathermy repeated if necessary. Cryosurgery may also be helpful. Lymphangioma of the upper lip should be dealt with by a lip shave and vermillion advancement and excision of muscle and cyst to get an acceptable size.

Recurrences usually appear within the first 9 months in about 10–15% of patients. The recurrence rate is higher with cavernous lymphangioma than with cystic hygroma.

Mid-line dermoid tumours

Pathology

In the head and neck there are three varieties of dermoid cyst [15].

(1) The *epidermoid cyst*, which has no adnexal structures, is lined by squamous epithelium and may contain cheesy keratinous material. This is the commonest variety.

(2) The *true dermoid cyst* which is lined by squamous epithelium and contains skin appendages such as hair, hair follicles, sebaceous glands and sweat glands. These are either congenital or acquired.

The congenital type derives from ectodermal differentiations of multipotential cells pinched off at the time of closure of the anterior neuropore. It therefore occurs along lines of fusion.

The acquired type is due to implantation of epidermis at the time of a puncture type of injury and is often solid with areas of cystic spaces containing sebaceous material.

(3) The *teratoid cyst* can be lined with squamous or respiratory epithelium and contains elements formed from ectoderm, endoderm and mesoderm – nails, teeth, brain, glands, etc. This is the rarest variety in the neck and is nearly always diagnosed in the first year of life. Less

than ten cases of teratoid tumours of the neck have been described in adults [16].

Twenty per cent of all dermoid cysts are found in the neck, and 30% in the head and face [17]. Dermoids form 28% of all mid-line cysts, and there is no sex predominance [18].

Clinical features

These cysts present as solid or cystic masses in the midline of the neck between the suprasternal notch and the submental region. They can also occur lateral to the submandibular gland. Pain-

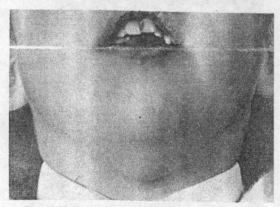

FIG. 22.3. A central suprahyoid mass in a 5-year-old child which on removal proved to be a dermoid cyst.

less swelling is the only symptom, but if the cyst is large, minor obstructive symptoms can occur.

About 20% of dermoids occur in the mouth [19], either deep to the mylohyoid (sublingual) or superficial to it (submental). They present in the second and third decades, but have probably been present since birth (Fig. 22.3).

Treatment

Complete excision is usually easy and should be done in all cases.

Thyroglossal duct cysts

The commonest mid-line neck cyst is a remnant of the thyroglossal duct. This cyst can occur anywhere in the area bounded by the foramen caecum above, the manubrial notch inferiorly and the anterior borders of the sternomastoid laterally [20].

Embryology

The thyroid anlage arises from the floor of the primitive pharynx midway between the first and second pharyngeal pouches. It becomes a hollow tube that soon loses its lumen to become solid as it migrates to the lower neck. The distal end divides into two portions which become the lobes of the thyroid gland; the stalk, if it persists, becomes the thyroglossal duct and pyramidal lobe. The duct atrophies at the sixth week, but persists at the top end as the foramen caecum. If it does not atrophy it remains as a persistent thyroglossal duct. Since the tongue develops later than the thyroid anlage, the thyroglossal duct is buried deep in the foramen caecum, and since the hyoid bone develops even later, the duct can run in front, behind and even through the bone.

Pathology

Men and women are equally affected. The age range is from 4 months to 70 years with a mean of $5\frac{1}{2}$ years. Ninety per cent are in the midline and 10% are to one side of the midline; of these 95% are on the left and 5% are on the right. Their site is as follows:

Prehyoid	75%
Thyroid cartilage level	15%
Suprahyoid	5%
Cricoid level	5%
Base of tongue	1%

The duct is always subcutaneous, and spontaneous fistula formation is rare. A fistula is usually the result of infection, attempted drainage of a misdiagnosed abscess, or inadequate removal of the hyoid. The cyst and the duct are lined by squamous epithelium, but thyroid tissue is rarely found in the wall.

Clinical features

Ninety-five per cent present with a painless cystic lump which moves on swallowing and protruding the tongue. The cyst is mobile in all directions and usually is transilluminable. If it is low in the neck the subcutaneous tract can often be seen. Five per cent present with tenderness and rapid enlargement due to infection.

Fistula is present in 15% of cases and is usually the result of a previous operation or an infection.

Suprahyoid cysts may be mistaken for a submental adenitis or a dermoid. Prehyoid cysts are nearly always dum-bell or bar shaped and can push the base of the tongue upwards causing

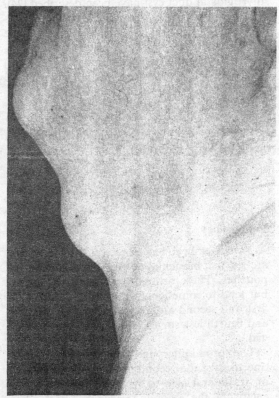

FIG. 22.4. A thyroglossal cyst presenting in front of the thyrohyoid membrane.

dysarthria. If the cyst is near the surface of the tongue base it must be distinguished from a lingual thyroid or a carcinoma. Cysts low in the neck must be differentiated from a thyroid adenoma by a thyroid scan. Other diagnoses to be considered are sebaceous cyst and lipoma (Fig. 22.4).

Some cases are asymptomatic; thyroglossal cysts are sometimes removed during a routine laryngectomy [21].

Treatment

Thyroglossal duct cyst should be removed including the central portion of the hyoid bone [22,

23]. An excellent description of the operative technique is given by Ward et al. [20].

Thyroglossal duct carcinoma

Sixty-six cases of thyroid carcinoma arising in a thyroglossal duct cyst have been described [24]. The tumour is always a papillary thyroid carcinoma. Most presented as benign cysts and the diagnosis was only made by histology.

There is a slight female preponderance (4:3) and the peak age incidence for women is 30–40 and for men 50–60 years. Only 10% had metastases compared to 40–50% for carcinoma arising in an ectopic thyroid.

The treatment is local excision followed by suppressive doses of thyroid.

Branchial cysts

Embryology

A 2-week embryo has on each side six branchial arches, five branchial clefts and five pharyngeal pouches. These arrangements are not parallel, but tend to come together at the sixth arch. The first and second arches are important, the third and fourth less so, and the fifth and sixth vestigial.

The second pharyngeal pouch forms the palatine tonsils; the second arch grows downwards on its lateral side to meet the fifth arch thus enclosing the second, third and fourth clefts forming the cervical sinus of His. By the sixth week the branchial apparatus has disappeared having formed the ear, tongue, hyoid, larynx, tonsils and parathyroids.

Theories of origin

The debate as to the origin of a branchial cyst reached a climax in the 1920s and 1930s [25–28]. There are four theories of origin of branchial cysts but because of the complicated development of the neck none has been proven by embryological investigation. Most of the theories have been an attempt to correlate clinical findings with known embryological facts and none can stand close scrutiny.

(1) *Branchial apparatus theory*. These cysts may represent remains of the pharyngeal pouches or branchial clefts or a fusion of these two elements [29]. When branchial cysts have an internal opening it is in the region of the tonsillar fossa indicating an origin from the second branchial pouch. Fistulae and sinuses from the second pouch would necessarily pass between the external and internal carotid arteries.

Origin from the third or fourth pouches is unlikely, as they would have to pass over the hypoglossal nerve to reach the skin and would be severed by the upward movement of that nerve during development.

A fourth arch tract would also have to pass below the subclavian artery on the right and the aortic arch on the left.

A third arch tract should have its internal opening in the piriform fossa and a fourth arch tract below this. These have never been described, so that origin from these pouches can be discounted.

Origin from the first pouch is possible because high branchial cysts have been described lying under the parotid gland with an internal opening between the bony and cartilaginous meatus. If the branchial apparatus theory were to be upheld one would expect a lot more cysts to have internal openings; it is a popular misconception that many branchial cysts have an internal opening. One would also expect more cysts to be present at birth. Not only has this only once been described [28] but the peak age incidence is in the third and fourth decades which is late for a congenital lesion (cf. thyroglossal duct cysts).

(2) *Cervical sinus theory*. This is an extension of the previous theory and considers that branchial cysts represent remains of the cervical sinus of His which is formed by the second arch growing down to meet the fifth. It is unlikely that this is true for those with an internal tract since this is closed by a fusion of its ectodermal lining from within towards the surface. This makes an internal opening difficult to achieve.

(3) *Thymopharyngeal duct theory*. Cysts may be a remnant of the original connection between the thymus and the third branchial pouch from which it takes origin [30]. The originator of this

theory presumed that the hyoid bone constituted the lower level of branchial derivatives. Not only is this false but a persistent thymic duct has never been described. Furthermore no branchial cyst has ever been described deep to the thyroid gland nor have there been any examples of tracts between the pharynx and the thymus.

(4) *Inclusion theories.* King stated that there was insufficient evidence to show that cysts arose from the branchial apparatus and suggested that the cyst epithelium arose from lymph node epithelium [31]. Others thought that cysts were the result of epithelial inclusion in lymph nodes [32]. The following facts support this theory:

(a) Most branchial cysts have lymphoid tissue in the wall and are found in the parotid and also the pharynx.

(b) The peak age incidence is later than expected for a congenital condition.

(c) A branchial cyst in a neonate is rare.

(d) This theory also explains why the large majority of branchial cysts have no internal opening or at best, a tract with an ill-defined termination. But a skin pit usually found in the lower neck does have a big tract, with no cysts in the tract and no internal opening. These pits are probably unconnected with branchial cysts and are probably due to malfusion in the development of neck skin.

In summary therefore, cysts with a proven internal opening are probably derived from the second or first branchial pouch, but the majority, without an internal opening, are probably due to epithelial remnants in lymph nodes. The lesion is therefore probably neither 'branchial' nor 'congenital'.

Clinical features

Sixty per cent occur in men and 40% in women; the peak age incidence is the third decade, the range being from 1–70 years. Two out of three are on the left and one in three are on the right. (Two per cent are bilateral.) Two-thirds are anterior to sternomastoid in the upper third of the neck and the remainder are in the middle and lower thirds, the parotid, the pharynx and the posterior triangle (Fig. 22.5).

The presenting features are:

Continuous swelling	80%
Intermittent swelling	20%
Pain	30%
Infection	15%
Pressure symptoms	5%

Seventy per cent are cystic on palpation and 30% are solid.

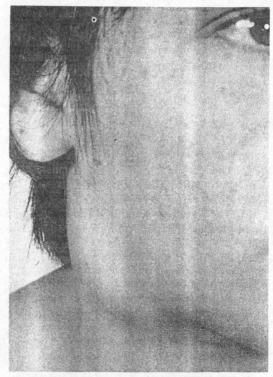

FIG. 22.5. A branchial cyst presenting in the classical site in the anterior border of the sternomastoid at the junction of the upper third and lower two-thirds.

Pathology

Cysts are usually lined by stratified squamous epithelium but may be lined by non-ciliated columnar epithelium. More than 80% have lymphoid tissue in the wall; this may be due to chronic infection or may indicate origin from a lymph node. The cyst contains straw coloured fluid in which cholesterol crystals can be found.

Treatment

Branchial cysts should be removed and a search made for a tract and an internal opening.

A carotid angiogram should be done to exclude a chemodectoma if there is direct or transmitted pulsation and the cyst feels solid.

Branchial fistulae and tracts should be dealt with by an elliptical excision of the pit and an initial dissection of the tract to as high a level as possible. A second skin incision should then be made at the highest level of dissection to complete the removal – the so called 'step-ladder' method.

Branchogenic carcinoma

Up to 1950 over 250 cases had been described. In that year Hayes Martin suggested that these were all metastatic deposits in a lymph node from an occult primary. He suggested four criteria that must apply if such a diagnosis is to be made [33].

(1) The carcinoma should be demonstrated as arising in the wall of a branchial cyst.

(2) The tumour should occur in a line running from a point just anterior to the tragus along the anterior border of sternomastoid to the clavicle.

(3) The histology should be compatible with an origin from the tissue found in branchial vestigia.

(4) No other primary should become evident in a 5-year follow-up.

Since then only fifteen cases of branchogenic carcinoma have been presented and of these only three fulfil Martin's criteria. Branchogenic carcinoma is therefore a real entity but extremely rare. Treatment is by radical neck dissection.

Laryngocoele

Pathology

In Britain the incidence is approximately 1 per $2\frac{1}{2}$ million population per year [34]. The sex incidence is 5:1 in favour of men and the peak age incidence is 50–60 years. Only one case has been reported in a neonate [35], but it is possible that this was a laryngeal cyst. Eighty-two per cent were in Caucasians. Eighty-five per cent are unilateral and 15% bilateral. They can be external (30%) where the sac arises from the laryngeal ventricle and expands into the neck through the thyrohyoid membrane, internal (20%) where it arises from the laryngeal ventricle and stays

within the larynx presenting in the vallecula, or combined (50%). Laryngocoeles are lined by columnar ciliated epithelium whereas simple laryngeal cysts are lined by squamous epithelium.

It has long been held that laryngocoeles are due to 'blowing' hobbies or jobs such as trumpet playing or glass blowing. A careful review of the published cases reveals at most four patients subject to these habits so that this theory appears to be untrue. Of more importance is the coexistence of a carcinoma or papilloma of the larynx which acts as a valve allowing air under pressure into the ventricle. External laryngocoeles can be found in 16% of laryngectomy specimens in laryngeal carcinoma as opposed to 2% in laryngectomy specimens for piriform sinus cancer [36]. The ventricle in these cases of laryngeal cancer was also significantly higher than that in patients with pharyngeal cancer due to increased air pressure consequent upon obstruction by the laryngeal carcinoma.

Lower animals have air sacs, e.g. the cheek pouch of monkeys, the fish pouch of pelicans, the tracheal sacs of emus, the syrinx of male quacking birds, etc. Lateral laryngeal sacs are well developed in certain anthropoid apes and are a means of enabling the animal to rebreathe while holding its breath for long periods.

Laryngocoeles in man therefore are almost certainly atavistic remnants corresponding to these lateral air sacs. On occasion they become manifest due to an increase in intralaryngeal air pressure due to blowing or coughing.

Clinical features

The commonest presenting features are hoarseness and a swelling in the neck. The third commonest symptom is stridor which can come on very suddenly over a period of a few days or even hours in a patient who had previously only mild symptoms for months or years. Other presenting symptoms are dysphagia, sore throat, snoring, pain or cough. Ten per cent present with infected sacs – pyocoeles – and because of the mixture of infection and air on the radiograph a diagnosis of gas gangrene is sometimes made. On palpation, the swelling, which is usually large and over the thyrohyoid membrane, can be emptied easily.

A plain radiograph of the neck is diagnostic

showing an air-filled sac. To diagnose smaller laryngocoeles one must keep the condition in mind and X-ray every patient with hoarseness since this is the commonest presenting symptom. This radiograph should be done with the glottis open since the detection rate falls markedly when the larynx is under tension [37] (Fig. 22.6). All patients with a laryngocoele should have a careful laryngoscopy to look for carcinoma.

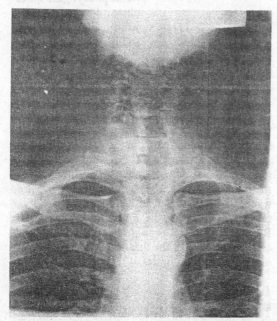

FIG. 22.6. Radiograph showing bilateral laryngocoeles.

Treatment

All laryngocoeles big enough to present in the neck should be removed. The most thorough method is to remove the superior half of the thyroid ala, after raising a perichondrial flap, to get at the neck of the sac. The ventricle is closed and the closure is reinforced by the perichondrial flap.

If the patient presents with a pyocoele this should be treated with antibiotics before surgery.

Internal laryngocoeles can be uncapped endoscopically; the scarring often stops recurrence. If they are large or recur a similar operation to that described above should be done to remove them.

INFECTIVE NECK LUMPS

Tuberculous cervical adenitis

Pathology

The condition is not common in USA or Europe, but it is still common in Asia and Africa. There are 32 000 new cases of tuberculosis (TB) in the USA each year and 5% of these (1600) get cervical lymphadenitis.

Where the incidence of TB is low primary infections are acquired later and so it is young adults who get TB nodes [38]. In Britain, the maximum age incidence is 5–9 years, but one in three is over the age of 25 [39].

The bacillus, which is usually the human variety, reaches the lymph nodes by direct drainage or by haematogenous spread. The incidence of coexisting pulmonary TB is less than 5%. In one series almost half of the tonsils removed showed evidence of TB, and it thus appeared that the tonsil was the source and that the cervical adenitis was precipitated by an attack of acute tonsillitis [39]. Once the bacillus has entered the host further exposure is not necessary to trigger off the adenopathy.

Clinical features

Most patients give a fairly long history and usually seek medical advice because the lumps have become painful. In Asia the presentation is different: 20% have discharging sinuses, 10% a cold abscess and 10% are adherent to the skin; in these patients all have a negative chest X-ray [40].

Ninety per cent are unilateral and 90% involve only one gland group, the commonest being the deep jugular chain followed by the nodes in the submandibular region and then those of the posterior triangle.

Diagnosis is by a positive tuberculin skin test, demonstration of AAFB in the biopsy and growth of *M. tuberculosis* from the biopsy. In the USA patients should also have histoplasmin and coccidioidin skin tests. The differential diagnosis is between lymphoma and metastatic cancer. The absence of a primary tumour in a young adult and the length of history usually makes the latter diagnosis improbable.

Treatment

The treatment is an excisional biopsy followed by 9–12 months of anti-tubercular chemotherapy. If the glands are very large and matted local removal is dangerous since the glands are often attached to the internal jugular vein. A functional neck dissection should then be done preserving the sternomastoid, accessory nerve, and jugular vein if possible [40]. In a child it is usually wise to remove and histologically examine the tonsils before removing the lymph glands.

If removal is not followed immediately by chemotherapy a sinus forms with persistent drainage and later ugly scars.

Sarcoidosis

Sarcoidosis presenting as cervical adenitis with no other manifestation of the disease is extremely rare. The neck glands are not often involved in this condition even when it is generalized. It is almost impossible therefore to make a pre-operative diagnosis, and a biopsy is always needed. The histological characteristic is the absence of caseation. Diagnosis may be confirmed by the Kveim skin test.

Neck space infections

Neck space infections are very rare and there is confusion about how many neck spaces there are: estimates vary from 13–20 [41–43]. A fascial space is an area of loose connective tissue bounded by dense connective tissue called fascia. It is a matter of opinion how thick connective tissue must be before it is called fascia and this is where the disagreement as to the number of spaces arises. Knowledge of the anatomy of the areas in which infection tended to collect was important in the pre-antibiotic days from the point of view of routes of spread, complications, and surgical drainage [43], but nowadays knowledge of three spaces will allow management of 90% of patients.

Anatomy

The spaces listed and described by Hollinshead [41] are as follows:

Below the hyoid   – carotid sheath
pretracheal space
retrovisceral space
visceral space
prevertebral space
Above the hyoid   – mandibular space
submaxillary space
masticator space
parotid space
Peripharyngeal area – retropharyngeal space
lateral pharyngeal space
submandibular space
Intrapharyngeal area – paratonsillar space

Nowadays abscesses usually only occur in the retropharyngeal, lateral pharyngeal and submandibular spaces.

Retropharyngeal space. This space lies between the pharynx and the posterior layer of the deep fascia which bounds the prevertebral space. It separates the pharynx from the vertebral column and extends from the base of skull to the posterior mediastinium as far as the bifurcation of the trachea. Anteriorly it connects with the pretracheal space so that infections can spread via this latter space to the anterior mediastinium. But mediastinitis due to a retropharyngeal abscess is rare [44]. In the infant this space contains one or two lymph nodes.

Lateral pharyngeal space. This is more commonly known as the parapharyngeal space; it lies lateral to the pharynx connecting with the retropharyngeal space posteriorly. Laterally it is bounded by the lateral pterygoid muscles and the sheath of the parotid gland. It extends from the base of the skull to the level of the hyoid bone where it is limited by the sheath of the submandibular gland. This sheath is also connected to the sheaths of the stylohyoid muscle and the posterior belly of the digastric muscle.

The carotid sheath is bounded anterosuperiorly by the pterygomandibular raphe and the spaces around the floor of the mouth anteroinferiorly.

This space is prone to infection because of its close connection to the tongue, teeth, parotid, submandibular gland and tonsils.

Submandibular space. This is bounded above by

the mucous membrane of the floor of the mouth and tongue and below by the deep fascia that extends from the hyoid to the mandible.

It is divided into two by the mylohyoid muscle and so the submandibular gland, which is wrapped around the mylohyoid muscle, extends into both parts of the space. The space superior to the mylohyoid muscle is called the sublingual space and contains the sublingual gland. The space inferior to the muscle is the submaxillary space which contains the submandibular gland. Anteriorly lies the submental space between the two anterior bellies of digastric.

Infections of this space are known as Ludwig's angina.

Clinical features and management

Retropharyngeal abscess

This abscess in infants is due to a lymphadenitis secondary to an upper respiratory tract infection. The child has a sore throat; examination shows a swelling behind an otherwise normal tonsil. The temperature is elevated to 101–102° F and the child is ill. The swelling may obstruct the posterior nares and push the soft palate down. Respiratory obstruction is an ever-present danger because a child's spine is short and his larynx is high. (In a 9-month-old infant, the epiglottis is at the level of the atlas.)

Radiographs of the neck show a large retropharyngeal swelling. Treatment is by incision and drainage in the tonsil position.

In an adult, a retropharyngeal abscess usually signifies a tuberculous infection of the cervical spine. It is of insidious onset with a low grade fever. Pus must be obtained to confirm the diagnosis which is also suggested on a radiograph of the cervical spine. Treatment is by antituberculous chemotherapy.

Parapharyngeal abscess

This is more common in adults than children. It is a complication of tonsillectomy or tonsillitis in about 60% of patients and a complication of infection or extraction of the lower third molar in a further 30%.

Infection of the petrous apex can rarely rupture directly into the space. Infection of the mas-toid tip can also enter the space via the digastric sheath.

There is fever and marked trismus because of involvement of the medial pterygoid muscle. The tonsil is pushed medially but looks normal. The most marked swelling is in the neck at the posterior part of the middle third of sternomastoid. Each patient should be given at least 48 hours treatment with an antibiotic, but by the time most patients have a swollen neck incision and drainage will be required.

Ludwig's angina

This is a rapidly swelling cellulitis of the floor of the mouth and submandibular space secondary to soft tissue infection, tonsillar infection and infection of the lower premolar and molar teeth. Over 80% of patients have dental disease, and in these patients the lower molars are set eccentrically with the roots closer to the inner than the outer side of the jaw, or the roots of the second and third molars may lie inferior to the mylohyoid line. Root abscesses of these teeth therefore drain into the submaxillary rather than sublingual space. This space may be affected with minimal discomfort from the tooth; pain comes from tension within the bone but if this gives way and drains there is no dental pain. In cases of dental origin the most usual organisms are *Streptococcus viridans* and *B. coli*.

When the infection spreads to the sublingual space the floor of the mouth becomes very swollen and appears as a roll of oedematous tissue rising to the level of the biting edge of the teeth. The tongue is elevated posterosuperiorly and respiratory obstruction is a danger. The patient is very ill with a temperature of over 101° F with pain, trismus and salivation.

Treatment is by antibiotics; incision and drainage should be postponed as long as possible because pus is seldom found.

Infectious mononucleosis

Pathology

This condition is probably caused by the Epstein–Barr virus although a similar disease can be caused by cytomegalovirus infection. It is infectious, common in young people and spread by personal contact such as kissing.

The disease is self-limiting, but it has been postulated that it is an atypical benign form of leukaemia. Atypical mononuclear cells derived from lymphocytes form 10–20% of white cells in the peripheral blood and infiltrate the spleen and lymph nodes (and occasionally the liver, brain, kidneys and bone marrow).

Clinical features

The presenting symptom is often a sore throat with high fever, anorexia and general malaise. The tonsils enlarge and are covered by exudate. The cervical lymph nodes are enlarged and rubbery. Skin rashes, mild jaundice, aseptic meningitis and peripheral neuropathies occur. Prolonged debility and depression often complicate recovery. More than 10% of mononuclear cells are found on the blood film, a monospot test is positive and a Paul Bunnel test is positive with a titre greater than 1:256. The latter test is positive in less than 80% of patients. Even in the absence of jaundice the serum bilirubin and aminotransferases may be raised.

Treatment

Antibiotics are contra-indicated, especially Ampicillin which often causes a skin rash in this condition. Patients should not be allowed back to work if there is persistent adenopathy to prevent relapse.

Brucellosis

Pathology

The host for the brucella organism is the cow for *B. abortus*, the pig for *B. suis* and the goat for *B. melitensis*. Man contracts brucellosis by contact or by consuming products from these animals. It is commonest in farmers, vets and abattoir workers.

Clinical features

The varied symptoms makes diagnosis difficult. Common symptoms are: an unexplained fever of the Pel–Ebstein type which continues for some weeks and subsides only to return a few weeks later, sweating, debility, fatigue, anorexia, sore throat and headache. Examination reveals neck node enlargement, hepatosplenomegaly and arthralgia. Diagnosis rests largely on suspicion and is confirmed by agglutination tests.

Treatment

The acute form responds to tetracycline, but the chronic form is resistant.

Toxoplasmosis

In a patient with all the clinical manifestations of infectious mononucleosis and a negative Paul Bunnel and monospot test, this diagnosis must be considered. It is due to infection with the small protozoon *Toxoplasma gondii*. Children can acquire it from their pets since infection is widespread among many domestic and wild animals in Europe and South America. Pregnant women can pass it on to the fetus causing death *in utero*, premature birth or congenital malformations including macular degeneration and ocular nystagmus. Diagnosis is made serologically or by lymph node biopsy.

The illness can last a few days or less commonly weeks or months.

Treatment is with pyrimethamine and a sulphonamide.

TUMOURS OF NEUROGENOUS ORIGIN

Peripheral nerve tumours

The neural crest differentiates into the Schwann cell and the sympathicoblast; this latter cell gives rise to paraganglionic cells from which arise chemodectomas and glomus jugulare tumours, and ganglionic cells from which arise benign and malignant ganglioma. The Schwann cell gives rise to the Schwannoma (neurilemmoma) and the neurofibroma (Table 22.1). Nerve tumours are rare, forming only about 1% of all head and neck tumours.

TABLE 22.1

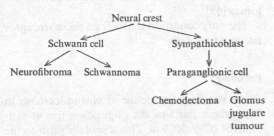

Pathology

The thin outer sheet of nerve is called the neurilemma and the inner sheath of Schwann is the neurolemma. Tumours arising from the inner nerve sheath are often called neurilemmomas which is wrong, as is neuronoma. The correct name is Schwannoma and this is clinically different from neurofibroma.

Peripheral nerve tumours are commoner in the head and neck than the rest of the body and are commonest in the lateral part of the neck. They arise from the cervical and brachial plexus and ninth to twelfth cranial nerves, but most commonly from the vagus within the carotid sheath. They are all commoner in women than men [45]. The differentiating features between Schwannoma and neurofibroma are shown in Table 22.2.

Histologically, *Schwannomas* show well-developed cylindrical bands of Schwann cells and delicate connective tissue fibres with a tendency toward pallisading of the nuclei about a central

TABLE 22.2. Showing differences between Schwannoma and neurofibroma

Schwannoma	Neurofibroma
Solitary	Usually occur as part of the syndrome of multiple neurofibromatosis
Never associated with von Recklinghausen's syndrome	Often associated with von Recklinghausen's syndrome
Painful and tender	Asymptomatic
Encapsulated	Non encapsulated
Seldom malignant	8% malignant

mass of cytoplasm (Verocay bodies). This is known as Antoni type A tissue whereas Antoni type B tissue is a loosely arranged stroma in which the fibres and cells form no distinctive pattern. These two types may be mixed with one preponderating. No neurites traverse the lesion.

Neurofibromas show a compact arrangement of spindle type cells arranged in streams and twists. They can present as cutaneous or subcutaneous masses or as a deep-seated plexiform neuroma involving major nerve trunks.

Other neurogenous tumours – ganglioneuroma, Schwannoma, glioma, meningioma, paraganglioma, neuronaevus – occur more often in patients with neurofibromatosis than in the general population. This suggests that neurofibromas are derived from a disseminated neuroblastoma or aberrantly migrating neural crest cells.

Gangliomas are also called ganglioneuromas; they are very rare. They usually arise from a cervical sympathetic ganglion, are firm, smooth, well encapsulated and microscopically contain ganglion cells and neurites. Twenty-five per cent are estimated to be malignant and these neuroblastomas grow relentlessly.

Post-operative neuromas are the result of amputation or trauma to the nerve. They are not true tumours but represent attempts by the damaged nerve to repair itself; the axis cylinders become enmeshed in Schwann cells and scar tissue. If this process becomes hyperactive the neuroma becomes clinically obvious and the patient experiences localized pain and tenderness.

Malignant change in nerve sheath tumours in the head and neck is very rare: only 1 sarcomatous change was described in a series of 303 of solitary nerve tumours [46]. But such change occurs in from 10–15% of patients with multiple neurofibromatosis. The only thing that differentiates a neurogenous sarcoma from a fibrosarcoma is its origin from a nerve trunk.

Surgery in neurofibromatosis does not predispose to sarcomatous change. Rapid growth suggests malignant change; pain and paraesthesia occur when a large nerve is involved. These tumours do not metastasize to regional lymph nodes, but to the lungs. Two in three recur locally and may metastasize later. Low-grade tumours grow slowly and anaplastic ones quickly.

Clinical features

These tumours enlarge slowly over a period of years with no symptoms and a painless neck mass as the only sign. While the tumour remains benign there is no interference with nerve function apart from pressure on the sympathetic chain which soon shows as a Horner's syndrome. Even if the tumour becomes malignant, the nerve may still function when the tumour reaches a large size. Diagnosis is from other lateral neck masses; an angiogram is usually required. If the tumour presents as a pharyngeal mass diagnosis is from other parapharyngeal space tumours such as deep lobe parotid tumours, minor salivary gland tumours, chemodectoma, lymphoma and hibernoma.

Treatment

The diagnosis of a solitary nerve tumour is made by excising it which is also the treatment.

The nerve with which the tumour is associated only becomes evident at operation in one patient out of four [47]. The nerve may be stretched over the capsule of the tumour or less commonly the tumour can be in the central core of the nerve with the fibres spread around it. Every effort should be made to preserve the nerve.

Post-operative neuromas must be excised to distinguish them from recurrent cancer.

The best treatment for malignant nerve tumours is *en bloc* excision of the area. Conley quotes a cure rate of 80% for well differentiated malignant Schwannoma but only 20% for the undifferentiated type [48].

Chemodectomas

Nests of non-chromaffin paraganglionic cells derived from the neural crest occur on the carotid bulb, the jugular bulb, in the cavity of the middle ear, and in the ganglion nodosum of the vagus nerve, the adventitia of the ascending aorta, the aortic, innominate and pulmonary arteries and in the ciliary ganglion of the orbit. Carotid body cells act as chemoreceptors so that it is suggested that tumours of these cells be called chemodectomas [49].

The only condition that affects chemoreceptor tissue is neoplasia.

Pathology

There is a high incidence of chemodectoma in Peru where most of the population live at altitudes of 2000–5000 m. This is probably due to the fact that chronic hypoxia at high altitudes leads to carotid body hyperplasia. A raised incidence has also been noted in other series from high altitude sites such as Colorado and Mexico City.

In other areas this tumour is rare: there have been just over 500 cases described in the literature.

The average age of presentation ranges from 35–50 years, the youngest reported case being 12 years [50–53]. The sex incidence is roughly equal.

There is a striking family history of up to 10% and also a tendency to bilateral tumours, tumours of other similar cells and phaeochromocytoma. Twenty-five per cent are bilateral in those with a positive family history compared to 30% in those with no family history [54].

The tumour is firmly adherent to the bifurcation of the common carotid artery, is globular or ovoid but seldom grows to more than 4–5 cm. The cut surface is homogenous, solid and grey-brown in colour.

Histology shows a marked similarity to the architecture of the normal carotid body: large uniform epithelioid cells surrounded by a vascular stroma. There are capillaries (shown by silver staining) in the fibrous septa between the cell nests. These tumours do not secrete.

Proven metastases are very rare, there being only thirty cases reported and not all of these stand scrutiny. There have been no reports of autopsies in which the death of the patient was attributed to a chemodectoma of the carotid body. Many of the cases claimed as malignant have in fact turned out to be due to metastases from a papillary carcinoma of the thyroid.

Clinical features

All patients present with a painless lump in the

neck which is palpable in the region of the carotid bulb. It is said to move from side to side but not up and down – this is not helpful because nearly all neck lumps in this area behave like that be they cystic or neoplastic.

There is always a long history varying from 4·5 to 7 yrs. This is helpful in differentiating a lump in this site from a lymphoma or a metastatic gland, but is compatible with a tuberculous gland or a branchial cyst. About 30% of patients have a pharyngeal mass pushing the tonsil medially and anteriorly; this mass should not be biopsied.

The normal site of growth of the tumour is from the inner aspect of the notch of the bifurcation of the carotid artery causing displacement and separation of the internal and external carotid arteries. If growth occurs mainly on the medial side (which is the usual side of origin) a pharyngeal swelling occurs with no lateral neck swelling. The tumour may grow up the vessels to the base of the skull.

The mass is firm and rubbery and usually demonstrates transmitted rather than expansile pulsation. A bruit may be present and the mass may decrease in size with carotid compression to refill in stages with each pulsation. Rarely patients complain of mild dysphagia or discomfort. Large tumours may involve the ninth, tenth, eleventh and twelfth cranial nerves and occasionally the sympathetic chain causing a Horner's syndrome.

Diagnosis

The diagnosis is usually erroneously made at an operation for biopsy of a neck mass. The diagnosis can be made provisionally on the history of a long standing neck mass in a young patient and on physical examination. Whenever it is suspected a carotid angiogram should be done for the following reasons:

(1) To see if there is separation of the internal and external carotid arteries with a tumour circulation in the mass. The feeding vessel arises from the external carotid or vertebral artery.

(2) To determine the extent of the tumour.

(3) To see if there is cross circulation. If the tumour is to be resected and the artery grafted it is essential to know about cross circulation so that the patient and the surgeon can balance the risk of the procedure against the possible benefits.

An angiogram nowadays in young fit people carries very little risk. The radiologist should use fast injection rates and rapid serial filming.

In the capillary phase there is an internal blush and the draining veins are usually dilated. The differentiation between chemodectoma and glomus vagale tumour is based only on the position of the tumour. The technique can be enhanced by the use of subtraction techniques. The investigation rules out the need for percutaneous aspiration biopsy which is dangerous and often unhelpful.

Treatment

From 1930–50 various reported series put the operative mortality rate at around 35% and the morbidity rate at 45% including frequent hemiplegia. It was concluded 'that it would seem doubtful whether anything more than a diagnostic biopsy should be done where tumours are without symptoms and growing slowly' [55]. With advances in arterial surgery, carotid bypass, hypothermia and a better understanding of the physiology of cerebral blood flow allowing better selection, the mortality from the operation has fallen dramatically. Although Westbury [52] states 'left alone, the patient runs the risks of a progressively enlarging tumour of uncertain innocence in the neck' most would now agree that the mere presence of a carotid body tumour does not justify an attempt at removal. The indications for removal [48] are:

(1) Tumours which are histologically and clinically malignant and which are resectable.

(2) Tumours growing aggressively.

(3) Patients in good health under 50 years of age with a small or medium sized tumour.

(4) Those tumours which have extended into the pharynx and palate and are interfering with swallowing, speaking and breathing.

Since no patient has died from the tumour the indications for surgery should be as conservative as possible.

It was originally thought that chemodectomas and all related tumours were radio-resistant, but some have now been shown to respond to radiotherapy. Radiotherapy should therefore be used in patients who should have surgery but who refuse, for poor risk patients, or in metastatic disease.

Glomus vagale tumours

This tumour is extremely rare [56]. It presents as a mass at the angle of the jaw, rather too high for a diagnosis of chemodectoma and too low for a diagnosis of a parotid neoplasm. Some cause pain and discomfort and a few a pharyngeal mass. Angiography shows an abnormal tumour circulation from the external carotid, at a higher location than that of a carotid body tumour.

After removal the patient will have a vocal cord paralysis in the cadaveric position and should be offered a teflon injection soon after the operation.

LYMPHOMA

Some of the most significant recent advances in the treatment of cancer have taken place in this condition in the last decade. It may present in any head and neck site, most commonly in the cervical lymph nodes, and the otolaryngologist will be involved in diagnosis including the biopsy. Here his involvement ends however because the accurate assessment of the staging and typing of the disease and its treatment is now done in most centres by a specialist multidisciplinary group.

The precise histological type is important and a simple classification on which treatment is based is shown in Table 22.3. The prognosis is closely linked to the histologic type.

Hodgkin's lymphoma

Table 22.4 shows the clinical staging of the disease. The best treatment is radiotherapy and all the investigations are designed to find the extent of the disease and whether or not it is technically possible to irradiate it all. If it is not possible then chemotherapy must be used. In general the prognosis is worst in elderly males with disease of mixed cellularity or lymphocytic depletion. It is best in younger women with lymphocytic predominant disease or nodular sclerosis.

Investigations
The investigations are as follows:

Blood count: This may show an eosinophilia and the ESR will be raised.

Chest radiograph: Tomography of the hilum may be especially helpful.

Gland biopsy: It is necessary to remove a whole gland and not do an incisional biopsy. Fixing the

TABLE 22.3

	New nomenclature	Old nomenclature
Hodgkin's lymphoma	Lymphocytic predominant	Paragranuloma
	Nodular sclerosis mixed cellularity	Granuloma
	Lymphocytic depletion	Sarcoma
Non-Hodgkin's lymphoma (N.H.L.)	Follicular lymphoma	Follicular lymphoma
	Well differentiated lymphocytic lymphoma Poorly differentiated lymphocytic lymphoma	Lymphosarcoma
	Histiocytic lymphoma	Reticulum cell sarcoma

gland in formalin spoils it for immunological studies so it is examined fresh. Frozen section diagnosis is unhelpful.

TABLE 22.4. Clinical staging of Hodgkin's disease (Ann Arbor)

Stage I	Involvement of a single lymph node region (I) or of a single extra lymphatic organ or site (I E).
Stage II	Involvement of two or more lymph node regions on the same side of the diaphragm (II) or localized involvement of extra lymphatic organ or site and one or more lymph node regions on the same side of the diaphragm (II E).
Stage III	Involvement of lymph node regions on both sides of the diaphragm (III) ± involvement of the spleen (III S) or localized extra lymphatic organ or site (III E).
Stage IV	Diffuse or disseminated involvement of one or more extra lymphatic organs or tissues, e.g. liver, marrow, pleura, lung, bone and skin.

Systemic symptoms = Weight loss, fever, sweating. If absent = 'A'. If present = 'B'.

Pedal lymphangiography: This assesses the spread to abdominal lymph nodes. The dye stays in the glands and so response to treatment can be gauged by radiography.

Staging laparotomy: The major benefit from this lies in detecting occult disease in small spleens. Clinical examination of the spleen is unhelpful; if the spleen is palpable there is only a 70% chance that it will be involved and conversely the spleen is impalpable in 50% of patients with Hodgkin's disease.

Bone marrow biopsy: This is done with a trephine of the iliac crest. If positive the disease is stage IV.

Treatment

This field is changing rapidly but currently the correct treatment is radiotherapy for localized disease plus pulsed multiple chemotherapy, e.g. MOPP (mustine, Oncovin (vincristine), prednisone, procarbazine) for disseminated disease. If the correct treatment is applied then over 80% of patients in the early stages of the disease survive 5 years.

Non-Hodgkin's lymphoma

The principles of management of non-Hodgkin's lymphoma are the same as for Hodgkin's disease. Histological typing is vital to assess the prognosis which is best with the follicular lymphoma and worst in histiocytic lymphoma. Staging the disease is also essential because all of the disease must be treated or else it will cause later symptoms in the untreated areas. The pattern of recurrence is not predictable as it is in Hodgkin's disease, making it difficult to know how extensive fields of radiotherapy should be. Localized disease is treated with radiotherapy and generalized disease is treated with chemotherapy.

References

[1] LERNHER A. (1843) Die Angebeorenen Zystem — Hygrome und die ihnen verwandten Geschwulste in anatomischer diagnostischer und therapeutischer Beziehung, p. 76. Giessen, Germany: G. G. Heger, Vater.

[2] SABIN F. R. (1901) On the origin of the lymphatic system from the veins and the development of the lymph heart and thoracic duct in the pig. *American Journal of Anatomy* **1**, 367.

[3] SABIN F. R. (1909) The lymphatic system in human embryos with a consideration of the morphology of the system as a whole. *American Journal of Anatomy* **9**, 43.

[4] DOWD C. N. (1913) Hygroma cysticum colli. *Annals of Surgery* **58**, 112.

[5] GOETSCH E. (1938) Hygroma colli cysticum and hygroma axillare. *Archives of Surgery* **36**, 394.

[6] LANDING B. H. & FARBER S. (1956) Tumours of the cardiovascular system. *Atlas of Tumour Pathology.* Washington, D.C.: Armed Forces Institute of Pathology.

[7] BILL A. H. & SUMNER, D. S. (1965) A unified concept of lymphangioma and cystic hygroma. *Surgery Gynecology & Obstetrics* **120**, 79.

[8] WARD P., HARRIS P. F. & DOWNEY W. (1970) Surgical approach to cystic hygroma of the neck. *Archives of Otolaryngology* **91**, 508.

[9] ANDERSON D. H. (1951) Tumours of infancy and childhood. *Cancer* **4**, 890.

[10] MOUSATTOS G. H. & BAFFES T. B. 1963) Cervical masses in infants and children. *Paediatrics* **32**, 251.

[11] BROOKS J. E. (1973) Cystic hygroma of the neck. *Laryngoscope* **83**, 117.

[12] WOODRING A. J. (1968) Cervical cystic hygroma: a review of the literature and report of an unusual case. *Annals of Otolaryngology, Rhinology & Laryngology* 77, 978.

[13] BROOMHEAD I. W. (1964) Cystic hygroma of the neck. *British Journal of Plastic Surgery* 17, 285.

[14] GROSS R. E. & GOERINGER C. F. (1939) Cystic hygroma of the neck. *Surgery Gynecology & Obstetrics* 87, 599.

[15] BATSAKIS J. G. (1971) Non-odontogenic and fissural cysts. *O.R.L. Digest* 33, 19.

[16] HAJDU S. I. & HAJDU E. O. (1967) Malignant teratoma of the neck. *Archives of Pathology* 83, 567.

[17] TAYLOR B. W., ERICH J. B. & DOCHERTY M. B. (1966) Dermoids of the head and neck. *Minnesota Medicine* 49, 1535.

[18] KATZ A. D. (1974) Midline dermoid tumours of the neck. *Archives of Surgery* 109, 322.

[19] SEWARD G. R. (1965) Dermoid cysts of the floor of the mouth. *British Journal of Oral Surgery* 3, 36.

[20] WARD P. H., STRAHAN R. W., ACQUARELLI M. *et al.* (1970) The many faces of cysts of the thyroglossal duct. *Transactions of the American Academy of Ophthalmology and Otolaryngology* 74, 310.

[21] BROWN P. M. & JUDD E. S. (1961) Thyroglossal duct cyst and sinuses: Results of radical (Sistrunk) operation. *American Journal of Surgery* 102, 494.

[22] SCHLANGE H. (1893) Ueber die Fistula colli congenita. *Archives für Klinische Chirurgie* 46, 390.

[23] SISTRUNK W. E. (1920) The surgical treatment of cysts of the thyroglossal tract. *Annals of Surgery* 71, 121.

[24] PAGE C. P., KEMMERER W. T., HAFF R. C. & MAZZAFERRI E. L. (1974) Thyroid carcinomas arising in thyroglossal ducts. *Annals of Surgery* 180, 799.

[25] BAILEY H. (1933) The clinical aspects of branchial fistulae. *British Journal of Surgery* 21, 173.

[26] FRASER J. E. (1923) The nomenclature of diseased states caused by certain vestigial structures in the neck. *British Journal of Surgery* 11, 131.

[27] FRASER J. E. (1926) The disappearance of the pre-cervical sinus. *Journal of Anatomy* 61, 132.

[28] RAVEN R. W. (1933) Pouches of the pharynx and oesophagus with special reference to the embryological and morphological aspects. *British Journal of Surgery* 21, 235.

[29] ASCHERSON F. M. (1832) De fistulis colli congenitis adjecta fissurarum branchialium in mammalibus avibusque historia succincta. 22 p. 4° Berolini, apund C. H. Jonas.

[30] WENGLOWSKI R. (1912) Ueber die Halsfisteln und Cysten. *Archives für Klinische Chirurgie*.

[31] KING E. S. J. (1949) The lateral lympho-epithelial cyst of the neck ('Branchial cyst'). *Australian & New Zealand Journal of Surgery* 19, 109.

[32] BHASKAR S. N. & BERNIER J. L. (1959) Histogenesis of branchial cysts; a report of 468 cases. *American Journal of Pathology* 35, 407.

[33] MARTIN H., MORFIT H. M. & EHRLICH H. (1950) Case for branchiogenic cancer (malignant branchioma). *Annals of Surgery* 132, 867.

[34] STELL P. M. & MARAN A. G. D. (1975) Laryngocoele. *Journal of Laryngology and Otology* 89, 915.

[35] HOLINGER P. H. (1961) Clinical aspects of congenital anomalies of the larynx, trachea, bronchi and oesophagus. *Journal of Laryngology and Otology* 75, 1.

[36] GERARD-MARCHANT R., MICHEAU C. & CACHIN Y. (1969) Epithélioma laryngé et laryngocèle pt. 1. Etudes anatomico-pathologique et statistique. *Annales d'Otolaryngologie (Paris)* 86, 431.

[37] MACFIE D. D. (1966) Asymptomatic laryngoceles in wind instrument bandsmen. *Archives of Otolaryngology* 83, 270.

[38] CANTRELL R. W., JENSEN J. H. & REID D. (1974) Diagnosis and management of tuberculous cervical adenitis. *Archives of Otolaryngology* 101, 53.

[39] WILMOT T. J., JAMES E. F. & REILLY L. V. (1957) Tuberculous cervical adenitis. *Lancet* 2, 1184.

[40] MULAY S. G. & HIRANANDANI L. H. (1970) A clinical study and the surgical management of two hundred and fifty cases of tubercular cervical lymphadenitis. *Journal of Laryngology and Otology* 84, 781.

[41] HOLLINSHEAD W. H. (1954) *Anatomy for Surgeons*, Vol. 1. London: Cassell and Company Ltd.

[42] GRODINSKY M. & HOLYOKE E. A. (1938) The fasciae and fascial spaces of the head, neck and adjacent regions. *American Journal of Anatomy* 63, 367.

[43] COLLIER F. A. & YGLESIAS L. (1937) The relation of the spread of infection to fascial planes in the neck and thorax. *Surgery* 1, 323.

[44] PEARSE H. E. (1938) Mediastinitis following cervical suppuration. *Annals of surgery* 108, 588.

[45] BATSAKES J. G. (1973) *Tumours of the Head and Neck*, p. 232. Baltimore: Williams & Wilkins.

[46] DAS GUPTA T. K., BRASFIELD R. D., STRONG E. W. & HAJDU S. I. (1969) Benign solitary schwannomas (neurilemmomas). *Cancer* 24, 355.

[47] KRAGH L. V., SOULE E. H. & MASSON J. K. (1960) Neurofibromatosis of the head and neck: cosmetic and reconstructive aspects. *Plastic and Reconstructive Surgery* 25, 565.

[48] CONLEY J. (1970) *Concepts in Head and Neck Surgery*. Stuttgart: Georg. Thieme Verlag.

[49] MULLIGAN R. M. (1950) Chemodectoma in the dog. *American Journal of Pathology* 26, 680.

[50] MORFIT H. M., SWAN H. & TAYLOR E. R. (1953) Carotid body tumours. *Archives of Surgery* 67, 194.

[51] PETTET J. R., WOOLNER L. B. & JUDD E. S. JR. (1953) Carotid body tumours (chemodectomas). *Annals of Surgery* 137, 465.

[52] WESTBURY G. (1960) Management of carotid body tumours. *British Journal of Surgery* 47, 605.

[53] WESTBROOK K. C., GUILLAMONDEGUI O. M., MEDELLIN H. & JESSE R. H. (1972) Chemodectomas of the neck. Selective management. *American Journal of Surgery* 124, 760.

[54] REVACK C. S., MORRIS S. E. ... ALEXANDER Q. H. (1971) Phaeochromocytomas and recurrent chemodectomas over a 25 year period. *Radiology* **100**, 53.

[55] LE COMPTE P. M. (1951) Tumours of the carotid body and related structures. *Atlas of Tumour Pathology*, sect. 4, fasc. 16. Washington D.C.: Armed Forces Institute of Pathology.

[56] WESTBURY H. (1967) Glomus intravagale tumours. *British Journal of Radiology* **40**, 148.

CHAPTER 23

Metastatic Neck Glands

Many carcinomas of the head and neck sooner or later metastasize to the lymph nodes of the neck which form a barrier that prevents further spread of the disease for many months. A carcinoma of the head and neck is assigned a stage which depends not only on the extent of the primary tumour (and the presence of distant metastases) but also on enlargement of the cervical lymph nodes. The current classification suggested by the UICC/AJC is shown in Table 23.1. This is a useful classification but is subject to some criticism. There is a great deal of observer error so that different observers only agree on the presence of palpable lymph nodes in about 70% of patients [1]. Furthermore the value of the a and b categories is doubtful since these categories depend on a clinical opinion as to whether tumour is present in a palpable node or not and must therefore be entirely subjective; previous reports [2] show that only 60% of palpable nodes contain tumour. Finally the progression from N0–N3 suggests that the prognosis diminishes in that order whereas the prognosis for bilateral nodes (N2) is usually much worse than that for fixed nodes (N3).

The approximate distribution of patients between the four categories N0–N3 is shown in Table 23.2. The four categories of the UICC/-AJC classification will be used as convenient headings to discuss various aspects of the management of metastatic nodes in the neck.

Patients with no palpable metastases (N0)

Over 40 years ago Blair & Brown [4] suggested that when an operation was carried out for a carcinoma of the mouth the glands in the neck should be cleared at the time without waiting for involvement to become evident, i.e. a so-called elective neck dissection.

The pathological argument supporting this concept is that some lymph nodes may be involved by tumour (occult nodes) and still be impalpable. The incidence of such occult nodes at various sites is given in Table 23.3 [5].

The value of prophylactic neck dissection is doubtful. A study of the subsequent course of several hundred patients with carcinomas of the larynx, hypopharynx and mouth, who were not submitted to prophylactic neck dissection showed that at all these sites only between 5 and 10% of the patients died of uncontrolled disease in the neck, the remainder either being cured, or dying of intercurrent disease, recurrence at the primary site or distant metastases [6–8]. The only patient who can theoretically be benefited by prophylactic neck dissection is the one who later dies of recurrent disease in the neck and it seems therefore that the maximum possible benefit in terms of increased survival rate is about 5–7%. Against this it must be remembered that the mortality rate of radical neck dissection is between 1 and 2% [9] so that the overall net improvement in 5-year survival figures which could theoretically be achieved by prophylactic neck dissection is reduced to around 5%.

It may be that elective neck dissection has some place in the patient who is unlikely to return for follow-up and has a tumour with a known high incidence of occult nodes such as the piriform fossa, whereas there can be little or no reason for doing the operation on a patient who can readily attend for follow-up and who has a tumour such as a laryngeal carcinoma where the incidence of occult nodes is small. In laryngeal carcinoma the incidence of occult nodes is in the region of 10–15% so that if all these patients are submitted to radical neck dissection 85–90% will suffer the increased morbidity and mortality associated with this operation to no purpose.

TABLE 23.1

N–Regional lymph nodes

N0–Regional lymph nodes not palpable
N1 – Movable homolateral nodes
    N1a – Nodes not considered to contain growth
    N1b – Nodes considered to contain growth
N2 – Movable contralateral or bilateral nodes
    N2a – Nodes not considered to contain growth
    N2b – Nodes considered to contain growth
N3 – Fixed nodes

Furthermore, it must be remembered that there is little evidence that a patient with a laryngeal carcinoma with no palpable nodes in the neck is better treated by radiotherapy [10] so that the issue of prophylactic neck dissection for laryngeal carcinoma scarcely arises in any case.

The issue therefore must remain open, and Conley's dictum (quoted by Reed & Miller, 1970) that 'there is at this time little evidence to indicate that routine elective neck dissection causes significant increase in survival and that careful follow-up and neck dissection when obvious metastases appear seriously lowers the cure rate' cannot be improved on [7].

All these arguments may in any case now be becoming superfluous because it appears that elective irradiation of the entire neck can sterilize the vast majority of occult nodes. Elective neck irradiation drastically reduced the recurrence in the same side of the neck in patients with carcinoma of the mouth, oropharynx, piriform fossa and supraglottic larynx [11]. In a further series of patients with carcinoma of the mouth, of those patients in whom the primary had been controlled by radiotherapy almost 30% later developed a metastasis in the neck, whereas no patient who had been subjected to elective neck

TABLE 23.2. Approximate incidence of lymph node metastases

N0	70%
N1	20%
N2	5%
N3	5%

TABLE 23.3. Incidence of occult nodes [5]

Supraglottic larynx	16%
Piriform sinus	38%
Base of tongue	22%
Transglottic	11%
Glottic with a fixed cord	3%

irradiation later developed a metastasis in the neck [12].

Unilateral neck glands (N1)

The standard operation for dealing with metastatic glands in the neck is that of radical neck dissection described by Crile in 1906 [13]; a further classical paper describing the indications, the technique and the complications was that of Hayes Martin [14]. It is generally accepted, at least by surgeons, that surgery is required to control lymph node metastasis in the neck since these have usually been thought not to respond to radiotherapy. Several radiotherapists have recently challenged this concept and control rates almost as good as those for surgery are now being claimed by some radiotherapists [15, 16]. It appears that small nodal metastases are more reliably sterilized than larger ones. Radiotherapy has the further advantage that if a node reappears after a course of radiotherapy a radical neck dissection can always be carried out, whereas radiotherapy can seldom be given with benefit for the usual diffuse recurrence which occurs after surgery. It remains to be seen whether radiotherapy can achieve better survival as distinct from the rather nebulous concept of 'control'.

Although the technique of radical neck dissection has been standard for many years several changes have taken place within the last 10 or 15 years, notably in the use of combined preoperative radiotherapy and surgery, in various technical modifications to reduce the incidence of complications, by way of extensions to the operation, and in the so-called functional neck dissection.

Preoperative radiotherapy

The vast majority of patients who die of head and neck carcinoma do so because of recurrence at the primary site or in the neck or at both. The causes of such recurrence could be tumour left behind at the periphery of the excision, implantation on raw surfaces at operation or squeezing of tumour emboli into veins and lymphatics during the operation. A small dose of radiotherapy (1000–2000 r) sterilizes about 98% of the cells in a tumour, thus in theory greatly reducing the chance of recurrence without at the same time increasing the chance of complications. Experiments in mice showed that preoperative radiotherapy did indeed increase the survival rate but whether this can be extrapolated to man is not certain [17].

Trials in man, which are open to some statistical objection, have shown a reduction of recurrence in the neck from approximately 35% to 70% [18, 19]. Whilst these results may indicate an improvement in survival rate and an improvement in the quality of life of the surviving patients what is certain is that preoperative radiotherapy does increase the complication rate [20]. Further work [21] suggests that careful selection of patients may define the place of preoperative radiotherapy. In a series of patients with tumours of the oropharynx, the supraglottic larynx and the hypopharynx, preoperative radiotherapy did not improve the control rate for a patient with a single ipsilateral node less than 3 cm in diameter but the recurrence rate was halved for multiple, fixed or bilateral nodes.

Prevention of complications

The incidence of major complications after radical neck dissection is quite high and can be as much as 20% [9]. Furthermore, between 1 and 2% of patients die of various complications of this operation. The major potentially lethal complications of radical neck dissection are wound breakdown and infection, necrosis of the skin flaps and rupture of the carotid arteries. It is also well known that these complications are increased by previous radiotherapy [22]. Two major modifications of technique have been introduced over the last 10 years to combat the major killing complications: modifications of the incision, and protection of the carotid sheath. The original incision introduced by Crile [13] for radical neck dissection was in the shape of a Y.

Many incisions introduced since, illustrated in Fig. 23.1, are basically similar. There are two principal departures from this: the double horizontal incision described by MacFee [23] and the half-H incision [24]. The MacFee incision (Fig. 23.2) consists of two horizontal incisions, one at about the level of the hyoid bone and one just superior to the clavicle with an intervening bridge of skin which is elevated to allow the neck dissection to proceed. Although some have opposed the use of this incision because it lengthens the time of the operation, many, including the author, have used this incision on many patients who have previously been irradiated, with very satisfactory results. A recent paper [29] shows that the blood supply of the skin of the neck is divided into two areas of distribution, one superiorly from the branches of the external carotid artery and one inferiorly from the branches of the subclavian artery. These two areas are divided by a watershed or an area of poor blood supply running in an antero-inferior direction from about the centre of the trapezius to the region of the medial end of the clavicle [25]. On theoretical grounds therefore it would seem advisable to use a ⊢ shaped incision, the horizontal limb running about the centre of the neck in the watershed and the vertical limbs running over the anterior border of the trapezius. Such an incision has proved to be satisfactory in patients who have been irradiated, although the access which it allows to the submaxillary compartment of the neck is limited.

In the patient who has been irradiated, particularly one in which a fistula is likely to form because a carcinoma in the larynx, pharynx or mouth has been resected, the carotid sheath should be protected. Two methods have been described. Muscle flaps [26] and free grafts of dermis [27]; the former method is safer than the latter. The favourite muscle to use is the levator scapulae which derives its blood supply from superiorly and anteriorly. At the end of the radical neck dissection it can therefore be divided at its inferior and posterior limits and be turned forward to be stitched over the carotid sheath, protection being completed by stitching the muscle graft to the posterior belly of the digastric superiorly and the remnant of the sternomastoid muscle inferiorly.

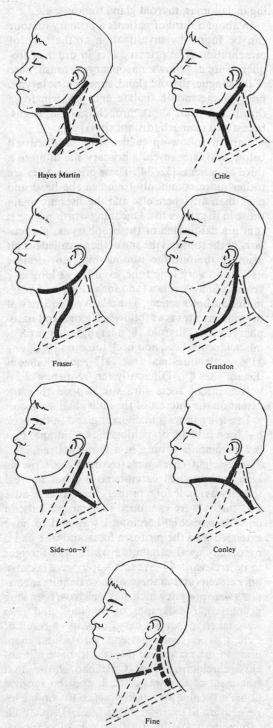

FIG. 23.1. Incisions for radical neck dissection.

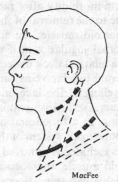

FIG. 23.2. The MacFee incision.

Extensions of radical neck dissection

Attempts have been made to widen the field removed by radical neck dissection particularly in an inferior direction into the superior mediastinum. Whilst the majority of head and neck tumours metastasize to the jugular system there are some tumours which are well known to metastasize to glands in the mediastinum notably those of the cervical oesophagus, the subglottic space and the thyroid gland. Sisson [28] has developed an operation for dissecting the superior mediastinum in safety based on a method previously described by Grillo for dealing with recurrences in the stoma after laryngectomy [29]. The principle of the operation is that a large bipedicled upper chest flap is developed, its superior incision being about at the level of the clavicle and its inferior incision being at the level of the xiphisternum. This skin flap is designed to protect the structures in the superior mediastinum which are exposed when the manubrium and the medial end of both clavicles are removed. The operation should be carried out in two stages not only for carcinomas at the sites detailed above but also for recurrence in the stoma after laryngectomy at the first stage the skin flap and muscle flap of the pectoral muscle are delayed; the pectoral muscle flap is laid over the mediastinum at the second external stage to protect the great vessels.

Functional neck dissection

Attempts have been made to reduce the morbidity after a radical neck dissection by the so-called functional, conservative techniques [30].

The long-term morbidity after radical neck dissection is due to the removal of three structures: the sternomastoid muscle, the accessory nerve and the internal jugular vein if both veins are removed in a bilateral neck dissection. Removal of both internal jugular veins can cause a very unsightly swelling of the face, in addition to a dangerous increase in intracranial pressure on rare occasions. In a functional neck dissection the entire aponeurotic system of the neck with its lymph nodes included is removed preserving the sternomastoid muscle, the accessory nerve and the internal jugular vein. Bocca reported 100 patients in whom he had carried out this procedure without a single recurrence in the neck, which forms a surprising contrast to other surgeons' reports of a recurrence rate of 20–30% after carrying out a more radical procedure [30].

It is of course well known that a restricted neck dissection of this type is indicated in papillary carcinoma of the thyroid gland, a tumour which does not rupture the capsule of the gland and therefore can be dealt with by a modified neck dissection, using a single transverse incision and preserving the sternomastoid muscle, the accessory nerve and the submaxillary space with sacrifice of the internal jugular vein [31].

One further problem to be discussed under the heading of a patient with a gland in one side of the neck is the pathology, diagnosis and treatment where a lymph gland in the neck is found to contain carcinoma but the primary site is apparently unknown ('occult primary').

The 'occult primary'

Several excellent reviews are available on this topic [32–34]. Cancer presenting with a gland in the neck is mainly a disease of men (men : women 4 : 1) with a maximum age incidence of 65 in men and 55 in women. The histology of the tumour obviously varies slightly depending on the interest of the surgeon but it appears that between one-third and one-half of all such nodes are replaced by squamous carcinoma, about a quarter by undifferentiated or anaplastic carcinoma and a similar number by adenocarcinoma if the supraclavicular nodes are involved, followed by a small number of miscellaneous tumours includ-

ing melanomas, thyroid gland tumours, etc.

In about a third of patients a primary tumour can be found by investigation at the time of presentation. The primary sites in order of frequency are as follows: nasopharynx, tonsil, base of the tongue, thyroid gland, supraglottic larynx, floor of the mouth, palate and piriform fossa (head and neck sites); bronchus, oesophagus, breast and stomach (distant sites) [34].

Careful follow-up, which will be discussed below, will later reveal a primary site in up to a third of patients [32, 34]. These primary sites are rather more commonly found in the head and neck than anywhere else and the sites are again those in the above list. One thing worth noting is that if a carcinoma of the oropharynx, particularly of the tonsil, is the site of the so-called occult primary tumour the tumour may not declare itself for a very long time, even for as long as 7 years in Shaw's series (and for as long as 6 years in this author's series). The relative frequency of the various sites is as follows [32]: oro and nasopharynx 23%, thyroid 18%, laryngopharynx 8%, miscellaneous head and neck tumours 10%, lung 21%, gastrointestinal tract 11%, miscellaneous distant sites 8%. Obviously the frequency of involvement of these sites will depend to some extent on the interest of the individual surgeon.

In earlier times a malignant gland in the neck has been called a branchiogenic carcinoma, that is a carcinoma arising in a branchial remnant. Twenty-eight cases were recorded by Crile as being a branchial carcinoma [35] but no real search was made for a primary tumour. The nose and throat were examined in some patients; in one the branchial carcinoma was said to have extended into the piriform fossa and one had a nasopharyngeal carcinoma which was thought to be irrelevant. Chest radiographs were taken in only eleven (and in three of these definite metastases were present which may well have been lung primaries); radiographs of the skull and jaws were taken in 'several cases' only. As a result of Crile's paper many patients with a malignant node in the neck were thought to have a branchial carcinoma; since Crile had shown that treatment of this was difficult and the survival poor, it became standard practice to confine investigation to excision of the node; if squamous carcinoma was found a diagnosis of branchial carcinoma was made, no primary tumour was looked for and little further was done.

Hayes Martin was the chief opponent of this policy and urged strongly that a biopsy should be the last investigation to be done and that a search for a primary tumour must be made [36, 37]. He showed that these tumours were virtually always secondary to a primary tumour of the head and neck which could be treated, although he stated that a branchial carcinoma might be a real entity [26].

Investigation

The steps to be followed in investigating such a patient are as follows [34]:

(1) Primary sites: head and neck	Inspection, palpation, radiology, endoscopy, biopsy, cytology, and supra-vital staining.
(2) Cervical lymph nodes	Inspection, palpation, pattern, level, aspiration, excision, morphology, histology.
(3) Other primary sites	General physical examination, radiology, laboratory tests, endoscopy, biopsy, cytology.

Endoscopy is to be meticulous and should include magnification particularly when examining the nasopharynx, the bronchi and the oesophagus. If no primary tumour is found a blind biopsy should be taken of the posterior wall of the fossa of Rosenmüller on the same side as the enlarged lymph gland, of the base of the tongue and of the piriform fossa on the same side. It is also preferable to remove the tonsil on the same side and have it examined by serial section.

Supra-vital staining with toluidine blue may be useful in showing up areas of abnormal epithelium in sites normally lined by squamous epithelium, but is of little value in sites such as the larynx which are normally lined in part by respiratory epithelium.

If the above regime of clinical examination and endoscopy does not provide an answer to the site of the primary tumour an aspiration biopsy should be carried out of the gland: reliable and positive results can be obtained by drill biopsy in 70–90% of patients [34].

If aspiration biopsy does not give a satisfactory answer excisional biopsy must be contemplated; such a biopsy must always excise the lymph gland entirely, and an incisional biopsy must never be carried out. Even then there may be serious consequences of excision including:

(1) Local and possibly general spread of the disease.

(2) Compromise of a subsequent neck dissection or irradiation.

(3) Additional scar tissue causing difficulty in accurate palpation.

(4) A false sense of security for the patient who feels that the lump has been removed.

It cannot be too strongly emphasized that excisional biopsy of a gland in the neck should seldom be necessary and Martin's statement [37] still holds true – 'an enlarged lymph node should never be excised as the first or even an early step in diagnosis', 'if, as a last resort, a cervical node must eventually be removed for diagnosis the operation must be performed by a surgeon who is able and willing to treat the primary cancer if it is later found somewhere in the head and neck.'

Management

In nearly all the series reported the treatment of the node with a truly occult primary has almost always been by radiotherapy. If the tumour is large and the biopsy shows a squamous carcinoma with rupture of the capsule, radiotherapy should be carried out. If one or more discrete glands in the upper part of the neck are involved a radical neck dissection should be carried out, whereas if there are one or more glands involved in the lower part of the neck radiotherapy is given; supraclavicular glands are not treated further on the presumption that they are secondary to a visceral carcinoma [32]. This policy provided a 34% survival at 3 years [32].

The main indications for removal of the neck nodes in the unknown primary are [34]:

(1) Where irradiation has failed, the nodes still being palpably involved, resectable and preferably on one side only.

(2) A single large well-defined and resectable neck mass 5 cm or more in diameter.

(3) Where biopsy raises suspicion of a primary tumour in the thyroid gland or a major salivary gland.

(4) In the very rare case of branchiogenic carcinoma.

In those patients where the primary tumour is

not found it is essential to repeat the search for a primary tumour at frequent intervals after the neck nodes have been treated. In a series of 1189 patients the primary lesion was later found in about 40%, whereas a further 40% died with metastatic disease and no evidence of a primary lesion. Of the survivors 16% showed no further evidence of any malignant disease at any time after treatment of the neck nodes [38]. The follow-up may need to be continued for a very long time, since the primary tumour, particularly if it is in the tonsil, may not appear for many years.

Bilateral neck glands (N2)

Bilateral neck glands are not common, occurring in about 5% of head and neck cancers overall, more commonly from tumours of the base of the tongue, the supraglottic larynx and the hypopharynx. The accuracy of clinical diagnosis is very high being 90% in one series [39]. It is generally agreed that the presence of bilateral neck glands is a very bad prognostic sign [40] and survival rates fall to about 5% in the presence of such an event [41, 42]. Despite this low survival rate many surgeons have advised staged [43] or simultaneous bilateral neck dissection.

For the last 10 years or more it has been appreciated that it may not be necessary to stage operation on the two sides so that it is possible to carry out neck dissection on both sides at the same sitting with reasonable safety, although the complication rate may be as high as two in three. Formation of fistulae, sepsis, skin slough and facial oedema, which tend to persist, are the most important complications, and the postoperative death rate is about 15% [39]. Half the patients died of uncontrolled local disease and a 5-year survival of 17% was achieved in this latter series. Unfortunately, the survival figures do not show the sites of the patients who survived. It is the author's distinct impression that patients with supraglottic carcinoma and bilateral neck glands have a reasonable prognosis, whereas nearly all other tumours particularly of the mouth, the oropharynx and the hypopharynx when associated with bilateral neck glands have an extremely bad prognosis and surgery probably does not influence the natural history of the disease [44]; it would therefore be interesting to

know if the long-term survivors in the above series had suffered from laryngeal carcinoma.

The most feared complication after bilateral neck dissection is probably increased intracranial pressure. It has been shown that tying one internal jugular vein produces a three-fold increase of the intracranial pressure, whereas tying the second side produces a five-fold increase; the intracranial pressure then tends to fall over about 8 days but not to normal. Furthermore the pressure falls quite rapidly within the first 12 hours so that if the patient can be got over this period he is probably out of immediate danger. The methods to be used to avoid this complication include [45]:

(1) Removal of CSF (which is dangerous).
(2) Keeping the patient in the sitting position.
(3) Avoiding dressings which compress the neck.
(4) Infusion of hypertonic glucose.

It should be noted that the treatment and prognosis for a patient in whom a gland appears on the second side of the neck some time later is quite different from the patient who suffers from bilateral neck glands at the time of presentation. In a series of 500 patients in whom a gland appeared on the opposite side of the neck (an invaded gland having been already dealt with on the ipsilateral side) the survival rate was almost 30% [46].

Fixed glands (N3)

The presence of fixed glands is an uncommon event occurring in about 5% of all patients with head and neck cancer. The word 'fixed' itself is one which is subject to individual interpretation and indeed very few glands are truly fixed [14]. A gland is unlikely to be fixed until it becomes very large, i.e. 6 cm or more in diameter and is rarely fixed when it is smaller than this [41]. It has generally been thought that the presence of fixed glands contra-indicates surgery [14], but this is probably not absolutely true. If the tumour is fixed to or invades the jugular vein the patient is almost certainly incurable, since nearly all patients will die of local recurrence and distant metastases or both [47], and it must therefore appear that such invasion is indeed a contra-indication to useful treatment.

Fixation to the base of the skull in the region of the mastoid process and to the brachial plexus is also almost certainly a contra-indication to treatment. Fixation to the skin is not necessarily a contra-indication and it is possible to resect the tumour with the overlying skin which is replaced with a deltopectoral flap. On occasion, this has produced long-term survival and certainly may give very helpful palliation [48].

A review of a small number of patients with fixed nodes being treated by preoperative radiotherapy and surgery showed that a few patients survived, but the only ones to do so were those in whom examination of the specimen after radical neck dissection showed that the tumour had been sterilized by radiotherapy; the remaining patients all died [49].

When a tumour invades the arterial tree resection of this vascular system has been described by Conley [50]: thirty-one patients underwent resection of the common carotid artery for carcinoma [50]. In seventeen, replacement was done by a vein graft, but the operative mortality was high (5/17). Despite this a few patients survived to live a useful life for periods up to 2 years. Six patients underwent anastomosis of the stumps of the internal and external carotid arteries. There were no postoperative deaths and two patients survived for long periods (3 and 5 years). Despite the occasional survivor reported by the highly skilled such as Conley, this technique does not appear to have become generally accepted.

References

[1] SAKO, K., PRADIER R. N., MARCHETTA F. C. & PICKREN J. W. (1964) Fallability of palpation in the diagnosis of metastasis to the cervical nodes. *Surgery, Gynecology and Obstetrics* 118, 989.

[2] NICHOLS R. T. & GREENFIELD L. J. (1968) Experience with radical neck dissection in the management of 426 patients with malignant tumours of the head and neck. *Annals of Surgery* 167, 23.

[3] LINDBERG R. (1972) Distribution of cervical lymph node metastases from squamous cell carcinoma of the upper respiratory tract and digestive tract. *Cancer* 29, 1446.

[4] BLAIR V. R. & BROWN J. B. (1933) Treatment of cancerous or potentially cancerous cervical lymph nodes. *Annals of Surgery* 98, 650.

[5] OGURA J. H., BILLER H. F. & WETTE R. (1971) Elective neck dissection for pharyngeal and laryngeal cancers. *Annals of Otology, Rhinology and Laryngology* 80, 646.

[6] JESSE R. H., BARKLEY H. T., LINDBERG R. D. & FLETCHER G. H. (1970) Cancer of the oral cavity. Is elective neck dissection beneficial? *American Journal of Surgery* 120, 505.

[7] REED G. F. & MILLER W. A. (1970) Elective neck dissection. *Laryngoscope* 80, 1292.

[8] FARR H. W. & ARTHUR K. (1972) Epidermoid carcinoma of the mouth and pharynx 1960–1964. *Journal of Laryngology and Otology* 85, 243.

[9] YARINGTON C. T., YONKERS A. J. & BEDDOE G. M. (1973) Radical neck dissection. *Archives of Otolaryngology* 97, 306.

[10] BRYCE D. P. (1972) The role of surgery in the management of carcinoma of the larynx. *Journal of Laryngology and Otology* 86, 669.

[11] FLETCHER G. H. (1972) Elective irradiation of subclinical disease in cancers of the head and neck. *Cancer* 29, 1450.

[12] MILLTON R. R. (1974) Elective neck irradiation for T × N0 squamous carcinoma of the oral tongue and floor of the mouth. *Cancer* 34, 149.

[13] CRILE G. (1906) Excision of cancer of the head and neck with special reference to the plan of dissection based on 132 patients. *Journal of the American Medical Association* 47, 1780.

[14] MARTIN H., DEL VALLE B. & EHRLICH H. (1951) Neck dissection. *Cancer* 4, 441.

[15] WIZENBURG M. J., BLOEDORN F. G., WEINER S. & GRACIA J. (1972) Treatment of lymph node metastases in head and neck cancer. *Cancer* 29, 1455.

[16] HENK J. M. (1975) Radiosensitivity of lymph node metastases. *Proceedings of the Royal Society of Medicine* 68, 85.

[17] POWERS W. E. & TOLMACH J. J. (1964) Pre-operative radiation therapy: Biological basis and experimental investigation. *Nature* 201, 272.

[18] HENSCHKE U. K., FRAZELL E. L., HILARIS B. S., NICKSON J. J., TOLLEFSEN H. R. & STRONG E. W. (1966) Value of pre-operative X-ray therapy as an adjunct to radical neck dissection. *Radiology* 85, 450.

[19] STRONG E. W., HENSCHKE U. K., NICKSON J. J., FRAZELL E. L., TOLLEFSEN H. R. & HILARIS B. S. (1966) Pre-operative X-ray therapy as an adjunct to radical neck dissection. *Cancer* 19, 1509.

[20] KETCHAM A. S., HOYLE R. C., CHRETIEN P. B. & BRACE K. C. (1969) Irradiation twenty four hours pre-operatively. *American Journal of Surgery* 118, 691.

[21] LINDBERG R. & JESSE R. H. (1968) Treatment of cervical lymph node metastases from the primary lesions of the oropharynx, supraglottic larynx and hypopharynx. *American Journal of Roentgenology* 102, 132.

[22] STELL P. M. (1969) Complications encountered in head and neck surgery. *Journal of Laryngology and Otology* 83, 671.

[23] MACFEE W. F. (1960) Transverse incisions for neck dissections. *Annals of Surgery* 157, 279.

[24] HETTER G. P. (1972) Neck incisions relative to the cutaneous vasculature of the neck. *Archives of Otolaryngology* **95**, 84.

[25] ROGERS J. H. & FREELAND A. P. (1976) Arterial vasculature of cervical skin flaps. *Clinical Otolaryngology* **1**, 325.

[26] SCHWEITZER R. J. (1962) Use of muscle flaps for protection of carotid artery after radical neck dissection. *Annals of Surgery* **156**, 811.

[27] CORSO P. F. (1963) Use of autogenous dermis for protection of the carotid artery and pharyngeal suture lines in radical head and neck surgery. *Surgery, Gynecology and Obstetrics* **112**, 37.

[28] SISSON G. A., EDISON B. D. & BYTELL D. E. (1975) Trans-sternal radical neck dissection. *Archives of Otolaryngology* **101**, 46.

[29] GRILLO H. C. (1966) Terminal or mural tracheostomy in the anterior mediastinum. *Journal of Thoracic and Cardiovascular Surgery* **57**, 422.

[30] BOCCA E. & PIGNATARO O. (1967) A conservative technique in radical neck dissection. *Annals of Otology, Rhinology and Laryngology* **76**, 975.

[31] ATTIE J. N., KHAFIF R. A. & STECKLIER R. M. (1971) Elective neck dissection in papillary carcinoma of the thyroid. *American Journal of Surgery* **122**, 464.

[32] JESSE R. H. & NEFF L. E. (1966) Metastatic carcinoma in cervical nodes with an unknown primary lesion. *American Journal of Surgery* **112**, 547.

[33] MACGOMB W. S. (1972) Diagnosis and treatment of metastatic cervical cancerous nodes from an unknown primary site. *American Journal of Surgery* **124**, 441.

[34] SHAW H. J. (1970) Metastatic carcinoma in cervical lymph nodes with occult primary tumour. *Journal of Laryngology and Otology* **84**, 249.

[35] CRILE G. & KEARNS J. E. (1935) Branchial carcinoma. *Surgery, Gynecology and Obstetrics* **60**, 703.

[36] MARTIN H., MORFIT H. M. & EHRLICH H. (1950) The case for branchiogenic cancer. *Annals of Surgery* **132**, 867.

[37] MARTIN H. (1961) Untimely lymph node biopsy. *American Journal of Surgery* **102**, 17.

[38] COMESS M. S., BEAHRS O. H. & DOCHERTY M. B. (1957) Cervical metastasis from occult carcinoma. *Surgery, Gynecology and Obstetrics* **104**, 607.

[39] MOORE O. S. & FRAZELL E. L. (1964) Simultaneous bilateral neck dissection. *American Journal of Surgery* **107**, 565.

[40] MOORE O. S. (1969) Bilateral neck dissection. *Surgical Clinics of North America* **49**, 277.

[41] SPIRO R. H., ALFONSO A. E., FARR H. W. & STRONG E. W. (1974) Cervical node metastasis from epidermoid carcinoma of the oral cavity and oropharynx. *American Journal of Surgery* **128**, 562.

[42] LEDERMAN M. (1967) Cancer of the pharynx. *Journal of Laryngology and Otology* **81**, 151.

[43] LECLERC G. & ROY J. (1932) La resection successive de deux jugulaires internes. *La Presse Medicale* 1382.

[44] STELL P. M. & GREEN J. T. (1976) Management of metastases to the lymph glands of the neck. *Proceedings of the Royal Society of Medicine.* **69**, 411.

[45] JONES R. K. (1951) Increased intracranial pressure following radical neck surgery. *Archives of Surgery* **63**, 599.

[46] FRAZELL E. L. & MOORE O. S. (1961) Bilateral radical neck dissection performed in stages. *Journal of Surgery* **102**, 809.

[47] DJALILIAN M., WEILAND L. H., DEVINE K. D. & BEAHRS O. H. (1973) Significance of jugular vein invasion by metastatic carcinoma in radical neck dissection. *American Journal of Surgery* **126**, 566.

[48] BAKAMJIAN V. Y., CERVINO L., MILLER S. & HENTZ V. R. (1973) The concept of cure and palliation by surgery in advanced cancer of the head and neck. *American Journal of Surgery* **126**, 482.

[49] SANTOS V. B., STRONG S., VAUGHAN C. W. & DITROIA J. F. (1975) Role of surgery in head and neck cancer with fixed nodes. *Archives of Otolaryngology* **101**, 645.

[50] CONLEY J. J. (1957) Carotid artery surgery in tumours of the neck. *Archives of Otolaryngology* **65**, 437.

CHAPTER 24

Tumours of the Nasopharynx

Because of its anatomical relationships, tumours arising in the nasopharynx may produce diverse clinical signs, and unless the clinician knows the anatomy of the surrounding structures it is difficult to understand the clinical signs and to relate these to the extensions of the disease. Furthermore, recent studies on the epidemiology and virology of a particular form of cancer (anaplastic carcinoma of this area) have yielded results which are of real significance in the fields of preventive and curative oncology.

Anatomy

Boundaries
The nasopharynx or post-nasal space is a cuboidal space lined by mucosa with transverse and vertical diameters of 4 cm and an anteroposterior diameter of 2 cm. The anterior boundary is formed by the posterior nasal choanae, the roof by the posterior inferior part of the sphenoidal sinus, basisphenoid and basiocciput bones which slope back to the vertical posterior wall. This is formed by the strong pharyngobasilar fascia overlying the anterior surface of the arch of the atlas and upper part of the body of the second cervical vertebrae. The pharyngeal tonsil or adenoid lies at the junction of the posterior wall and roof. The lateral wall is formed by the internal or pharyngobasilar lamina of the pharyngeal fascia, and the superior constrictor muscle. Between the upper border of the muscle and the base of the skull (sinus of Morgani) the levator palati muscle and the cartilaginous Eustachian tube pass, enveloped by the internal and external layers of the pharyngeal fascia. The Eustachian tube, roughly triangular in shape with its apex superior, opens into the nasopharynx approximately 1 cm behind the posterior end of the inferior turbinate. The posterior margin forms a prominent projection on the lateral wall of the nasopharynx (torus tubarius). The mucosa covering the less prominent anterior margin merges with the posterior border of the soft palate.

The lateral recess of the nasopharynx, or fossa of Rosenmüller, an epithelial lined cleft which may exceed 1 cm in depth, lies immediately behind the torus. The roof of the fossa is related to the foramen lacerum and the floor of the carotid canal in the petrous temporal bone. Anteroinferiorly the fossa is bounded by the epithelium covering the Eustachian tube and the levator palati muscle, and the posterior wall is formed by the mucosa covering the pharyngobasilar fascia. Inferiorly the nasopharyngeal space opens into the oropharynx so that the floor is formed by the dorsal aspect of the soft palate which is the only mobile boundary.

Histology
At birth, the cavity is covered solely by columnar ciliated epithelium but between the ages of 10 and 80 years patches of squamous epithelium become evident, usually surrounded by areas of transitional or intermediate epithelium. About 80% of the posterior wall is covered by squamous epithelium and after the age of 10 years approximately 60% of the total mucosal surface is stratified squamous [1]. The cause of the change in the lining from the pseudo-stratified columnar ciliated epithelium of infancy to a predominantly stratified squamous epithelium of adult life is not known, but it may be due to a metaplastic transformation [2]. Mucous and serous secreting glands are scattered throughout the mucosa and melanin pigmentation may be found in the basal cells of all three types of epithelium.

Lymphatic drainage

In addition to the mass of lymphoid tissue constituting the adenoid, masses of lymphoid tissue are situated in the fossa of Rosenmüller and about the pharyngeal orifice of the Eustachian tube. Numerous smaller masses of lymphoid tissues are scattered throughout the submucosa. These, together with the lingual and palatine tonsil, constitute Waldeyer's ring. These masses of lymphoid tissue drain to lymph nodes in the retrostyloid compartment of the parapharyngeal space or directly into the upper deep cervical nodes. Rouvière described an intensive submucosal plexus of lymph vessels which drains into medial and lateral retropharyngeal lymph nodes [3]. The medial retropharyngeal nodes lie on either side of the midline posteriorly between the internal and external layers of the pharyngeal fascia (Weintraub's space) but are inconsistent and often disappear in adult life. The main lymph nodes are the lateral retropharyngeal nodes on each side. These lie high up in the retrostyloid compartment of the parapharyngeal space near the base of the skull anterior to the lateral mass of the atlas. These lymph glands, often referred to as the *Nodes of Rouvière*, lie adjacent to the ninth and tenth, eleventh and twelfth cranial nerves, the superior cervical ganglion, the internal carotid artery and the internal jugular vein. Metastatic growth in these nodes may involve the adjacent nervous and vascular structure as well as the arch of the atlas, the atlanto-occipital joint and the occipital bone near the joint and the foramen magnum. Efferent vessels pass to the nodes of Rouvière from the nasopharyngeal submucosal plexus. These nodes drain into the posterior triangle and upper deep cervical nodes which also receive vessels direct from the nasopharynx.

The parapharyngeal space

The clinical presentation of many pathological processes involving the head and neck area are determined by both the behavioural characteristics of the disease and the structures affected. A disease may grow by expansive spread into contiguous natural cavities and by local expansive pressure, destroy adjacent structures. A rapidly growing proliferating lesion is more likely to spread by infiltration through the preformed pathways formed by fascial planes. A knowledge of the parapharyngeal fascia and the anatomy of the parapharyngeal compartments provides an explanation of many perplexing clinical symptoms and signs associated with some diseases of the nasopharynx. Lederman has summarized the work of some French anatomists on the parapharyngeal fascia [4] and describes:

(1) an *internal layer* or the pharyngobasilar fascia which lies beneath the mucosa covering the superior constrictor muscle, and at the upper margin of this muscle splits to enclose the Eustachian tube and levator palati muscle;

(2) an *external layer* or pharyngeal portion of the bucco-pharyngeal fascia which extends upwards on the outer side of the superior constrictor muscle and splits to enclose the tensor palati muscle lying external to the Eustachian tube and levator palati.

The parapharyngeal space lies between the nasopharynx and the inner surface of the angle and ascending ramus of the mandible and is subdivided into three compartments by the styloid process and its muscles and by fascial expansions from the carotid sheath to the prevertebral fascia and posterolateral pharyngeal wall (Fig. 24.1).

The boundaries and major structures in each of the three compartments are as follows.

(1) *The pre-styloid compartment*. The roof of this space includes the foramen ovale, foramen spinosum and the under surface of the greater wing of the sphenoid. The medial wall is formed by the bucco-pharyngeal fascia covering the tensor palati and superior constrictor muscle. The lateral boundaries include the lateral pterygoid muscle, the deep lobe of the parotid and the medial pterygoid muscle. The floor is formed by the fascia investing the submandibular gland which stretches from the hyoid bone to the mandible (Fig. 24.2). This compartment is traversed by the inferior dental, lingual and auriculotemporal nerves and by the internal maxillary artery.

Direct access to this space may be made inferiorly through the floor, or superiorly by reflecting the temporalis muscle. The retrostyloid compartment and its contents are easily accessible through this compartment particularly if the mandible is first divided posterior to the last molar tooth.

(2) *The retrostyloid compartment.* The carotid sheath and vessels, the last four cranial nerves, the cervical sympathetic nerves and many lymph nodes are situated within this compartment.

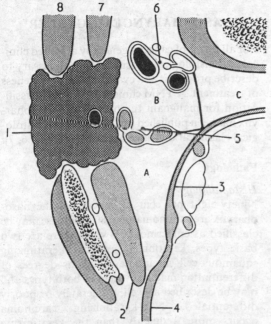

FIG. 24.1. Horizontal section through the parapharyngeal space (after Rouvière and Lederman). A, Pre-styloid compartment; B, retrostyloid compartment; C, retropharyngeal compartment; 1, parotid gland; 2, medial pterygoid muscle; 3, superior constrictor muscle; 4, buccinator muscle; 5, styloglossus, stylopharyngeus and stylohyoid muscles; 6, carotid sheath, vagus nerve, internal jugular vein and sympathetic chain; 7, digastric muscle; 8, sternomastoid muscle.

(3) *The retropharyngeal compartment.* This separates the nasopharynx from the prevertebral muscles and contains lymph nodes, in particular the lateral retropharyngeal node of Rouvière.

Examination

Indirect examination with a suitable mirror may allow an adequate inspection of the nasopharynx. A local anaesthetic spray to the nose and soft palate reduces the patient's anxiety, and facilitates examination. The entire area should be inspected and in particular the roof and sphenoid

vomer junction area as well as both fossae of Rosenmüller. In suitable circumstances biopsies may be taken with a Luc's or Tilley–Henckel forceps introduced through the anterior nares. A Stortz nasopharyngolaryngoscope which can be

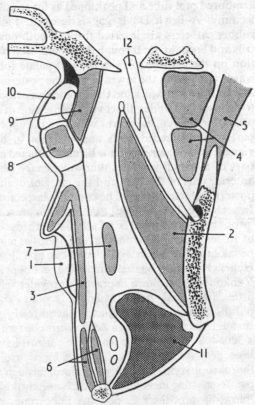

FIG. 24.2. Coronal section through pre-styloid compartment (after Rouvière and Lederman) showing relationship to base of skull, submandibular gland and the oronasopharynx. 1, tonsil; 2, medial pterygoid muscle; 3, superior constrictor muscle; 4, lateral pterygoid muscle; 5, temporalis muscle; 6, middle constrictor and hyoglossus muscles; 7, digastric muscles; 8, levator palati muscle; 9, tensor palati muscle; 10, Eustachian tube; 11, submandibular salivary gland; 12, inferior dental nerve.

used in the clinic with local anaesthetic allows a detailed examination of the fossae of Rosenmüller, the roof of the nasopharynx and the margins of the posterior choanae. A flexible instrument may be used through which the nasopharynx may be photographed [5]. In some patients a full and adequate inspection requires a general anaesthetic which will also allow a tumour, if present, to be biopsied or 'proof biopsies' to be taken from selected areas.

Examination under anaesthesia

The patient is anaesthetized through an armoured oral tube and positioned as for tonsillectomy. A Boyle-Davis gag is inserted. Fine rubber catheters are inserted through both nostrils and brought out through the mouth. Retraction on the catheters draws the soft palate forwards and allows the lower part of the posterior and both lateral walls and the Eustachian orifice to be inspected under direct vision. Insertion of a warm, large laryngeal mirror will allow the upper part of both lateral walls and the roof to be viewed. If the examination is being conducted as part of a search for an unknown primary, the anterior part of the roof and the margins of the posterior choanae should be carefully inspected. In such cases if an obvious tumour is not present 'proof biopsies' should be taken from both fossae of Rosenmüller and from the roof. Biopsies may be taken under vision with a small Luc or Tilley–Henckel forceps passed through the nose. A Yankauer's speculum, in practice, provides very little additional help. Magnified views and photographs may be obtained, either directly or through the mirror using a Zeiss microscope with a 300–400 mm objective lens. Five patients have been described in which a positive biopsy from the nasopharynx was only obtained through a palate-splitting incision [22] but it is usually possible to inspect the nasopharynx fully using the method described above. Taking multiple deep biopsies from the roof, posterior wall and fossae of Rosenmüller, even though the surface mucosa appears normal is usually sufficient to exclude or confirm a primary carcinoma in the nasopharynx.

Radiological examination

Lateral soft tissue radiography may demonstrate a tumour, and submentovertical views may indicate bone erosion. Particular attention should be paid to the pterygoid plates and the bony outlines of the carotid foramen, foramen ovale, foramen lacerum and foramen spinosum. If the third, fourth, fifth or the sixth cranial nerves are involved sagittal tomograms may demonstrate erosion of the sella turcica and sphenoid. If the patient presents with a lesion of the last four cranial nerves, radiographs may demonstrate bone erosion of the arch and transverse process of the atlas, and the bone about the jugular foramen and occipital condyle.

NASOPHARYNGEAL CANCER

For all forms of cancer a generally accepted clinical and histological classification is necessary to describe prognosis and evaluate the effectiveness of treatment. A TNM clinical descriptive classification for malignant tumours of the nasopharynx has been published by the UICC and histological classifications have been published [2, 6, 7].

Pathology

Histopathology

Ninety-eight per cent of cancers of the nasopharynx are carcinomas and 80% of these may be classified as epidermoid of which there are two basic types, keratinizing and non-keratinizing squamous cell carcinomas. Various degrees of differentiation may be evident in both types and may be described as well, moderately or poorly differentiated. Non-keratinizing carcinoma occurs more frequently than the keratinizing type and in both types poorly differentiated forms are most usual. Terms such as anaplastic, undifferentiated, transitional cell, embryonal cell have been used to describe variants of the poorly differentiated non-keratinizing (non-glandular) carcinoma. In the past, rich infiltration of lymphocytes in some cases of anaplastic or poorly differentiated carcinoma led to the concept that the 'lymphoepithelioma' represented a special carcinoma particular to the nasopharynx. Various forms of 'lymphoepithelioma' were described and different theories were developed to describe the role and character of the lymphoid component. But it is now generally accepted that the lymphocytes are evident in the cancer because it has developed in an area naturally rich in lymphoid tissue.

The minor salivary and seromucinous glands of the nasopharyngeal mucosa may give rise to adenocarcinomas, which may or may not be mucous secreting and present with or without an adenoid cystic pattern.

Rare mesenchymal tumours such as lympho-sarcoma, reticulosarcoma, fibrosarcoma, mixo- and liposarcoma have been reported as occurring in the nasopharynx [2, 4]. These tumours rarely arise from the mucosal surfaces. Lymphomas may involve the structures of Waldeyer's ring and recognition may be important in staging and treatment.

Epidemiology

The epidemiology of the most common cancer of the nasopharynx, the anaplastic or poorly differ-entiated non-keratinizing squamous carcinoma, infiltrated in varying degrees by lymphocytes, has recently aroused the interest of oncologists for two reasons [8]:

(1) the possibility that the Epstein–Barr virus (EBV), a DNA herpes type virus may have a causative role; and

(2) suggestive evidence that genetic factors determine susceptibility to this disease. A certain inherited genetic profile involving the HL-A sys-tem has been shown to be associated with this disease.

Nasopharyngeal carcinoma is rare in the Cau-casian peoples of Europe, India and America. In populations of European origin the relative fre-quency of this disease is less than 0·3% in men and 0·2% in women. These rates are very much lower than those reported from Chinese com-munities living in China, particularly in the Southern provinces and also in emigrant Chinese communities in South-East Asia and the Amer-icas. Rates, higher than those from European, but lower than Chinese registries, have been reported from parts of Africa (Kenya and Tuni-sia). But nowhere in the world does the disease have the significance than it has in Kwangtung and in the city of Canton in South China where this disease is the most common cancer in men, constituting 56·9% of all cancers occurring in that sex [9].

Site of origin

If the tumour is large and exophytic it may be impossible to determine the point of origin apart from noting which wall of the nasopharynx is most affected. Small tumours often involve the fossa of Rosenmüller. In patients presenting with enlarged neck nodes and where the nasopharynx is being examined as part of the search for the primary growth, if tumour is not obvious in the nasopharynx 'proof biopsies' should be taken from the roof of the cavity immediately behind the nasal septum, from the fornices above the torus, and from both fossae of Rosenmüller. The less common well differentiated non-keratinizing carcinomas usually present as localized ulcera-tive growths whereas the common anaplastic carcinomas usually but not always appear as a large exophytic tumour filling the nasopharynx. In a minority of patients the primary growth in the nasopharynx may not be immediately obvious on inspection, and the presence of the lesion may require 'proof biopsies' from multiple sites.

Spread

Lymphoid tumours of the nasopharynx are char-acterized by symptoms arising from the presence of the local tumour and regional lymph node involvement, whereas carcinomas may metasta-size to the regional nodes and beyond, and also affect local structures by direct extension. A dis-tinct pattern of spread is not associated with any particular type of carcinoma and erosion of the skull base occurs as frequently with poorly differ-entiated tumours as with the more differentiated forms. Direct lateral spread of the tumour may take place through the sinus of Morgani, between the upper border of the superior con-strictor muscle and the skull base; the parapha-ryngeal space may also be invaded by direct exten-sion through the superior constrictor muscle (Fig. 24.2). The carcinoma may extend super-iorly along the carotid artery and enter the skull through the carotid canal. Lederman has stressed that this is the most likely manner in which the middle cranial fossa is invaded [4]. Though the foramen lacerum lies at the apex of the fossa of Rosenmüller it is filled with fibrocar-tilage, a structure extremely resistant to malig-nant invasion, but a malignant growth entering the skull along the path of the carotid artery could easily involve the cavernous sinus, the third, fourth, fifth and sixth cranial nerves and the bone of the middle cranial fossa. This area might also be affected by growth spreading upwards from the pre-styloid compartment of the parapharyngeal space along the fifth division of the trigeminal nerve through the foramen ovale (Fig. 24.2). The tumour may also extend anteriorly through the posterior choanae to involve the nose or through the posterior ethmoidal cells into the orbits.

Clinical features

Anatomical relationships are of major importance in understanding the clinical features of nasopharyngeal carcinoma. For convenience, symptoms may be classified as rhinological, otological, laryngopharyngeal, and pain in the face and head.

Rhinological
A tumour in the nasopharynx may obstruct one or both nasal airways. Epistaxis may be due to bleeding from the tumour or from erosion of the surrounding tissues. Attempts by the patient to relieve the irritation of the tumour in the nasopharynx by hawking may lead the patient to cough out blood-stained sputum.

Otological
The commonest symptom is conductive deafness which may be associated with a retracted tympanic membrane and a serous exudate into the middle ear or an otitis media. This form of deafness may be due to a fungating tumour obstructing the Eustachian orifice or due to tumour infiltrating into and about the levator palati muscle. This muscle takes origin from the floor of the Eustachian tube and the tube is opened by contraction of the muscle. The motor nerve to this muscle is supplied through the pharyngeal plexus and this also may be affected by tumour infiltration. Cartilage is extremely resistant to tumour infiltration and the tube itself is rarely eroded by malignant growth or by an associated perichondritis. Pain in the ear may arise following tubal obstruction or the pain may be referred to the ear from tumour extension into the pre-styloid compartment of the parapharyngeal space involving the third division of the trigeminal nerve or from involvement of the glossopharyngeal and vagus nerves in the retrostyloid compartments.

Ophthalmological
Symptoms may result from tumour infiltrating

the skull base either as an extension along the carotid artery or through the foramen ovale at the apex of the pre-styloid compartment. The trunks of the second to the sixth cranial nerves may be affected, adjacent to or in the cavernous sinus. Symptoms indicating involvement of the fourth and sixth cranial nerves and the second and third divisions of the trigeminal are usually the earliest neurological indications of extension of disease outside the nasopharynx. Tumour invasion of the orbit with displacement of the globe and occulomotor paresis may occur from extension of the tumour through the cavernous sinus and superior orbital fissure. Alternatively the orbit may be invaded by extracranial spread from the pterygopalatine fossa or through the posterior ethmoid. Spread to involve the orbit may progress to proptosis of a fixed blind eye. Horner's syndrome indicating a cervical sympathetic paralysis is not uncommon and if associated with a paresis of the ninth, tenth, eleventh and twelfth cranial nerves on the same side, the lesion may be due to compression of the nerves by a metastasis in the lateral retropharyngeal node of Rouvière.

Laryngopharyngeal
Limitation of soft palate movement may be due to tumour infiltration of the soft palate, its musculature or their nerves (vagus through the pharyngeal plexus, and from the third division of the trigeminal). This may lead to voice changes and difficulties in swallowing. Extension of tumour into the prestyloid compartment of the parapharyngeal space may lead to trismus due to tumour infiltrating the pterygoid muscles. The motor branch of the trigeminal may be affected. Infiltration or compression of the ninth and tenth cranial nerves may result in hoarseness, dyspnoea and dysphagia. Involvement of the cranial nerves about the jugular foramen may be bilateral and life threatening.

Pain in the face or head
The commonest cause of facial pain is trigeminal involvement. Any or all of the three branches may be involved. Pain in areas supplied by the second division is a common presenting symptom. Glossopharyngeal involvement leads to pain in the throat and pharynx, and pain may be

referred to the ear (via the nerve of Jacobson. Cervical node metastases may stretch the cervical plexus or compress the brachial plexus and cause pain in the head, neck, shoulder or arm. Shoulder drop may result from compression or infiltration of the accessory nerve in the retrostyloid compartment or in the neck.

Diagnosis

Patients with nasopharyngeal carcinoma may present in the first instance with symptoms relating to:

(1) enlarged metastatic neck nodes without cranial nerve involvement (45%);

(2) symptoms arising from cranial nerve paresis and enlarged neck nodes (45%);

(3) cranial nerve lesions without neck gland metastases (5–10%).

Patients initially presenting only with neck node metastases may be suspected of suffering from a tubercular adenitis or from a reticulosis and those presenting with cranial nerve lesions from a neurological or ophthalmic condition. Godtfredson reviewed the ophthalmological and neurological syndromes associated with malignant diseases of the nasopharynx that were described in the period 1864–1927 [10]. Though clinical awareness may raise a suspicion that a patient is suffering from a nasopharyngeal cancer the absolute diagnosis is dependent on a positive biopsy taken from the nasopharynx.

Radiological investigation

This is used mainly to investigate possible bone erosion of the middle cranial fossa floor, and has been described earlier. If the patient complains of neck pain on head movement, the basi-occiput and arch of the atlas should be investigated. Metastases beyond the neck is a late phenomenon in this disease but patients should have regular and periodic chest radiographs.

Late metastases to ribs, lumbar and thoracic vertebrae may cause severe bone pain, the nature of which will be established by a radioactive isotope bone scan. An ultrasound liver scan may be of help if metastases to that organ are suspected.

Treatment

Surgical control of carcinoma of the naso-

pharynx is probably impossible because of the relative inaccessibility of the primary site. A radical neck dissection of involved cervical lymph nodes, which may be bilateral, should include the parapharyngeal lymphatics (and in particular the nodes of Rouvière) and this in practice is impossible. High dose mega voltage external irradiation is at present the treatment of choice [4], and there is evidence that the results of this treatment are improved if given synchronously with multiple drug chemotherapy [11]. The axillary lymph nodes receive afferents which drain from the skin of the back of the neck and in patients with cervical metastases there may be advantages in adopting 'mantle' type fields so that the axillae and mediastinum are included in the fields of irradiation.

The results of treatment are influenced by the clinical state on presentation. Lederman has noted that 90% of patients presenting with cranial nerve lesions died with uncontrolled cancer and the prognosis was not altered by the presence or absence of regional lymph node metastases [4]. The best results may thus be expected if the disease is confined to the mucosa of the nasopharynx. A 54% 5-year survival rate has been quoted for patients whose disease was confined to the nasopharynx; 40% in those with cervical metastases and only 16% in those presenting with neurological symptoms [12]. The histological classification of the tumour may significantly affect the response to radiotherapy, the more poorly-differentiated tumours having a better prognosis than the well-differentiated squamous carcinomas [13]. This is in complete contrast to the results published by Lederman, who noted a 20% 10-year survival in patients with a well-differentiated carcinoma whereas in those with anaplastic carcinoma the rate fell to 9·9% [14].

Though the factors enumerated above influence the results of treatment large series indicate only a 15–16% 5-year survival [4, 15].

NASOPHARYNGEAL ANGIOFIBROMA

Pathology

Theories regarding the origin and histogenesis of

this tumour relate to its site of origin and histological appearance. Batsakis [7] cites Ringertz, who suggested that these tumours originate from the ventral periosteal layer of bones developed from the embryonal occipital plate (basilar process of the occiput, body of sphenoid, medial pterygoid processes, region of the foramen lacerum and the pterygopalatine fossae), and Schiff who thought that the structural similarity of these tumours to the cavernous tissue of the turbinates might indicate a common origin, the tumour arising from a displaced or ectopic focus of developing cells. Harrison [16] quoted the work of Osborne which suggested that the tumours were either hamartomas or arose from remnants of fetal erectile tissue. This tumour is highly vascular, non-encapsulated and locally destructive, occurring in the nasopharynx or posterior nares most frequently in males in the age group 7–21 years. Harrison has stressed that these growths are not limited to the nasopharynx and suggested the bony area about the superior margin of the sphenopalatine foramen as the site of origin. The tumour is not confined to males but females have a significantly lower incidence, and though the prefix 'juvenile' has been used to describe this tumour, it is not restricted to adolescents. The tumour is histologically benign, composed of fibrocysts with numerous wide and thin-walled vessels surrounded by mature connective tissue, so that the microscopic appearance may vary from an erectile-like tissue or cavernous haemangioma to that of a myxomatous fibromatosis. The tumour is locally invasive but non-infiltrating. It is not common and it has been estimated that this growth forms 0·5% of all neoplasms of the head and neck.

Clinical features

The highest incidence occurs in the 13–16 age group and patients present with symptoms of:

(1) *nasal obstruction*, which may be severe and associated with deformity of the palate, alveolus and face;

(2) *epistaxis* which may be severe;

(3) symptoms and signs arising from invasion of the base of the skull, i.e. visual and oculomotor defects.

Diagnosis

Inspection of the nasopharynx reveals a round, perhaps lobulated, firm deep-red tumour, which may extend forward into one or both nares.

The radiological appearances are stated to be definitive and have been well described [17, 18]. Erosion of the skull base is common (Fig. 24.3) and in many cases the tumour may invade and extend far more widely than the presenting symptoms suggest. Bone erosion is usually demarcated by a well-delineated bone margin. Anterior bowing (displacement) of the posterior wall of the maxilla is considered to be the most consistently typical feature of this tumour on plain films. A presumptive diagnosis made on the history, clinical examination and plain films may be confirmed without biopsy by carotid angiography. The appearances are typical and consistent, the salient diagnostic points being the anterior displacement of the internal maxillary artery (Fig. 24.4) and the demonstration of the tumour circulation by films of the late capillary and venous phases of the angiograms (Fig. 24.5). These films may also demonstrate the major feeding vessels and as the blood supply may be bilateral, angiograms of both carotid systems are advisable.

Though the diagnosis may be suggested by the clinical presentation and the angiographic appearances if biopsy is considered necessary prior arrangement should be made to manage a possible severe resultant haemorrhage. Cranial base erosion is common in these lesions and there are no hard and fast rules regarding operability. Though the tumour may extend through a breach in the skull base (20%) it does not grow through the dura and the decision that operative removal can be undertaken depends on the surgeon's capability and the particular presentation of each case.

Treatment

Because of the difficulties and dangers of severe haemorrhage associated with removal of these tumours, other less hazardous and 'appropriate' forms of management have been advocated and tried, but the best treatment is still total removal.

Radiotherapy is no longer used as the primary

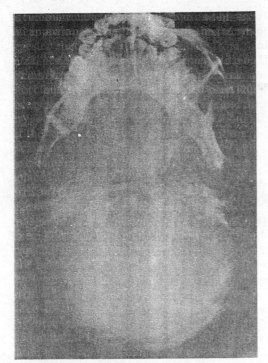

FIG. 24.3. Submentovertical radiograph of a 14-year-old boy with a large nasopharyngeal angiofibroma. The posterior border of the tumour can be seen extending backwards into the nasopharynx. The posterior and medial walls of the left maxillae, the hard palate and the posterior ethmoids and sphenoidal sinus were destroyed by pressure of the expanding tumour. The boy was blind in the left eye and vision on the right side was impaired but improved following removal of the tumour.

form of treatment and there is no unanimity regarding its value, but though it is not curative it may reduce vascularity and may be of value in the management of residual tumours not accessible to surgery. Other adjuncts to surgical removal include:

(1) *Cryotherapy* which may be of value in the management of small lesions confined to the nasopharynx [19].

(2) *Arterial ligation.* Preoperative angiography demonstrates the major feeding vessels and on these appearances a decision regarding the possible value of internal maxillary or external carotid ligation may be made. Interference with the external carotid arterial system should be bilateral to be effective and temporary, so that postoperative angiography is possible and also to reduce the risk of any residual tumour developing an arterial supply from the internal carotid system [18].

(3) *Embolization techniques* utilizing Silastic beads or Gelfoam particles to occlude selectively the arterial supply may be of value [20, 21], but the facilities for this adjuvant are not universally available.

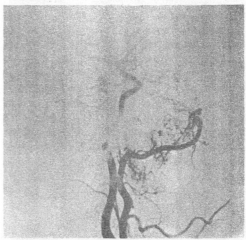

FIG. 24.4. Subtraction film of left carotid angiogram of patient whose SMV radiograph is shown in Fig. 24.3. The internal maxillary artery is enlarged and displaced forwards and downwards. The blood supply from this artery to the tumour is demonstrated.

(4) *Hormonal therapy.* Oestrogens and testosterones have been advocated but there is no real proof of their value. In addition undesirable side effects may develop in the adolescent.

Surgery

The optimum approach will depend on the extent of the tumour as defined by clinical examination and study of X-ray films and angiograms. Various approaches have been described, the most widely used being the transpalatine approach described by Wilson [22] but this is not ideal for every case. Harrison has suggested that a lateral rhinotomy gives good access to the maxillary antrum, lateral nasopharynx and sphenoidal sinus area [16]. Bocca has developed a transpharyngeal approach [23]. Biller [24] and Boles & Dedo [25] have indicated some routes by which the different extensions of this tumour may be adequately demonstrated. Bleeding may be severe and an adequate quantity of blood should be available (i.e. not less than 2000 ml). A reasonably wide surgical exposure will make total tumour removal easier. Large tumours may have lobular extensions which may make division of

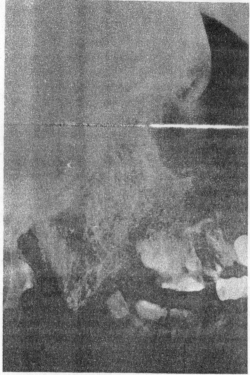

FIG. 24.5. Lateral radiograph taken during the late capillary/venous phase of carotid angiogram shown in Fig. 24.4. This demonstrates the richness of the vascular supply.

the tumour necessary as removal proceeds. Careful preoperative study of the plain X-ray films and the angiograms will demonstrate the extensions of the tumour. Blunt finger and instrument dissection usually reveal an easy plane of cleavage. When the main bulk of the tumour has been removed, the arrest of immediate bleeding with a temporary pack will allow the tumour bed to be inspected and any remaining tumour fragments to be removed. A BIPP pack is useful to control any residual bleeding and this may be left in place for a week or 10 days.

With modern surgical techniques a tumour

recurrence rate should be less than 3%. Symptoms relating to a recurrence are usually evident in the first 12 months, and are rare after 2 years [7]. It is suggested that angiograms should be repeated 9 months after the primary surgery [24]. Ideally, if residual tumour is present, it should be resected but if that is considered impossible irradiation may reduce the rate of growth.

CHORDOMAS

Pathology

These tumours arise from vestigial remnants of the notocord and are most likely to appear in those areas of great developmental upheaval where the segmental pattern of the embryo is extensively modified and small 'rests' are separated from the main body of the notocord. These rests have been demonstrated in the region of the clivus, the submucosa of the nasopharynx and pharynx and in the bodies of the second and third cervical vertebrae. As the notocord is enclosed within the bodies of the primitive vertebrae chordomas may develop *in any part of the spine* but more than one-third occur at the base of the skull [7]. Five hundred cases of this tumour have been reported [26], 39% of which were cranial or spheno-occipital. The lesions occur more often in men than women and the peak age period is between 20 and 40 years for the cranial tumours, but sacrococcygeal lesions become evident later. Chordomas presenting into the nasopharynx are usually covered with an intact and non-ulcerating mucosa.

Clinical features

The most constant symptoms associated with spheno-occipital chordomas are fronto-occipital headaches and visual disturbances. The patient may also complain of nasal obstruction, a sense of fullness in the nose and deafness. There may be associated neuro-ophthalmological and otological symptoms with signs of cranial nerve involvement. The trigeminal, facial and acoustic nerves may be affected and with a large intracranial extension hypophyseal and bulbarpontine symptoms and signs may be evident. High cervical chordomas may protrude into the lower naso-pharynx and extend downwards to distort the pharynx and displace the larynx. These tumours may cause dysphagia, dysphonia and dyspnoea. On occasions cervical chordomas may be palp-able in the neck behind the posterior border of the sternomastoid muscle. Pain may be severe due to involvement of the spinal cord or nerve roots.

Diagnosis

The outstanding radiographic feature of the anterior and ventrally presenting spheno-occipi-tal and cervical chordomas is extensive bone des-truction and a nasopharyngeal soft tissue mass. Submentovertical and lateral cervical tomo-grams define the extent of the tumour and areas of calcification may be evident.

Though there are no absolute or specific histo-logical features in chordomas, certain micro-scopic features are constant and diagnostic [7]. Microscopically the tumour is lobulated but un-encapsulated or has a pseudo-capsule and has a mucoid translucent appearance, and part of the tumour may be removed by suction. The tumour grows round structures such as nerves and blood vessels.

Treatment

The site of these tumours, and the stage at which symptoms are produced and a diagnosis is made, makes complete surgical removal difficult if not impossible. There has, to date, been no report of total removal of an intracranial chordoma. The prospect of cure for these tumours is poor but the tumour may grow slowly and patients may sur-vive for years. High voltage radiotherapy may be of value as the primary form of treatment [27]. In the author's limited experience radiotherapy fol-lowed by apparent total tumour removal has not altered the poor prognosis.

RARE TUMOURS

Cysts arising from Rathke's pouch and second branchial cleft remnants

Developmental cysts of the nasopharynx are slow growing and are usually symptomless until nasal respiration is obstructed. Midline cysts may originate from remnants of Rathke's pouch and branchogenic cysts usually involve the lateral wall of the nasopharynx and the adjoining soft palate. These are derived from the inner end of the second branchial cleft [28, 29]. Marsupiali-zation, aspiration and the injection of sclerosing fluids have been used in treatment, but excision is preferable. A transpalatine approach [22] may be indicated and total removal should be the aim. Before surgery, radiographs taken after an opaque medium has been injected into the cyst may help to define the extent and ramifications of the cyst as occurs in the lateral branchogenic cysts. Ectopic normal pituitary tissue is often found in the mucoperiosteum of the nasopharyn-geal roof behind the vomer sphenoid articula-tion, and this is thought to be the origin of the rare extrasellar chromophobe adenoma occur-ring as a nasopharyngeal mass [30] and unrelated to an intracranial tumour.

Dermoid cysts and teratomas

These tumours are not common. Three types have been described. An epidermoid cyst is lined by simple squamous epithelium, has a fibrous wall and no adnexal structures. A dermoid cyst is lined with epithelium and contains skin-asso-ciated appendages, such as hair and sebaceous glands. The teratomas and teratoid cysts contain tissues of ectodermal, mesodermal and endoder-mal origin. All three types may contain kera-tinous material. In the head and neck area the epidermoid variety is the most common, the der-moid next in frequency and the teratoid cyst or teratoma is rare. The pathogenesis of these lesions is uncertain. It has been suggested that the epidermoid and dermoid cysts are due to an enclavement of epithelium on closure of embryonic processes, such as occurs in the de-velopment of the orbit, nose and mouth where these cysts are most frequently encountered. The origin of teratomas and teratoid cysts is more complex. The hairy polyp of the nasopharynx is the most common. Eighty-nine cases have been reported [31]. The condition is usually diagnosed at birth and the tumour may be pedunculated and present through the mouth (Fig. 24.6). It may originate from the roof or posterior wall of the nasopharynx. Females are more frequently affected and other developmental abnormalities of the palate or skull are not unusual, and the base of the teratoma may be connected with neurological tissue through a perforation in the bony skull base.

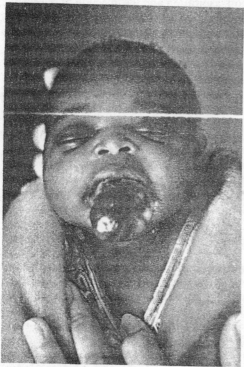

Fig. 24.6. Eighteen-hour-old African female baby with a pedunculated teratoid cyst of the nasopharynx. The tumour stalk originated high on the posterior nasopharyngeal wall. The child survived removal of the tumour by a cutting snare applied to the base of the pedicle.

The size of the tumour determines the clinical presentation. If large, interference with respiration and feeding difficulties will be evident, and if pedunculated the tumour may be evident in or through the mouth. Small tumours may not be diagnosed for many years and may erroneously be classified as nasopharyngeal fibromas.

The severity of the symptoms and the general fitness of the patient determine the urgency of treatment. If the child appears otherwise healthy, the obstructing tumour may be removed by using a cutting snare to cut the pedicle or if the tumour is sessile it may be avulsed by passing a grasping forceps behind the soft palate. These procedures are best performed under general anaesthesia. A tracheostomy may be indicated. No operative deaths or recurrences were noted in the eighty-nine patients reported [31].

Extramedullary plasmacytoma

The head and neck is the site most frequently involved by these tumours, and was the site in 90% of 250 cases reviewed [32]. The incidence is 0·04 per 100 000 population [33]. Fourteen (63·4%) of twenty-two cases involved the head and neck area, and in four the nasopharynx was the primary site.

The tumour presents as a non-ulcerating mass and may be lobulated. There may be an associated lymphadenopathy. The diagnosis is established by biopsy and by excluding general medullary involvement. Treatment is by chemotherapy and radiotherapy.

Rhabdomyosarcoma

The nasopharynx is the primary site in 10% of these myogenic neoplasms [7]. This is a neoplasm of the first decade of life. The presenting symptoms are those associated with a mass in the nasopharynx. The embryonal or botryoid form is the most common and is characterized by rapid local growth and a tendency for early metastases. Treatment is by radiotherapy and chemotherapy [34].

References

[1] ALI M. Y. (1967) Distribution and character of the squamous epithelium in the human nasopharynx. In *Cancer of the Nasopharynx*, eds. Muir C. S. & Shanmugaratnam, K., pp. 138–46. UICC Monograph Series Vol. 1. Copenhagen: Munksgaard.

[2] YEH SHU (1962) A histological classification of carcinomas of the nasopharynx with a critical review as to the existence of lymphoepitheliomas. *Cancer* **15**, 895.

[3] ROUVIÈRE H. (1938) *Anatomie des lymphatiques de l'homme*. Anatomy of the human lymphatic system. A compendium translated from the original by Tobias M. J. Ann Arbor, Michigan: Edwards Brothers, Inc.

[4] LEDERMAN M. (1961) *Cancer of the Nasopharynx: Its Natural History and Treatment*. Springfield, Illinois: Charles C. Thomas.

[5] SILBERMAN R. D., WILF H. & TUCKER J. A. (1976) Flexible fiberoptic nasopharyngolaryngoscope. *Annals of Otology, Rhinology and Laryngology* 85, 640.

[6] PEREZ C. A., ACKERMAN L. V., MILL W. B., OGURA J. H. & POWERS W. E. (1969) Cancer of the nasopharynx–factors influencing prognosis. *Cancer* 24, 1.

[7] BATSAKIS J. G. (1974) *Tumours of the Head and Neck: Clinical and Pathological Consideration.* Baltimore: Williams and Wilkins Company.

[8] CLIFFORD P. (1976) Epidemiology of some human cancers: (1) Nasopharynx. In *The Scientific Foundations of Oncology,* eds. Symmington T. & Carter R. L., Chap. 25. London: William Heinemann Medical Books Ltd.

[9] CLIFFORD P. (1970) A review on the epidemiology of nasopharyngeal carcinoma. *International Journal of Cancer* 5, 287.

[10] GODTFREDSON E. (1944) Ophthalmologic and neurologic symptoms of malignant nasopharyngeal tumours. Copenhagen: Munksgaard.

[11] CLIFFORD P. (1975) Combined modality therapy in head and neck cancer. In *Cancer of the Head and Neck,* eds. Chambers R. G., Janssen de Limpens A. M. P., Jaques D. A. & Routledge R. T. Amsterdam, Oxford: Excerpta Medica; New York: American Elsevier Publishing Co. Inc.

[12] LITTLE J. B., SCHULTZ M. D. & WANG C. C. (1963) Radiation therapy for cancer of the nasopharynx. *Archives of Otolaryngology* 77, 621.

[13] BLOOM S. M. (1969) Cancer of the nasopharynx: a study of ninety cases. *Journal of Mount Sinai Hospital* 36, 277.

[14] LEDERMAN M. (1975) Malignant tumours of the nasopharynx. In *Cancer of the Head and Neck,* eds. Chambers R. G., Janssen de Limpens A. M. P., Jaques D. A. & Routledge R. T. Amsterdam, Oxford: Excerpta Medica; American Elsevier Publishing Co. Inc.

[15] SHEDD D. P., VON ESSEN C. F., CONNELLY R. R. & EISENBERG H. (1968) Cancer of the pharynx in Connecticut, 1935–1959. *Cancer* 21, 706.

[16] HARRISON D. F. N. (1976) Juvenile postnasal angiofibroma – an evaluation. *Clinical Otolaryngology* 1, 187.

[17] HOLMAN C. B. & MILLER W. E. (1965) Juvenile nasopharyngeal fibroma – roentgenologic characteristics. *American Journal of Roentgenology, Radium Therapy and Nuclear Medicine* 94, 292.

[18] SESSIONS R. B., WILLS P. I., ALFORD B. R., HARRELL J. E. & EVANS R. A. (1976) Juvenile nasopharyngeal angiofibroma: radiographic aspects. *Laryngoscope* 86, 2.

[19] SMITH M. F. W., BOLES R. & WORK W. P. (1964) Cryo-

[20] ROBERTSON G. H., BILLER H., SESSIONS D. G. & OGURA J. H. (1972) Presurgical internal maxillary artery embolization in juvenile angiofibroma. *Laryngoscope* 82, 1524.

[21] SOLIS O., ROBERTSON G. & WEBER A. L. (1976) Juvenile nasopharyngeal angiofibroma. *Annals of Otology, Rhinology and Laryngology* 85, 415.

[22] WILSON C. P. (1957) Observations on the surgery of the nasopharynx. *Annals of Otology, Rhinology and Laryngology* 66, 5.

[23] BOCCA E. (1971) Transpharyngeal approach to nasopharyngeal fibroma. *Annals of Otology, Rhinology and Laryngology* 80, 171.

[24] BILLER H. F., SESSIONS D. G. & OGURA J. H. (1974) Angiofibroma: a treatment approach. *Laryngoscope* 84, 695.

[25] BOLES R. & DEDO H. (1976) Nasopharyngeal angiofibroma. *Laryngoscope* 86, 364.

[26] UTNE J. R. & PUGH D. A. (1955) The roentgenologic aspects of chordoma. *American Journal of Roentgenology* 74, 593.

[27] WRIGHT C. (1968) Nasopharyngeal and cervical chordoma – some aspects of their development and treatment. *Journal of Laryngology and Otology* 82, 1337.

[28] MILLS C. P. (1955) A midline cyst of the nasopharynx. *Journal of Laryngology and Otology* 69, 215.

[29] BADRAWY R., SAJWAT F. & FAHMY S. (1974) Cysts of the nasopharynx. *Journal of Laryngology and Otology* 88, 571.

[30] CHESSIN H. & SMITH H. (1976) Chromophobe adenoma manifesting as a nasopharyngeal mass. *Archives of Otolaryngology* 102, 631.

[31] FOXWELL P. B. & KELHAM B. H. (1958) Teratoid tumours of the nasopharynx. *Journal of Laryngology and Otology* 72, 647.

[32] BOOTH J. B., CHEESMAN A. D. & VINCENTI N. H. (1973) Extramedullary plasmacytomata of the upper respiratory tract. *Annals of Otology, Rhinology and Laryngology* 82, 709.

[33] PAHOR A. L. (1977) Extramedullary plasmacytoma of the head and neck, parotid and submandibular salivary glands. *Journal of Laryngology and Otology* 91, 241.

[34] DONALDSON S. S., CASTRO J. R., WILBUR J. R. & JESSE R. H. (1973) Rhabdomyosarcoma of head and neck in children – combination treatment by surgery, irradiation and chemotherapy. *Cancer* 31, 26.

CHAPTER 25

Diseases of the Oropharynx

TONSILLITIS

Follicular tonsillitis

This disease remains localized to tonsillar tissue and is only moderately contagious.

The streptococcus is the most frequent causal agent; the betahaemolytic streptococcus group A is the most aggressive organism and is responsible for the articular and renal complications. The pneumococcus may also be responsible, and during the course of the last 10 years the proportion of Gram-negative organisms (coliforms, proteus and pseudomonas) has steadily increased, but it is necessary to take account of the fact that the yield on culture of the streptococcus or the pneumococcus is very low, whereas the Gram-negative bacteria grow very easily. An initial culture therefore still has considerable value.

The initial symptoms of tonsillitis, both local and general, do not differ from those of erythematous pharyngitis. The tonsils are enlarged, very red and studded with an exudate which is white and later grey and which can easily be detached with a cotton wool probe. This picture can extend to the other collections of pharyngeal lymphoid tissue. There is always a painful adenopathy of the jugulodigastric gland. The white blood count is usually raised at around 10–12 000 leucocytes/mm^3.

Complications are rare with peritonsillar abscess being commonest and arthritis, endocarditis and glomerulonephritis being much less frequent than in former days.

A swab should be taken for culture and sensitivity, since this may eventually be required if the tonsillitis is prolonged or if complications arise.

Treatment with antibiotics is mandatory in patients who have previously had rheumatism or who have chronic nephritis or valvular disease of the heart; it is wise, however, to use them in most patients. The best antibiotic to start treatment with is penicillin which is successful for the majority of cases of tonsillitis due to the streptococcus or the pneumococcus; if the patient is allergic to penicillin it is best to use erythromycin. If the responsible organism is Gram-negative broad spectrum antibiotics (ampicillin, cephalosporin) should be used. If the antistreptolysin titre remains elevated after the tonsillitis has healed this indicates that the cause of the pharyngitis was streptococcal and that treatment with penicillin should be prolonged. In recurrent cases it is often necessary to remove the tonsils.

Peritonsillar abscess

If an acute infection of the tonsil extends beyond the capsule into the peritonsillar space then an abscess will result.

This disease usually occurs in the adolescent or the young adult between 20 and 35 years of age. It tends to recur and the following local anatomical factors predispose to this: a deep tonsillar fossa due to the extent of the pillars, intratonsillar crypts not connecting with the pharynx, and scars due to a previous incomplete tonsillectomy.

The abscess is most commonly sited anteriorly. The abscess pushes the tonsil medially, inferiorly and posteriorly and tends to point anteriorly through the anterior pillar. A posterior abscess is rarer and pushes the tonsil anteriorly.

Several organisms may be responsible but the haemolytic streptococcus is most common.

The course of the disease is slow; it begins with unilateral pharyngeal pain, severe otalgia and spasms of pain felt during swallowing. The fever is moderate (38–38·5°) and the local signs are not marked during the first few days.

The following signs declare themselves about the third to fourth day; intense pain, almost complete dysphagia, rhinolalia, trismus of varying severity and deterioration of the general condition. A blood count shows a leucocytosis of 15–30 000/mm³. The unilateral pharyngeal swelling becomes very extensive and in an anterior abscess occupies the superior part of the anterior pillar and a large proportion of the soft palate. The tonsil is displaced and often covered by soft exudate and there is usually a painful adenopathy of the jugulodigastric gland.

The abscess takes 5–8 days to accumulate and ruptures spontaneously between the fifth and tenth day if it is not incised.

It is rare for peritonsillar abscesses to cause complications but oedema of the palate or of the larynx can occur and can cause dyspnoea.

Diagnosis is sometimes difficult because of the severity of the trismus but is usually easy to make because all the symptoms are unilateral. The following three possibilities should be borne in mind; pseudophlegmonous pharyngitis (unilateral), a lymphoma of the tonsil or a parapharyngeal abscess which is rare.

The treatment is incision through the anterior or posterior pillar respectively. It is preceded by aspiration to confirm the presence of pus and to guide the site of incision; this causes almost immediate relief of the pain and of the general symptoms. Treatment with antibiotics is only effective early in the disease but it can assist in diminishing the extent of the inflammatory process. Steroids should only be used for extensive oedema.

A peritonsillar abscess almost always recurs and so it is therefore necesssary to remove the tonsils 5–6 weeks later.

Chronic tonsillitis

Chronic infection can often be found in large cryptic tonsils, in small sclerosed tonsils and in the tonsillar remnants left behind by incomplete tonsillectomy.

The streptococcus is the most common causative organism.

In the adult, chronic tonsillitis usually manifests itself in one of two ways.

(1) Chronic caseous tonsillitis, characterized by the presence of crypts full of white concretions, the product of maceration of food debris. This type of local infection is not accompanied by suppuration and does not lead to complications. It is treated by cleaning of the crypts and minor manoeuvres destined to facilitate their drainage.

(2) Chronic suppurative tonsillitis is characterized by the presence of pus when the tonsils are squeezed. The tonsils often appear normal, and are normal in size or even appear small. The disease is not usually accompanied by cervical adenopathy. Although it may be the starting point of a peritonsillar abscess it does not usually cause generalized signs.

While some patients may prefer to avoid tonsillectomy in adult life and take antibiotics on an episodic basis, the most usual treatment is tonsillectomy when the disease has become recurrent in character.

Lingual tonsillitis

The muscular mass of the posterior third of the tongue is covered by lymphoid tissue, the lingual tonsil.

Embryologically the base of the tongue is constituted by two lateral processes, the second and third branchial arches; their union with an anterior process which becomes the mobile part of the tongue produces a pharyngeal invagination which takes the form of a cellular cord, the thyroglossal duct leading from the foramen caecum to the isthmus of the thyroid gland; this canal ultimately disappears.

The median thyroid anlage may not migrate inferiorly so that the body of the thyroid gland remains entirely within the base of the tongue and also some elements of the thyroglossal duct can persist and give rise to thyroglossal duct cysts.

Simple hypertrophy of the lingual tonsil does not usually cause symptoms; it often develops after removal of the palatine tonsil and the adenoids.

Acute lingual tonsillitis is relatively frequently associated with a palatine tonsillitis and it is seen in isolation in patients who have had their tonsils removed. It should be remembered and looked for with a mirror in patients with the symptoms of pharyngitis in whom examination with the tongue depressor apparently shows no abnormality of the oropharynx.

An abscess of the base of the tongue is fairly rare; this abscess develops in the cellular peritonsillar tissue. It causes a mid-line dysphagia, nasal speech and protrusion of the tongue. Antibiotics are required and occasionally incision, which is never easy to carry out.

These conditions must always be differentiated from:

(1) *Ectopic lingual thyroid* which is not rare, particularly in women; in the majority of cases the thyroid gland is not found in its normal situation. It presents as a midline tumour the size of a walnut, dull red in colour, slightly blue, situated posterior to the foramen caecum. It does not usually cause symptoms but can occasionally be injured by the slight trauma of swallowing and can then cause excessive bleeding which is difficult to treat.

An ectopic thyroid gland is subject to all the diseases to which the normal gland in the normal position is subject, such as tumours, hypothyroidism, etc. The diagnosis is made by biopsy and scanning with ^{131}I. Rarely it is necessary to carry out partial excision of the ectopic thyroid or to transplant it on a pedicle.

(2) *Cysts* at the base of the tongue develop from remnants of the thyroglossal duct and are situated in the midline; they are very rare in contrast to the thyroglossal cysts which develop in the midline of the anterior part of the neck.

PHARYNGITIS

Acute pharyngitis

This is a seasonal disease which is very contagious, producing epidemics of greater or lesser severity, and which is often viral in origin. While primarily affecting the tonsil it usually involves the entire pharyngeal mucosa. The onset is sudden with general ill health, rigors, painful dryness of the throat followed by referred pain to the ear on swallowing. The fever is of varying severity depending on the amount of tissue in-

volved, the pathogenicity of the offending organism and the resistance of the host. There is seldom any cervical lymphadenopathy. The disease follows a short course usually resolving spontaneously in 3 or 4 days without complications. It takes one of three forms.

(1) Influenzal pharyngotonsillitis, which is due to the influenzal or orthomyxoviruses causing a high fever and severe generalized symptoms such as malaise, headache and myalgia.

(2) Seasonal erythematous pharyngotonsillitis which is due to the adenovirus; this virus is characterized by both a complement fixation reaction and a neutralization reaction from pharyngeal or conjunctival secretions. The course of the disease is less severe but as well as the pharynx, the larynx, trachea and conjunctiva are also affected.

(3) Erythematous bacterial pharyngotonsillitis is caused by the streptococcus and is the least common form. It is characterized by cervical lymphadenopathy. An allergy of the pharyngeal mucosa must be excluded as should an early scarlet fever.

The treatment of all these forms is symptomatic with rest, hot drinks and analgesics. Local measures such as mouthwashes are ineffective but good for the morale of the patient. Antibiotics are of no value unless a bacterial cause is suspected.

Chronic pharyngitis

Chronic pharyngitis is very frequent because of the permanent irritation suffered by the pharynx both in the child and the adult by the inhalation of vapours, dust and smoke, the swallowing of liquids and solids and contact with bacteriological agents. Two main clinical pictures occur.

Catarrhal pharyngitis
In this condition the mucosa of the pharynx is red, dotted with hypertrophic lymphoid follicles, particularly posterior to the posterior pillar and by granulations corresponding to the dilated mucosal glands. The clinical picture varies depending on whether the disease is primarily congestive or hypertrophic.

In the adult, mucopurulent chronic pharyngitis is fairly rare and is usually secondary to nasal or sinus infection. The common form is the catarrhal one which is extremely common over the age of 40. It occurs constantly in the smoker and in the chronic alcoholic, these two vices often going together, but it can also be due to industrial pollution, inclement weather and misuse of the voice. Clinical examination always shows reddening of the pharynx and a hypertrophic and granular appearance. The mucosa is always hypersensitive so that the examination is often difficult.

Chronic congestive pharyngitis, because of the symptoms it causes, such as cough, is one of the most frequent reasons for consulting an otolaryngologist.

Treatment consists in persuading the patient to give up the responsible agent such as alcohol or tobacco, and perhaps modifying the working conditions. Local or general treatment may produce partial and often temporary improvement.

In the infant, chronic pharyngitis is of the congestive type with abundant secretion of mucus and hypertrophy of the lymphoid follicles. Its cause is infection often secondary to a chronic infection of the adenoids or the nasal sinuses. Adenoidectomy and treatment of the chronic sinusitis often leads to healing of the chronic pharyngitis but this does not always occur because allergic factors often accompany the infection.

A specific chronic pharyngitis is seen in some children who have undergone adenoidectomy and tonsillectomy and who later present with a compensatory hypertrophy of the lingual tonsil and of the lymphoid follicles of the posterior wall of the pharynx which are subject to chronic inflammation.

Atrophic pharyngitis

This disease is often the final stage of congestive or hypertrophic pharyngitis and manifests itself by dryness of the pharynx. The lymphoid follicles and the mucosal glands are atrophic and there is sometimes crusting. The submucosal cellular tissue tends to disappear and the muscular tissue scleroses. The mucosa is dry and loses its shiny appearance. In advanced cases crusting and ozaena can occur.

Atrophic pharyngitis can also be secondary to radiotherapy for head and neck tumours. It is often very extensive and causes considerable disability. All the secretory elements are lost so that it is necessary to constantly humidify the pharynx especially during eating which may otherwise be impossible.

Diphtheritic pharyngitis

This disease has now become exceedingly rare but it is possible that cases may be seen in the future as public attitudes to childhood immunization become lax. It is characterized by a pseudomembranous pharyngitis which is the primary lesion of a generalized illness caused by the spread of a neurotropic toxin.

In its common form, usually seen in a child, the early symptoms are insidious and the signs modest; examination shows pearly white spots which become yellow and adhere to the mucosa and then extend progressively. The pharyngitis is accompanied by extensive lymphadenopathy and by a mucopurulent coryza. There is only a mild fever but the child suffers from malaise.

Some cases of diphtheritic pharyngitis are classified as 'malignant' from the beginning and are characterized by the extension of the false membrane to the entire pharynx, and sometimes to the larynx, and by the seriousness of the general upset (haemorrhages, renal involvement and cardiac disorders). This disease is generally fatal within 10–12 days.

The diagnosis is usually easy but the disease can be confused with certain pharyngeal manifestations of the leukaemias or infectious mononucleosis. It is established by bacteriological examination of a culture. The differential diagnosis from the pseudodiphtheritic bacillus of Hoffman is sometimes difficult.

The treatment of the common form is to give serum by a single intramuscular injection of 10–20 000 units in the child and 30–50 000 in the adult with antibiotics (penicillin G or erythromycin). The antibiotics sterilize the local lesion but only the serum can exert any effect on the general toxic manifestations. Treatment with steroids is given if the local inflammatory reaction is extensive.

The dose of serum and antibiotics should be greatly increased in the malignant form and the patient should be looked after in an intensive care unit so as to be able to manage the effects of the toxin on the general condition.

In every case vaccines are given several weeks later; even if there is a rapid cure the malaise persists for a long time.

Scarlet fever

The pathogenic agent is the betahaemolytic streptococcus type A. The pharyngitis constitutes both the portal of entry of this exanthematous fever and the first sign of the disease.

Its clinical picture is typical: a sudden onset with a fever of 39–40° C, headache, vomiting, tachycardia, abdominal pain, intense dysphagia, a diffuse erythematous pharyngitis contrasting with the white appearance of the dorsum of the tongue, the so-called strawberry tongue. The blood count shows a leucocytosis of 20 000/mm³ often with an eosinophilia of 5–8%. The exanthem appears the following day making the diagnosis easy.

There is usually a rapid resolution of the condition with antibiotics and complications are rare. Local complications that used to cause much concern were mastoiditis, sinusitis and cervical adenitis. General complications such as arthritis and nephritis are now almost unknown.

Vincent's angina

Vincent's angina is a unilateral ulcerative pharyngitis which evolves in two stages, the first being pseudomembranous and the second ulcerative.

The causative agents are a fusiform bacillus and a spirochaete acting together. This association is not specific and can commonly be isolated from the mouth and more particularly from the gingivodental area but in this case it is associated with other microbial agents. The confirmation of a fusiform organism without any other organisms is therefore still valuable but culture of these organisms is very difficult.

This unilateral ulcerative pharyngitis is seen particularly in adolescents and young adults and often in patients who suffer a chronic gingivo-

dental infection. It does not appear to be infectious.

The disease begins insidiously with practically no fever and declares itself by a unilateral dysphagia. Examination in the early stages shows a friable false membrane localized to the tonsil on one side only, sometimes with a palpable jugulodigastric gland. Several days later ulceration appears which is usually circumscribed, fairly deep, irregular and covered by a yellowish exudate, but the tonsil remain soft to palpation.

The course of the disease is relatively slow and tends to resolve in about 10 days even in the absence of any treatment. Penicillin or antibiotic mouthwashes shorten the natural course of the disease.

Other causes of acute pharyngitis

Other infective diseases can be accompanied by pharyngitis: *typhoid fever* in which there may be ulceration of the anterior pillars, *tularaemia, erysipelas* and *measles*. The pharyngotonsillitis due to *syphilis* and *tuberculosis* is now of extreme rarity.

Gangrenous pharyngitis is a very rare disease which can appear as an incidental finding during the course of severe diabetes, serious renal insufficiency, agranulocytosis or leukaemia. The causal agent is an anaerobic bacteria, usually the anaerobic streptococcus which is always associated with a pyogenic bacteria particularly the haemolytic streptococcus.

The generalized upset is very severe with a pyrexia of 40–41° C, prostration, hypotension and diarrhoea; the breath is foetid and the tonsils and the pharynx are covered with brownish haemorrhagic spots.

Treatment consists of massive doses of antibiotics; usually penicillin (penicillin G or ampicillin), but erythromycin and tetracyclines may also be used. This treatment is not always effective and does not always prevent a rapid downhill course and death.

Pharyngeal manifestations of blood disorders

Pharyngitis due to agranulocytosis and leucopenia
These diseases are characterized by a consider-

able decrease in the number of polymorphonuclear leucocytes in the peripheral blood. Pharyngeal manifestations are very frequent when their absolute number falls below 1000/mm³.

Whether the cause is a pure acute agranulocytosis or a pancytopenia associated with a decrease of the red cell count and of the thrombocytes besides the granulocytes, the first symptoms are pharyngeal accompanied by fever. The dysphagia rapidly becomes intense, the breath foetid and the pharynx and later the mouth are covered first by a false membrane and then by necrotic hollowed-out ulcers which bleed, in the case of the pancytopenias, and which extend rapidly. The general health is profoundly affected. There is little reactive lymphadenopathy.

Bacteriological examination shows commensal organisms only and the diagnosis is made on the blood count and a bone marrow biopsy.

The history may show that the cause is sensitivity to a drug, usually amidopyrine, but also phenylbutazone, antipyrines, chloramphenicol, sulphonamides and antithyroid drugs such as thiouracil, and chlorpromazine. In pancytopenia occupational exposure to agents such as benzine or the cytotoxic drugs may be responsible. The development of chemotherapeutic agents for cancer has considerably increased the frequency of medullary aplasia and their pharyngeal manifestations if the dose given is too great or the timing of administration is incorrect.

Treatment of pharyngitis due to agranulocytosis is often successful; massive doses of antibiotics are given with steroids, together with blood transfusions including platelets and white cells in the case of a pancytopenia.

The pharyngitis of infectious mononucleosis

Pharyngitis is one of the most important symptoms of this disease but is not absolutely constant. However it is usually the first symptom and is often preceded by a period of malaise and moderate fever. The pharyngitis may not even manifest itself for 2–3 weeks.

The pharyngitis is usually follicular and has no distinguishing characteristics; however, a pseudomembranous form can be seen which is actually ulceronecrotic. The dysphagia is of variable intensity. Enlarged cervical glands are constantly seen; they are firm, slightly painful and can affect any part of the cervical chain but often the supraclavicular region. The general signs are usually moderate but malaise is constant and prolonged. Bacteriological examination of the pharyngeal secretions shows commensal organisms only.

The diagnosis is confirmed by a blood count which shows an inversion of the ratio of white cells and the presence of abnormal monocytes, and by the Paul–Bunnell reaction, which changes slowly and which often must be repeated two or three times.

The course is benign and prolonged for 2–4 weeks and followed by a period of malaise. Symptomatic treatment is usually satisfactory in the common form but if there is super-added infection, antibiotics and steroids (30–50 mg of prednisone per day for 8–10 days) can be prescribed.

It should be recalled that the aetiology of infectious mononucleosis is not known with certainty but is suspected to be of viral origin (the Epstein–Barr virus); the infection is transmitted direct particularly through saliva.

Pharyngitis in the haemorrhagic disorders

Thrombocytopenic purpura usually only causes petechiae or ecchymoses on the mucosa of the soft palate or the tonsil; sometimes bullae with a bloodstained outline and rarely an extensive haematoma can occur.

In haemophilia large haematomas of the pharynx can occur but are rare. This haematoma should of course not be incised and a tracheostomy should be done for dyspnoea.

The pharyngitis of acute leukaemia

This disease occurs mainly in infants and adolescents and is sometimes accompanied by pharyngeal manifestations, either an erythematous, a pseudomembranous, or an ulceronecrotic pharyngitis, but this is far from being constant. The pharyngitis is often accompanied by an extensive gingivostomatitis. Many of the lymph glands in the neck are enlarged.

Diagnosis is made by haematological examination; examination of the nose and throat is of little importance.

Vesicular and ulcerative lesions of the oropharynx

These lesions usually accompany the dermatoses but can occur in isolation affecting both the oropharynx and oral cavity and are considered in Chapter 26.

TUMOURS OF THE OROPHARYNX

Anatomy

The anatomical boundaries of this area have been laid down clearly by the UICC and AJC. According to this classification the oropharynx extends from the junction of the hard and soft palates to the level of the floor of the vallecula, and consists of the following areas:

(1) Anterior wall (glosso-epiglottic area).
(a) Tongue posterior to the vallate papillae (base of tongue or posterior third);
(b) vallecula;
(c) anterior (lingual) surface of epiglottis.
(2) Lateral wall – tonsils, faucial pillars and glossotonsillar sulci.
(3) Posterior oropharyngeal wall.
(4) Superior wall – inferior surface of soft palate and uvula.

Two further points of surgical anatomy require emphasis. The retromolar trigone is a sort of no-man's-land since in some classifications (e.g. MacComb and Fletcher) this structure is part of the oropharynx, and in others it is not. Because the retromolar trigone is included as part of the oral cavity in the UICC/AJC definition tumours of this area should *not* be included in oropharyngeal tumours.

Secondly there is often a tendency to regard tumours of the anterior (lingual) surface of the epiglottis and the vallecula as laryngeal tumours. They behave in a similar way to such tumours and are treated in a similar way, but it should be remembered that these structures are part of the oropharynx.

Pathology

There is evidence that carcinoma of the oropharynx is much more common in North America than in the United Kingdom: According to

Rolander [1] 12 000 new cases of carcinoma of the tonsil are seen in the USA annually, a rate of 60 per million. Comparable figures for the United Kingdom are difficult to obtain, but it is likely that cancer of the pharynx is roughly equal in incidence to cancer of the larynx, of which 1000 cases occur annually in the UK. Since 40% of pharyngeal cancers affect the oropharynx, the incidence of this tumour is thus of the order of 8 per million. A similar proportionate incidence can be deduced from Ledermann's figures [2].

The pathology of malignant tumours of the oropharynx is dictated by the anatomical and histological characteristics of this region.

The mucosa is squamous in type over the tonsillar fossae, the soft palate, the base of the tongue and the posterior wall of the pharynx. This explains why 85–90% of tumours are squamous in type.

The submucous tissue, particularly of the soft palate, has a large number of salivary glands which are mucous in type; from these arise the 5–10% of adenoidcystic carcinomas of this area.

There are extensive collections of lymphoid tissue in the palatine and lingual tonsils from which arise the 5–10% of malignant lymphomas. In this respect it is important also to note the particular radio-curability of the carcinomas of this region which develop in contact with lymphoid tissue (the so-called lymphoepithelioma).

The situation of the oropharynx at the crossroads of the respiratory and digestive tracts explains the main symptom which is pain on swallowing. The symptoms are unilateral in cancers of the tonsil and bilateral in cancers of the soft palate, the base of the tongue and the posterior wall of the pharynx.

In addition to squamous carcinomas, adenoidcystic carcinomas and malignant lymphomas, other malignant tumours occur, but are rare: Hodgkin's disease, chronic lymphocytic leukaemia, plasmocytomas of the tonsil (which may be isolated or may arise during the course of multiple myelomatosis), malignant melanomas of the palate, mesenchymal sarcomas and finally the very exceptional metastases to the tonsil of carcinomas of the thyroid gland and the kidney.

Tumours of the oropharynx are staged under the UICC/AJC scheme, with the following conditions:

(1) The classification applies only to carcinoma.

(2) There must be histological verification of the disease.

(3) The extent of disease must be assessed clinically, radiographically and endoscopically.

The following TNM classification is then recommended:

TlS Pre-invasive carcinoma (carcinoma *in situ*).

T0 No evidence of primary tumour.

T1 Tumour limited to one site.

T2 Tumour extending into two sites.

T3 Tumour extending beyond oropharynx.

The N and M systems are the same as in other head and neck sites.

Tumours of the tonsil

This is one of the most frequent carcinomas of the upper respiratory tract.

Squamous carcinoma

This constitutes 85–95% of all cancers of the tonsil. It occurs particularly between 50 and 70 years of age. Men form 90% of the total and are very often chronic alcoholics or very heavy smokers.

The initial symptom in two patients out of three is unilateral dysphagia and sore throat which is often not severe, and in one case out of three the appearance of a cervical gland.

The tonsillar tumour is usually ulcerating and infiltrating and painful and hard to palpation. When it is small the only signs may be limited infiltration, minor ulceration and simple erythematous hypertrophy of one faucial pillar, all of which require careful investigation. As soon as the diagnosis is suspected the following steps must be taken:

(1) The extent of the tumour should be confirmed by digital palpation, inferiorly towards the tonsilloglossal sulcus and the tongue, anteriorly towards the floor of the mouth, the anterior faucial pillar and the internal surface of the cheek, posteriorly towards the posterior pillar

and the lateral wall of the pharynx and superiorly towards the soft palate.

(2) Examination of the cervical lymph nodes. Three patients out of four have palpable nodes, which are bilateral in 10–20% of cases, and most often affect the jugulodigastric gland. The glands are hard and are either mobile or already fixed to the deep plane. Their size and site should be noted on a diagram. The existence of a palpable gland does not necessarily indicate neoplastic infiltration because 20–25% of palpable glands are not histologically invaded.

(3) Classification of the tumour into one of the categories by the TNM classification of the UICC and AJC.

(4) A search is undertaken for a second cancer of the upper respiratory tract, which is found in 15–20% of patients either at the time of first examination or later.

(5) Assessment of the general health is performed as is a search for metastases which are present in 6% of cases.

(6) Biopsy of the tonsil usually shows a squamous carcinoma which may be well or poorly differentiated. In rare cases other varieties of carcinoma are found: lymphoepithelioma, carcinoma with a sarcomatous stroma, carcinoma with pseudocystic metastatic glands.

The diagnosis is usually easy to make even before the biopsy is done, but tuberculosis and Vincent's angina should be borne in mind as should a tumour originating in the parapharyngeal space pushing the tonsil medially without invading it; this may be a tumour of the deep lobe of the parotid gland or a large neurogenic tumour.

Treatment
The treatment is principally by radiotherapy because these tumours are particularly curable by cobalt or the linear accelerator. The radiotherapy should encompass the oropharynx and the entire lymph gland area of both sides. The dose is 7000–7500 rads in 7–8 weeks. If there are no glands palpable in the lower half of the neck only 5000 rads is given at this level.

Excision is reserved for recurrence of the tumour after failed radiotherapy. Excision should be extensive consisting of the commando operation with resection of the angle of the jaw and immediate repair of the pharynx as necessary. A radical neck dissection is indicated if there are cervical gland metastases.

Chemotherapy may be a useful adjunct using systemic treatment for 6 months to 1 year after the end of radiation but this has not yet been confirmed.

Cobalt therapy provides a 5-year survival rate of 35% falling to 12% at 10 years due to the later development of other cancers of the upper respiratory tract.

Non-Hodgkin's lymphomas

These consisted of what were formerly known as lymphosarcomas and reticulum cell sarcomas and constitute 5–15% of tumours of the tonsil; they can occur at any age and even in children. Men are affected about 60% of the time [3].

The early symptoms are the same as those of a carcinoma but the appearance of the tonsillar tumour is different; the entire tonsil is hypertrophic, the mucosa is red with some necrotic ulceration.

The investigations are as follows:

(1) A search for other tumours of Waldeyer's ring which are observed in 10–20% of cases.

(2) A search for palpable cervical nodes which are found in 60–80% of cases, being bilateral in 20–50% of cases. They are firm but not hard and may form a mass of multiple glands.

(3) A tonsillar biopsy and cytological examination of a smear or a needle biopsy of a cervical gland.

(4) General examination for tumour in sites outside the head and neck; examination of other glands, full blood count, a bone marrow biopsy and lymphangiography. The examination is usually carried out under the supervision of a lymphoma team, and confirms whether the disease is still localized or is disseminated.

Localized disease is treated by teletherapy with cobalt to a dose of 4000–5000 rads followed by chemotherapy; disseminated disease is treated by chemotherapy followed by radiotherapy to the neck and possibly to the subdiaphragmatic area.

Results of treatment of local and regional metastases in the neck gives a prognosis of 40% survival at 5 years.

Tumours of the soft palate

Squamous carcinoma

This forms 75–95% of carcinomas of the soft palate; over 90% of the patients are men and are often heavy smokers and drinkers.

The first symptom is dysphagia which is often felt in the midline and is not lateralized; it therefore gives little cause for concern. The tumour sometimes manifests itself by a cervical node.

There are three sites of predeliction: an ulcero-infiltrating form on the uvula, an irregular tumour which shows little tendency to ulcerate or infiltrate on the inferior margin of the soft palate, an exuberant superficial or localized erythematous area on the anterior surface of the soft palate.

Investigations include the following:

(1) Confirmation of the extent of the tumour by digital palpation and by examination of the nasopharynx with a mirror. Extension occurs laterally towards the faucial pillars and the tonsils, superiorly towards the lateral wall of the nasopharynx and, uncommonly, anteriorly on to the hard palate.

(2) Examination for enlarged cervical nodes. About 50% of the patients have palpable glands when first seen, usually of the jugulodigastric gland. They are less often bilateral (13% of the cases) which indicates how infrequently the tumour is midline.

(3) Classification by the TNM system.

(4) A search for a second carcinoma of the upper respiratory tract, which is particularly frequent and occurs in 8–35% of cases in published series.

(5) Assessment of the general health.

(6) Radiological examination of the palate in the anteroposterior plane and by sagittal tomograms and assessment of possible involvement of the posterior surface of the palate.

(7) Biopsy.

Diagnosis is usually easily made and poses the same problem as for that of carcinoma of the tonsil.

Treatment
This is essentially by radiotherapy and similar to that for carcinoma of the tonsil.

However, endocurie therapy using ^{192}Ir can be used alone or preferably combined with tele-cobalt therapy for tumours which are small in volume, particularly those of the uvula.

It should be noted that there are a few indica-tions for surgical excision after failed radio-therapy: either a limited excision (removal of the uvula) or more extensive (excision of the entire soft palate). In the latter case reconstructive sur-gery generally gives mediocre results, and a pala-tal prostheses can adequately close the communi-cation between the oro- and nasopharynx.

The results are of the order of 20–30% survival at 5 years; some publications claim 64% but these are selected series.

Salivary tumours

These present 3–24% of carcinomas of the soft palate according to various published series. Whether the tumour is a pleomorphic adenoma, an adenoidcystic carcinoma or a mucoepider-moid tumour (which is the rarest), they all have certain characteristics in common: minimal symptoms, no involvement of the mucosa over a long period, and a long natural history.

Mixed tumours occur between 20 and 50 years of age. Their natural history is very long covering 5, 10 or even 20 years and they do not cause symptoms although they often become very large. These tumours are oval in shape, regular with clear margins and are covered by normal mucosa. The tumour should be differentiated from a mixed tumour of the deep lobe of the parotid gland. Treatment is excision by the oral route. Recurrence is unusual; malignant degen-eration can eventually occur but this is excep-tional [4].

Adenoidcystic carcinomas have a similar clini-cal history; but once they attain a certain size the tumour is more papillary, the mucosa covering it becomes erythematous and then ulcerates. Recurrence after excision is frequent and repeated.

The treatment of adenoidcystic carcinomas depends on the size. Small tumours are managed by extensive excision and tumours which are moderate or large in size are treated by combined radiotherapy and surgery in which the excision is followed by irradiation to 7000 rads.

Tumours of the posterior wall of the pharynx

These tumours are rare and have a disastrous prognosis. They are almost always squamous carcinoma (98% of cases) and usually affect the posterior wall of the oro and hypopharynx.

The presenting symptoms are dysphagia, which may be in the midline or lateralized, or sometimes a cervical node; tumours of the pos-terior wall of the pharynx usually have an ulcer-ated, excavated surface surrounded by a greater or lesser infiltrated zone. The lesion is always in the midline and symmetrical in extent but may sometimes be bigger on one side.

Investigations are as follows.

(1) Confirmation of the superior extent of the tumour into the nasopharynx, its inferior exten-sion into the hypopharynx and its lateral exten-sion towards the posterior faucial pillars which for a long time constitute the limits of the tumour.

(2) Radiological examination (plain films and contrast films) which confirm the inferior extent. The vertebral bodies behind are almost never invaded and the retropharyngeal space for a long time remains free of involvement by tumour.

(3) A search for cervical nodes which occur in 75% of patients (bilateral in 15–20%). These usually occur in the jugulodigastric gland.

(4) Biopsy.

(5) Assessment of the general health.

The diagnosis is easy and the only rare differ-ential diagnosis to be considered is tertiary syphilis.

Treatment

Treatment usually consists of radiotherapy to the pharynx and the cervical area to a dose of 7000 rads. The results are usually very bad giving a 5-year survival of 3–15%.

Excision should be carried out if possible but only for tumours which are small or medium in size, which are not often seen. The best technique of excision is via the intra-oral route using sus-pension laryngoscopy; a tracheotomy is done. The results in the long-term in these cases are appreciably better.

Tumours of the base of the tongue

These tumours are of moderate frequency but

are only half as frequent as cancers of the mobile portion of the tongue. In France these tumours nearly always affect men (97% of cases in our material) but this is not so striking in other countries.

Squamous carcinoma of the base of the tongue

This constitutes 95% of cancers of this region.

The symptoms appear late and are not marked. Vague but persistent sore throat, a sensation of a foreign body in the midline, and sometimes a cervical lymph node.

Examination with a tongue depressor is not usually sufficient to demonstrate the tumour and examination should be carried out with the mirror and by palpation with a finger.

Investigations include the following.

(1) Confirmation of the extent of the tumour which is often very large at the first examination: Anteriorly towards the mobile part of the tongue, laterally towards the tonsillolingual sulcus and the tonsils and posteriorly towards the glosso-epiglottic fold.

(2) A search for cervical lymph nodes which are found in 75% of patients being bilateral in 50% of patients. They generally affect the jugulo-digastric node.

(3) A search for a second cancer of the upper respiratory tract which is seen in 6% of patients in our material.

(4) Radiological examination (plain films and sagittal tomograms with and without contrast media) which allows differentiation between proliferative forms and those with deeper ulceration of the base of the tongue; the latter have a very poor prognosis.

(5) Assessment of the general health.

(6) Biopsy which is occasionally difficult: an excision into the mucosa is sometimes necessary in the infiltrating forms.

The diagnosis is simple and the differential diagnosis is from lingual thyroid, abscess and cyst.

Treatment

The treatment is exclusively by radiotherapy to the oropharynx and both sides of the neck; 7500 rads are given, but the results are mediocre. The survival at 5 years is between 7 and 31%.

Excision is rarely done because it is either relatively limited and ineffective or very extensive and mutilating requiring total laryngectomy and glossectomy plus reconstruction.

Malignant glandular tumours

These tumours, principally adenoidcystic carcinomas, constitute 3% of tumours of the base of the tongue. They are multilobed, grow slowly and cause little pain; they ought to be treated by combined radiotherapy and surgery. They may recur on several occasions.

Malignant lymphomas

Lympho- and reticulum cell sarcomas constitute 2% of all cancers of this region. Their frequency is less than the other malignant lymphomas of Waldeyer's ring, but their treatment and clinical course are the same.

References

[1] ROLANDER T. L., EVERTS E. L. & SHUMRICK D. A. (1971) Carcinoma of the tonsil: a combined therapy approach. *Laryngoscope* 81, 1199.

[2] LEDERMAN M. (1967) Cancer of the pharynx. *Journal of Laryngology and Otology* 81, 151.

[3] BRUGERE J., SCHLIENGER M., GERARD-MARCHANT R., TUBIANA M., POUILLART P. & CACHIN Y. (1975) Non-Hodgkin's malignant lymphomata of the upper digestive tract. *British Journal of Cancer* Supplement 2, 31, 435.

[4] SPIRO R. H., KOSS L. G., HAJDU S. I. & STRONG E. W. (1973) Tumours of minor salivary gland origin. *Cancer* 31, 117.

CHAPTER 26

Diseases of the Oral Cavity

BENIGN LESIONS OF THE ORAL MUCOSA

The oral mucosa is lined by stratified squamous epithelium. It is exposed to many irritants and is often injured or infected, but being well vascularized it usually heals quickly. Diseases of the oral mucosa can be divided in three groups: benign, pre-malignant and malignant. Some of the lesions that will be discussed are actually not mucosal lesions but originate in the deeper structure of the oral soft tissues.

Ulcers

Traumatic ulcer

A traumatic ulcer is commonly caused either by biting the cheeks or lips or by the use of extremely hot drinks and spices. A sharp edge of a broken tooth and poorly fitting dentures are other common causes. After elimination of the possible cause a traumatic ulcer should heal within a week. If not, a biopsy is indicated to rule out the possibility of a *malignant* or a *specific* ulcer.

Aphthous ulcer

An aphthous ulcer of the oral mucosa is common; multiple, painful lesions may be scattered throughout the oral cavity. The aetiology is unknown. An immune deficiency may be the cause of this disease, affecting about 20% of the population sometime during their life. Stress has been suggested as a possible promoting factor. Non-smoking patients seem to be affected more than heavy smokers, but this statement has never been proven. Some patients have frequently occurring, multiple ulcers, while others may occasionally suffer from one or two ulcers. The lesions usually measure a few millimetres, but

much larger ulcers may occur (Fig. 26.1). The aphthous ulcer is surrounded by a small erythematous zone. Spontaneous healing takes place in 1–2 weeks. The larger the ulcer, the longer the healing time, which in some cases may be 1–2 months. The diagnosis of an aphthous ulcer is a clinical one. The histologic features of an aphthous ulcer are those of a non-specific ulcer and in the very early stage large numbers of lymphocytes can be seen. Only the larger aphthous ulcer may leave a visible scar. There is no medicament or mouthwash available to promote healing of these ulcers and antibiotics are of no use. Steroids applied topically may be useful but should be used only for very severe cases.

Herpetiform ulcer

A herpetiform ulcer may look like an aphthous ulcer, but in herpes the ulcers are much more widespread. In addition, the patient will have fever, loss of appetite and general malaise, which is not the case in aphthous stomatitis.

White lesions

Some of the following lesions are not really white, but are included in this group because of their similar clinical presentation.

Fordyce's granules

These are heterotopic sebaceous glands, occurring in the oral mucosa. Clinically, the granules are either spread as pin-point sized lesions or fused together as plaque-like configurations; they have a yellowish-white appearance and are elevated above the surface of the oral mucosa. The most common sites are the buccal mucosa, the retromolar area and the inner sides of the lips.

Fordyce's granules rarely occur in the floor of the mouth, the tongue and the palate. The 'lesions' are asymptomatic and can be seen in almost every patient. Histologically, sebaceous glands can be seen without the presence of hair follicles. Pathologic changes in these sebaceous glands are exceptional and no treatment is required.

Papilloma

A papilloma is uncommon in the mouth. A virus is believed to be the cause but this has never been proven. The appearance is a white, cauliflower-

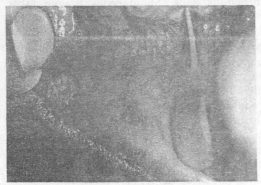

FIG. 26.1. Two aphthous ulcers at the right side of the lower lip.

like hyperplastic lesion of the mucosa. The differential diagnosis should include verrucous carcinoma, especially when the buccal mucosa is involved. Histologically, exophytic finger-like projections can be seen, formed by squamous epithelial cells. Malignant degeneration seldom occurs in an oral papilloma. The treatment consists of surgical removal.

Papillomatosis of the palate

This is characterized by multiple, red papillomas of the palate, almost always occurring in patients with ill-fitting dentures. The histology may show pseudo-epithelial hyperplasia and acinar and ductal metaplasia in the underlying salivary gland structures, but true malignant degeneration does not seem to occur. The clinical aspect of a verrucous carcinoma or a malignant salivary gland tumour may be similar to that of papillomatosis. A biopsy is thus required if there is the slightest doubt about the nature of a papillary lesion.

Focal epithelial hyperplasia (Heck's disease)

This is a rather rare condition characterized by multiple papillomatous swellings of the oral mucosa and the lips, especially of the lower lip. The cause is probably a virus of the papova group. Originally this disease was thought to be limited to an Indian tribe, but cases have been reported now from all over the world. Treatment is not required since these lesions disappear spontaneously, usually in about 6–12 months.

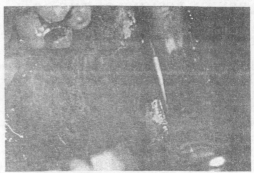

FIG. 26.2. Lichen planus of the cheek mucosa, reticular type.

Lichen planus

Lichen planus often presents as an intra-oral disease without accompanying skin lesions. The buccal mucosa, the lower lip, the gingiva and the border of the tongue are the sites of predilection. Quite often the lesions are arranged in a symmetrical way, affecting both sides of the oral cavity. The lesions may cause pain, which may be severe. Several types of lichen planus are being recognized, the reticular type and the erosive type being the most common (Fig. 26.2).

The diagnosis of lichen planus can usually be made by clinical judgement. In case of doubt a biopsy is very helpful because of the pathognomonic histologic features. Treatment is usually symptomatic; sometimes spontaneous regression occurs. Lichen planus is not a premalignant disorder [1], although some authors claim that a malignant transformation occurs in 1–2% of patients with lichen planus.

Pemphigus

Pemphigus and its many subdivisions can occur in the mouth; Nikolsky's phenomenon is one of the characteristic clinical findings. Histologically a suprabasilar split in the surface epithelium is one of the pathognomonic features.

Candidiasis or moniliasis

Candidiasis or moniliasis usually presents as white, multiple plaque-like lesions of the mucosa which can be scraped off rather easily. In the acute type the patient has fever and loss of appetite. Involvement by *Candida albicans* has been described in leukoplakia, median rhomboid glossitis and diseases of the lips. Treatment consists of the use of fungicides by local application or as a mouthwash.

Submucosal lesions

Fibroma

The soft tissue *fibroma* occurs often in the mouth, but is usually a reactive hyperplastic lesion rather than a neoplasm. The initial stage is probably a pyogenic-granuloma type of lesion, i.e. a non-specific reactive swelling due to trauma or other irritating factors. The line of occlusion along the buccal mucosa and the borders and the tip of the tongue are the most favourite sites. In patients wearing dentures, fibrous hyperplastic swellings may occur along the borders of the dentures. A fibroma presents as a pedunculated growth above the mucosal surface. Ulceration is very uncommon. The consistency may range from soft to very firm. The colour is usually the same as the surrounding tissue. There is no typical clinical picture and almost any benign or malignant tumour may present as a fibroma-like lesion. Treatment consists of excision.

Haemangioma

A haemangioma in the mouth usually represents a benign, congenital lesion. Most of the lesions probably are merely hamartomas. Clinically a haemangioma can be a flat or elevated lesion and may be either red or bluish. The lips, the tongue, the floor of the mouth and the buccal mucosa are the most common sites. *Hereditary haemorrhagic telangiectasia* (Rendu–Osler–Weber disease) is a special type of haemangioma, characterized by multiple pin-point lesions scattered throughout the skin and the oral mucosa. The *encephalotrigeminal angiomatosis* (Sturge–Weber disease) is another special, congenital form of haemangioma. One of the characteristic findings in this disorder is the extent of the lesions up to or just across the midline of the face and the oral cavity. Histologically, several subclassifications of haemangiomas are recognized, like cavernous haemangioma, capillary haemangioma and haemangioendothelioma. Haemangiomas hardly ever become malignant and many of the haemangiomas undergo spontaneous regression before puberty. When treatment is required, surgery, embolization, sclerosing agents or cryotherapy may be useful, depending on the size and the site of the lesion.

Lymphangioma

Lymphangioma in the mouth is usually also a hamartoma; the tongue is the most common site. Correct diagnosis is important since treatment differs from that of haemangiomas. Sclerosing agents and radiotherapy are not suitable for the treatment of a lymphangioma.

Lipoma

An oral *lipoma* is uncommon. The lesion manifests itself as a non-ulcerative encapsulated lesion and the overlying mucosa sometimes shows a yellowish texture. Histologically the tumour cells look like normal fat cells. The cells of the buccal fat pad can, therefore, be misinterpreted as part of a lipoma. Fibrolipomas and angiolipomas are variants of the lipoma. The change into a liposarcoma can be very gradual. The treatment of a lipoma consists of conservative excision; recurrences are uncommon.

Muscle lesions

Both *leiomyoma* and *rhabdomyoma* are very rare in the mouth; a few cases of both have been reported in the tongue and the floor of the mouth.

Neurogenous lesions

Traumatic neuroma is a reactive lesion rather

than a neoplasm and seldom occurs in the mouth. Clinically the lesion may manifest itself as a small submucosal nodule. The microscopic features are quite characteristic. Treatment consists of removal along with a proximal portion of the involved nerve. When multiple neuromas are found in the oral mucosa the possibility of a neuropolyendocrine syndrome (Sipple's syndrome) should be considered.

Neurofibroma. In patients affected by neurofibromatosis a neurofibroma may occur in the mouth. The clinical features of these submucosal nodules are not pathognomonic and a biopsy is required to make the diagnosis. Malignant transformation has been reported.

Neurilemmona or *Schwannoma* is not an exceptional oral tumour: it is a slow-growing tumour that is otherwise asymptomatic. The tongue is the most common site in the mouth. The microscopic features are rather typical, Verocay bodies being one of the characteristic findings. Treatment is excision. Malignant degeneration of a Schwannoma is extremely rare.

Cystic lesions

Benign lymphoepithelial cyst

The benign lymphoepithelial cyst can occur in the mouth, the floor being the most common site [2]. The clinical appearance is of a small, greyish-white nodule shining through the overlying mucosa. This cyst, when located in the oral mucosa may represent a so-called oral tonsil. In a doubtful case, an excisional biopsy can be done.

Epidermoid and dermoid cysts

The epidermoid and dermoid cysts are probably derived from epithelial cells enclosed during the development of the mandibular and hyoid branchial arches. The cyst may present either as an extra-oral, submental swelling or as a swelling of the floor of the mouth. The lumen is lined by squamous epithelium. When appendages are present like sebaceous glands and hair follicles the term *dermoid cyst* is applied and, in the absence of such structures, the term *epidermoid cyst* is used. Treatment consists of removal [3].

Nasolabial cyst

The nasolabial cyst is located in the soft tissue and, therefore, can hardly be detected on a radiograph. Synonyms used for this cyst are naso-alveolar cyst and Klestadt's cyst [4]. The origin of the epithelial lining is the subject of discussion and is believed to be either from epithelium trapped in the naso-optic groove or from the lower part of the nasolacrimal duct. There seems to be a predilection for women and the mean age is about 40 years. The histologic features are not pathognomonic. Treatment consists of removal.

Heterotopic oral gastrointestinal cyst

This is a choristomatic cyst that rarely occurs in the mouth but, when it does, the tongue and floor of the mouth are the most common sites [5]. The cyst is usually discovered shortly after birth. The lumen of the cyst may be partially or totally lined by gastric or intestinal mucosa. Excision is the treatment of choice.

Specific tongue lesions

Median rhomboid glossitis

The median rhomboid glossitis is a lesion of the tongue characterized by a reddish, rhomboid shaped area, devoid of lingual papillae, immediately anterior to the foramen caecum (Fig. 26.3). The lesion is usually interpreted as a developmental disturbance. More recently the cause of median rhomboid glossitis has been questioned and the role of *Candida albicans* has been and still is the subject of several studies [6, 7]. Most patients are not aware of this condition, which is harmless and does not require treatment, although application of a fungicide can give a good result. A biopsy may be necessary to rule out any other disease.

Lingual thyroid

This is a rather rare lesion of the tongue, predominantly occurring in women [8]. In some of these patients the lingual thyroid tissue is the only active thyroid tissue. Carcinoma arising in a lingual thyroid has been described. The lesion usually presents on the posterior surface of the tongue, and may cause dysphagia. When a lingual thyroid is suspected, a thyroid scan should be done to see whether the normal thyroid gland is present.

Lingual osseous choristoma

Lingual osseous choristoma is rather rare, occurring in the region of the foramen caecum [9].

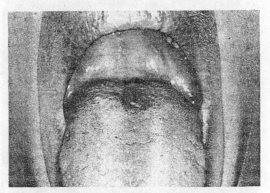

FIG. 26.3. Median rhomboid glossitis in a 46-year-old woman, perhaps caused by *Candida albicans* infection.

Geographic tongue

The geographic tongue is a common condition which is often overlooked. Large or small areas of the dorsal surface of the tongue show atrophy of the filiform papillae, resulting in a smooth, red mucosal surface in which the fungiform papillae become visible as little red elevations. The borders of the smooth area will usually be accentuated by a 'marginal' hypertrophy of the filiform papillae (Fig. 26.4). In a matter of weeks or months the area becomes normal again and the lesion may then become visible somewhere else on the tongue. The cause is unknown but stress has been suggested. Patients are usually not aware of this condition.

Recently, similar pictures have been described on the oral mucosa and for this condition the term geographic stomatitis has been proposed. Not so much is known about the microscopic picture of geographic tongue. A psoriaform picture has been mentioned in the description of the microscopic aspect.

Geographic tongue is a harmless lesion not requiring treatment.

Hairy tongue

Hairy tongue is a common, but still not completely understood, condition of the tongue, characterized by a hairy, black-brown or yellow aspect of the dorsal surface of the tongue. Micro-organisms may play a role as well as changes in

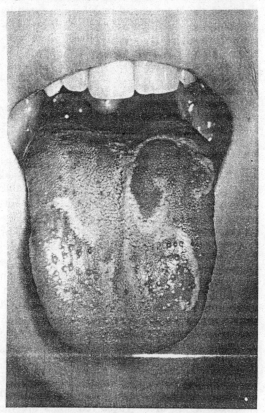

FIG. 26.4. Typical appearance of a geographic tongue in a 26-year-old woman. Notice the bright fungiform papillae in the erosive area, which are normally outgrown by the filiform papillae (white areas).

the physiologic movements of the tongue. Smoking seems to be a promoting factor. Treatment consists of mechanical cleaning of the tongue with a toothbrush twice or more a day, starting at the posterior end of the tongue and moving gently towards the tip. Good results are usually seen within a week.

Fissured tongue

Fissured tongue is characterized by numerous grooves in the surface of the tongue. It is probably an acquired abnormality since it is mainly seen in middle-aged and older people. Fissured tongue can occur in the Melkersson–Rosenthal syndrome, facial paralysis and cheilitis granulomatosa being the other two classic manifestations; it is a harmless condition. Secondary infection can occur as a result of accumulation of debris in the grooves and may be prevented by good oral hygiene and, if necessary, by additional brushing of the tongue.

PREMALIGNANT LESIONS OF THE ORAL MUCOSA

Leukoplakia

Leukoplakia of the oral mucosa can be defined as a white patch that cannot be scraped off and that cannot be classified as any other diagnosable disease. The term leukoplakia has a purely clinical meaning without any histopathologic correlation. Chronic irritation, either mechanical or chemical, is supposed to be the main cause. Whether or not *Candida albicans,* found in many cases of leukoplakia, plays a role in the initiation or aggravation of leukoplakia is not known. Leukoplakia is mainly found in middle-aged and older people. The buccal mucosa, especially near the commissure, and the borders of the tongue are the sites of predilection. Nicotinic stomatitis is a leukoplakia-like lesion in which smoking, especially of a pipe, produces a whitening of the palate with many little red spots dispersed throughout the area. These red spots are the inflamed ducts of salivary glands. About 5% of

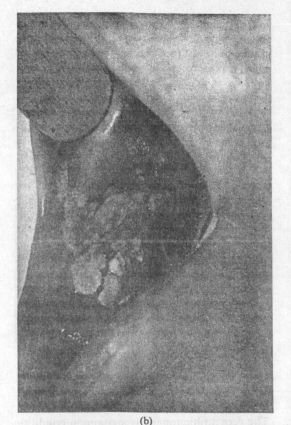

(b)

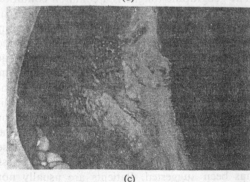

(c)

FIG. 26.5. Leukoplakia: (a) simplex type, in a 68-year-old woman, cause unknown; (b) verrucous type, of the buccal mucosa; (c) erosive type, of the buccal mucosa.

all oral leukoplakias ultimately transform into a squamous cell carcinoma.

The clinical aspect of leukoplakia is of some help in predicting the chance of malignant transformation. Three types of leukoplakia are recognized (Fig. 26.5a, b, c): leukoplakia simplex, ver-

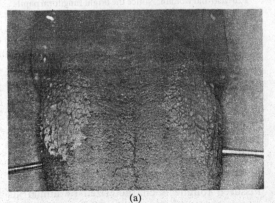

(a)

rucous leukoplakia and erosive leukoplakia. The latter type is also called 'speckled leukoplakia'. Malignant changes are much more common in the erosive type and are very rare in the simplex (the smooth, not indurated, homogenous) type of leukoplakia.

Several histologic changes can produce a leukoplakia. Hyperkeratosis, acanthosis, acantholysis, basal cell hyperplasia and pseudo-epitheliomatous hyperplasia may all result in a white aspect of the oral mucosa. None of these conditions can be considered as premalignant. The same is true for the loss of architecture and an increase in the number of mitotic figures. It is almost impossible to predict a malignant change just from the microscopic features, with the possible exception of a carcinoma *in situ*. Leukoplakia may undergo spontaneous regression when the cause, for instance smoking, is withdrawn [10]. A small single leukoplakia patch can easily be removed, but the large patch is a challenge. The clinical impression and the microscopic examination of one or more biopsies must indicate whether the leukoplakia should be treated or not. Besides surgical excision, cryosurgery may be very useful. Radiotherapy should not be used because of the risk of malignant transformation. A fungicide may be helpful to eliminate the candida. A close follow-up is mandatory.

Other premalignant lesions

Erythroplakia

The term erythroplakia should only be used to describe a reddish change of the mucosa that cannot be explained on the basis of any known disease entity. It has been stressed in recent years that erythroplakias should be considered as premalignant which in some cases may even prove to be malignant [11, 12, 13].

Pigmented lesions

An oral *nevus*, presenting as a localized brown-black discoloration of the mucosa (Fig. 26.6) should be considered as a premalignant lesion requiring excision [14, 15]. Occasionally an oral

nevus actually represents a malignant melanoma.

Most blue-black pigmented lesions in the mouth represent amalgam particles introduced into the tissue by the dentist when extracting or restoring a tooth. In some cases this pigmentation can be shown on a radiograph.

Racial pigmentation is a common and harmless condition in the mouth, especially along the gums. This diffuse type of pigmentation can sometimes also be seen in white patients.

Diffuse pigmentation of the oral mucosa can

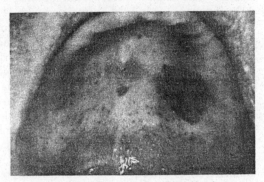

FIG. 26.6. A large pigmented area in the palatal mucosa of a 49-year-old man. Most likely diagnosis: nevus or even malignant melanoma.

also be seen in *Addison's disease* and in the *Peutz–Jeghers syndrome*.

Submucous fibrosis

This is a condition almost exclusively occurring in south-east Asia. For unknown reasons hyalinization takes place in the lamina propria, resulting in atrophy of the overlying epithelium [16]. The oral mucosa becomes stiff and even trismus can occur. There is no known treatment. It has been suggested that carcinomas are likely to develop in the atrophied epithelium often enough to consider this condition to be premalignant.

MALIGNANT NEOPLASMS OF THE ORAL MUCOSA

Most oral soft tissue malignancies are squamous cell carcinomas; soft tissue sarcomas are very rare. Malignant salivary gland neoplasms do occur (see Chapter 33). Malignant lymphomas of the mouth are rare, as are malignant melanomas. Metastases can occur in the jawbones, but are extremely rare in the soft tissues.

Squamous cell carcinoma

Pathology

Cancer of the mouth is fairly common in Europe and the USA, constituting 2–5% of all human cancers. The highest incidence (amounting to 40% of cancers) is in India, associated with the widespread habit of chewing a quid composed of areca-nut, tobacco, lime and betel leaves and with the habit of reverse smoking. In Western countries consumption of alcohol and tobacco are considered to be causes. Exposure to solar rays and other atmospheric conditions are accepted as an important cause of cancer of the lip that is most prevalent among men in rural areas. There is little support for the theory that syphilis predisposes to tongue cancer. Irritation by sharp edges of teeth or poorly fitting dentures may be a cause. Apart from these extrinsic factors, intrinsic changes of the mucosa as a result of anaemia or avitaminosis, for example, may be important; usually a combination of various factors is present. In about half of these patients there is no indication of the cause.

Oral cancer is a disease of the middle-aged and elderly. The sex ratio is different for the various sites within the oral cavity. Overall, women are less afflicted than men but the difference is not as great as, for example, in carcinoma of the larynx. For instance, the incidence of carcinoma of the tongue (the most common site in the mouth when the lip is excluded) is similar for both sexes. Fifty years ago the incidence was much higher in men; there is no explanation for this change in the sex ratio.

Most squamous cell carcinomas of the mouth are well or moderately differentiated, poorly differentiated squamous cell carcinoma and undifferentiated carcinoma being rare.

In 5–10% of patients a second primary tumour develops later in life; the majority of these are found in the mouth, pharynx, larynx, oesophagus and lung. These patients must be followed up for life, paying special attention to the upper air and food passages and the lungs.

Clinical features

Squamous cell carcinoma may develop anywhere in the mouth, but over 75% of cancers develop in the gutters between the inferior alveolar arch and the tongue (the so-called drainage area of the mouth) which make up only 20% of the total mucosa of the mouth. Carcinoma of the lateral border of the tongue is the most frequent site and accounts for half of all intra-oral cancers (Fig. 26.7). Cancer of the dorsum of the tongue, on the other hand, is extremely rare. In over 90% of

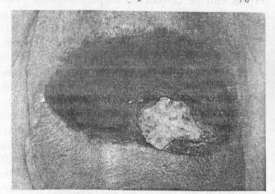

FIG. 26.7. Carcinoma of the lateral border of the tongue of a 67-year-old woman.

cases the lesion is infiltrating, usually presenting as an ulcer with rolled up margins (Fig. 26.8); at times extension of the tumour may be mainly submucous with only very slight ulceration, which is hard to detect. Exophytic papillary growths are rare. Quite often there is leukoplakia in the vicinity of the tumour and at times entirely separate primary multiple cancers are observed.

The patient generally seeks medical or dental care because he has noted a mass or ulcer in the oral cavity. Occasionally the only complaint is that the denture is ill-fitting, when it was not before, or that teeth are loosening. Only rarely is there a history of bleeding. The lesion may be painful, especially when touched. This pain may be referred to the ear on the affected side as a result of involvement of the lingual nerve. Occasionally the patient is referred because of a mass in the neck without any symptoms of a primary tumour in the mouth, but this is more common with cancer of the pharynx.

Oral cancer has a strong tendency to metastasize to the regional lymph nodes. Haematogenous spread is uncommon even in advanced disease. The incidence of cervical metastasis is different for the various sites of the primary tumour in the mouth. The overall incidence is highest for carcinoma of the tongue (well over half) and lowest for cancer of the hard palate (less than 10%); in these figures are included

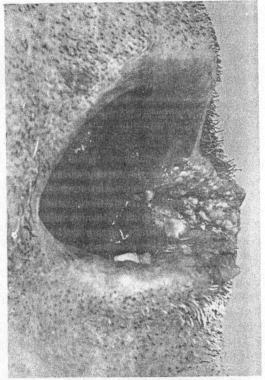

FIG. 26.8. Ulcerating squamous-cell carcinoma of the buccal mucosa in a 72-year-old man.

metastatic nodes appearing during follow-up in patients who seemed to have been cured of their primary. The incidence rises sharply as the size of the primary increases. Especially in carcinoma of the anterior part of the floor of the mouth and carcinoma of the tongue, bilateral neck metastases are quite common. A significant correlation between the histologic grading of the tumour and the incidence of neck node metastasis has never been shown.

Investigation and diagnosis

Inspection under adequate illumination is indis-

pensable to arrive at a proper diagnosis. It seems hard to break the average doctor of the habit of only depressing the tongue in order to look at the tonsils. One must inspect all of the oral mucosa. By asking the patient to put out his tongue or by grasping the tongue with a swab, inspection of the important drainage area is facilitated. By so doing one can also detect fixation of the root of the tongue or involvement of the hypoglossal nerve. The patient is then told to put the tip of his tongue on his hard palate, and the undersurface of the tongue is examined. Any suspicious area or any area that does not permit adequate inspection should be palpated with the forefinger. Bimanual palpation can be applied to the cheeks. The induration of a carcinoma is seldom unrecognized by palpation which is the best clinical method of assessing the extent of the tumour. In advanced tumours it may at times be very hard to evaluate the extent due to pain and trismus; examination under general anaesthesia is then indicated. Palpation of the neck is an essential part of the routine examination; bimanual palpation with one finger in the mouth of the submental and submaxillary glands is emphasized.

Knowledge of the likely areas of nodal spread in the neck for each individual site [17] helps the investigator to detect the smaller nodal metastases. If the tumour is close to the mandible or the maxilla radiographs of these structures are indicated.

A biopsy is taken to establish the diagnosis. When the lesion is ulcerating this is easily done by spraying the area with pantocaine 0·5% and taking a piece of tumour with a forceps. Taking an adequate biopsy from the margin rather than from the necrotic centre of the tumour helps the pathologist to make a proper diagnosis. Only in the rare case where there is no obvious ulceration is an incisional biopsy indicated, under either general anaesthesia or a peripheral nerve block. Local infiltration anaesthesia should always be avoided because of the risk of metastases due to a rise of tissue pressure. Aspiration biopsy is only rarely indicated.

A short comment must be made about oral cytology because the widespread application of this diagnostic tool has made such a tremendous contribution to the earlier diagnosis of carcinoma of the female genital tract. The situation in the mouth is very different. Most oral lesions are readily accessible, so that a specimen of tissue can be easily obtained. The costs are high whereas the frequency of oral cancer is low in comparison to that of cancer of the cervix, so that its routine use as a screening method is not warranted.

Classification

The importance of an accurate description of the lesion in the patient's record and the routine use of diagrams in which the extent is recorded cannot be overemphasized. A retrospective analysis will furthermore be facilitated by the routine application of site-specific computerized data forms.

The need for a clinical staging system based on the best possible estimate of the extent of disease before treatment, has been recognized by both the UICC (Union Internationale Contre le Cancer) and the AJC (American Joint Committee on cancer staging and end results reporting). For this purpose the mouth is considered to extend from the vermilion borders of the lips to the junction of the hard and soft palate above and the line of the circumvallate papillae below and is divided into the following specific sites: lips (upper and lower), buccal mucosa, lower and upper alveolar ridge, retromolar trigone, floor of mouth, hard palate and anterior two-thirds of tongue. Definition of 'T' categories of oral cavity carcinoma is as follows:

T1S   Carcinoma *in situ*;
T1   Tumour 2 cm or less in greatest diameter;
T2   Tumour greater than 2 cm but not greater than 4 cm in greatest diameter; and
T3   Tumour greater than 4 cm in greatest diameter.

The following regional node classification is applicable to all malignant head and neck tumours:

N0   Regional lymph nodes not palpable;
N1*   Movable homolateral nodes;
N2*   Movable contralateral or bilateral nodes; and

* For N1 and N2 categories connotations a and b may be added, indicating, respectively, nodes not considered to contain growth and nodes considered to contain growth.

N3   Fixed nodes.

It seems important to note that the AJC has recently proposed a more elaborate nodal staging system including both the size and the number of involved homolateral nodes; moreover, a T4 category is added to the staging of the primary tumour. As yet this system has not been approved by the UICC but it is hoped that it will find universal acceptance.

Treatment policy

Treatment of cancer in general and of the mouth in particular demands a multidisciplinary approach. Apart from the ablative and reconstructive surgeon and the radiotherapist, a dental colleague with a profound knowledge of the problems involved should participate in the team; at times the help of a medical oncologist is needed. Treatment policy differs among the large cancer clinics, reflecting not only the controversy during the last 50 years over surgery versus radiotherapy, but also the available facilities and expertise in a particular institution; chemotherapy has only in the last decade come into the picture.

The behaviour of these tumours with regard to their metastases to regional lymph nodes is of the utmost importance in establishing any plan of therapy. If nodes are palpable, therapy should encompass both the primary tumour and the regional node areas. Since palpable metastases in the neck are not eliminated by radiotherapy (excluding the highly radiosensitive undifferentiated malignancies which are extremely rare in the mouth) the argument is in favour of surgery, that is surgery of the *en bloc* composite type. When there are no palpable nodes on admission the problem is far more complex and many factors should be taken into account.

Treatment of the primary tumour will be discussed first. In general it can be said that T1 lesions and early T2 lesions can be treated with either surgery or radiotherapy alone. The larger T2 and the 'smaller' T3 lesions are best dealt with by surgery. The massive T3 lesions carry a poor prognosis and even very radical surgery often proves inadequate. For these advanced lesions, therefore, the principle of combination therapy should be applied [18].

Radiotherapy, particularly interstitial radiation using iridium or radium needles, either alone or combined with external megavoltage beam, has proved to be effective in treating the smaller primary tumours (up to 3 cm in greatest dimension). Radionecrosis of the mandible is a serious risk of radiation for lesions of the mouth. When the bone is invaded by cancer or when the lesion is fixed to the bone or approaches the bone closely, it is generally agreed that such therapy should not be used [19]. Furthermore, limitations to interstitial therapy are set by the anatomical relationships. Radiotherapy is thus to be considered in carcinoma of the tongue and of the buccal mucosa when the lesion measures less than 3 cm in its greatest dimension.

If radiotherapy is successful there will be little alteration in the patient's functional capacity, but the direct sequelae of radiotherapy are usually underestimated. Many older patients tolerate surgery better than radiation. Even if the pain and difficulty in swallowing produced by radiotherapy is only temporary, the resulting malnutrition is usually not readily overcome. Loss of function after surgery for lesions up to 3 cm is minimal, whereas it is socially acceptable for the larger tumours when reconstructive surgery is used. Besides, surgery has the great advantage that it allows pathological examination of the resected specimen, so that an opinion can be obtained as to whether the procedure has been adequate. After radiotherapy, on the contrary, it is often not easy to determine whether radiation has completely eliminated the primary tumour. The irradiated area may remain permanently indurated and repeated biopsies may not help in deciding on the true nature of the induration. When nodes later appear in the neck, the surgeon is faced with the unhappy choice of performing only the neck dissection and hoping for the best, or performing an *en bloc* removal of the primary site with radical neck dissection. Surgery of the composite type after a full course of radiotherapy carries a high risk of complications.

As mentioned above, massive T3 lesions are probably best dealt with by combinations of radiation and surgery or chemotherapy and surgery, the radiation or chemotherapy being administered first. The aims of such pre-operative radiation or chemotherapy are to increase the margins of uninvolved tissue by sterilizing the periphery of the tumour and reduction of the risk of implantation metastasis within the surgical field and that of iatrogenic metastasis beyond the head and neck. The choice between radiation and chemotherapy very much depends on the expertise available in a particular centre. We favour chemotherapy over radiotherapy because the toxic effects of chemotherapy on the healthy tissues in the mouth are reversible, whereas those of radiotherapy are not. This is vital with respect to the extensive reconstruction required to rehabilitate the patient adequately after the major surgery required for such advanced disease. Moreover, chemotherapy is usually much better tolerated by the patient than radiotherapy.

There has been a long-standing discussion about the indications for an elective radical neck dissection. This discussion is, furthermore, complicated by the more recent evidence [20] that elective irradiation of the neck might also be adequate in eliminating microscopic nodal disease. No set rules can be given as lymph nodes are not palpable. The incidence of metastasis for a specific cancer must first be known. If not more than 10% of all patients with a given malignancy develop a nodal metastasis, as is the case in carcinoma of the hard palate, there is not much indication for prophylactic neck dissection. An entirely different problem arises in carcinoma of the tongue and floor of the mouth (as the commonest lesion in the mouth) with an overall incidence of neck metastasis of at least half, varying according to the size of the primary tumour. In lesions at these sites, measuring over 3 cm, the need for treating the neck in the absence of palpable metastases is generally accepted. In lesions measuring less than 3 cm in their greatest dimension we have a 'wait-and-see' policy and perform a neck dissection when nodes become palpable during follow-up. Such a policy is only justifiable when frequent follow-up visits can be guaranteed which is no problem in a country where patients never live far away from the centre where they have been treated. Moreover, this policy is not as conservative as would appear on the surface, because if the neck must be entered to remove the primary tumour, at least a partial neck dissection is carried out *en bloc*, e.g. for anterior floor of the mouth lesions. This is based on the principle that if a dissection were to be needed later on in such a case, the presence of scar tissue would not permit the performance of a clean anatomical procedure.

An alternative to elective neck dissection is elective irradiation of the neck. Although such irradiation may prove valuable in eradicating microscopic disease in the neck, it has yet to be shown that the results are as good as those of elective neck dissection. From our own experience it has become apparent that such elective irradiation of the neck is not easily tolerated by the older patient. An important argument in favour of radiotherapy is that neck dissection leads to more mutilation.

There are situations in which post-operative radiotherapy and/or chemotherapy is indicated or might be considered. When the pathologist reports that the excision was inadequate and further surgery is impracticable, or metastatic tumour in the neck is extending beyond the confines of the nodes, post-operative irradiation is indicated. Post-operative chemotherapy might be of value in patients with a high risk of haematogenous metastasis, e.g. those in whom the neck specimen contained multiple metastatic nodes with capsular rupture and tumour emboli in lymphatics.

Finally, it should be remembered that some patients with very advanced disease or of very old age are probably best not or only palliatively treated. This is particularly true if the ensuing mutilation would not be compatible with a socially acceptable life, for instance when a total glossectomy would be necessary to excise the lesion adequately.

Principles of surgery

Although descriptions of operative techniques are not within the scope of this book, it seems useful to indicate some general principles of surgery for carcinoma of the oral cavity.

It is very helpful to cauterize, before embarking on the resection of the tumour, any ulcerative surface of the lesion and indeed to continue this procedure well into macroscopically healthy tissue. The risk of implantation metastasis will thus be reduced. Secondly, the bulk of the tumour

having been taken away, a much clearer view of the field is obtained. When experience with cauterization has been gained, it will be appreciated that this procedure gives much more accurate information about the extent of the tumour than do inspection and palpation because even the smaller offshoots of the tumour appear as small white points in the red muscle during the procedure of coagulation. After irrigation with a cytotoxic solution the coagulated area is excised with a margin of 1 cm surrounding tissue.

Good exposure as for all surgical procedures is of prime importance. Whenever the mouth opening is considered insufficient for adequate removal of the tumour either the lower lip or the upper lip is divided in the midline in zig-zags and a cheek flap raised on the side of the lesion. Especially in patients with heavy mandibles it may be advantageous to section the mandible stepwise in the midline and swing the whole flap of bone and soft tissue laterally and upwards.

Many times the question comes up as to whether the mandible can be preserved and a marginal resection safely be carried out or whether the continuity of the mandible has to be sacrificed. For this problem no set rules can be given, the decision not only being dependent upon the relationship of the tumour to the mandible but also on the height and the thickness of the mandible. The mylohyoid muscle marks a very important plane in regard to this particular problem.

After major surgery for oral cavity carcinoma, defects of the soft tissues, the mandible and/or the maxilla may result. A basic requirement for their successful reconstruction is careful preoperative planning, that often includes close cooperation with a prosthodontist. In general, midline defects pose far greater problems than do lateral defects. In lateral soft tissue defects the use of pedicled skin flaps probably has been a little overemphasized, whereas the use of delayed split skin grafting in that particular situation has not received the attention it deserves. Anterior floor-of-mouth defects need to be reconstructed primarily to retain a functional tongue remnant. Local, regional and distant flaps such as a tongue flap, nasolabial flaps, cervical flaps, a deltopectoral or a forehead flap can all be used to this end; the ultimate choice depends on the particular patient and defect and the preference of the surgeon [21]. Mandibular reconstruction is to be considered vital in anterior arch defects and ideal in lateral defects. The continuity is best restored with an autogenous cortico-cancellous bone graft from the iliac crest, carried out as a secondary procedure [22]. Maxillary defects need prosthetic closure [23].

Prognosis

The prognosis of carcinoma of the mouth depends on many factors such as site of origin, TNM staging, method of treatment, etc. It is disappointing to note that too many patients still have advanced local regional disease on admission, considering the easy accessibility of the mouth to diagnosis both by patient and doctor. This seems to be the main reason that the overall 5-year survival figures are still below 50%.

Other malignant tumours

Soft tissue sarcoma

Soft tissue sarcomas do not have any clinical features that differ from carcinoma although the lesion usually develops somewhat faster. The age of the patient may be less and even infants may be affected by an oral soft tissue sarcoma [24]. The prognosis of oral sarcomas used to be very gloomy. Results seem to have improved with combined treatment.

Lympho-proliferative lesions

Recently a group of lympho-proliferative lesions, probably representing a stage of a *malignant lymphoma,* have been reported on the palate [25]. These lesions may present as unilateral or bilateral soft tissue swellings of the palate, usually at the junction of the hard and soft palate. Early removal or radiotherapy may be indicated but not enough data are available yet to make a firm statement about the treatment of this lesion.

Malignant melanomas

Malignant melanomas in the mouth are extremely rare [26]. The palate and the upper alveolar ridge are the sites of predilection (Fig. 26.9). Although mucosal melanomas are predomina-

tely a disease of middle age, they do occur in the younger age groups. As mentioned earlier these intra-oral melanomas often develop from a pre-existing nevus. Wide excision is the preferred method of treatment. Although the prognosis is poor in comparison to that of skin melanoma, the disease at times runs a very protracted course. Treatment of recurrences, therefore, may be of great palliative value.

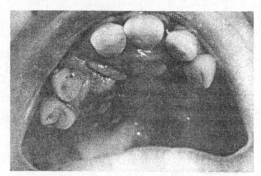

FIG. 26.9. Melanoma of the palate in a 56-year-old woman.

TUMOURS AND TUMOUR-LIKE CONDITIONS OF THE MINOR SALIVARY GLANDS

Congenital and developmental lesions of the minor salivary glands are very rare, as are inflammatory lesions. The most common pathologic conditions are formed by the mucous retention phenomenon, the sialoliths and the neoplasms.

Mucous retention phenomenon

The mucous retention phenomenon may occur at several sites, the lower lip being the most common [27]. The lesion presents as a soft, bluish swelling; the exact cause is unknown but obstruction of an excretory duct has been suggested as the most likely and in the lower lip the term mucocoele is applied. Mucocoeles in the upper lip and on the palate are extremely rare and should, clinically, be looked on with suspicion. Microscopy of a mucous retention phenomenon shows accumulation of mucus surrounded by a wall of connective tissue which may be lined by epithelium. Treatment consists of removal. Incomplete removal readily leads to a recurrence.

Sialolith

A sialolith in the duct of the submandibular gland is a common finding, but a sialolith in a minor salivary gland is rather rare. Clinically, a small submucosal nodule may be palpated, usually in the cheek. A radiograph of the soft tissues may be helpful in making a pre-operative diagnosis.

Necrotizing sialometaplasia

From studies of cadaver tongues it is known that squamous sialometaplasia can occur, and is harmless. Sialometaplasia has also been described on the palate, even resulting in ulceration of the overlying mucosa. This so-called necrotizing sialometaplasia is still a somewhat debatable lesion. Since it may mimic, clinically, a malignant ulcer, careful examination and a proper biopsy are necessary. Necrotizing sialometaplasia does not require treatment and healing usually takes place in 1–2 months [28, 29].

Minor salivary gland tumours

These may occur at any age, but are most often seen in people between their thirties and sixties. There is no significant sex or race predilection. No proven aetiological factors are known, although trauma and extraction of a tooth have been suggested as possible causes. A salivary gland tumour in the oral cavity most often presents as a slowly growing, non-ulcerative, asymptomatic swelling [30]. When dealing with a submucosal swelling the possibility of a salivary gland tumour is very often not included in the differential diagnosis. A correct clinical diagnosis of a minor salivary gland neoplasm is made in only 10% of the cases. One should also realize that about 50% of the minor salivary gland tumours are malignant and that there are no clinical aspects to indicate whether a minor salivary gland tumour is benign or malignant.

The most common location is the soft palate and the posterior part of the hard palate. The upper lip, the cheeks, the tongue, the floor of the mouth and the retromolar area are less frequently involved. A salivary gland tumour in the lower lip is extremely rare. In the palate a wrong tentative diagnosis of palatal abscess, mucous

retention cyst, median palatal cyst or fibroma can be made. A small firm nodule in the upper lip or the cheek is often misdiagnosed clinically as a mucocoele (Fig. 26.10). Mucocoeles seldom occur in the cheek or upper lip and are almost exclusively limited to the lower lip. Other tentative diagnoses that have been made in this location are sebaceous cyst, sialolith, fibroma, lipoma, haemangioma and lymphangioma.

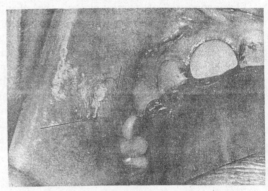

FIG. 26.10. Submucosal swelling in the upper lip. Diagnosis: pleomorphic adenoma.

Many salivary glands can be found in the tongue, especially in the dorsum of the tongue around the foramen caecum. Salivary gland tumours in this area are rare and can clinically be misinterpreted as granular cell myoblastoma, osteoma, osteochondroma, median rhomboid glossitis, lingual thyroid, thyroglossal duct cyst and fibroma. Salivary gland tumours of the floor of the mouth can clinically be misdiagnosed as a mucous retention cyst, a mucous plug in the Wharton's duct, a dermoid cyst or a mesenchymal neoplasm.

Diagnostic procedures

Only in small, circumscribed tumours of the lips, the cheek, the tongue and the floor of the mouth, is a wide excisional biopsy the correct procedure. For locations on the palate an excisional biopsy would in itself entail a major procedure. Therefore, an incisional biopsy should be carried out prior to treatment. Because of the difficulties in histological typing of salivary gland tumours one should not rely on fresh-frozen sections to obtain a diagnosis. In the case of a salivary tumour of the palate, tomographs should be taken before the final treatment in order to detect a possible destruction of the underlying bone and to reveal a possible antral or nasal involvement.

Pathology

The histology of salivary gland tumours is varied. The same types of tumour that occur in the major salivary glands can be found in the minor glands with the difference that the adenolymphoma is very rare and the adenoid cystic carcinoma is very common.

The percentages of benign versus malignant tumours reported in the literature show a wide range. Spiro et al. [31] reported 88% of tumours to be malignant, while Crocker et al. [32] described malignancy in only 32%. This difference can partly be explained by the different types of hospital in which the research was done. Another reason may be a different interpretation of the microscopic picture, which is a very real problem in typing salivary gland tumours.

Controversial opinions are given about the value of grading a mucoepidermoid tumour in respect to the type of treatment. According to Eversole et al. [33] and Melrose et al. [34], low and intermediate grade mucoepidermoid tumours can be cured by a rather conservative surgical procedure. On the other hand Lentrodt and Hafke stated 'It is not correct to delimit the excision on the basis of the histological picture, since this criterion has proven unreliable' [35].

The acinic cell tumours can be either benign or malignant but information about these is scarce.

Treatment

Surgery is the preferred method of treatment. The margin of healthy tissue to be included in the specimen depends on the histologic type of the tumour. Adenoid cystic carcinoma especially is known for its perineural and intraosseous extension far beyond the clinical margins of the lesion. In some cases even wide excision may not be adequate. Although salivary gland tumours generally are more or less radio-resistant, radiotherapy has been proven to be effective in eradicating microscopic disease left in situ at operation.

DISEASES OF THE JAWS

Osteomyelitis and osteoradionecrosis

Osteomyelitis

Most lesions of the jaws are odontogenic lesions such as the periapical granuloma and odontogenic cysts. These lesions are rather well localized, but widespread changes may occur as, for instance, in osteomyelitis.

Osteomyelitis of the jaws occurs most often in the mandible as the result of a tooth extraction or an odontogenic infection, usually of periapical nature. Osteomyelitis may be either chronic or acute. Specific micro-organisms may be involved, but usually are not. Osteomyelitis of the jawbones can either produce a very dense, sclerotic type of bone or cause suppuration of bone, accompanied by fistulae either on to the skin or into the mouth; sequestration may occur. Osteomyelitis is usually found in the middle-aged or elderly patient, except for the rare type of blood-borne osteomyelitis that can occur in babies and infants. Osteomyelitis can be asymptomatic or can cause recurrent episodes of mild or severe pain, with or without recurrent swellings [36].

Fever can occur in acute exacerbations. The radiograph may vary from a dense, diffuse radiopaque picture to a radiolucent one and may or may not show sequestration (Fig. 26.11). The histologic features do not seem to have any typical aspects and can be confused with other inflammatory and non-inflammatory lesions of the jaws. Treatment of osteomyelitis can be very difficult. Every possible causative factor should be eliminated. In general, curettage or removal of sequestrae should be done very gently. The value of antibiotics before or after operation or alone without surgery is still not known. The same uncertainty exists about the value of treating these patients with hyperbaric oxygen [37]. The subdivisions of osteomyelitis are so many and the particular problems in the patients are so diverse, that comparison of the data of different authors is almost impossible.

Osteoradionecrosis

This is a type of osteomyelitis caused by radiation of the jaw or its surrounding tissues. The blood supply is altered, resulting in a bone prone to infection. A simple extraction of a tooth, either of the maxilla or mandible, can lead to extensive inflammation comparable with the course of osteomyelitis. Once a patient has undergone radiotherapy to the head and neck, the possibility of osteoradionecrosis should be borne in mind for the rest of his life. If dental surgery is unavoidable, prophylactic antibiotics and gentle manipulation are obligatory. If possible, such surgery should be anticipated and performed before the radiotherapy is started [38].

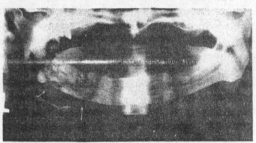

FIG. 26.11. Destruction of the mandible by osteomyelitis in a 55-year-old man, 2 months after removal of an impacted wisdom tooth. (Courtesy of Dr. J. L. Becker, The Netherlands.)

Exostoses

Torus palatinus
One of the most common localized swellings is the torus palatinus, a bony protuberance in the midline of the palate. The lesion is not a true tumour but the cause is unknown. The torus palatinus can be unilobular or multilobular. Ulceration of the overlying mucosa does not occur. Patients are usually unaware of this condition and the diagnosis is based on clinical judgement. Removal of the torus is indicated only if an upper denture cannot be made properly (Fig. 26.12).

Torus mandibularis
The torus mandibularis is a lesion similar to the torus palatinus and is often symmetrically located on the lingual sides of the bicuspid areas. When a lower denture needs to be constructed, surgical removal of the tori may be indicated.

Multiple exostoses
These can occur on the bucco-alveolar aspect of

the maxilla, usually in older patients. The cause is unknown, although some form of chronic irritation is most likely. Surgery is only indicated in exceptional cases.

Tumours and tumour-like lesions

All tumours and tumour-like lesions that can occur in the skeleton may also affect the jaws,

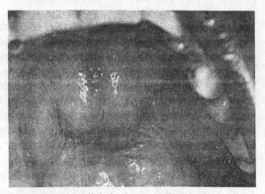

FIG. 26.12. Multilobular bony swelling on the palate. Unknown duration. Diagnosis: torus palatinus.

and therefore, do not need special attention in this chapter, except for a few conditions with unique features.

Osteopetrosis
The benign type is found in the jaws. Expansion of the bone may occur and pain and facial paralysis may be the result of narrowing of the cranial foramina. The jaw may become densely sclerosed, preventing normal eruption of the teeth. Also the teeth may be affected. Minor trauma to the jaw can cause a serious osteomyelitis due to the diminished vascularity of the bone [39].

Paget's disease
This disease can be either polyostotic or monostotic and usually occurs in patients above the age of 40 years. The disease may affect the jawbones and can cause considerable expansion, usually of the maxilla [40]. It is quite exceptional to diagnose the disease from an initial lesion of the jaw. Hypercementosis of the teeth may be a characteristic finding in the polyostotic form.

Fibrous dysplasia

Fibrous dysplasia quite frequently occurs in the jaws, usually as a monostotic lesion [41]. The use of the term monostotic is somewhat debatable for a lesion in the upper jaw, because many of these lesions extend either into the zygomatic bone, the frontal bone or into the floor of the orbit. The term facial fibrous dysplasia has been used in these cases instead. The disease, the cause of which is unknown, usually starts in childhood or early adult life. The most common finding is an asymptomatic, bony swelling, most often at the buccal aspect of the alveolar ridge. The teeth may be displaced. Depending upon the stage of the disease the radiograph may show a variety of pictures and may be either radiolucent or radiopaque, showing a ground-glass appearance. The lesion is usually not well circumscribed. The age of the patient, the history of a slow developing bony lesion and the radiographic aspects may together lead to a reliable diagnosis of fibrous dysplasia, but a biopsy is still important.

In a patient with a fibrous dysplastic lesion of the jaw, the question arises whether, in the absence of any other clinical sign or symptom, to refer the patient for a skeletal survey to rule out the polyostotic variant of the disease. The question seems to be of academic interest since positive findings have hardly ever been reported.

The treatment of fibrous dysplasia is a challenge. Removal of all or part of the lesion before adulthood almost always leads to a recurrence, often in a matter of months. A radical excision of affected bone of the maxilla is hardly ever possible because of the extent and diffuse spread of the lesion. Radiotherapy is not indicated.

Unfortunately there are no histologic criteria that can be used to predict the clinical behaviour of fibrous dysplasia. Most lesions halt spontaneously and finally even show some regression. The most reasonable approach seems to be to observe the patient and to wait until the lesion does not show any progression. In some patients, repeated corrective operations may be required for aesthetic reasons.

Spontaneous malignant degeneration is rare even after multiple operations.

When dealing with a polyostotic type of fibrous dysplasia, Albright's syndrome should be remembered.

Giant cell granuloma

This lesion is of unknown origin and most often occurs in the mandible. The lesion may present as an asymptomatic swelling of the jaw; sometimes the teeth become mobile. The radiograph shows a rather well circumscribed, sometimes multilobular, lucency [42].

The radiographic differential diagnosis includes: ameloblastoma, aneurysmal bone cyst, central haemangioma, central odontogenic myxoma, traumatic or haemorrhagic bone cyst and even focal osteoporotic bone marrow defect.

Histologically, the lesion is characterized by numerous multinucleated giant cells in fibrous connective tissue. The mitotic activity of the stromal cells may be quite marked; occasionally islands of bone are found within the lesion, but inflammatory cells are usually absent. This microscopic picture is indistinguishable from the so-called brown tumour occurring in hyperparathyroidism. In every patient with a central giant cell lesion of the jaw, additional investigations should be done to rule out hyperparathyroidism. From a histologic point of view the classification of the central giant cell lesion as a granuloma rather than a neoplasm seems hardly justified, but clinical experience has shown that these lesions do not behave like neoplasms and can be adequately treated by thorough curettage. Recurrences, however, may occur.

Osteoma

An osteoma rarely occurs in the jaws but when it does, the differentiation between it and other fibro-osseous lesions can be difficult, both by radiography and histopathology.

Chondroma

This almost never occurs in the jaws [43]. When cartilage is seen in histologic sections of the jaw bone, except in the mandibular joint region, the diagnosis of chondrosarcoma or chondroblastic osteosarcoma should be considered.

Sarcoma

The *reticulum cell sarcoma* of bone, the *Ewing sarcoma*, the *osteosarcoma* and the *chondrosarcoma* may affect the jaw as a primary site. None of these neoplasms has typical signs or symptoms, except the osteosarcoma which may show a 'sunray' aspect on radiography. Because these tumours are rare, a correct clinical diagnosis can almost never be made.

Metastatic tumours

Metastatic tumours in the jaws are usually situated in the angle of the mandible. The most common primary sites are the breast, the lung and the kidney. Clinical symptoms may consist of anaesthesia of the lower lip, local swelling or an increased mobility of one or more teeth in the affected area. The radiograph usually shows a rather ill-defined radiolucency. Occasionally sclerosing metastases can be seen. The metastatic lesion in the jaw is only rarely diagnosed before the primary tumour [44].

Diseases of the temporomandibular joint

The temporomandibular joints can cause a number of typical symptoms such as pain (within the joint or radiating to the forehead, the occipital or cervical region), clicking sounds during movements of the mandible, limitation of the movement of the mandible and even complete locking of the jaws, especially in the early morning. The radiograph may show changes of the surface of the condylar head or heads, which is called *arthrosis deformans*. The cause of this condition is probably a neuromuscular dysfunction due to malocclusion or unbalanced dentures. Treatment consists of improvement of the occlusal balance. Only in very severe cases is surgery of the joint indicated [45].

True luxation of the joint, requiring manual reposition, is rather rare. If it recurs frequently, surgery is indicated. Several procedures are possible, varying from techniques designed to increase the steepness of the articular eminence to limit the mobility of the condylar head, to techniques meant to eliminate the articular eminence completely, thereby providing an easy way back for the condyle.

Cysts and tumours very rarely originate in the condyle. In fractures in the condylar region a disturbance of the mandibular growth may occur, as well as ankylosis of the joint. Immobilization of such fractures should not last for more than 2–3 weeks. Good post-operative exercises

and professional guidance are essential to prevent these complications.

DENTAL DISEASES

Dental caries

Aetiology

Dental caries is a disease of civilized life, caused by an increased intake of refined carbohydrates. In the western world almost the whole population is affected by this disease, whose exact cause is not fully understood. The chemico-parasitic theory proposed by Miller in 1890 is still well accepted. Miller stated that several micro-organisms in the mouth can produce acids from carbohydrates in the food and that these acids, mainly lactate acids, cause decalcification of the enamel and finally also of the dentine. The production of acids takes place in the 'plaque', a tenacious membrane-like structure that sticks to the tooth surface. The plaque is made up of mucines, desquamated cells from the oral mucosa and micro-organisms. After the initial attack, micro-organisms can invade the altered tooth structure and destroy the remaining organic parts.

Carbohydrates are important but the role of micro-organisms is less clear, although their presence is essential, as shown by experiments in germ-free animals. Several types of micro-organisms take part in the production of acid on the tooth surface. Some of these, like *Str. mutans,* also affect the plaque, causing prolonged exposure of the tooth surface to the acids.

The role of the saliva is still debatable, but there is a marked increase in caries in the complete absence of saliva in patients with atrophy of the salivary glands after radiotherapy to the head and neck—the so-called 'radiation caries'.

Heredity may be important but is hard to evaluate.

Clinical features

The first sign of dental caries is a white, chalky appearance of the enamel, the surface remaining smooth and intact. If the lesion is treated at this stage, it may be reversible and remineralization may occur. In the next stage the enamel surface breaks down and a cavity can be detected by using an explorer or, at a more advanced stage, can be seen. Caries of the 'interdental' or proximal surfaces can be diagnosed by radiographs. Tissue breakdown and accumulation of debris cause a brown discoloration. Dental caries if untreated almost always destroys not only the enamel but also the dentine, and finally damages the pulp of the tooth. When caries is limited to the enamel portion of the tooth the patient does not experience pain but as soon as the dentine is involved, irritating toxins and waste products readily reach the pulp and cause pain.

Caries often starts as a very small area at the enamel surface and later undermines the enamel widely. Apparently healthy teeth can then suddenly fracture under minor chewing or biting forces, so that the patient believes that the disease originated within the tooth.

Caries is usually aggressive in patients under the age of twenty. In extreme cases this is called 'rampant caries'. Above the age of 20–25 years new lesions are less common. Sometimes a small cavity may not progress; this is called 'arrested caries'. Besides primary caries (caries in a previously intact tooth surface), secondary caries may occur at the margins of fillings. Residual caries is the dental decay that occurs when a filling has been placed in a previous insufficiently excavated cavity.

Treatment and prevention
Dental caries can be prevented by avoiding excessive intake of refined carbohydrate, but most patients are unwilling to do this. Caries can also be prevented by fluoridation of the drinking water in a concentration of 1–2 parts per million, which is safe and which reduces the incidence of caries by up to 60%, when used from birth to early childhood. The fluoride is built into the enamel of the tooth during its formation by an exchange of the hydroxy-group of the apatite crystals, forming a less acid-soluble structure. Once the formation of enamel has been completed and after the tooth has erupted, the importance of continued exposure to fluoride decreases for that particular tooth. In spite of the proven effectiveness and safety of fluorides added to the drinking water, many objections have been raised, not only questioning the medical safety of these fluorides, but also debating the moral rights of adding 'medicines' to the public drinking water.

Alternative methods are tablets of fluoride taken from early childhood until adult age and also topical application of fluoride solutions once or twice a year by a dentist. All this is not going to do much good, however, unless the rules of proper diet are obeyed. Good oral hygiene, brushing the teeth at least twice a day, does help to prevent caries, but not as much as we would like to believe. The addition of fluorides to toothpaste is beneficial, but again, the effect of the fluoride is not so great once the enamel has been formed and calcified.

Radiation caries can be prevented by meticulous dental care and proper treatment planning.

Periodontal diseases

The supporting tissues of the teeth are called the periodontium and consist of the gingiva (gums), the alveolar bone, the cementum layer of the tooth and the periodontal ligament between the alveolar bone and the cementum. The periodontal ligament is mainly made up of a network of interlacing fibres holding the tooth tightly in its socket and at the same time providing it with a cushion to accomodate the biting and chewing forces applied to the teeth.

Gingivitis and periodontitis

Aetiology
Most periodontal diseases are inflammatory. Gingivitis is a chronic, non-specific disease affecting most people to a greater or lesser degree. Many causes can be thought of, but none can be considered as the only aetiologic factor. Non-specific micro-organisms are involved, whose toxins irritate the gingival tissues when debris accumulates along the gums.

The formation of calculus on the tooth-surface promotes gingivitis, but the exact mechanism of the calculus formation is not known. Some patients accumulate calculus very quickly, while others with comparable oral hygiene do not. Smoking seems, for reasons not well understood, to promote gingivitis. Malocclusion of the teeth is by some considered to be a major cause of gingivitis, but in general this is not believed to be true.

Malnutrition, drugs, diabetes mellitus, allergy, endocrine disturbances, pregnancy, heredity and psychic phenomena can all be listed as secondary, promoting factors of periodontal disease, not primary.

Acute gingivitis is uncommon. Synonyms for this disease are Vincent's angina and 'trench mouth'. *Borrelia vincentii*, a spirochaete, and a fusiform bacillus are found in large numbers in these patients and were once considered to be the specific cause of this type of gingivitis. These micro-organisms, however, can also be found in many healthy mouths. A more accepted cause is a lowered resistance to infection. In this way the endemic pattern of the disease in soldiers living in the trenches in World War I can be understood. The disease has never been proven to be contagious. If not treated properly the inflammation does not remain limited to the gums, but attacks the other parts of the periodontium, particularly the periodontal ligament and the alveolar bone. When the alveolar bone resorbs, the attachment of the gingival tissue to the tooth lowers concurrently. This may lead to the formation of a 'pocket', a non-physiologic space between the gingiva and the tooth, which in its turn may lead to further tissue damage and possible abscess formation.

As soon as the destruction of alveolar bone becomes visible on a radiograph or is visible by exposing the root surface of a tooth, the term gingivitis is replaced by periodontitis. The causes of periodontitis are the same as those of gingivitis.

Clinical aspects

Gingivitis usually runs a chronic course. Although the disease may start in childhood, symptoms usually do not appear until the gingivitis has progressed to periodontitis. It then appears to be a disease affecting people of 35 years and older, but it is not.

The most common finding in *chronic* gingivitis is a slight, generalized, erythematous swelling of the gums and a tendency to bleed on touching the tissues. Pain is uncommon, as are fever and general malaise.

In *acute* gingivitis pain can be very prominent; the patient usually has a moderate fever, the cervical lymph nodes may be enlarged and the patient can be very ill. A striking foetor often makes it possible to diagnose acute gingivitis when the patient enters the office. Most patients affected by acute gingivitis are between the age of 15 and 25 years.

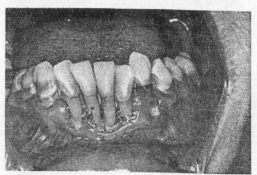

FIG. 26.13. Severe chronic periodontitis in a 42-year-old woman.

In *periodontitis* the patient may have additional complaints of a bad taste, due to a purulent discharge from the tissues. In a more advanced stage of periodontitis the teeth become mobile as a result of loss of alveolar bone and destruction of the periodontal ligament (Fig. 26.13).

Finally, the patient loses his teeth due to this inflammatory, preventable disease and not as the result of an inevitable physiologic process, as so many patients seem to believe.

The differential diagnosis is from the following conditions:

Herpetic gingivo-stomatitis can mimic acute gingivitis closely but it does not cause the penetrating odour and is seldom limited to the gingival structures.

Periodontal disease can be the first sign of *leukaemia*. When a generalized soreness or bleeding of the gums cannot be readily explained on the basis of poor oral hygiene, one should be very suspicious of an underlying blood disorder.

Lichen planus, especially the atrophic or erosive type, may mimic periodontal disease, but can usually be differentiated from it by close examination. Other lesions of lichen planus elsewhere in the mouth help in making the diagnosis.

The diagnosis of gingivitis and periodontitis is almost always based on clinical judgement and does not require a biopsy.

It can be difficult to differentiate between a periapical abscess and a periodontal abscess. A positive vitality test of the tooth usually rules out a periapical lesion due to pulp necrosis and is in favour of a periodontal abscess.

Treatment

Gingivitis and periodontitis can never be cured by mouthwashes. Penicillin is also useless, except in some extreme circumstances. The only way to solve the problem is by eliminating the causative factors.

Chronic gingivitis should be treated by removal of all calculus, by correcting overhanging fillings and by eliminating other possible causes. All this is not going to do much good unless the patient is taught how to brush his teeth and how to maintain proper oral care.

In acute gingivitis, mechanical cleaning with instruments and brushing the teeth is extremely painful and also carries the risk of inducing sepsis. Mouthwashes can be prescribed, applied as many times a day as possible. In very ill patients antibiotics may be administered to prevent secondary infections. The patients should be followed daily and the causative factors should be treated as soon as the acute stage has regressed.

In many cases of periodontitis proper oral hygiene and removal of all possible causes will result in a clinically acceptable, healthy periodontium. It is important to know that alveolar bone, once lost, never regrows. One can only try to prevent further breakdown. In some patients surgical correction of the gums (gingivectomy) and recontouring of the alveolar bone can be helpful in improving the local anatomy and promoting better cleansing of the gums.

A dentist or an oral surgeon is often asked for advice on patients with blood disorders complicated by periodontal disease. In these patients oral hygiene must be meticulous in order to reduce the inflammatory changes. Telling these patients not to brush their teeth because it may cause bleeding is poor advice, since it only worsens the problem.

Periodontosis

The term periodontosis has often been misused to describe an advanced stage of periodontitis in which one or more teeth become loose. Periodontosis is a rather uncommon periodontal disease affecting patients before the age of 25, and women more often than men. The cause is unknown, although many authors believe that a nutritional deficiency or a metabolic disease is responsible. Inflammation does occur in this disease, but seems to be a secondary phenomenon rather than a primary one. Pockets form, usually around a single tooth in a dentition that is very well looked after, and that does not show plaque or calculus accumulation. The tooth usually becomes loose and starts to drift. A radiograph may show a diffuse resorption of the alveolar bone. Widening of the periodontal ligament of a single tooth may indicate a sarcoma.

A syndrome has been described in which severe periodontosis of some or all the teeth occurs in early childhood. These patients also have keratotic lesions of the palmar and plantar surfaces. The aetiology is unknown [46].

In all patients with unexplained looseness of one or more teeth, malignant tumours should be included in the differential diagnosis.

Since the cause of periodontosis is not known, not much can be done to prevent the disease. Treatment is also difficult and consists of eliminating secondary factors such as calculus and debris. The prognosis for teeth affected by periodontosis is poor and extraction of the tooth or teeth is often inevitable.

Resorption of the alveolar ridges

Resorption of the alveolar ridges occurs when teeth have been extracted. In some patients this process occurs rapidly, while in others the bone loss is very gradual. The speed with which the bone is resorbed may be influenced by the patient's previous periodontal status; the patient's age also seems to be important. The younger the patient at the time of extraction of the teeth, the faster the resorption proceeds. In severe cases, especially in the lower jaw, surgical correction may be required for a denture. The operation may consist either of a lowering of the buccal and lingual muscular attachments to the jaws or of a subperiostal bony implant inserted on top of the residual alveolar ridge.

Fibromatosis gingivae

Ideopathic fibromatosis gingivae is a generalized hyperplastic change of the gingival tissues whose cause is not known. The gums are swollen, but are a normal, pink colour and feel firm on palpation. Fibromatosis gingivae may even occur before the teeth have erupted and may disturb or prevent normal eruption of the teeth. Corrective surgery may be necessary.

Fibromatosis gingivae in epileptics using phenytoin is a distinct entity. In this type of fibromatosis gingivae all the teeth may become covered by fibrous masses (Fig. 26.14).

Secondary infection, resulting in gingivitis and finally in periodontitis, may occur. Surgery is often needed to uncover the frontal teeth, not for functional but for aesthetic reasons. Meticulous oral hygiene can prevent recurrences.

Fibromatosis gingivae should not be confused with multiple exostoses that sometimes occur on the buccal aspects of the maxillary ridge.

A rather remote possibility is generalized swelling of the gums due to amyloid deposits.

Localized gingival swellings

A *pyogenic granuloma,* a localized, non-specific inflammatory lesion, can occur on the gingiva usually at the interdental papilla. The lesion is called by some authors epulis granulomatosa, or, in a more mature, sclerosed stage, epulis fibrosa. Pyogenic granuloma is sometimes seen during pregnancy and may regress partially or even disappear post partum. In pregnant women the terms epulis gravidarum and 'pregnancy tumour' have been used. It requires a lot of clinical experience and self confidence to just watch a gingival growth in a pregnant woman, without taking a biopsy, as is so often recommended. Why take a risk? A biopsy, taken under local anaesthesia, will not harm the patient or the fetus and may well reveal a wrong clinical diagnosis.

In *Crohn's disease* (regional enteritis), a localized erythematous swelling of the gingiva may occur

and can even lead to the diagnosis of the gastro-intestinal lesions.

A *peripheral giant cell granuloma* appears as a bluish, localized swelling on the gingival tissue. This can also be the appearance of a peripheral haemangioma. The exact nature of this lesion is unknown. It does not behave as a true neoplasm, does not metastasize, but may recur when not

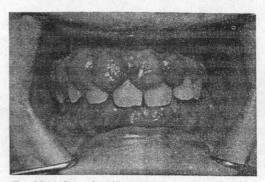

FIG. 26.14. General swelling of the gingiva due to the use of an anti-epileptic drug. (Courtesy of Dr. W. A. M. van der Kwast, The Netherlands.)

excised completely. The numerous giant cells may be derived from osteoclasts since these lesions often occur during the shedding of the teeth in which there is a physiological resorption of the deciduous teeth. The peripheral giant cell granuloma can also occur in the mucosa of edentulous maxillary or mandibular ridges, which does not support the previously suggested origin of the giant cells.

A *peripheral fibroma* of the gingiva is considered by some to be the healing stage of a pyogenic granuloma, a reactive gingival lesion; others consider this lesion to be of odontogenic origin and use the term peripheral odontogenic fibroma; yet others describe this lesion as a *peripheral ossifying* or *cementifying fibroma,* reflecting the presence of bone or cementum in some of these lesion – even dentine formation has been described. Simple excision is usually sufficient.

The *gingival cyst,* a rare swelling occurring on the gingiva, is an odontogenic cyst usually limited to the lower bicuspid region. A primary carcinoma or a soft tissue sarcoma of the gingiva is rare, but should be included in the list of possible diagnoses; metastases to the gingiva are very rare. A localized gingival swelling always demands a preoperative intraoral radiograph to rule out bone destruction or alteration. Central bone lesions may sometimes present as a localized swelling of the gingiva.

Odontogenic cysts

Cystic lesions lined by epithelium derived from the odontogenic apparatus are quite common in the mouth. Most of these cysts lie within the bone; many cause no symptoms and may reach a large size before being detected.

The odontogenic epithelium is derived from the oral mucosa and the lining of the odontogenic cyst almost always consists of stratified squamous epithelium, but the odontogenic epithelium has the potential to change into mucus-producing cells and may even give rise to a salivary gland tumour within the jaws, especially the mandible. Other tumours that may arise in the lining of an odontogenic cyst are an ameloblastoma and, rarely, a squamous cell carcinoma. Odontogenic cysts should therefore be removed and examined microscopically.

The most common odontogenic cyst is the *apical* or *radicular cyst*. The radicular cyst develops at the apex of a tooth and is the response to a non-vital pulp (Fig. 26.15). A radicular cyst may cause no symptoms for a long time until secondary infection takes place, although slight expansion of the jaw may occur. In spite of the equal incidence of caries in the deciduous and the permanent dentition, radicular cysts rarely occur in children. Radiography almost always shows a unilobular, well-circumscribed radiolucency around the apex of a tooth. A radicular cyst can never be diagnosed on the radiographic findings alone, but should be confirmed by microscopic examination. The epithelial lining of the radicular cyst is stratified squamous epithelium. Carcinomas or ameloblastic changes in this lining are very uncommon. Removal of the cyst is not always necessary. Proper root canal treatment may be effective in dealing with a small cyst but a large one should be enucleated; the tooth in-

volved can be treated by either apicoectomy or extraction. When the tooth is extracted, part or all of the cyst may be left behind. An unknown proportion of these residual cysts resolve, but others continue to expand, to be detected many years later.

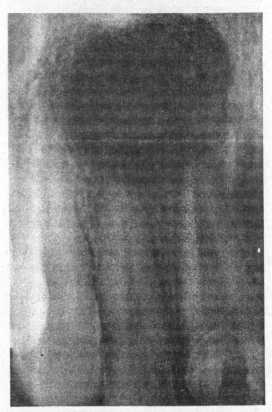

FIG. 26.15. Large, well-circumscribed radiolucency at the apices of the upper and lateral right incisor. The most likely cause is the non-vital central incisor. Microscopic examination showed the presence of a (radicular) cyst.

The *dentigerous* or *follicular cyst* is produced by cystic changes in a tooth follicle of an impacted tooth. The cyst seems to be limited to the permanent dentition and usually occurs in association with a lower wisdom tooth or an upper canine. The radiograph usually shows an unilobular, well-circumscribed radiolucency around the crown of the impacted tooth (Fig. 26.16). Microscopically a squamous epithelial lining may be seen, but some of the follicular cysts show the characteristics of a keratocyst. Removal of the impacted tooth and the cyst is required, since the epithelial cells of this cyst may transform into an ameloblastoma, a salivary gland tumour (most often a mucoepidermoid carcinoma) or a squamous cell carcinoma.

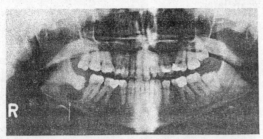

FIG. 26.16. Impacted lower right wisdom tooth surrounded by a well-circumscribed radiolucency. Besides a follicular cyst, a keratocyst or even an ameloblastoma should be taken into account.

Other cysts which may occur include the *odontogenic keratocyst,* in which the superficial layers of the epithelium flatten and produce keratin, filling the lumen with a white cheesy material, the *primordial cyst,* a rare cyst which develops from the epithelium of a tooth bud before enamel or dentine forms, the *eruption cyst,* seen in the soft tissue above the crown of an erupting tooth, and, very rarely, the *gingival cyst,* the *keratinizing and calcifying odontogenic cyst* and the *botryoid odontogenic cyst.*

Odontogenic tumours

Tumours derived from odontogenic structures are usually located within the jaws. Most of these tumours are benign and many simply represent hamartomas rather than neoplasms. Rather than discussing all odontogenic tumours [47], only the most important ones will be described.

Odontoma

The term odontoma implies an odontogenic neoplasm, but this term is now restricted to a benign odontogenic malformation. An odontoma is usually discovered as an incidental finding on a radiograph and is often located at or between the apices of the teeth and can occur anywhere in the jaw. In the compound odontoma, dental tissues

(enamel, dentine and cementum) are laid down in an orderly, tooth-like structure. In the complex odontoma the dental tissues are arranged in a disorderly pattern.

The remote possiblity of the presence of an ameloblastic odontoma (odonto-ameloblastoma), a lesion acting like an ameloblastoma, should always be considered and this is one of the reasons why an odontoma should be removed and examined microscopically.

Cementoma

Cement and bone can show a remarkable histologic resemblance and this explains part of the confusion in the classification of the cementomas.

The *benign cementoblastoma* is the only true neoplasm of this group and is almost always found around and attached to the root of a lower bicuspid or molar tooth; expansion of the jaw may occur. Radiographically a well-demarcated radiopaque structure surrounded by a radiolucent zone is seen. Microscopically massive areas of cementum are seen, showing numerous reversal lines. This picture can be indistinguishable from an osteoblastoma, an osteoid osteoma or even an osteosarcoma.

Periapical cemental dysplasia can hardly be considered as an odontogenic tumour. It would be more appropriate to classify this lesion in the category of fibrous dysplastic or fibro-osseus lesions of the jaws.

The lesion most often occurs at the apices of the lower front teeth and shows a strong predilection for middle-aged Negro women; the cause is unknown but trauma has been suggested. The lesions cause no symptoms and are usually incidental findings on the radiographs. Depending on the stage of development and the degree of calcification, rather diffuse periapical radiolucencies are seen, showing different degrees of central radiopacities. Especially in the early radiolucent stage, these apical rarefactions can be misinterpreted as periapical granulomas or cysts, and the vitality of one or more teeth may, unnecessarily, be sacrificed by the dentist. No treatment is necessary.

The *cementifying fibroma* can occur in the mandible as well as the maxilla. In its early stage the lesion presents as a well-demarcated radiolucency. With time, increasing amounts of radiopaque structures can be seen in the centre and this finally results in a dense, sclerotic mass surrounded by a thin radiolucent band. The cementifying fibroma is, in contrast to the benign cementoblastoma, not connected with the root of a tooth. Removal and confirmation of the diagnosis by microscopic examination is required. The lesion does not tend to recur.

The *gigantiform cementoma* is an ill-understood entity described as multiple cemental lesions occurring in the jaws of Negro women. It has been suggested that this lesion is a type of fibrous dysplasia of the jaws, but more recently an inflammatory origin has been proposed [48]. It is a benign condition that probably should be left alone.

Ameloblastoma

The most important odontogenic tumour is the ameloblastoma. The term ameloblastoma depicts the histologic resemblance of the tumour cells to ameloblasts. The tumour cells, however, do not form enamel matrix. The cells may be arranged either in follicles with a stellate reticulum-like structure centrally, or in strands and cords. The ameloblastoma occurs in both sexes with equal frequency; the mean age is about 30 years. The tumour shows a strong predilection for the lower-third molar region (Fig. 26.17). Most ameloblastomas are located within the jawbone and quite often show a radiolucency; there can be a marked expansion of the jaw. In spite of the destructive growth, the inferior alveolar nerve and the mental nerve are seldom affected. Many histologic subdivisions of the ameloblastoma are recognized, none of which has clinical implications. Ameloblastomas behave aggressively locally but rarely metastasize. Metastases of ameloblastoma, usually in the lung, cannot be distinguished histologically from a non-metastasing ameloblastoma. Some only use the term malignant ameloblastoma for ameloblastomas that have metastasized.

The treatment of ameloblastoma is controversial. It is said that an ameloblastoma of the mandible may be treated by conservative surgery, avoiding, if possible, loss of continuity of the mandible but this is a dangerous statement, since insufficient data are available to support this opinion. Patients may benefit from having the continuity of the mandible saved, even if they must undergo multiple operations for their local

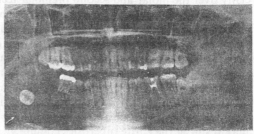

FIG. 26.17. An impacted lower wisdom tooth surrounded by a large radiolucency, causing resorption of some of the adjacent teeth. Microscopic examination showed an ameloblastoma. (Courtesy of Dr. H. P. Meynen, The Netherlands.)

recurrences. On the other hand, recurrences are much more difficult to treat. In any event, long-term follow-up is necessary since recurrences may appear after 10 or more years. Ameloblastomas of the maxilla behave more aggressively and should therefore be excised by radical surgery, if possible. Radiotherapy has not been proven to be of much value in the treatment of ameloblastomas. Little is known about the place of chemotherapy in the treatment of ameloblastoma. Ameloblastic carcinomas and ameloblastic sarcomas have been reported, but are very rare.

The dentinoma, the adenomatoid odontogenic tumour, the ameloblastic fibroma, the calcifying epithelial odontogenic tumour and the odontogenic myxoma are all very rare lesions that will not be discussed further.

ORO-ANTRAL FISTULA

Pathology

Most oro-antral fistulae follow dental extractions but may also follow gun-shot wounds, fractures of the maxilla or maxillary sinus operations. Less commonly, a fistula develops spontaneously as the result of erosion by a neoplasm of the maxilla.

Predisposing causes

The intervening bone between the apices of the teeth and the antrum is normally quite thin, especially over the molar and second premolar teeth where the tooth roots as a rule cause visible indentations on the antral floor; occasionally, however, the bone may be totally absent with the mucosa of the antrum being in direct contact with the dental apices. A well-developed antrum is sometimes associated with abnormal pneumatization of the maxillary tuberosity. If this situation exists then the removal of an upper 8 tooth may result in the entire tuberosity coming away attached to the tooth.

Pathological conditions of the alveolar bone or teeth also constitute important aetiological factors. Localized sclerosis of bone may lead to difficulties during dental extraction partly on account of the brittle nature of the bone and partly due to ankylosis between the teeth and alveolus. A similar problem is encountered in relation to teeth with tortuous roots. In some instances the dental apices act like claws and grip the surrounding bone like a vice. This frequently causes trouble in the case of the first molar tooth, the three roots of which enclose a triangular area of bone which is extremely thin and especially liable to separate when the tooth is removed.

At the other extreme, softening and erosion of the alveolar bone may result from inflammation, especially in connection with the apices of the teeth; an apical abscess may develop, erode inwards and finally rupture through the antral mucosa so that a fistula is inevitable if the overlying unhealthy tooth is extracted. A similar situation may be encountered in malignant erosion of the maxillary antrum.

The liability to fistula formation appears to increase in proportion to the amount of force required but a minor degree of trauma may be sufficient to cause a fistula in the presence of any of the anatomical or pathological abnormalities already outlined. A fistula commonly follows the search for retained root fragments after a tooth has been broken. The palatal root of the first molar is particularly liable to breakage and subsequent attempts at its removal frequently lead to fistula development. The root may be displaced between the alveolus and the antral mucous membrane and the latter is liable to perforation by an elevator or other instrument inserted to remove the root.

Natural healing of a fistula

Most fistulae if left undisturbed will heal spontaneously. The defect becomes filled with blood clot which acts as a framework and glues the damaged fragments together. A rapid healing reaction takes place with organization of the blood clot and replacement by fibrous tissue; the mucosal integrity is finally restored by proliferation of surface epithelium from the torn edges of the mucosa on both the antral and buccal aspects of the fistula. This process of 'primary' healing will normally occur provided blood clot fills the defect and remains undisturbed.

If for any reason clot fails to form in sufficient quantity, or forms and subsequently disintegrates, spontaneous healing is interrupted and the exposed tissues become raw, swollen and granular. In the case of a small fistula they may become adherent over the defect and healing by fibrous and epithelial repair may eventually occur – 'secondary' healing. In larger fistulae there is a marked tendency for the mucosa to grow down the tract instead of bridging the gap, the oral and antral mucosal surfaces eventually becoming united to form a completely epithelialized tract which has then no further tendency to close.

'Primary' healing may fail to occur for various reasons:

(1) In the presence of a very large fistula the blood clot may be unstable or insufficient in quantity to cover the defect.

(2) The rapid development of infection causes the blood clot to disintegrate.

(3) Vigorous attempts at probing the fistula or the excessive use of mouthwashes or syringing may result in detachment of the blood clot.

(4) Failure of a fistula to heal without an obvious reason suggests the possibility of underlying malignant disease.

Diagnosis

The creation of an oro-antral fistula is frequently obvious at the time of dental extraction. In other instances, however, the dentist is quite unaware of the existence of the condition and the patient returns for one or more of the following reasons. He may notice that air or fluid can be sucked through the fistula or that a denture fitted after dental extraction lacks the normal properties of retention. The patient may complain also of a purulent discharge in the nose or mouth which frequently has a foul smell or taste. In doubtful cases, the diagnosis can be established by passing a probe through the tooth socket into the antrum. A 'pseudo-fistula' – an alveolar opening ending blindly in a dental cyst – may cause difficulty in diagnosis and in order to differentiate it from a true fistula it may be necessary to inject fluid through the fistula to demonstrate a communication between the antrum and nose.

Radiological examination is essential in all cases. Retained root fragments, foreign bodies or infections of the maxillary sinus may thus be demonstrated. A contrast medium is helpful in confirming the presence of a fistula in a doubtful case.

The incidence of oro-antral fistula is almost certainly higher than is recognized. Doubtless many fistula escape diagnosis following dental extraction and heal spontaneously without complications. Over-zealous probing of a tooth socket merely to establish the diagnosis should not be attempted since a fistula may be created where none previously existed or blood clot sealing a fistula may be dislodged and the healing process interrupted.

Treatment policy

The important factors in determining the treatment policy are, first, the length of time the fistula has been present and, secondly, the presence or absence of maxillary sinus infection.

1. Recent fistula
This is a fistula seen within 24 hours of onset. It is usually non-infected and, to stop infection supervening, it should be closed surgically. In many instances, the dentist can suture the wound himself at the time of extraction but if it is too large then removal of the bony edges of the socket and a rotation flap closure is usually successful. If a fistula is small and there is a good blood clot a trial of conservative treatment with antibiotics and decongestants can be given. If this fails, however, then the results of surgical closure will not be as good as they would have been with primary closure.

2. Intermediate fistula
After 24 hours the traumatized tissues are granular and friable and a low grade infection is invariably present. Sutures will tend to cut out and so a conservative regime is followed. The blood clot should not be disturbed and the patient is put on to an antibiotic for at least 2 weeks. He is instructed not to blow or suck through the fistula and if possible the fistula should be covered by a prosthetic appliance. If the antrum is infected it should be washed out or an intranasal antrostomy performed. If healing has not occurred in 8 weeks it must be treated as a 'late' fistula.

3. Late fistula
Spontaneous closure is impossible in a late fistula because the tract has epithelialized and so it must be closed surgically in two layers. The epithelial tract is incised circumferentially around the margins of the fistula and turned inwards. The bare area is then covered by a mucoperiosteal flap of adjacent buccal mucosa. Palatal flaps may also be used but they tend to lack the elasticity of the buccal mucosa.

If there are retained roots these should be removed at the same time and it may be necessary to open the antrum to recover them. Adjacent teeth often cause problems in closure and it is nearly always necessary to remove one adjacent tooth if the fistula goes up towards its roots.

By the time a fistula is 'late' there will almost always be chronic infection of the antrum which militates against healing. Thus a radical antrostomy should be performed at the same time as fistula closure.

References

[1] REISMAN R. J., SCHWARTZ A. E., FRIEDMAN E. W. & GERRY R. G. (1974) The malignant potential of oral lichen planus – diagnostic pitfalls. *Oral Surgery* **38,** 227.

[2] GIUNTA J. & CATALDO E. (...) vmphoepithelial cysts of the oral mucosa. *Oral Surgery* 37, 77

[3] MEYER I. (1953) Dermoid cysts (dermoid) of the floor of the mouth. *Oral Surgery* 8, 1149.

[4] ROED-PETERSEN B. (1969) Nasolabial cyst: a presentation of five patients with a review of the literature. *British Journal of Oral Surgery* 7, 84.

[5] HARRIS C. N. & COURTEMANCHE C. (1974) Gastric mucosal cyst of the tongue: case report. *Plastic and Reconstructive Surgery* 54, 612.

[6] RUSSELL C. & JONES J. H. (1975) The histology of prolonged candidal infection of the rat's tongue. *Journal of Oral Pathology* 4, 330.

[7] COOKE B. E. D. (1975) Median rhomboid glossitis; candidiasis and not a developmental anomaly. *British Journal of Dermatology* 93, 399.

[8] MONROE J. B. & FAHEY D. (1975) Lingual thyroid; case report and review of the literature. *Archives of Otolaryngology* 101, 574.

[9] McCLENDON E. H. (1975) Lingual osseous choristoma; report of two cases. *Oral Surgery* 39, 39.

[10] PINDBORG J. J., JØLST, O., RENSTRUP G. & ROED-PETERSEN B. (1968) Studies in oral leucoplakia: a preliminary report on the period prevalence of malignant transformation in leucoplakia based on a follow-up study of 248 patients. *Journal of the American Dental Association* 76, 767.

[11] TROIT J. R. & REDDY J. (1972) Benign and malignant erythroplasia. *Journal of Canadian Dental Association* 38, 225.

[12] MASHBERG A., MORISSEY J. B. & GARFINKEL L. (1973) A study of the appearance of early asymptomatic oral squamous cell carcinoma. *Cancer* 32, 1436.

[13] SHAFER W. G. (1975) Oral carcinoma *in situ. Oral Surgery* 39, 227.

[14] KING O. H., BLANKENSHIP J. P., KING W. A. & COLEMAN S. A. (1967) The frequency of pigmented nevi in the oral cavity. *Oral Surgery* 23, 82.

[15] TRODAHL J. N. & SPRAGUE W. G. (1970) Benign and malignant melanocytic lesions of the oral mucosa: an analysis of 135 cases. *Cancer* 25, 812.

[16] PINDBORG J. J., POULSEN H. E. & ZACHARIAH J. (1967) Oral epithelial changes in thirty Indians with oral cancer and submucous fibrosis. *Cancer* 20, 1141.

[17] LINDBERG R. (1972) Distribution of cervical lymph node metastases from squamous cell carcinoma of the upper respiratory and digestive tracts. *Cancer* 29, 1446.

[18] MOORE C., FLYNN M. B. & SCOTT R. M. (1975) *Cancer of the Head and Neck*, eds. Chamber R. G., Janssen de Limpers A. M. P., Jaques D. A. & Routledge R. T., p. 120. Amsterdam. Excerpta Medica.

[19] HARROLD CH. C. (1971) Management of cancer of the floor of the mouth. *American Journal of Surgery* 122, 487.

[20] FLETCHER G. H. (1972) Elective irradiation of subclinical disease in cancers of the head and neck. *Cancer* 29, 1450.

[21] LEE S. E. & WILSON J. S. P. (1973) Carcinomas involving the lower alveolus, an appraisal of past results and an account of current management. *British Journal of Surgery* 60, 85.

[22] SNOW G. B., KRUISBRINK J. J. & VAN SLOOTEN E. A. (1976) Reconstruction after mandibulectomy for cancer. *Archives of Otolaryngology* 102, 207.

[23] KRUISBRINK J. J. & VAN STEENBERGEN F. D. (1975) *Cancer of the Head and Neck*, eds. Chamber R. G., Janssen de Limpens A. M. P., Jaques D. A. & Routledge R. T., p. 168, Amsterdam: Excerpta Medica.

[24] FARR H. W. (1971) Soft part sarcomas of the head and neck. *American Journal of Surgery* 122, 714.

[25] TOMICH C. E. & SHAFER W. G. (1975) Lymphoproliferative disease of the hard palate: a clinicopathologic entity – a study of 21 cases. *Oral Surgery* 39, 754.

[26] ENEROTH C. M. (1975) Malignant melanoma of the oral cavity. *International Journal of Oral Surgery* 4, 191.

[27] CATALDO E. & MOSADOMI A. (1970) Mucoceles of the oral mucous membrane. *Archives of Otolaryngology* 91, 360.

[28] ABRAMS A. M., MELROSE R. J. & HOWELL F. V. (1973) Necrotizing sialometaplasia; a disease simulating malignancy. *Cancer* 32, 130.

[29] DUNLAP C. A. & BARKER B. F. (1974) Necrotizing sialometaplasia; report of five additional cases. *Oral Surgery* 37, 722.

[30] CHAUDRY A. P., VICKERS R. A. & GORLIN R. J. (1961) Intraoral minor salivary gland tumours. *Oral Surgery* 14, 1194.

[31] SPIRO R. M., KOSS L. G., HAJDU S. I. & STRONG E. W. (1973) Tumours of minor salivary origin; a clinico-pathologic study of 492 cases. *Cancer* 31, 117.

[32] CROCKER D. J., CAVALARIS C. J. & FINCH R. (1970) Intraoral minor salivary gland tumours. *Oral Surgery* 29, 60.

[33] EVERSOLE L. R., ROVIN S. & SABES W. R. (1972) Mucoepidermoid carcinoma of minor salivary glands: report of 17 cases with follow-up. *Journal of Oral Surgery* 30, 107.

[34] MELROSE R. J., ABRAMS A. M. & HOWELL F. V. (1973) Mucoepidermoid tumors of the intraoral minor salivary glands: a clinicopathologic study of 54 cases. *Journal of Oral Pathology* 2, 314.

[35] LENTRODT J. & HAFKE G. (1974) Beitrag zur Klinik und insbesondere zur Dignität der Mukoepidermoidtumoren der Speicheldrüsen. *Deutsche Zahnartzliche Zeitschrift* 29, 615.

[36] KHOLSA V. M. (1970) Current concepts in the treatment of acute and chronic osteomyelitis: review and report of four cases. *Journal of Oral Surgery* 28, 209.

[37] MAINOUS E. G., HART G. B., SOFFA D. J. & GRAHAM G. A. (1975) Hyperbaric oxygen treatment of mandibular osteomyelitis in osteopetrosis. *Journal of Oral Surgery* 33, 288.

[38] GUTTENBERG S. A. (1974) Osteoradionecrosis of the jaw. *American Journal of Surgery* 127, 326.

[39] DYSON D. P. (1970) Osteomyelitis of the jaws in Albers–Schönberg disease. *British Journal of Oral Surgery* **7**, 178.

[40] COOKE B. E. D. (1956) Paget's disease of the jaws: fifteen cases. *Annals of the Royal College of Surgeons, England* **19**, 223.

[41] GOLD L. (1955) The classification and pathogenesis of fibrous dysplasia of the jaws. *Oral Surgery* **8**, 628, 725, 856.

[42] WALDRON C. A. & SHAFER W. G. (1966) The central giant cell reparative granuloma of the jaws. *American Journal of Clinical Pathology* **45**, 437.

[43] KRAGH L. V., DAHLIN D. C. & ERICH J. B. (1960) Cartilaginous tumours of the jaws and facial regions. *American Journal of Surgery* **99**, 852.

[44] MEYER I. & SHKLAR G. (1965) Malignant tumors metastatic to mouth and jaws. *Oral Surgery* **20**, 350.

[45] GREENE C. S. & MARKOVIC M. A. (1976) Response to nonsurgical treatment of patients with positive radiographic findings in the temperomandibular joint. *Journal of Oral Surgery* **34**, 692.

[46] GIANSANTI J. S., HRABAK R. P. & WALDRON C. A. (1973) Palmar–plantar hyperkeratosis and concomitant periodontal destruction (Papillon–Lefèvre syndrome). *Oral Surgery* **36**, 40.

[47] PINDBORG J. J., KRAMER I. R. H. & TORLONI H. (1971) Histologic typing of odontogenic tumours, jaw cysts and allied lesions. *International Histological Classification of Tumours, No. 5*, World Health Organization, Geneva.

[48] WALDRON C. A., GIANSANTI J. S. & BROWAND B. C. (1975) Sclerotic cemental masses of the jaws (so-called chronic sclerosing osteomyelitis, sclerosing osteitis, multiple enostosis and gigantiform cementoma). *Oral Surgery* **39**, 590.

CHAPTER 27

Diseases of the Hypopharynx

GLOBUS HYSTERICUS

This is a common condition, which unfortunately suffers from having been mislabelled. Patients with this condition are virtually never hysterical. Although they are often anxious, they do not necessarily suffer from an anxiety neurosis.

Pathology

It is said that the symptom is caused by spasm of the cricopharyngeal sphincter but it is not really known if this is true, although EMG of the muscle shows increased activity [1]. A careful radiological study of 307 patients with this symptom [2] showed completely negative clinical and radiological findings in two patients out of three. The remainder showed a variety of lesions of the foregut, extending as far as the stomach, the commonest being hiatus hernia. One patient in five also showed an osteophyte of the cervical spine.

Clinical features

The patient is usually a middle-aged woman who complains of difficulty in swallowing – this discomfort is felt when swallowing saliva, and is in fact relieved by swallowing food; it is always felt in the midline just above the suprasternal notch. There are no other symptoms of throat disease – no hoarseness, sore throat, otalgia, etc. The patient appears well and has not lost weight.

Examination of the larynx, pharynx and neck is entirely normal. Careful questioning, either at the first visit or perhaps later, shows that the patient often has a real cause for anxiety. The effect of strong emotion on the throat is recognized by popular sayings – 'choking with rage', 'heart in my mouth', etc. Furthermore, the patient is often anxious specifically about his throat. Close questioning often reveals that a friend or relative has recently died of a 'cancer of the throat'.

Investigations

A lateral radiograph of the soft tissues of the neck provides a good screening technique for these patients (Fig. 27.1). If the pharyngeal soft tissue shadow posterior to the trachea is narrower than the body of the vertebra behind it, the patient can reasonably be reassured that there is no organic disease present and be reviewed 2–3 weeks later. If the symptoms persist for more than 3 weeks a barium swallow and meal and an oesophagoscopy must be done.

Treatment

The best and often the only treatment necessary for this disease is strong reassurance that the patient does not have any serious disease including cancer. There is indeed little other treatment available, except perhaps antacids if the symptom is clearly associated with reflux oesophagitis. Patients should not be given tranquillizers – the fewer patients introduced to this habit the better.

SIDEROPENIC DYSPHAGIA

It appears better to give this disease a name, rather than to indulge in a sterile argument over priorities. The syndrome was first described in Britain in 1919 by Paterson and Brown-Kelly and by Vinson in the USA in 1922 [3–5]. Brown-Kelly described a condition of dysphagia in anaemic women, with atrophic glossitis, and fissuring of the corners of the mouth. Paterson, at the same meeting of the Royal Society of Medicine, also reported women with spasmodic dysphagia and glossitis.

Aetiology

It is thought by some that the changes in the pharynx are caused by the iron deficiency anaemia but as the web usually persists despite

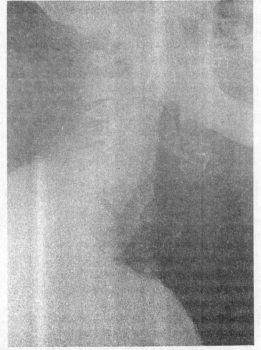

FIG. 27.1. Normal lateral soft tissue radiograph of the neck.

attempts at correction of the anaemia, and since the vast majority of anaemic women do not suffer from this syndrome, this hypothesis appears to be unlikely.

Pathology

The mucosal lining of the entire upper digestive tract is smooth and atrophic, and a high proportion of these patients develop a web, which is usually in the post-cricoid space, but may be in the upper oesophagus. In addition a high proportion have atrophic gastritis.

Clinical features

The disease begins about the age of 30, and its maximum age incidence is 60. 90% of the patients are women.

Dysphagia is the presenting symptom. Clinical examination shows the fissuring of the corners of the mouth, glossitis, splenomegaly and occasionally koilonychia.

Additional conditions

Many of these patients [6] show other conditions, the commonest being thyroid disease, malignant disease and rheumatoid arthritis. It might be thought that autoimmunity is thus a possible cause but this has been disproved [7].

Investigations

Laboratory studies confirm a hypochromic anaemia in 60% of the patients, with the haemoglobin being less than 12 g/100 ml [8]. The serum iron is also low in approximately 70% of patients. Serum B_{12} may be low in 10% of patients and be associated with macrocytic anaemia. Tubeless gastric analysis shows achlorhydria in three patients out of four.

Barium swallow shows a post-cricoid web in three out of four patients and in 20% there are two webs [8]. One patient in four may have an upper oesophageal stricture, and occasionally a carcinoma is found (Fig. 27.2).

Oesophagoscopy shows the smooth atrophic pharyngeal mucosa and the web when present. Post-cricoid carcinoma is also looked for.

Treatment

The anaemia is treated by parenteral iron until the serum iron reaches normal levels and the patient is advised to take a soft diet. Thereafter the patient should take iron orally until repeated checks of the haemoglobin show that it is stable. The stricture is dilated at oesophagoscopy.

It is important to keep these patients under observation since about 10% later develop a post-cricoid carcinoma [9].

TRAUMA AND FOREIGN BODIES

Foreign bodies in the hypopharynx are reasonably uncommon; large round objects such as coins usually impact at the upper and lower oesophageal sphincters, but small sharp objects such

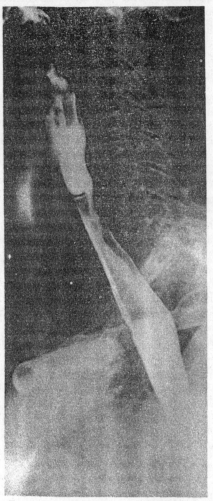

FIG. 27.2. Radiograph of a post-cricoid web.

as fish bones may occasionally impact in the piriform fossa. They cause discomfort in the throat, which is well localized by the patient. They can usually be seen on mirror examination, but plain radiographs of the neck are seldom helpful; the vertical line demonstrated by the posterior part of the vertical plate of the cricoid cartilage, which is the first part of this cartilage to calcify, should not be confused with a foreign body. These foreign bodies are removed by endoscopy under general anaesthetic.

Trauma to the hypopharynx may be open or closed. The pharynx may be involved in external open injuries, such as cut throat wounds or stabbings. If the patient survives, which is unusual, the tear is repaired.

Mucosal lacerations of the pharynx occasionally occur at the same time as blunt trauma to the larynx. They are dealt with in the acute phase, at the same operation as the larynx, and are repaired by suturing.

Trauma to the hypopharynx may occur during oesophagoscopy, the area of the cricopharyngeal sphincter being compressed over the cervical spine during introduction of the oesophagoscope which is said to occur in 1% of oesophagoscopies. This injury is not usually diagnosed until the patient recovers from the anaesthetic. Pain is felt locally or in the ears, unlike the pain of oesophageal perforation which is felt in the back. There may be also spasm of the strap muscles of the neck. The patient is also not usually so shocked as the patient who has suffered an oesophageal perforation. Surgical emphysema of the neck is almost always found (Fig. 27.3).

Investigations consist of plain radiographs which demonstrate air in the soft tissues of the neck and broadening of the retrotracheal space. A barium swallow should not be done but a little gastrografin may be used to outline the perforation.

Perforation of the hypopharynx should be treated conservatively [10]. The patient is treated by tube feeding, a broad spectrum antibiotic and fluid replacement. If the patient's general condition deteriorates or if the temperature rises an abscess has probably formed and should be drained via an external approach.

Many of these patients develop a fistula which virtually always closes spontaneously, and some develop a stricture. The mortality of perforations in this region is low compared to those of the thoracic oesophagus.

PHARYNGEAL DIVERTICULUM

Pathology

Diverticulae of the pharynx are uncommon;

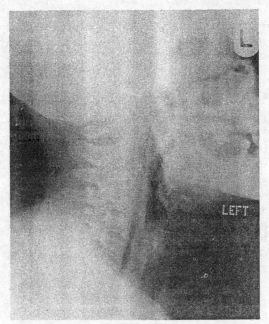

FIG. 27.3. Emphysema of the pharyngeal tissues due to perforation of the pharynx by a foreign body.

much the commonest is the pulsion diverticulum of the posterior wall arising in the so-called Killian's dehiscence. Other diverticulae are very rare, but can be classified as follows [11].

Congenital

(a) *Lateral:* Congenital diverticulae occur through the branchial clefts and have thus been recorded arising above the superior constrictor muscle, between the middle and inferior constrictor, and below the inferior constrictor. These are all exceedingly rare [12].

(b) *Posterior:* Can present as large diverticulae causing symptoms in infancy (rare) or may be occult, small diverticulae arising in infancy but not causing symptoms until early adult life.

Acquired

(a) *Posterior:* The well-known pulsion diverticulum.

(b) *Lateral:* Pharyngocoeles, arising from the piriform fossa, and said to occur in trumpeters and glass blowers.

Aetiology

The cause of pulsion diverticulae is unknown. They always arise posteriorly, through a relatively unsupported part of the posterior pharyngeal wall known as Killian's dehiscence (Fig. 27.4) bounded superiorly by the oblique fibres of the thyropharyngeal part of the inferior constrictor and inferiorly by the transverse fibres of the cricopharyngeal part of this muscle.

It is thought that these pouches are caused by some disorder of swallowing, more particularly of the cricopharyngeus, and the alternate explanation that they are congenital and grow gradually throughout life does not seem to have been entertained seriously.

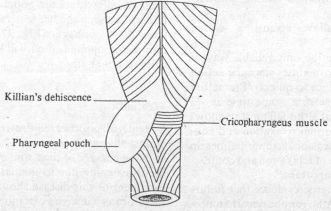

Killian's dehiscence

Cricopharyngeus muscle

Pharyngeal pouch

FIG. 27.4. Anatomy of a pharyngeal pouch.

It is thought that the disorder of swallowing occurs in the sphincteric zone caused by the cricopharyngeus; there is here a zone of elevated pressure, which falls in response to swallowing.

The zone measures between 2 and 6 cm but the width of the band of maximum pressure is usually only 1 cm. The inferior constrictor and the oblique part of the cricopharyngeus contribute to the proximal part of the pressure zone, and the circular upper oesophageal fibres to the distal part.

The sphincter is always closed and its resting pressures vary between 15 and 60 cm H_2O. The sphincter opens naturally during swallowing but may also open during vomiting, belching, regurgitation and retching. The sphincter normally opens by relaxation which is usually accompanied by laryngeal elevation. Relaxation lasts less than 1 second and is followed by a contraction producing pressures of 70–100 cm H_2O and lasting 2–4 seconds. The sphincter opens in anticipation of the bolus arriving and before maximum pharyngeal pressures have been reached.

Electrical recording of cricopharyngeal activity demonstrates inhibition of reflex activity for several hundred milliseconds at the onset of swallowing which would be impossible in smooth muscle.

The abnormalities of the cricopharyngeal sphincter, based on manometric studies can be divided into:

(1) spasm;

(2) delayed onset of relaxation;

(3) premature contraction which shortens relaxation;

(4) a second swallow against a closed sphincter.

Pressure studies are the only reliable way of discovering these abnormalities since the action of swallowing takes place so quickly. Premature contractions can be seen at some time in all patients, indicating that although most swallows are associated with normal relaxation and contraction, there are occasional abnormalities in the temporal sequence of relaxation and contraction which could be important.

There is no manometric evidence that failure to relax ever occurs. A larger pharynx than normal has been described with pharyngeal pouches, and is thought to be caused by incomplete emptying of the pharynx, leaving behind residual material, and by a second swallow meeting a closed sphincter [13].

Clinical features

Pulsion diverticulae are usually only seen in the elderly. They cause long standing dysphagia for food, halitosis, regurgitation of undigested food, weight loss, and recurrent chest infections due to aspiration of food and saliva; hoarseness is rare and is usually due to involvement of the recurrent laryngeal nerve by a carcinoma arising in the pouch. The latter event has certainly been recorded, but it is not clear whether a carcinoma occurs any more commonly than would be expected to arise by chance.

Examination of the pharynx shows retained secretions in both piriform fossae. The well-known swelling low on the left side of the neck is rarely seen.

Investigations

Occasionally an air bubble in a pouch is demonstrated by a lateral plain film of the neck, but the classical investigation is a barium swallow which demonstrates the pouch (Fig. 27.5). The lower end of the oesophagus should also be examined since it is said that many of these patients also have a hiatus hernia.

Oesophagoscopy should be carried out to exclude the presence of carcinoma. The instrument usually enters the pouch, and anterior to this will be seen the bar separating the pharynx from the oesophagus (Fig. 27.6). The opening into the oesophagus itself will be seen with difficulty or not at all.

Treatment

Virtually all pouches require treatment since they almost all cause symptoms, which become worse with the passage of time, and eventually become life-threatening due to inhalation of food. The treatment of this disease should be approached therefore as if it were a carcinoma. Two possibilities are available: endoscopic diathermy coagulation [14] of the bar between the pouch and the

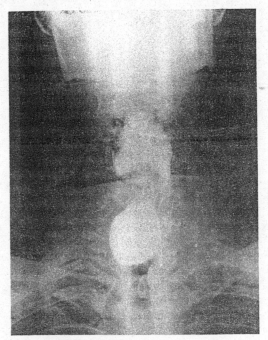

FIG. 27.5. Radiograph of a pharyngeal pouch.

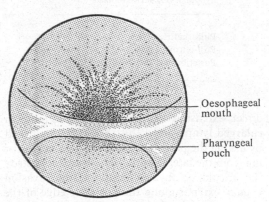

Oesophageal
mouth

Pharyngeal
pouch

FIG. 27.6. Endoscopic appearance of a pharyngeal pouch.

oesophagus, which appears to be the best treatment for the frail and very elderly, and excision via an external approach, which is probably better for younger, fitter patients but has a high complication rate, notably fistula formation, paralysis of the recurrent laryngeal nerve, recurrence and stenosis of the pharynx.

TUMOURS OF THE HYPOPHARYNX

Surgical anatomy

The hypopharynx extends from the hyoid bone superiorly to the lower border of the cricoid cartilage inferiorly, and consists of three parts: the post-cricoid area, the piriform fossae and the posterior wall (Fig. 27.7). The boundaries of these areas have been defined precisely by the UICC for the purpose of tumour classification (Table 27.1) [15].

The distribution of tumours among these areas varies in different series, but the approximate site incidence of hypopharyngeal carcinoma is as shown in Table 27.2 [16].

This site distribution varies between different countries and even within countries. Thus, true post-cricoid carcinoma is very rare in the USA and in continental Europe. Furthermore, the incidence varies within England and Wales, being commoner in South Wales for instance than in London; approximately 400 hypopharyngeal carcinomas occur per year in England and Wales.

Histology

Benign tumours of the hypopharynx are virtually unknown. Malignant tumours, as would be expected in an area lined by squamous epithelium, are virtually all squamous carcinomas. Unlike tumours of the oropharynx and nasopharynx, squamous carcinomas of the hypopharynx are usually moderately differentiated [17].

Rare tumours include the fibrolipoma, the leiomyosarcoma and the malignant synovioma but the only uncommon tumour of importance is the pseudo-sarcoma. This is a polypoidal tumour consisting of a stroma which has the appearance of a sarcoma covered by a layer of squamous carcinoma. The sarcomatous element rarely metastasizes, and the carcinomatous part does so late, to the lymph nodes of the neck. The 'sarcomatous' element is thought to be an unusual stromal reaction to squamous carcinoma and is not truly malignant. These tumours are not particularly aggressive and localized removal without sacrificing the pharynx and larynx is usually

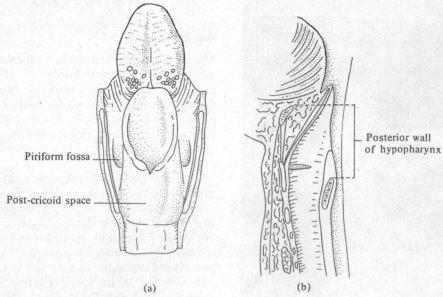

Fig. 27.7. Anatomical divisions of the hypopharynx.

TABLE 27.1

(1) *Piriform sinus* – Extends from the pharyngoepiglottic fold to the upper end of the oesophagus. It is bounded laterally by the thyroid cartilage and medially by the lateral surface of the aryepiglottic fold and the arytenoid and cricoid cartilages.
(2) *Pharyngo-oesophageal junction* (post-cricoid area) – This site lies posterior to the larynx. It extends from the level of the arytenoid cartilages and connecting folds to the inferior border of the cricoid cartilage.
(3) *Posterior pharyngeal wall* – Extends from the level of the floor of the vallecula to the level of the cricoarytenoid joints.

TABLE 27.2. Relative site incidence of hypopharyngeal carcinoma

Piriform fossa	55%
Post-cricoid space	40%
Posterior pharyngeal wall	5%

sufficient to control the disease for long periods [18].

Surgical pathology of squamous carcinoma

Local spread

Tumours of the piriform fossa can be subdivided into those affecting the lateral and those affecting the medial wall. Tumours arising on the lateral wall extend through the thyrohyoid membrane to invade the carotid sheath or the cricothyroid membrane to invade the thyroid gland. A palpable neck mass in this disease may be direct extension of the tumour and not an enlarged lymph node: this should be confirmed by asking the patient to swallow. Tumours arising from the lateral wall often invade or destroy the cricoid or thyroid cartilage; the invasion usually extends along the posterior edge of the thyroid lamina. Tumours of the medial wall rapidly invade the aryepiglottic fold and false cord, structures rich in lymphatics, and pass through these to invade and fix the vocal cord, causing hoarseness [19].

The vocal cord is often paralysed in tumours arising on the medial wall. The cause may be:
(1) infiltration of the posterior cricoarytenoid muscle;
(2) invasion of the cricoarytenoid joint;
(3) invasion of the recurrent laryngeal nerve [20, 21].

Larger growths in which it may be difficult to

decide whether the tumour arose laterally or medially may spread as follows:

(1) across the upper part of the post cricoid area to the opposite piriform fossa;

(2) over the pharyngoepiglottic ligament to the base of the tongue.

Larger tumours arising on the medial wall invade the supraglottic larynx, but the pattern of spread is not the same as in supraglottic carcinoma, in that these tumours spread downwards within the paraglottic space below the level of the ventricle.

These tumours behave like oesophageal tumours and show significant submucosal spread of 10 mm on average [22].

The local spread of post-cricoid carcinoma has not been so well studied. It has been known for a long time that these tumours in the late stages invade the pre-vertebral fascia. Vocal cord paralysis is also fairly common (approx. 10%) and is usually due to extension of the tumour outside the oesophagus to invade the tracheo-oesophageal groove. Because of the close proximity of the thyroid gland to the cervical oesophagus invasion of this latter gland is said to occur commonly.

Submucosal extension averages 5 mm [22] and these tumours also tend to invade the thin tracheo-oesophageal wall. In addition to involvement of the deep cervical chain there is a high incidence of involvement of the paratracheal nodes. On this account some surgeons have advocated mediastinal dissection but as enlarged nodes in the tracheo-oesophageal groove can be removed by finger dissection from above, it is probably unnecessary.

Lymph node metastases

Cancer of the hypopharynx has a notorious propensity to metastasize to the lymph nodes of the neck, and indeed an involved node may be the presenting symptom, particularly of tumours of the piriform fossa. The incidence of lymph node metastases in hypopharyngeal carcinoma approximates to the figures shown in Table 27.3.

Staging

Squamous carcinomas have been staged by the joint UICC/AJC report and the full classification should be consulted for details [15]. In principle,

tumours of the hypopharynx are divided into three T categories: T1 is a tumour localized to one site within the hypopharynx, T2 is a tumour extending to another site within the hypopharynx, and T3 indicates extension to neighbouring structures, notably the larynx and the soft tissues of the neck. One disadvantage of this system is that spread to the cervical oesophagus

TABLE 27.3. Incidence of lymph node metastases

	Total	Unilateral	Bilateral
Piriform fossa	65%	60%	5%
Post-cricoid space	20%	15%	5%
Posterior pharyngeal wall	55%	*	*

* Figures not given because the numbers are too small.

is not mentioned but this is the common direction of spread of post-cricoid tumours which are thus difficult to stage. A classification based on size for these latter tumours would probably be more realistic. N and M have the usual connotations.

Aetiology

Several supposed causes of hypopharyngeal cancer have been found.

1. Sex

Cancer of the post-cricoid space is the only head and neck cancer which is more common in women, the sex ratio being about 3 : 1. This proportion is reversed for piriform fossa tumours. This may be related to the fact that anaemia is commoner in women.

2. Geography

The incidence of the tumour varies between countries and inside countries and this has been referred to above.

3. Anaemia

Sideropenic dysphagia first described by Paterson and Brown-Kelly [3, 4] is often associated with post-cricoid carcinoma [9]: Between one and two-thirds of patients with post-cricoid carcinoma have a history of this syndrome [23]. The risk for an individual patient with the Paterson–Kelly syndrome is small, of the order of 2%; the anaemia is not necessarily microcytic but may be macrocytic [8].

4. Blood groups

There is some evidence that this disease is commoner in patients with blood group O [24].

5. Smoking and drinking

Inevitably heavy smoking and drinking have been said to be aetiological factors of pharyngeal cancer [25]. Accurate statistics about drinking habits are difficult to collect since the moderate drinker usually loses count after the first few drinks, and the heavy drinker seldom admits to drinking at all.

There is some evidence that heavy smoking is commoner in patients with pharyngeal cancer [25], but this must be interpreted with great caution since the incidence of pharyngeal cancer has not increased during this century, despite the enormous increase in tobacco consumption, and despite the fact that a higher proportion of the population now survive into the cancer age group.

6. Radiation

In the 1920s and 1930s there was a vogue, particularly in the north-west of England, for treating thyrotoxicosis with small doses of radiotherapy at weekly intervals for several months. This appears to have been quite effective, particularly when one remembers that surgical treatment of thyrotoxicosis at that time was an adventure with a significant mortality. A small proportion of these patients are now developing a pharyngeal carcinoma, with an average latent interval of 25 years [26].

Investigation

Patients with tumours of the hypopharynx require more careful assessment than any other carcinoma of the head and neck, because such a high proportion of these tumours are inoperable.

History

In addition to the history of local disease, i.e. dysphagia for food, sore throat, hoarseness and otalgia and loss of weight, it is important to ask about the general health, particularly for previous operations, medications, and previous radiotherapy for thyrotoxicosis.

Examination

The mouth is examined for dental sepsis, and for the condition of the oral mucous membrane, which may be atrophic suggesting that the patient suffers from a form of the Paterson–Brown-Kelly syndrome.

The hypopharynx is next examined. A tumour of the piriform fossa can almost always be seen, and some idea of its local extent can be obtained.

The larynx is also examined for local invasion of the supraglottic structure and immobility of the vocal cords.

Post-cricoid tumours are not usually seen although if the tumour is very large there may be visible involvement of the piriform fossa, or of the posterior surface of the arytenoids. Usually the tumour is not visible but retained secretions may be seen in the piriform fossa. It is also very important to see if the vocal cords move.

The neck is then examined carefully for enlarged lymph nodes; usually these are felt in the upper deep cervical chain. It is also very important to move the larynx from side to side over the vertebral column for two reasons:

Laryngeal crepitus is lost in patients with post-cricoid carcinoma.

To assess fixation to the pre-vertebral fascia.

A general medical examination particularly of the cardiorespiratory system is also carried out.

Laboratory tests

A routine full blood count, blood urea and blood sugar are done. The serum proteins are almost always low in this disease, as is the serum potassium, and both these deficits need to be corrected before operation.

Radiology

The following radiographs are used routinely. Plain lateral soft tissue films of the neck (Fig. 27.8) and a barium swallow are performed in every case. They are needed not only to help in the differential diagnosis of patients with globus hystericus but also to define the extent of a pharyngeal tumour.

Radiology is mandatory if tumours are to be staged under the UICC classification. Furthermore, radiology is of great practical importance in defining the lower limit of a post-cricoid tumour, which may often be difficult or impossible to assess by oesophagoscopy.

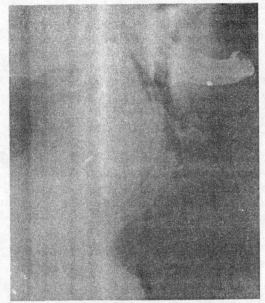

FIG. 27.8. Plain lateral soft tissue radiograph of the neck in a patient with a post-cricoid carcinoma.

Plain lateral films demonstrate any widening of the retrotracheal soft tissues. If the width of these soft tissues is greater than that of the vertebra behind, an oesophagoscopy must be done.

Endoscopy

The purpose of an endoscopy in a patient with a hypopharyngeal carcinoma is the assessment of the extent of the disease; obtaining a biopsy specimen is a minor part of the exercise.

In a patient with a carcinoma of the piriform fossa the following points are noted:

(1) Spread of the tumour into the upper end of the post-cricoid space (indicating that a total pharyngolaryngectomy will be necessary).

(2) Spread of the tumour to or beyond the midline of the posterior wall (also indicating that a total pharyngolaryngectomy will be necessary).

(3) Involvement of the larynx, which is interesting but not important.

(4) Spread of the tumour superiorly over the pharyngoepiglottic ligament into the base of the tongue which can be felt better than seen, and which indicates extensive and possibly incurable disease.

In a post-cricoid carcinoma the following points require attention.

(1) The lower extent of the tumour, measured with reference to the incisor teeth. This is needed to decide whether the tumour is operable, and to decide what method of pharyngeal replacement is to be used. It may be difficult to introduce an oesophagoscope through such a tumour, in which case it may be possible to introduce a bronchoscope over a bougie after dilating the tumour carefully and leaving a filiform bougie within the lumen.

(2) The upper end of the tumour, and extension into the piriform fossa (for staging of the tumour).

(3) The mobility of the pharynx over the prevertebral fascia, which is assessed by palpation.

Treatment

Perhaps the most important point to emphasize is that one patient in four with a hypopharyngeal carcinoma is untreatable and identification of this group is very important. The following factors make a tumour of the hypopharynx untreatable:

(1) Poor general condition and advanced age. Absolute statements about either of these cannot be given, and individual judgement must be exercised. But major surgery should seldom be advised for patients beyond their early seventies.

(2) Fixation of the tumour to the pre-vertebral fascia.

(3) Fixation of the vocal cord in post-cricoid carcinoma.

(4) Bilateral neck glands; treatment does not affect the natural history of the disease in the presence of involved glands on both sides of the neck, and certainly surgery only makes the patient more miserable.

(5) Distant metastases.

(6) Refusal by the patient.

In practice the patient who is not treated usually shows more than one of these unfavourable factors.

Combined surgery and radiotherapy

One of the most recent fashions in the treatment of head and neck cancer has been to administer pre-operative irradiation in order to reduce local recurrence by implantation and dissemination by veins and lymphatics [27]. The concept is attractive but there is general disagreement on the dose, different authorities using doses ranging from 1000 R to 5500 R. Furthermore, despite the claims of some authors, there is little evidence either from controlled prospective trials or from matched retrospective studies to show that combined treatment improves survival rates [28].

Since pre-operative radiotherapy increases the morbidity, a controlled trial is needed to establish whether it improves survival.

Radiotherapy

The largest series of patients to receive curative radiotherapy alone is that of Lederman who showed that patients without enlarged lymph nodes (the minority) stood a 20% chance of surviving 5 years when treated with radiotherapy [17]. However, in the presence of enlarged nodes the cure rate was negligible – less than 5%. Radiotherapy therefore should be reserved for the patient without enlarged nodes, and with a small tumour. Conversely, surgery will be needed as the primary form of treatment for large tumours with enlarged cervical nodes and for tumours which recur after radiotherapy.

Management of lymph nodes

For the patient with secondarily involved lymph nodes the operation of radical neck dissection has stood the test of time [29]. More recently, many surgeons have advocated prophylactic neck dissection, that is, radical neck dissection in the absence of palpable lymph nodes, on the grounds that, though impalpable, some may be histologically involved. No evidence has been produced from prospective controlled trials that

this procedure improves the patient's chances of survival, and the issue remains 'not proven'.

Resection of the primary tumour

The operation advised obviously depends on the site of the primary tumour.

Posterior pharyngeal wall tumours usually require a total pharyngolaryngectomy but Ogura and his colleagues [30] showed that it is usually unnecessary to sacrifice the larynx. Such tumours can be removed by a lateral pharyngotomy; the resultant defect is filled by a split skin graft stitched over the pre-vertebral fascia. Preliminary results indicate that this operation is satisfactory, and has the enormous advantage of preserving the voice.

Tumours of the piriform fossa may require laryngectomy and partial pharyngectomy or total pharyngolaryngectomy. Supraglottic laryngectomy, removing the affected part of the pharynx and the suprastructure of the larynx, but preserving the patient's vocal cords and hence his voice, has been described [31]. However, pathological studies have repeatedly shown that most of these tumours invade the larynx making the operation highly dangerous [20]. It appears that there is little or no place for this operation at least in the United Kingdom in the treatment of piriform fossa tumours, and because of invasion of the larynx the latter should always be removed. It is not necessary always to do a total pharyngectomy. Indeed, in the author's series, it was possible to preserve enough pharyngeal mucosa in two patients out of three for closure of the defect, in the same manner as after total laryngectomy for laryngeal carcinoma. The patient is thus spared the problem of a pharyngeal reconstruction. When this is not possible (usually because the tumour has invaded the post-cricoid space) a total pharyngolaryngectomy with pharyngeal reconstruction is necessary.

Tumours of the post-cricoid region should be treated surgically. A total pharyngolaryngectomy is required with resection of part of the oesophagus if the tumour extends into the cervical oesophagus, which it usually does.

Pharyngeal repair

The methods of pharyngeal reconstruction made necessary by a pharyngolaryngectomy will now be discussed. The development of the operations historically falls broadly into three phases.

Cervical oesophagectomy was first carried out by Czerny in 1877 [32], but it was not until 1942 that Wookey described a reliable method of reconstruction of the pharynx [33]. A large *laterally based cervical skin flap* was raised and, at the end of the operation, the upper end of the flap was sewn round the orostome and the bottom edge round the oesophagostome, leaving a gutter open laterally which was closed 3 weeks later. This operation gained a bad reputation, probably because it was used in circumstances in which Wookey said it would not work. The repair often did not succeed at the first attempt, and further operations to close the fistula were necessary, often resulting in the formation of a stricture. These staged operations imposed a long hospital stay on the patient, often up to 1 year or even more, and, when Ranger showed that the 1-year survival after pharyngolaryngectomy at that time was only 40% it became obvious that a more reliable and speedy method of replacing the pharynx, preferably at the time of excision, was necessary [34].

Several of these operations were described in the 1950s; the pharynx being replaced at the primary operation with various *visceral loops*, either on a pedicle or as a free revascularized graft. The only methods still in use appear to be transposed colon [35, 36] and stomach [37, 38].

Revascularized loops of small bowel have been tried without success. It is said that they will probably be successful when microvascular techniques are developed to provide reliable anastomoses. This is almost certainly an illusion, however, for pharyngeal cancers are inevitably heavily infected, and this would militate against the success of such repairs.

The use of a transposed viscus, colon or stomach, was a tremendous step forward. The pharynx could be excised and replaced at the same operation; the patient began to swallow food within a few days of operation and went home within 2–3 weeks of operation. Furthermore, there was no limit to the amount of oesophagus which could be removed: it was not

needed for the pharyngeal repair and thus there was no anxiety about recurrence in the oesophageal stump. Unfortunately, the hospital mortality was high: 40% in many reported series. This is hardly surprising when one considers that these operations demand simultaneous dissection in the neck, thorax and abdomen. Many of those who survived the operation lived only for another year or so before dying of metastases. Hence the long-term survival was short – 10% in Ranger's original series [34]. Initial enthusiasm gave way to gloom, and many surgeons came to regard these procedures as a form of palliation: the prospect of cure receded rapidly.

During this time several other methods were being tried, including replacement of the pharynx by a plastic tube sewn in at the time of operation [39]. The tube has recently been modified, being now covered by Silastic to encourage in-growth of the patient's tissues.

The third significant advance in this field came in 1965 when Bakamjian showed that the pharynx could be replaced primarily with a *deltopectoral skin flap* [40]. After the pharynx and larynx have been removed at the excisional operation, the flap is raised and tubed with its skin surface inwards; the end of the tube is then anastomosed to the orostome and the oesophageal stump is anastomosed end to side to the lower part of the tube. A temporary fistula is left where the pedicle emerges from the neck and is closed 3 weeks later by division and return of the flap. Skin repair of the pharynx imposes a longer stay in hospital on the patient than visceral repair, but not as long as the original secondary forms of skin repair. This operation provides a 5-year cure of about 35%.

After-care and follow-up

As in all patients with malignant disease of the head and neck careful after-care and follow-up of these patients is required. The following points require attention.

Adjustment of medication. Operations for cancer of the hypopharynx often require a total thyroidectomy. The parathyroid glands are therefore almost always removed in addition and replacement therapy both for the thyroid and parathyroid glands is required. This will usually need to be supervised by a physician interested in this field, but as a rough guide thyroxin 0·1 mg daily, calciferol 50 000 units daily and calcium supplements such as calcium Sandoz will be required.

Rehabilitation of speech. A very much smaller proportion of patients develop artificial speech after pharyngolaryngectomy than after straightforward total laryngectomy. There are several factors mitigating against the development of 'oesophageal speech' after such an operation: many of these patients are women who do not like oesophageal speech because the voice sounds masculine; the reconstructed pharynx is without a nerve supply and is relatively stiff and thick, and so does not vibrate well. For all these reasons and perhaps more, only about 10% of patients develop artificial voice after pharyngolaryngectomy; the remainder may need to be helped with one of the mechanical electronic devices which are held on the neck, or may be helped by implantation of a prosthesis such as the Voice-Bak.

Detection of recurrence. These patients should be followed up to detect recurrence, particularly in the glands of the neck if a radical neck dissection has not been carried out. As most of these recurrences occur within the first year the patient should be followed up at monthly intervals during that period and thereafter at longer intervals such as every 3 months. A recurrence within the pharynx may also be detected but is rarely treatable with any hope of success.

Terminal care. As the overall survival in hypopharyngeal cancer is at best in the region of 35%, at least two patients out of three with this disease will require terminal care. This is usually the responsibility of the surgeon, whose main task in addition to providing moral support for the patient and his family is to ensure that the patient is free of pain. Operations for pain relief such as transcutaneous cordotomy or division of nerve roots are seldom applicable or successful in this condition; since the terminal period is usually short, of a few weeks only, the best treatment is morphine which should be given in doses which are large enough and given at sufficiently frequent intervals to ensure that the patient is constantly free of pain.

References

[1] DeWeese D. D. & Saunders W. H. (1913) *Textbook of Otolaryngology*, p. 125. St. Louis: Mosby.

[2] Malcolmson K. G. (1968) Globus hystericus vel pharyngis. *Journal of Laryngology* 82, 219.

[3] Paterson D. R. (1919) A clinical type of dysphagia. *Journal of Laryngology* 34, 289.

[4] Kelly A. B. (1919) Spasm at the entrance to the oesophagus. *Journal of Laryngology* 34, 285.

[5] Vinson P. P. (1922) Hysterical dysphagia. *Minnesota Medicine* 5, 107.

[6] Chrisholm M., Ardran G. M., Callender S. T. & Wright R. (1971) A follow-up study of patients with post cricoid webs. *Quarterly Journal of Medicine* 40, 421.

[7] Chrisholm M., Ardran G. M., Callender S. T. & Wright R. (1971) Iron deficiency and auto-immunity in post cricoid webs. *Quarterly Journal of Medicine* 40, 421.

[8] Jacobs A. & Kilpatrick G. S. (1964) The Paterson–Kelly syndrome. *British Medical Journal* 1, 79.

[9] Jones R. F. McN. (1961) The Paterson–Brown-Kelly syndrome. Its relationship to iron deficiency and post cricoid carcinoma. *Journal of Laryngology* 74, 529 (I), 544 (II).

[10] Leading Article (1972) Traumatic perforation of the oesophagus. *British Medical Journal* 1, 524.

[11] Korkis B. (1958) *Recent Advances in Otolaryngology*, 3rd ed., p. 375. London: Churchill.

[12] Wilson C. P. (1962) Pharyngeal diverticulae, their cause and treatment. *Journal of Laryngology and Otology* 76, 151.

[13] Earlam R. (1976) *Clinical Tests of Oesophageal Function*. London: Granada.

[14] Dohlmann G. & Mattson O. (1960) The endoscopic operation for hypopharyngeal diverticula. *Archives of Otolaryngology* 71, 744.

[15] UICC (1973) *TNM Classification of Malignant Tumours*, p. 20. Geneva: UICC.

[16] Dalley V. M. (1968) Cancer of the laryngopharynx. *Journal of Laryngology and Otology* 82, 407.

[17] Lederman M. (1967) Cancer of the pharynx. *Journal of Laryngology and Otology* 81, 151.

[18] Baker D. C. (1959) Pseudosarcoma of the larynx. *Annals of Otology, Rhinology and Laryngology* 68, 471.

[19] Ogura J. H. (1955) Surgical pathology of cancer of the larynx. *The Laryngoscope* 65, 867.

[20] Kirschner J. A. (1975) Piriform sinus cancer: A clinical and laboratory study. *Annals of Otology, Rhinology and Laryngology* 84, 793.

[21] Olofsson J. & Van Nostrand A. W. P. (1973) Growth and spread of laryngeal and hypopharyngeal carcinoma with reflections on the effect of pre-operative irradiation. *Acta Otolaryngologica*. Supplement 308.

[22] Harrison D. F. N. (1970) Pathology of hypopharyngeal cancer in relation to surgical management. *Journal of Laryngology and Otology* 84, 349.

[23] Ahlbom H. E. (1937) Pradispanierende Faktoren fur

Platten epittial karzinomin mund hals und Speiserohre. *Acta Radiologica* 18, 163.

[24] STELL P. M. & KELL R. A. (1970) Blood groups and hypopharyngeal cancer. *The Lancet* 2, 819.

[25] VINCENT R. G. & MARCHETTA F. (1963) The relationship of the use of tobacco and alcohol to cancer of the oral cavity, pharynx or larynx. *American Journal of Surgery* 106, 501.

[26] SOM M. L. & NUSSBAUM M. (1969) Surgical theory of carcinoma of the hypopharynx and cervical oesophagus. *Otolaryngologic Clinics of North America* 2, 631.

[27] GARRETT M. (1959) Eight further cases of radiation induced cancer. *British Medical Journal* 1, 1329.

[28] BRYCE D. P. (1972) The role of surgery in the management of carcinoma of the larynx. *Journal of Laryngology and Otology* 86, 669.

[29] CRILE G. (1906) Excision of cancer of head and neck. *Journal of American Medical Association* 47, 1780.

[30] OGURA J. H., WATSON R. K. & JUREMA A. A. (1960) Partial pharyngectomy and neck dissection for posterior hypopharyngeal cancer. *The Laryngoscope* 70, 1523.

[31] OGURA J. H., SALTZSTEIN S. L. & SPJUT H. J. (1961) Experience with conservation surgery in laryngeal and pharyngeal carcinoma. *The Laryngoscope* 71, 258.

[32] CZERNY V. (1877) Neue operationen: Vorlaufige Mittheilung. *Zentralblatt zur Chirurge.* 4, 433.

[33] WOOKEY H. (1942) The surgical treatment of carcinoma of the pharynx and upper oesophagus. *Surgery, Gynecology and Obstetrics* 75, 499.

[34] RANGER D. (1964) Replacement surgery for post-cricoid carcinomas. *Proceedings of the Royal Society of Medicine* 57, 1099.

[35] GOLIGHER J. C. & ROBIN I. G. (1964) Use of left colon for reconstruction of pharynx and oesophagus after pharyngectomy. *British Journal of Surgery* 51, 663.

[36] FAIRMAN H. D., HADLEY S. K. J. & JOHN H. J. (1964) Pharyngolaryngectomy and colonic reconstruction. *British Journal of Surgery* 52, 283.

[37] ONG G. B. & LEE T. C. (1960) Pharyngogastric anastomosis after oesophago-pharyngectomy for carcinoma of the hypopharynx and cervical oesophagus. *British Journal of Surgery* 48, 193.

[38] LE QUESNE L. P. & RANGER D. (1966) Pharyngolaryngectomy with immediate pharyngogastric anastomosis. *British Journal of Surgery* 53, 105.

[39] STUART D. W. (1966) Surgery in cancer of the cervical oesophagus: plastic tube replacement. *Journal of Laryngology and Otology* 80, 382.

[40] BAKAMJIAN Y. (1965) A two stage method for pharyngo-oesophageal reconstruction with a primary pectoral skin flap. *Plastic and Reconstructive Surgery* 36, 173.

CHAPTER 28

Tumours of the Larynx

PATHOLOGY

Tumours of the larynx may be benign or malignant but true benign tumours constitute 5% or less of all laryngeal tumours. The relative incidence is shown in Table 28.1.

Benign tumours

Papillomas

True papillomas are much the commonest benign laryngeal tumour. They can be divided into two types, the juvenile which is multiple and usually regresses after puberty, and the adult which is usually single and does not undergo spontaneous resolution.

The juvenile papilloma occurs mainly on the true and false cords and the anterior commissure but often extends into the subglottic space, the trachea, bronchi and epiglottis. It has often been thought that these lesions are not true tumours but are an abnormal tissue response to an initiating, viral factor. However, electron microscopy has failed to reveal inclusion bodies. Malignant change may occur in a juvenile papilloma but *only* if the patient has been irradiated. The hallmark of the juvenile papilloma is its multiple nature and notorious propensity to recur.

Although there are no histological differences between an adult and a juvenile papilloma the former rarely recur after local removal.

Haemangiomas

These occur almost exclusively in the subglottic space of infants and are dealt with elsewhere (p. 533).

Cartilaginous tumours

This term is used deliberately to emphasize the fact that there is no clear cut histological or clinical distinction between chondromas and chondrosarcomas. Of those reported in the literature 20% have been considered to be malignant. This is a distinctly male disease (5:1) occurring between the ages of 40 and 60. Seventy per cent of cartilaginous tumours arise from the cricoid cartilage, 20% from the thyroid, and most of the remainder from the arytenoid. Clinically these tumours are smooth and encapsulated, and radiographs often show mottled calcification.

Irrespective of the histological appearances these tumours grow and extend locally, and require removal with a good margin. Local or distant metastases have been recorded very rarely.

Neurogenous tumours

These include Schwannomas and neurofibromas, although laryngeal involvement in multiple neurofibromatosis is unusual. These tumours usually occur in the aryepiglottic fold. Malignant variants have not been recorded.

Granular cell myoblastoma

This uncommon lesion which may not be a true tumour but a degenerative disease of mature striated muscle cells may occur in the larynx. The vast majority arise within the substance of the vocal cord and cause hoarseness. The most important point about these tumours is that the overlying epithelium may show the appearances of pseudoepitheliomatous hyperplasia, and if the clinician and the pathologist are unaware of this, unnecessary radical surgery may be advised.

TABLE 28.1. Benign tumours of the larynx (modified from Friedmann)

	%
Papilloma	85
Adenoma	5
Chondroma	5
Miscellaneous (granular cell myoblastomas, lipomas, haemangiomas, neurofibromas)	5

Plasmacytoma

About 25% of extramedullary (primary or soft tissue) plasmacytomas occur in the larynx, but they are none the less rare. They are usually single and in appearance vary from polypoid to sessile. Lymph node metastases can occur, and ultimately a small proportion develop disseminated medullary disease.

Malignant tumours

Squamous carcinoma forms the vast majority of malignant laryngeal tumours. This is rather surprising in an organ lined largely by respiratory epithelium and presumably indicates that squamous metaplasia is common. The relative incidence of malignant tumours is shown in Table 28.2.

Squamous carcinoma

Frankly invasive squamous carcinoma is usually

TABLE 28.2. Incidence of malignant tumours (modified from Ferlito)

	%
Squamous cell carcinoma	85
Carcinoma-in-situ	3
Verrucous carcinoma	3
Undifferentiated carcinoma	5
Adenocarcinoma	0·5
Miscellaneous carcinomas (adenoid cystic, spindle cell, etc.)	1·5
Sarcomas (including reticulosis)	2

moderately to well differentiated and the incidence of lymph node metastases and survival depends on this degree of differentiation. The incidence of lymph node metastases varies from 10% for well differentiated tumours to 20% for moderate differentiation to 50% for poorly differentiated tumours. The survival at 5 years also falls from 80% for well differentiated tumours to 20% for poorly differentiated tumours.

Carcinoma of the larynx may arise from the supraglottic, glottic or subglottic areas. The definition of these three areas is given in Table 28.3.

TABLE 28.3. Carcinoma of the larynx

Regions	Sites
1. Supraglottis	
Epilarynx (including marginal zone)	Posterior surface of suprahyoid epiglottis (including the tip) Aryepiglottic fold Arytenoid
Supraglottis (excluding epilarynx)	Infrahyoid epiglottis Ventricular bands (false cords) Ventricular cavities
2. Glottis	Vocal cords Anterior commissure Posterior commissure
3. Subglottis	

Approximately 90% of laryngeal carcinomas occur in men, with a peak age incidence between 55 and 65. For reasons which are not fully explained the disease is becoming commoner in women and in the earlier years of life.

Supraglottic carcinoma

The proportion of laryngeal tumours affecting the supraglottic space varies between 60% and 15% but 40% appears to be a reasonable figure for the UK and 30% for North America. For some unexplained reason the incidence is much higher in Continental Europe.

Supraglottic carcinoma is staged as shown in

Table 28.4. The commonest supraglottic carcinoma is that occurring on the infrahyoid epiglottis. These tumours nearly always (90%) invade the fenestrae in the cartilage and about 50% invade the thyroid cartilage anteriorly or along its upper lateral edge. About half of these tumours also invade the pre-epiglottic space, either by spreading through the fenestrae, or more commonly by destroying the thyro-epiglottic ligament and passing through the resulting breach into the pre-epiglottic space.

The latter space is bounded by the hyoepiglottic ligament, the epiglottis and the quadrangular membrane and the thyrohyoid ligament. It is continuous laterally with the paraglottic space. Tumours of the base of the epiglottis involve the pre-epiglottic space frequently but the paraglottic space virtually never. It is thus safe to carry out a horizontal supraglottic laryngectomy.

A small proportion, perhaps 5% or less, of these tumours extend inferiorly to invade the floor of the ventricle or the vocal cords.

Carcinoma of the lateral part of the supraglottic space, i.e. of the ventricular bands, is much less common. These tumours tend to spread superficially on the mucosal surface to the laryngeal surface of the epiglottis and to the aryepiglottic fold. More important however is spread into the paraglottic space.

This space is bounded by the thyroid ala, the conus elasticus, the quadrangular membrane and the anterior reflection of the piriform mucosa; it embraces the ventricles and saccules. Involvement of this space is inferred from radiography or clinical examination which shows oedema or swelling increasing the distance between the piriform fossa and the false cord. Radiographic reversal of the subglottic contour is due to inferior paraglottic extension of disease. Extension to this space can occur in tumours of the false cord or of the ventricle (the only mucosa embraced by this space) and in tumours of the glottis and of the medial wall of the piriform fossa. This is the cause of vocal cord fixation seen in the latter tumours.

Lymph node metastases are classified in the usual way (N0=no palpable nodes, N1=palpable nodes on one side of the neck, N2=palpable nodes on both sides of the neck and N3=fixed nodes). Lymphatic spread occurs via the superior lymphatic pedicle which accompanies the superior laryngeal artery and nerve, to the immediately adjacent upper deep cervical nodes.

The supraglottic portion of the larynx is derived from the buccopharyngeal anlage (arches III and IV), whereas the glottic and subglottic portions derive from the pulmonary anlage (arch VI). Thus each major component possesses an independent lymphatic circulation.

The incidence of lymph node metastases is shown in Table 28.5.

Glottic carcinoma

The proportion of carcinomas affecting the glottis also varies in different series, but 60% would be a reasonable estimate for North America and 50–55% for the UK. Glottic carcinoma may be divided into those small tumours which arise on one vocal cord and remain localized to it for long periods and those tumours, often called transglottic, which involve a large part of the

TABLE 28.4. TNM Classification

T – Primary tumour

Supraglottis

T1S Pre-invasive carcinomas (carcinoma-*in-situ*)
T1   Tumour limited to the region with normal mobility
       T1a Tumour confined to the laryngeal surface of the epiglottis or to an aryepiglottic fold or to a ventricular cavity or to a ventricular band
       T1b Tumour involving the epiglottis and extending to the ventricular cavities or bands
T2   Tumour of the epiglottis and/or ventricles or ventricular bands, and extending to the vocal cords, without fixation
T3   Tumour limited to the larynx with fixation and/or destruction or other evidence of deep invasion
T4   Tumour with direct extension beyond the larynx, i.e. to the piriform sinus, the postcricoid region, the vallecula or the base of the tongue

TABLE 28.5. Supraglottic carcinoma: lymph node metastases (modified from Till *et al.*)

	%
N0	65
N1	20
N2	7·5
N3	7·5

laryngeal surface crossing the vocal cord, and which are extensive when first seen. These tumours are *not* a later stage of smaller tumours but probably represent a wide field malignant degeneration.

Glottic carcinomas are classified according to the UICC as shown in Table 28.6.

It should be noted that tumours may also arise from the posterior third of the glottis, i.e. that part of the glottis lying over the vocal process. For some reason such tumours are omitted from the classification of laryngeal tumours by the UICC.

Glottic carcinomas arise on the vocal cord and spread along the cord in Reinke's space, that space immediately beneath the laryngeal epithelium, i.e. superficial to the thyroarytenoid muscle, and bounded superiorly and inferiorly by the junction of the columnar and squamous epithelium.

These tumours may spread superficially into the neighbouring supra or subglottic areas in about 10% of patients. The tumour may also spread across the anterior commissure to the

TABLE 28.6. TNM Classification

Glottis

T1S Pre-invasive carcinoma (carcinoma-*in-situ*)
T1 Tumour limited to the region with normal mobility
    T1a Tumour confined to one cord
    T1b Tumour involving both cords
T2 Tumour extending to either the subglottic or the supraglottic regions (i.e. to the ventricular bands or the ventricles) with normal or impaired mobility
T3 Tumour limited to the larynx with fixation of one or both cords
T4 Tumour extending beyond the larynx, i.e. into cartilage, the pyriform sinus, the postcricoid region or the skin

opposite cord. Invasion of the intrinsic laryngeal muscles is common, notably the thyroarytenoid muscle.

Small glottic tumours do not invade cartilage but larger ones may involve the arytenoid cartilage, or the thyroid cartilage at the anterior commissure. Once a carcinoma extends more than 1 cm inferior to the free edge of the vocal cord it may invade the cricoid cartilage.

Tumours limited to the glottis without fixation virtually never transgress the conus elasticus.

If a glottic carcinoma involves the anterior commissure and extends subglottically it is close to the cricothyroid membrane and escapes by this route early and often. This appears to be related to the close proximity of the mucosa to the thyroid ala at the anterior commissure and to the presence of the anterior commissure tendon. The latter tendon is formed by the fusion of the two vocal ligaments anteriorly to form a tendon which is inserted into the thyroid cartilage. Tumour may spread along this route to invade the anterior supraglottic, the glottic and subglottic larynx in the mid sagittal plane.

There is an anterior-inferior subglottic wedge which separates the inferior paraglottic portions of the larynx. The mucosa over this wedge lies in a coronal plane whereas the mucosa over the lateral portions lies in the sagittal plane. The superior limit of this wedge is the anterior commissure. The mucosa of this area overlies the cricothyroid membrane which is pierced by branches of the superior thyroid artery. This provides an escape route for the carcinoma and explains the grave prognosis of tumours involving this area.

The larger transglottic tumour is one which crosses the ventricle to invade two or three regions of the larynx although the tumour may have originated in the ventricle. This tumour invades the paraglottic space; it is an aggressive tumour which almost always invades the laryngeal framework and emerges from the laryngeal framework between the thyroid and cricoid cartilages at the cricothyroid membrane.

Transglottic tumours also extend posteriorly through the cricoarytenoid joint to involve the pharyngeal mucosa overlying this area, an important surgical point.

Lymph node metastases are rare in true glottic

tumours, but occur in about 30% of transglottic tumours as follows:

N0	70%
N1	20%
N2	5%
N3	5%

Distant metastases are rare, as in all forms of laryngeal carcinoma, occurring in less than 1% of patients when first seen.

Subglottic carcinoma

Subglottic carcinoma is uncommon in all published series, forming 5% or less of the total; indeed subglottic extension of a glottic carcinoma is as common as true subglottic carcinoma.

These tumours are classified as shown in Table 28.7.

True subglottic carcinoma is usually unilateral, virtually always ulcero-fungating (i.e. not exophytic as are many epiglottic carcinomas), it quickly invades the perichondrium of the thyroid and cricoid cartilages and always extends to and frequently through the cricothyroid membrane.

These tumours virtually always spread through the conus elasticus to the glottic region where the margins of the tumour tend to invade the intrinsic muscles of the true cord, producing the effect of a thickened and fixed cord, but not invading the free margin of the mucosa.

True subglottic carcinoma usually presents with stridor, as distinct from subglottic spread of a glottic tumour which usually causes hoarseness. Vocal cord fixation occurs in about 30% of both groups; 20% of true subglottic tumours have lymph node metastases, against only 5% of the group with subglottic spread.

Unusual tumours

Verrucous carcinoma

This tumour was first described in the mouth but may also involve the supraglottic area. It is a relatively non-aggressive tumour, which seldom metastasizes to the neck or generally; it is radio resistant and furthermore, radiotherapy may induce transformation to anaplastic carcinoma. It

should be treated surgically, therefore, since this form of treatment gives very good results. The characteristics of the tumour are as follows:

(1) The tumour epithelium is unusually well differentiated keratinizing squamous epithelium arranged in compressed invaginating folds.

(2) The tumour has a warty papillary surface.

(3) The clefts between adjacent papillary folds can be traced to the depths of the tumour.

TABLE 28.7. TNM Classification

Subglottis

T1S Pre-invasive carcinoma (carcinoma-*in-situ*)

T1 Tumour limited to the region with normal mobility

  T1a Tumour limited to one side of the subglottic region and not involving the undersurface of the cord.

  T1b Tumour extending to both sides of the subglottic region and not involving the undersurface of the cords

T2 Tumour involving the subglottic region and extending to one or both cords

T3 Tumour limited to the larynx with fixation of one or both cords

T4 Tumour extending beyond the larynx, i.e. into the post-cricoid region, the trachea or the skin

---

(4) The tumour infiltration is on a broad basis with pushing margins against a stroma containing a prominent inflammatory reaction.

(5) The usual cytological and infiltrating growth pattern of squamous carcinoma is absent.

Adenocarcinoma

True adenocarcinoma is a very uncommon lesion in the larynx. The tumour is confined mainly to men, is generally large on presentation and about half the patients have lymph node metastases. Distant metastases are also fairly common, and the prognosis whatever the treatment is poor.

The salivary adenocarcinomas, mainly adenoid cystic carcinoma, are probably equally as common; they behave in the same way as these tumours elsewhere.

Spindle cell carcinoma (pseudosarcoma)

This interesting tumour is polypoidal, with a

stroma of dysplastic spindle cell material (the pseudosarcomatous element) covered by a squamous cell carcinomatous component. This tumour is probably of epithelial origin and the sarcomatous element is probably an unusual proliferative response to the carcinoma.

Much the commonest site of origin is the vocal cord. About 20% of these tumours metastasize to the cervical glands; contrary to what is often said both histological elements may metastasize.

This tumour is treated surgically; it is becoming clear that the prognosis is not as good as was once thought.

Sarcomas

Although the reticuloses can occur very rarely in the larynx, the only sarcoma of any frequency is the fibrosarcoma. This is a predominantly male disease (4:1). Most of the tumours arise from the anterior part of the vocal cords, but rarely metastasize to the cervical glands.

These tumours spread by vascular routes or locally by infiltration along the local muscle and fascial planes. Different histological grades are recognized and the prognosis is strongly influenced by these grades.

Paraganglioma

Paragangliomas, or chemodectomas, of the larynx have been recorded rarely. They have nearly all arisen from the arytenoid region, recur repeatedly, ultimately metastasize widely and are characterized by the marked pain which they produce.

INVESTIGATIONS

History

Ask about hoarseness and its duration, sore throat, dysphagia, pain in the ear, difficulty in breathing, haemoptysis and loss of weight. Dysphagia and pain in the ear generally indicate that the tumour has spread to the pharynx, usually the piriform fossa by spreading over the aryepiglottic fold. It is surprising how rarely a laryngeal tumour causes haemoptysis, compared to a bronchial carcinoma.

Ask also about the general health, the patient's family and his occupation.

Examination

A routine examination of the mouth, nose and throat should be carried out, looking for sepsis and the uncommon second tumour elsewhere in the upper respiratory tract. The laryngeal tumour is noted and its extent delineated. The mobility of the vocal cords must also be determined carefully.

The neck is then examined carefully to look for enlarged lymph nodes, particularly in the upper part of the deep cervical chain. The larynx itself is examined for tenderness and widening.

A general physical examination is also carried out.

Radiology

The purpose of radiology of the larynx in tumours is to determine:

(1) The site of the lesion.
(2) The character of the lesion.
(3) The size of the lesion.
(4) The upper and lower limits of the lesion.
(5) The mobility of mobile structures: the true cords, false cords and epiglottis.
(6) The distensibility of the distensible structures: the ventricle and piriform fossa.
(7) Involvement of adjacent structures.
(8) Erosion of the cartilaginous framework.

Several radiological techniques are used to achieve the above:

Plain films.
Tomograms.
Laryngograms.
Xerograms.

Plain lateral films show the upper and lower extent of large supraglottic or subglottic tumours respectively, but are otherwise of little help in defining the limits of a tumour. But these films are helpful in showing destruction of the thyroid cartilage and in delineating the pre-epiglottic space. The thyroid cartilage calcifies in an irregular manner, but as a rule it begins to calcify at about the age of 30, beginning along its inferior and anterior border; the anterior border particularly has a characteristic figure-of-eight appearance, the vocal cord and thyroepiglottic ligaments being inserted into the waist of the figure-of-eight so that destruction of the cartilage should be looked for particularly at this point. Later the superior border of the thyroid cartilage and the cornua calcify leaving one, or more usually two, oval defects in the centre of the cartilage which should not be confused with erosion by tumour.

The maximum definition of plain films is 6–8 mm; the quality of such films is best at 150–200 kV with added filtration, for example 1 mm brass.

Tomograms give a more accurate assessment of the extent of the tumour, with a maximal definition of 3 mm.

Laryngography is a double contrast technique in which the laryngeal structures are outlined by a radio-opaque dye, double contrast being provided by the air in the larynx and pharynx. The patient is prepared with atropine to dry the throat, the throat is sprayed with local anaesthetic, and the tumour is then outlined by instilling a radio-opaque dye such as dionosil into the larynx. The larynx can then be screened for movement to show the mobility of the vocal cords, and spot films are taken in the anteroposterior and lateral plains at rest, during phonation and during the Valsalva manoeuvre. This technique should be carried out before a biopsy is done since the latter produces oedema which distorts the picture. This technique delineates laryngeal tumours accurately but is slightly tedious and time consuming to perform and should probably not be used for all patients with laryngeal carcinoma; however, it is very useful in patients for whom a partial vertical or horizontal laryngectomy is being considered to elucidate the following points:

(1) The mobility of the vocal cords (these may not be seen either because of over sensitivity of the throat or because of a large overhanging supraglottic tumour);

(2) The lower extent of an epiglottic carcinoma, particularly with reference to its relation to the anterior commissure of the vocal cords; and

(3) The superior and inferior limits of a tumour on one vocal cord when a partial vertical hemilaryngectomy is being considered.

Xerography is a relatively new technique in which conventional X-ray beams are used but the film is printed on a plate charged with selenium; the process is thus electrostatic rather than photochemical. The film which is produced is a positive rather than a negative and the main advantage of this technique is that soft tissues stand out very clearly compared to the bone. Anteroposterior films of the larynx are of little value because of the overlying cervical spine but a soft tissue mass is well shown on the lateral film provided it projects beyond the framework of the laryngeal cartilages. Erosion of the thyroid cartilages is shown better by this technique which is also extremely useful in the assessment of a patient with a stenosis of the cervical trachea. The main disadvantage of this technique is the relatively large dose of irradiation used.

The relative value of these techniques is shown in Table 28.8.

Endoscopy

An endoscopy is carried out for two reasons:

To obtain a biopsy; and

To assess the limits of the tumour so that a rational decision may be made as how best to treat the patient.

Endoscopy may be carried out either under local anaesthetic, which is preferred in the USA, or under general anaesthetic, which is preferred in the United Kingdom; neuroleptanalgesia may also be used. If the operation is to be carried out under general anaesthesia an anaesthetist interested and experienced in this technique is required. Special techniques are necessary to deliver the anaesthetic in such a way that there is still room available for the surgeon to see the larynx, since the laryngeal airway may be restricted because of the size of the tumour. Insufflation techniques, using a small tube which lies in the posterior part of the larynx and high flow rates, have generally proved to be satisfactory.

The techniques of microlaryngoscopy have been well described by Kleinsasser and have established a well deserved place in the treatment of benign laryngeal lesions such as laryngitis, vocal cord nodules, Reinke's oedema and so

TABLE 28.8 Comparative diagnostic value of three methods of laryngeal radiology

	Lateral soft tissue radiograph	Frontal tomograms	Contrast laryngograms
A. Characteristics	Static	Static	Dynamic
B. Anatomical abnormalities			
(1) Tumour mass			
(a) small lesion	−	?	+
(b) infiltrative lesion	+	+	+ +
(c) Exophytic lesion	+	+	+ +
(2) Mucosal irregularity	−	−	+
C. Functional abnormalities			
(a) Mobile structures	−	−	+
(b) Distensible structures	−	−	+
D. Specific areas			
(a) Anterior commissure	−	−	+
(h) Inferior margin of true cord	−	?	+
(c) Subglottic space	+	+	+
(d) Base of epiglottis	?	−	+
(e) Area distal to a bulky supraglottic tumour	?	−	+
(f) Pre-epiglottic space	+	−	?
(g) Thyroid cartilage	+	?	?

forth, but the value of microlaryngoscopy in assessment of a patient with laryngeal carcinoma is doubtful. Certainly many experienced laryngeal surgeons assess a laryngeal carcinoma using a laryngoscope and the naked eye.

An ordinary laryngoscope is first used to assess the extent of the tumour looking for extension of particular tumours in particular directions. In a tumour of the epiglottis it is vital to know if the tumour extends below the free edge of the false cord on to the true cords and particularly if the true cords are affected at the anterior commissure, the commonest site at which this occurs. It is also important to know whether an epiglottic tumour extends over the aryepiglottic folds into the piriform fossa or erodes through the epiglottis to involve its lingual surface.

Tumours of the false cords often invade or involve the true cords and this must also be looked for.

It is extremely important to know whether a tumour on the true vocal cord extends posteriorly on to the vocal process or anteriorly to or across the anterior commissure. Extension of such a tumour superiorly into the floor of the ventricle and inferiorly into the subglottic space is also important. Extension in these two directions, particularly the latter, is best assessed by an anterior commissure laryngoscope. Tumours of the subglottic space should be assessed to see if they involve the true vocal cords which they almost always do, but the most important point is their inferior limit, which is important in assessing whether they can be removed surgically.

After assessing the extent of the tumour a large biopsy is taken from the growing part of the tumour. Biopsies taken from the central core of the tumour may show necrotic material only, and biopsies taken from the edge of the tumour may merely show hyperplastic epithelium which will necessitate the inconvenience of a further biopsy or at worse may lull the clinician and the patient into a false sense of security. Further biopsies are also taken of suspicious areas and areas where it is important to exclude extension, such as the lingual surface of the epiglottis in carcinomas of this latter structure.

Other investigative techniques such as mediastinoscopy and transconioscopy have not been generally accepted. In the latter technique a tele-scope is passed through a cannula piercing the crico-thyroid membrane. This allows the inferior surface of the vocal cords to be seen.

TREATMENT

Ninety-five per cent of patients with laryngeal carcinoma are suitable for treatment. The contra-indications to treatment include distant metas-tases (1%), possibly very advanced age and poor general condition (although a small glottic car-cinoma may be worth treating by radiotherapy in a reasonably fit ninety-year-old), refusal by the patient, and finally very advanced disease. The chance of 5-year survival of the patient with a large tumour with a fixed vocal cord, and bila-teral or fixed glands in the neck is only 5%. It is doubtful if the extensive surgery required in such a patient is justifiable against such long odds.

Both radiotherapy and surgery are available for the treatment of the remaining tumours. Practice differs between the USA, where surgery is offered to many patients, and Europe, where most patients are treated primarily by radio-therapy. It seems that the decision in favour of one or the other is based more on local enthu-siasm than on any evidence that one form of treatment is better than another. Combined treatment – that is, a course of radiotherapy of varying dosage followed by surgery – has given very good results in the hands of a few, but is not widely used and indeed recent careful controlled trials have shown that preoperative radiotherapy does not increase the survival in head and neck cancer, but does increase the complication rate.

The most important factor in deciding treat-ment is the presence of enlarged nodes in the neck; these usually indicate that the patient should be treated primarily by surgery. With this in mind the various sites will now be discussed with a suggestion of what should be done at each site.

Supraglottis

For the patient with a reasonably small tumour with no nodes in the neck (T1a and T1b, T2), the results of radiotherapy are as good as those of surgery. If the patient has a gland in the neck (N1 or N2) surgery should be advised. For tumour limited to the epiglottis or the aryepiglottic fold (T1a or T1b, N1 or N2) it is unnecessary to sacrifice the whole larynx and a supraglottic laryngectomy should be advised provided the patient is young (say below 65) and fit, and in particular does not suffer from chronic chest disease.

Larger tumours (T2 and T3) with nodes in the neck should be treated by a total laryngectomy and radical neck dissection; recurrences after radiotherapy should also be treated by total laryngectomy–supraglottic laryngectomy should not be carried out in a patient who has been irradiated. The largest tumours of all, particu-larly when associated with bilateral or fixed glands, are seldom cured and it is doubtful if surgery is justified.

Glottis

Small tumours (T1a and T1b) should be treated by radiotherapy, if a good radiotherapy service is available. Primary surgery, using one of the forms of partial vertical hemilaryngectomy such as the lateral or fronto-lateral techniques, or by cordectomy, gives results which are no better than standard radiotherapy and should only be advised where good radiotherapy is not avail-able. Recurrence of such a tumour after radio-therapy can be treated by a vertical hemilaryn-gectomy provided that the cord remains mobile, there is no supraglottic spread, there is not more than 10 mm of subglottic spread below the free edge of the vocal cord and there is no appreciable spread across the anterior commissure or into the vocal process; perhaps most important of all the surgeon must have seen the patient before he was irradiated and know that these criteria applied before the radiotherapy.

Larger, T2, tumours with supra or subglottic spread are treated by radiotherapy if no glands are present. Recurrence is more likely, so that careful follow-up is needed, and a total laryngec-tomy should be carried out if the tumour recurs.

Fixation of the vocal cord is classified as a T3 lesion, but there are in fact two types of glottic tumour with a fixed cord: The small tumour confined to the vocal cord which is fixed, and the large tumour affecting two or three of the regions of the larynx (transglottic tumour) with a fixed cord. The former should be treated by radiotherapy and careful follow-up, and the latter by total laryngectomy.

This is a suitable place to discuss the management of the patient who presents with stridor. This is usually caused by a large transglottic growth, but is also the commonest presenting symptom of a subglottic carcinoma which is uncommon of whatever size. If a tracheostomy is done and the patient is later treated by radiotherapy or by surgery, with or without excision of the track of the tracheostomy, one patient in four will die of a soft tissue recurrence around the stoma. The best treatment therefore is 'emergency' laryngectomy usually carried out within 24 hours of presentation. This operation usually passes surprisingly without incident: It is easy to persuade the patient that his larynx is now not only valueless but indeed a threat to his life, and the post-operative course is often surprisingly smooth.

Subglottis

A true subglottic carcinoma presents most commonly with stridor which is the commonest symptom in two patients out of three with this disease. Because the disease is so uncommon it is difficult to know what is best to advise for the patient. Certainly if the patient does not require a tracheostomy because of stridor, and does not have enlarged lymph glands in the neck (which only occur in 20% of patients) all the evidence is that the chance of survival by radiotherapy is at least as good as that by surgery with the added advantage that the patient keeps his voice. Surgery on the other hand should be advised for a patient with enlarged glands in the neck, and also of course for a tumour which recurs after radiotherapy. If the patient presents with stridor probably the best treatment is emergency laryngectomy, because of the danger of recurrence in the track of a tracheostomy, as explained above, but this matter is not proven at this time. The value of pre-operative radiotherapy in this disease is also unknown; additional techniques such as mediastinal dissection after resection or all or part of the manubrium and infraglottic partial laryngectomy have not been generally accepted.

After care and follow-up

Patients who have been treated for laryngeal carcinoma either by radiotherapy or by surgery must be followed up:

(1) To detect a recurrence of the tumour within the larynx or in the lymph glands of the neck.

(2) To detect any complications of treatment such as perichondritis after radiotherapy, inhalation after partial laryngectomy or stricture of the pharynx after total laryngectomy.

Recurrences after radiotherapy are treated by total laryngectomy for a recurrence within the larynx or by radical neck dissection for a recurrence in the glands. The sole exception to this is that a carcinoma confined to one vocal cord which remains mobile can be treated by vertical hemilaryngectomy, provided that the tumour was confined to these limits before it was treated by radiotherapy, and that the surgeon who is to carry out the operation saw the patient himself before the patient was treated by radiotherapy.

Perichondritis can be divided clinically into two forms, those with foetor and those without. Patients without foetor are usually found to have oedema of the larynx, which will settle with steroids and rest of the larynx, and tracheostomy if necessary. More severe cases in which there is foetor, pain referred to the ear and difficulty in swallowing will be found not only to have oedema but also ulceration of the larynx and in addition to inflammation of the cartilaginous structures of the larynx are also usually found to have a recurrence of the carcinoma which may well be bound up in fibrous tissue and be difficult to prove by biopsy. These patients should usually be treated by laryngectomy in which the pharynx is closed but the skin wound is left widely open and is only closed by a secondary suture when the infection has been controlled.

A fairly high proportion (20%) of patients who have undergone supraglottic laryngectomy later develop *recurrent chest infections*, some of which are accompanied with permanent radiological changes in the lungs. These complications should be watched for and treated appropriately.

Strictures of the pharynx should be very uncommon after total laryngectomy; they are treated by oesophagoscopy and dilation.

Recurrences after surgery are generally untreatable although a few may respond to radiotherapy, and for a time, with relief of pain, to the newer kinetic regimes of chemotherapy.

A very important part of the rehabilitation of a patient after total laryngectomy is the *restoration of his voice*. This may be done by teaching the patient oesophageal speech or by various artificial devices.

Oesophageal speech is much the best method of laryngeal speech since the patient can use it at all times and no artificial devices which must be carried are needed. Although the voice achieved by this method can be very good it is naturally never as good as the normal voice and many women dislike it because it sounds gruff and masculine. However, many men who need their voice for their work have returned to work by the use of this method. The principles of oesophageal speech are that air is passed into the oesophagus either by swallowing or by pressing with the tongue and is then regurgitated so that it causes the cricopharyngeus or other pharyngeal structures to vibrate producing a sound which is modulated by the articulating mechanism in the usual way. It is thought that a development of good oesophageal voice depends on the following factors: sex, age (elderly patients sometimes do not bother to develop this type of voice), motivation, intelligence, local factors in the pharynx such as scarring, the formation of diverticulae and the shape of the pharynx (a wide pharynx is thought to be necessary) and the condition of the oesophagus (if the patient has a hiatus hernia he may find it difficult to control the air stream in the oesophagus). It is difficult to assess how many patients develop satisfactory oesophageal voice, and although more than 90% may do so if given intensive treatment this is not the usual figure. Certainly very good results can be obtained by keeping the patient in hospital until he has developed satisfactory speech and giving him lessons two or three times a day; this system is used in the Netherlands with extremely good results, but in countries with limited facilities, particularly in the UK where this is not possible, the results are not nearly so good and probably not more than half develop really satisfactory speech. For other patients various artificial devices are available; these can be divided basically into two types: various external machines which produce a sound which the patient can then modify by articulation, and various artificial devices to provide a tracheopharyngeal fistula to conduct air from the trachea into the pharynx where vibrations are set up as in oesophageal speech.

The various artificial devices which produce sound include the Cooper–Rand electronic speech aid, the Servox transcervical vibrator, the Tait oral vibrator mounted on a dental plate, and the Bart's vibrator. Most of these devices consist of a machine held to the patient's throat which produces a buzzing sound. The theory is that the patient then modifies the sound by articulation to produce intelligible speech; in practice the noise produced is monotonous, metallic and often scarcely intelligible.

The alternative is some form of tracheopharyngeal fistula to allow air to be passed from the trachea into the pharynx to produce vibration. The main problem of this method is the leakage of secretions and food into the trachea, and maintenance of the fistula. Various valvular devices have been developed, e.g. the Taub Voice-Bak prosthesis, which are designed to overcome these difficulties.

Further reading

The original sources for this chapter can be found in the following monographs:

ALBERTI P. W. & BRYCE D. P. (1976) *Centennial Conference on Laryngeal Cancer.* New York: Appleton-Century-Crofts.

EDWARDS N. (1976) The artificial larynx. *British Journal of Hospital Medicine* 16, 145.

FERLITO H. (1976) Histological classification of larynx and hypopharynx cancers. *Acta Otolaryngologica* Supplement 342.

KLEINSASSER O. (1968) *Microlaryngoscopy and Endolaryngeal Microsurgery. Techniques and Typical Cases.* Philadelphia: Saunders & Co.

OLOFSSON J. & NOSTRAND A. W. P. (1973) Growth and spread of laryngeal and hypopharyngeal carcinoma. *Acta Otolaryngologica* Supplement 308.

TILL J. E., BRUCE W. E., ELWAN A., TILL M. J., NIEDERER J., REID J., HAWKINS N. V, & RIDER W. D. (1975) A preliminary analysis of end results for cancer of the larynx. *Laryngoscope* 85, 259.

CHAPTER 29

Laryngeal Trauma and Stenosis

LARYNGEAL FRACTURES

Surgical anatomy

The mandible protects the larynx against direct frontal injury except when the head is extended. Crushing injuries to the larynx force it against the cervical spine and fracture the cricoid and thyroid cartilages. These cartilages resist fracture but when displacement occurs severe injury to the laryngeal structures will result. Significant disruption of function may result from acute injury or from extensive scarring of the larynx.

The thyroid alae fused together anteriorly serve as an elastic spring to maintain the posture of the vocal cord [1] (Fig. 29.1). The elasticity of the thyroid cartilage decreases later in life as it calcifies and thus it may more readily fracture. This elasticity also allows for an inward bending and elastic recoil from a direct blow which may cause other injuries in the absence of cartilagenous fracture such as dislocation of the arytenoid accompanied by extensive laceration of the vocal cord. Fracture of the thyroid alae with displacement disturbs laryngeal function disproportionately to the extent of the fracture itself. Loss of the spring action of the intact alae causes shortening of the vocal cords, loss of their tension and weakening of the voice.

The glottis and supraglottis are frequently damaged by direct force to the neck resulting in thyroid cartilage fracture. The subglottis is surrounded by the cricoid ring (Fig. 29.2) which is very strong and is much less often fractured. The common injury of the subglottis is cricotracheal separation with associated fracture of the anterior crura of the cricoid cartilage which will produce significant stricture if untreated. The recurrent laryngeal nerves may be injured by the tearing force of cricotracheal separation or by

dislocation posteriorly of the inferior cornu of the thyroid cartilage.

Less commonly, fractures of the posterior plate of the cricoid cartilage occur, often in company with other injuries. Such fracture may displace the cricoarytenoid articulation intact and interrupt normal vocal cord movement. In other cases, perichondritis and chondritis may result producing intraluminal granulations and later scar tissue. Scarring may reduce the glottic or subglottic lumen or bind the arytenoid cartilages so that the vocal cords are immobilized in the midline.

Diagnosis of laryngeal injury

A laryngeal injury must be diagnosed in the acute phase. The patient with injury to the larynx will usually be seen in the emergency room and will also have multiple injuries to other systems. Laryngeal fractures are often associated with multiple facial fractures, head injuries, fractures of the cervical spine and crush injuries to the chest. The patient may be unconscious and, as a result, may have already had a tracheotomy.

The management of life-threatening injuries must take precedence but, when the type of injury that the patient has received is likely to have damaged the larynx, a healthy suspicion of laryngeal injury must be maintained until a proper examination can be made.

The absolute indications for open reduction of the larynx at the appropriate time are an external laryngeal deformity or the presence of loose cartilaginous fragments in the lumen of the pharynx, or larynx. Stridor, haemorrhage, subcutaneous emphysema and lacerations of the pharynx suggest the need for exploration, but conservative therapy may successfully manage

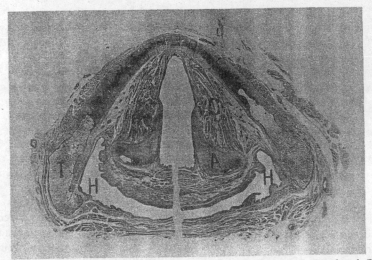

FIG. 29.1. A horizontal whole-organ section of the larynx at the level of the vocal cord. The vocal cords (VC) insert into the thyroid alae at the anterior commissure. The thyroid alae (T) relate closely to the arytenoids (A) and hypopharynx (H).

such complications with preservation of the laryngeal function.

When the appropriate indications are present, laryngeal displacement should be managed by exploration and reconstitution of the fractured cartilaginous segments about an indwelling stent (Fig. 29.3). It may be necessary to delay the appropriate repair for 1–2 weeks to allow for the management of the more demanding acute and life-threatening injuries.

The diagnosis and management of individual injuries will now be considered.

The diagnosis of acute laryngeal injury in the presence of an open wound where the injury is obvious is not difficult. As soon as local infection can be controlled and if other conditions allow, the wound should be thoroughly explored, debrided and the structure of the larynx reconstituted about an indwelling stent.

The diagnosis of chronic laryngeal scarring is

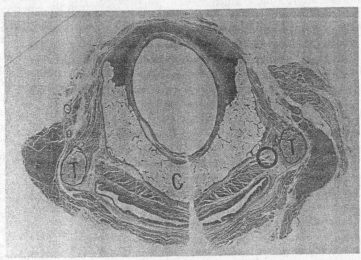

FIG. 29.2. A whole-organ section of the larynx at the level of the cricoid cartilage. Note the circular complete cartilaginous and bony ring of the cricoid (C) and the relationship of the recurrent laryngeal nerve (circled) to the cricoid and the thyroid cartilages (T).

made as the symptoms of stridor and hoarseness bring the patient to seek aid from his physician. Indirect laryngoscopy, laryngeal and tracheal tomography with or without contrast media are essential to determine the extent and site of the stenosis so that proper management can be planned. Early diagnosis of laryngeal injury is essential if the late results of scarring and stenosis are to be avoided.

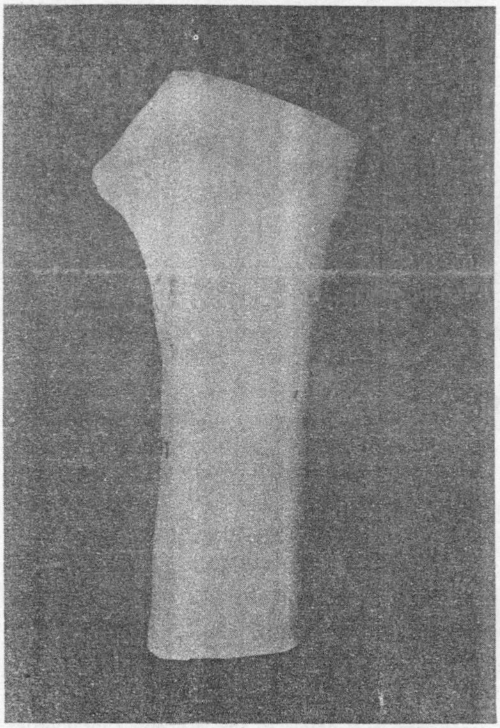

Laryngeal fractures are classified into four types:

(1) Supraglottic fractures.
(2) Glottic fractures.
(3) Cricotracheal separation.
(4) Combined comminuted fractures.

Supraglottic fractures

Pathology

Supraglottic fractures result from a force directed posterosuperiorly acting against the mid portion of the thyroid alae. If a sagittal section of the human larynx is examined (Fig. 29.4) a relatively weak point is noted at the junction of the laryngeal ventricles anteriorly just superior to the attachment of the vocal cords to the thyroid alae. Fracture at this point may be minor or major. In

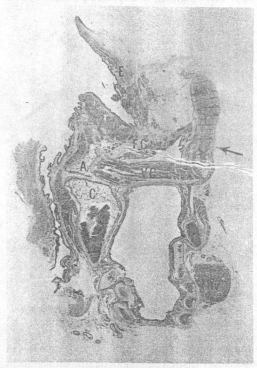

Fig. 29.3. A cadaver-moulded Silastic laryngeal stent ideally suited for the support and shaping of laryngeal displacements.

Fig. 29.4. A whole-organ sagittal section of the larynx to demonstrate the area of weakness at the site of the arrow, which coincides with the type of fracture seen in supraglottic laryngeal fractures.

both cases, the superior fragment is displaced superiorly and posteriorly (Fig. 29.5).

In extreme cases, there is complete posterior displacement of the supraglottic structures completely obstructing the airway. In minor injuries, this displacement will be slight and its recognition may be difficult.

Diagnosis

The diagnosis of supraglottic laryngeal fracture is made on suspicion of such an injury when the force acting on the neck is an appropriate one. In men the prominence of the thyroid alae or 'Adam's apple' can be clearly seen; flattening of this anatomical landmark is then diagnostic of the injury.

In women the diagnosis is not so obvious. When the fracture and displacement is extreme, the diagnosis can be made by indirect laryngoscopy. The epiglottis is displaced posteriorly and

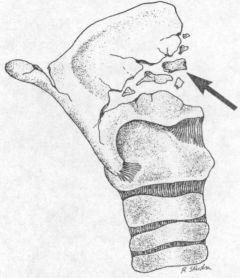

FIG. 29.5. Supraglottic fracture and displacement. The force acting in the direction of the arrow displaces the supraglottic structures posteriorly and superiorly.

superiorly when the tongue is depressed. The posteriorly displaced epiglottis and supraglottic structures lie over the vocal cords which cannot be seen. Respiratory obstruction may result.

In the minor conditions displacement of the epiglottis may be recognized only by direct laryngoscopy. Even so, the diagnosis may not be easy as the blade of the laryngoscope lifts the epiglottis forward out of the way as the anterior commissure is exposed. But if the laryngoscope is not advanced into the larynx completely, this posterior displacement can be readily recognized. In major displacements, there is tearing and bleeding from the displaced supraglottic structures; later scarring reduces the antero–posterior diameter of the airway at the supraglottic level.

Lateral tomography and xerography are very useful in identifying posterior displacement of the supraglottic structures.

Treatment

Exploration of the supraglottic fracture in the acute phase reveals the visor-like deformity of the fracture (Fig. 29.6). This may be closed by displacing the superior segment inferiorly and

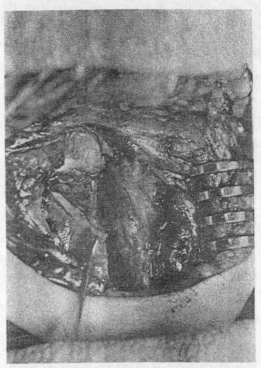

FIG. 29.6. In this operative picture, the skin hook at the vocal cord level points to the visor-like supraglottic displacement of the fractured thyroid ala.

anteriorly, and resuturing it to the inferior segment of the thyroid ala. A stent must be inserted during the initial post-operative period to hold the superiorly displaced supraglottis in place.

If the displacement is a major one and there is difficulty in reconstituting the supraglottis in its proper position, a lateral pharyngotomy should be done and the displaced supraglottic structures removed as in a modified supraglottic laryngectomy. As this is a benign condition, only displaced structures need to be removed and the operation need not be as extensive as that for carcinoma.

In the chronic condition, replacement of the posteriorly displaced laryngeal fragments is very difficult because of scarring. These patients should be treated by supraglottic laryngectomy. Sometimes posterior displacement of the epiglottis is so slight that diagnosis is difficult until the larynx is exposed by lateral pharyngotomy. Removal of the epiglottis itself may be sufficient in minor chronic conditions, but in extensive ones removal of the aryepiglottic fold will also be required.

Supraglottic laryngectomy for major displacement of the supraglottic structures is a remarkably effective procedure and does not produce difficulties in swallowing. When a supraglottic laryngectomy is done for a benign condition, there is also an abundance of pyriform sinus mucous membrane to cover the remaining denuded areas.

Lateral glottic fractures

Pathology

Lateral glottic fracture is the commonest injury resulting from direct trauma; the fracture is vertical and the posterior vertical segment of the thyroid ala on the side involved is displaced posteriorly and medially (Fig. 29.7). This results in a characteristic step deformity which can be palpated externally. In some patients the lateral thyroid ala is not fractured but is merely severely sprung medially and posteriorly. The same soft tissue injury may result.

Diagnosis

Laryngoscopy shows tearing of the fibres of the vocal cord and often dislocation of the arytenoid on the involved side; the arytenoid may be denuded of its epithelium. The displacement of the arytenoid may result from dislocation of the cricoarytenoid joint, or from fracture of the cricoid cartilage with displacement of the fractured portion carrying the arytenoid with it.

Free cartilage is not commonly seen in the airway in this type of fracture and diagnosis may be difficult. Minor degrees of this fracture are often missed and only later does the scarred immobile cord draw the attention of the laryngologist to the injury. Because of the lack of the

spring action of the thyroid ala, on the fractured side, there may also be a reduction in the airway so that mild stridor may be one of the presenting symptoms. Radiology is not as helpful in lateral as in supraglottic fractures.

Treatment

In the acute stage when the diagnosis can be made by external palpation or laryngoscopy

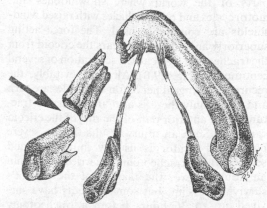

FIG. 29.7. Lateral glottic fracture. The force acting in the direction of the arrow displaces or fractures the thyroid ala which results in damage to the glottis and arytenoid.

open reduction is indicated to wire the posterior segment of the thyroid ala back in place. In the chronic state, replacement of the fractured thyroid cartilage is very difficult or impossible.

It may not be possible to correct the injury to the vocal cord. The tears in the vocal cord itself and the injury to the recurrent nerve are probably irreversible with resulting cord fixation. If the arytenoid has been grossly displaced it should be removed. The displaced arytenoid may prevent approximation of the vocal cords and cause hoarseness; its removal may then result in a satisfactory improvement of the voice.

In severe lateral glottic fractures where the airway is embarrassed, and in the chronic state where replacement of the fragment is not possible, a modified form of vertical hemilaryngectomy should be done. The displaced, scarred vocal cord and cartilage are removed. Such a procedure is necessary to obtain an adequate airway although the voice will not be normal thereafter. Methods to improve the voice after such an injury by injection of Teflon to the vocal cord or by augmenting it with muscle or cartilaginous grafts are not usually successful because of the inevitable scarring in the glottic region.

Cricotracheal separation

Pathology

This injury is becoming more common in those parts of the world where snowmobiles and motorcycles and other vehicles with raised windshields are commonly used. The force acting superiorly and posteriorly tears the cricoid from the trachea and may cause a separation of several centimetres (Fig. 29.8). Almost inevitably, the recurrent laryngeal nerves on both sides are torn and commonly there is also an associated fracture of the anterior part of the ring of the cricoid cartilage. Such an injury results from a severe blow, and stridor is usually immediate and severe. Unless tracheotomy is carried out within an hour or two, the chances of the patient's survival are slim, but some patients have survived up to 36 hours before a tracheotomy became imperative.

Diagnosis

The diagnosis is usually made by the surgeon who carries out the tracheotomy into the open distal segment of the trachea.

If diagnosis is not made at the time of tracheotomy, difficulty with extubation leads to direct laryngoscopy where a loss of continuity between the trachea and the subglottis will be noted. Tomography demonstrates the gap between the trachea and the cricoid ring (Fig. 29.9). The type of injury and the history of the stridor are helpful in reaching a proper diagnosis.

Ultimately, if extubation is impossible and the diagnosis is otherwise confused, exploration provides the correct diagnosis.

Treatment

The trachea must be sutured back to the cricoid cartilage as early as possible. In the acute phase, an indwelling prosthesis is not necessary. If a

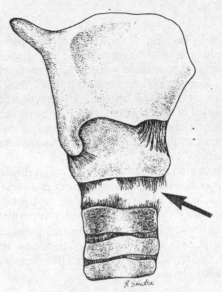

FIG. 29.8. Cricotracheal separation. This is the only common traumatic injury to the trachea. The trachea is torn from the cricoid cartilage and is displaced inferiorly. Often there is associated cricoid cartilage fracture.

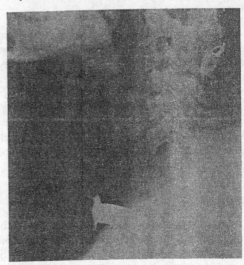

FIG. 29.9. A lateral tomogram of larynx and trachea demonstrating a complete subglottic stenosis and a distal displacement of the trachea into the superior mediastinum.

prosthesis is used to strengthen the suture line, it may be removed in 3 weeks if there is no infection.

In the chronic state, where the trachea and the cricoid cartilage have been allowed to heal in the separated position, management is much more difficult. The trachea has retracted into the superior mediastinum from which it must be freed to approximate it to the larynx. There is also a complete stricture of the subglottis usually with fracture of the cricoid cartilage at the laryngeal level.

At surgical exploration, the trachea is found in the mediastinum and tracheotomy will complicate the freeing up of the tracheal segment. The trachea should be approached distal to the thyroid gland so that the normal plane surrounding the trachea in the superior mediastinum can be identified and dissected proximally, and the tracheal remnants be identified and freed from surrounding scar. The blood supply of the trachea will be affected if too much of the tracheal wall needs to be mobilized to approximate it to the larynx. The trachea should be dissected until two or three intact and viable rings are identified. Further separation will probably result in ischaemic necrosis of the proximal segment of the freed trachea.

The degree of the stenosis of the larynx is determined. The recurrent laryngeal nerves are certainly damaged so that they need not be avoided. It will probably be necessary to excise the anterior ring of the cricoid cartilage and a portion of the posterior plate in order to reach a level above the scarred and stenosed mucous membrane. A laryngeal drop should then be done so that the greater part of the gap between the trachea in the superior mediastinum and the subglottis is closed by this method rather than by elevating the trachea. Anastomosis can then be carried out by suturing the thyroid alae anteriorly and the posterior ring of the cricoid posteriorly to the first tracheal ring. It is wise to insert an indwelling stent for about 5 or 6 weeks. This supports the suture line and the lumen which is otherwise uneven. During this period, a distal tracheotomy must be maintained.

Complications

There are two complications of this type of injury:

(1) The recurrent laryngeal nerve is severed and the paralysed vocal cords cause respiratory obstruction.

(2) Associated tears in the anterior wall of the oesophagus with a tracheo-oesophageal fistula.

The vocal cords may lie in the median position or may be sufficiently abducted to allow respiration and a reasonable voice. It is unwise to correct the position of the vocal cords either by injection or by lateralization until about 6 months after the injury as their relative positions may change over this period of time.

Rupture of the anterior wall of the oesophagus is a commonly associated injury when the trachea is separated from the cricoid cartilage. This complication is very serious as aspiration through the fistula is incompatible with life. The diagnosis of such a fistula is usually not difficult as the patient aspirates and coughs up food. If there is any doubt, a thin barium swallow readily demonstrates the fistula.

The management of this complication is the same in the acute or chronic state. The trachea must be separated from the oesophagus and the fistula identified. The wall of the oesophagus can then be repaired; the repair must be supported by a rotated muscle graft using the sternothyroid muscles if they are available. These can be sutured anterior to the oesophageal wall over the fistula and then the trachea is brought superiorly and anastomosed to the cricoid cartilage anterior to the rotated muscle graft. A laryngeal drop reduces strain on the oesophageal wall and assists healing. It is also wise to support this repair by an indwelling laryngeal stent left in place for the usual length of time.

Combined comminuted fractures

Pathology

In this type of laryngeal fracture, there is fragmentation both of the thyroid alae and the anterior ring of the cricoid cartilage to varying degrees (Fig. 29.10).

Diagnosis

The diagnosis is not difficult as the fracture is often compound and the force has obviously been great. There is external deformity of the laryngeal framework and disruption of the laryngeal structure so that stridor is a very early and

urgent symptom. There are usually also associated lacerations of the pharynx, and dysphagia.
Combined comminuted fracture is frequently
associated with other severe head injuries or fractures; primary repair must often be delayed until
these emergencies have been managed.

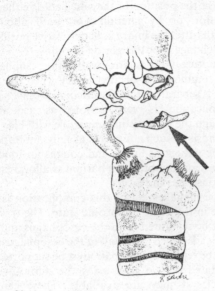

FIG. 29.10. Combined frontal comminuted fracture.
There are multiple fractures with displacement of the
larynx and cricoid cartilage. The trachea is often displaced from the cricoid cartilage.

Treatment

In the acute phase, open exploration of the
larynx and the cervical trachea is essential. There
will usually be major comminution of the cartilaginous fragments and it may not be possible to
reconstruct the larynx primarily. But if sufficient
fragments are available, they should be carefully
replaced about an indwelling laryngeal stent
which must extend from the tracheotomy below
to above the level of the glottis. The stent is left in
for at least 6 weeks. When the stent is removed 6
weeks after operation the state of the repair must
be assessed, to determine whether an adequate
airway has been obtained.

In the chronic state, there may be complete
stenosis of the laryngeal lumen and, in severe
cases no glottic structures will be identifiable.
The stenosis may be extensive and may involve

several tracheal rings. A wide exposure and complete exploration of the stenosis is indicated.
Sometimes it may be possible to reconstruct
the fragmented and distorted cartilage, excise
the scar and either anastomose the larynx to the
trachea, after removing the scarred area, or
reconstitute the cartilage about an indwelling
stent.

In severe cases, the extent of the destruction of
the larynx and cervical trachea may make excision of the scar with direct anastomosis impossible. The only alternatives are then a permanent
tracheotomy or reconstruction of the trachea
using isografts.

Reconstruction of the trachea and laryngeal
structures to provide an adequate lumen is a
long, complicated and extremely difficult procedure which is not often successful. A great
number of prosthetic materials have been used
for reconstruction but the only universally successful material is isogenic tissue, either bone
cartilage or skin. A combination of skin flaps
with a plastic material has been used successfully
as a composite graft [2].

The principle of the operation is to form a
trough connecting the trachea below with the
larynx and pharynx above, and to build up the
lateral walls of the trough to obtain an adequate
anterior posterior diameter, and then to close the
trough with a lid which will not collapse with
respiration [3].

LARYNGEAL STENOSIS

Pathology

Injury to the laryngeal glottis and supraglottis
from indwelling endotracheal tubes and cuffs
(Fig. 29.11) is not common but the subglottic
area is often injured. The sites of injury are
shown in Figs. 29.12 and 29.13.

Shortly after the development of the respiratory failure unit and the universal use of positive
pressure respiration, it became apparent that significant and very serious damage to the larynx
and trachea was often produced by the therapeutic methods used. The size of tube inserted
through the larynx into the trachea, the amount
of cuff pressure used, and the movement of the

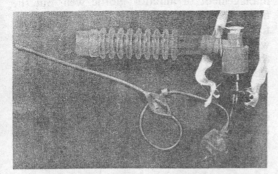

FIG. 29.11. Cuffed inflatable tracheotomy tube with connector to the respirator.

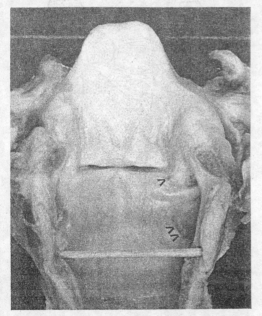

FIG. 29.12. Ischaemic necrosis of subglottis. The larynx is opened from its posterior aspect to illustrate ulceration overlying the arytenoid (arrow) and separate ulceration overlying the cricoid posteriorly (double arrow). The ulceration illustrated is typical of that produced by an endotracheal tube in that all of the areas of ulceration occur posteriorly. Ulceration secondary to the cuff pulled up into the subglottic region would be circumferential in distribution.

tube because of its attachment to the respirator, were the significant factors causing damage. Correction of these over the past few years has reduced the numbers of severe injury. Such injuries have not been completely eradicated because of unavoidable problems associated with the management of these very sick patients. Very often the patients are extremely debilitated and are hypotensive or have periods of hypotension during their treatment. Moreover, high levels of cuff pressure may, at times, be necessary in order to ventilate the lungs adequately.

The major efforts to prevent injury to the larynx and trachea have been in the development of specially designed cuffs which prevent ischaemic necrosis of the mucosa of the tracheal wall. These cuffs are flabby and need only be inflated to very low pressures. Better attachments from the tube to the respirator have been developed to prevent movement from being transmitted to the larynx or trachea. Early tracheotomy to replace endotracheal tubes has resulted in reduction in the number of subglottic stenoses. Better techniques for the surgical formation of the tracheostome have prevented stenosis at this level. Constant attention to the problem of possible laryngeal and tracheal damage has also reduced these injuries. The management of infection, care with suction through the tracheotomy and endotracheal tubes and careful regulation of the inflation of the cuff have all played their part in the recent reduction of laryngo-tracheal injury.

Diagnosis

Injury to the mucosa of the larynx or trachea as a result of an indwelling endotracheal tube with or without an inflated cuff must be identified early. Diagnosis requires a routine examination of the larynx and the subglottic region of all patients at risk at the time of extubation and later at regular intervals for 8–12 months. Only in this way will the diagnosis be made promptly and the extent of the scarring be accurately identified.

Management

Supraglottis

The supraglottis is rarely significantly damaged by endotracheal tubes but abrasion of the mucosa with ulceration may sometimes cause granulomas involving the false cords and the aryepiglottic folds. These granulomas may be removed but if left untreated they often become pedunculated and may disappear or be coughed up.

Glottis

The glottis may be damaged by indwelling endotracheal tubes with or without cuffs. Three clinical entities are seen.

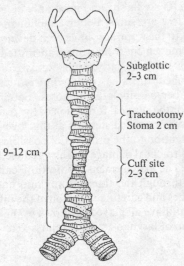

Intubation with P.P.R.

- Subglottic 2–3 cm
- Tracheotomy Stoma 2 cm

9–12 cm

- Cuff site 2–3 cm

FIG. 29.13. The three sites of laryngotracheal injury and stricture are demonstrated diagrammatically. In each case the length of stricture usually encountered is noted. A combination of any two of these areas of stricture will represent a maximum amount of trachea to be excised so that primary anastomosis can be carried out.

Anterior glottic web

An anterior glottic web may result from injury to the anterior commissure in which the mucous membrane of both vocal cords is damaged and the commissure is denuded. This lesion is also seen as a result of a fracture of the thyroid alae involving the anterior commissure. The anterior glottic web may be slight and can be ignored, or may be severe and extend sufficiently far posteriorly to cause respiratory difficulty (Fig. 29.14).

Treatment

Various methods have been devised for the management of anterior glottic web, but the most successful is an anterior laryngeal keel interposed between the two vocal cords after the web has been incised. The keel is fastened to the thyroid alae externally and is left in place for 4–6 weeks. This method of correction is almost always successful. The web is usually of considerable depth so that the function of the vocal cords is interfered with and the voice rarely returns to its previous quality.

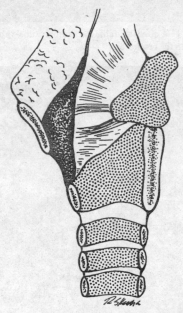

FIG. 29.14. A sagittal diagram to demonstrate the distribution of the usual anterior commissure web. Note the extent of the scarring.

Posterior glottic web

A posterior glottic web results from ulceration produced by an endotracheal tube lying posteriorly in the larynx (Fig. 29.15). The resulting scar contracts and eventually prevents free movement of the arytenoids so that the cords become fixed in the midline (Fig. 29.16). This type of web is difficult to see indirectly or even directly, unless the clinician suspects it. Rarely the web is a band uniting the tips of the vocal processes of the arytenoids with intact mucous membrane posteriorly extending into the subglottis.

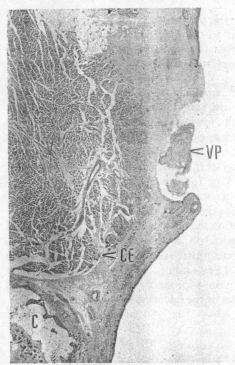

FIG. 29.15. Ulceration of the arytenoid. Coronal section of an intubated larynx taken at the level of the vocal process of the arytenoid. The photomicrograph illustrates marked necrosis of the mucosa and submucosal tissues surrounding the vocal process (VP) which now appears as a dead sequestrum of cartilage. The underlying vocalis muscle (V) is unaffected by the process. The conus elasticus (CE) and the upper margin of the cricoid cartilage (C) are clearly shown. H & E ×15.

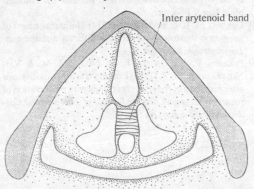

FIG. 29.16. Bilateral ulceration with loss of mucosa into the posterior commissure or between the two arytenoids may result in a posterior glottic web which ultimately fixes both cords to the extent of producing significant airway obstruction.

Treatment

Management of the posterior laryngeal scar is difficult. It may be excised and an indwelling laryngeal stent left in place for several weeks, but the scarring frequently recurs sufficiently to immobilize the cords. Exploring the larynx through a thyrotomy is more effective. The scar is excised making sure that the arytenoids are not damaged and the subsequent denuded area is covered by a mucous membrane rotation flap from the hypopharynx [4]. An indwelling laryngeal stent is then necessary to ensure healing of the rotation flap and to prevent recurrence of scar.

Arytenoid dislocation

Arytenoid dislocation is not usually caused by the tube itself, but very often damage and dislocation may occur by the improper insertion of the tube.

The diagnosis is not difficult as the displaced arytenoid can be seen by indirect examination.

Treatment

The dislocated arytenoid is removed endoscopically or by thyrotomy. This immobilizes one vocal cord which should be fixed in the midline so that the quality of the voice is not impaired.

Subglottis

Pathology

The subglottis is involved in a third of all cases of damage to the trachea and larynx as a result of indwelling endotracheal tubes. It is particularly prone to injury because of the rigidity of its walls. The degree of injury may vary from slight localized mucosal necrosis and scarring without limitation of laryngeal movement or interference with respiration, to complete circumferential ischaemic necrosis of the mucous membrane and cartilage of the cricoid ring with subsequent complete stenosis and fixation of the vocal cords.

Diagnosis

Unless suspicion of such an injury has resulted in routine examinations of the subglottis following extubation, the diagnosis of this injury is usually delayed until stridor develops. Direct laryngoscopy reveals a circumferential subglottic stenosis. If injury to the cricoid ring is diagnosed early after extubation, prevention of subsequent stenosis may be possible by skin grafting supported by an indwelling laryngeal stent.

The extent of a significant subglottic stenosis must be determined to plan appropriate management. Direct and indirect laryngoscopy, laryngeal tomography and laryngography determine the position of the stenosis in relation to the vocal cords and to the trachea. Despite all the diagnostic methods available accurate delineation of the site of the stenosis is not easy and very often will not be obtained without exploration.

Treatment

The affected area is excised and a direct anastomosis of the trachea to the subglottic structures is done.

In minor cases, where the scarring is neither lengthy nor completely circumferential, excision of the scar and skin grafting supported by an indwelling stent may be sufficient, or a keel may be used to break the circumferential scar and provide sufficient airway.

When the scarring is extensive and involves the circumference of the subglottis and perhaps also the first ring or two of the trachea, excision and anastomosis is the method of choice [5]. If the subglottic stenosis is secondary to the use of an indwelling tube with a cuff, the recurrent laryngeal nerves are not likely to be damaged and must be identified and preserved. Once the nerves have been identified the scarred areas of the cricoid and trachea can be removed and direct anastomosis achieved.

The subglottic scarring may be proximal to the cricoid-thyroid joint which is usually considered to be the upper limit of excision. Under these circumstances, it may be possible to core out the posterior plate of the cricoid cartilage and thus allow the trachea to be brought up proximally almost to the level of the vocal cords without disturbing the cricoid joints or the recurrent laryngeal nerves [6].

Complications

The most common complication of the anastomosis following excision of a subglottic stenosis is restenosis of the suture line. This may occur up to 1 or 2 years; its management depends on its severity. If the patient can be followed closely an indwelling tube such as a Montgomery T tube often arrests the stenotic process.

When the vocal cords have been mobile before operation the recurrent nerves must be identified and spared during the operation. After operation the cords move well but may eventually become fixed. The cause of this late complication is not known but is probably scarring of the laryngeal muscles or the cricothyroid joint.

References

[1] FINK B. RAYMOND (1975) *The Human Larynx: a functional study.* New York: Raven Press.
[2] FRIEDMAN WM. H., BILLER H. F. & SOM M. L. (1975) Repair of extended laryngotracheal stenosis. *Archives of Otolaryngology* **101(3),** 152.
[3] BRYCE D. P. & LAWSON V. G. (1967) The 'trough' method of laryngotracheal reconstruction. *Annals of Otology, Rhinology and Laryngology* **76,** 793.
[4] MONTGOMERY W. W. (1973) Glottic stenosis. In *Surgery of the Upper Respiratory System,* pp. 565–96. Philadelphia: Lea & Febiger.
[5] GERWAT M. B. & BRYCE D. P. (1974) The management of subglottic stenosis by excision and direct anastomosis. *Laryngoscope* **84,** 940.
[6] PEARSON F. G., COOPER J. D., NELEMS J. M. & VAN NOSTRAND A. W. P. (1975) Primary tracheal anastomosis after resection of the cricoid cartilage with preservation of recurrent laryngeal nerves. *Journal of Thoracic and Cardiovascular Surgery* **70,** 806.

CHAPTER 30

Vocal Cord Paralysis

Surgical anatomy and physiology

The course of the recurrent laryngeal nerves is described in anatomical texts. Variations in their course are described elsewhere [1–3] and are summarized in Fig. 30.1.

The glottis consists approximately of 60% membranous vocal cord and 40% vocal process and medial border of arytenoid body. Stimulation of the recurrent and superior laryngeal nerves results in adduction of the arytenoids which meet completely in the midline leaving a tiny chink between the membranous cords anteriorly due to the slightly more medial position of the vocal processes. As the column of air passes up from the trachea the Bernouilli effect occurs. The pressure between the cords drops, pulling in the mucosa to fill the small gap. This complete closure causes a sharp rise in the subglottic air pressure which increases until a column of air passes between the mucosal folds causing them to close again. The repetition of this mechanism causes mucosal vibration in the larynx, and sound.

The laryngeal nerves merely adduct the laryngeal muscles in phonation and contrary to the view put forward by Husson [4] they do not supply synchronous impulses to open and close the cords actively with each vibration. This *coup par coup* theory has been disproved.

Pathophysiology

Vocal cord paralysis may be unilateral or bilateral, complete or incomplete, abductor or adductor. It is probably better to describe the lesion in terms of what the vocal cord cannot do if paralysed and so only the terms abductor and adductor paralysis should be used.

The cord may be in the median, paramedian or cadaveric position. Since the cords do not assume the 'cadaveric position' after death it has been suggested that this be changed to 'intermediate'.

The difference between the median and paramedian positions is so subjective that 'paramedian' only should be used.

All theories about the position which the vocal cords assume after a paralysis of the nerves are compromised by the fact that it is impossible to record the position accurately. Such inaccurate observations may explain the incorrect theories and also the apparent inconsistencies in other theories.

The difference between the paramedian and cadaveric positions is only to the order of 2–3 mm and this is reported laryngoscopically – an endeavour fraught with inaccuracy. The small variations can be due to atrophy or scarring of the cords or arytenoids, or be due to compensation and rotation of the normal cord.

Semon's law
The first and best known theory depended on the observation that abductor fibres in the recurrent laryngeal nerves are more susceptible to pressure than the adductor fibres. This concept has been supported by many experimental studies but the theory is not totally accepted because it has so many clinical inconsistencies. The theory was first propounded by Rosenbach [5] and Semon [6] but is usually known as Semon's Law. It states that 'In the course of a gradually advancing organic lesion of a recurrent nerve or its fibres in the peripheral trunk of the recurrent nerve, three stages can be observed.

'In the first stage, only the abductor fibres are damaged; the vocal cords approximate in the midline and adduction is still possible.

405

'In the second stage, additional contracture of the adductors occurs so that the vocal cords are immobilized in the median position.

'In the third stage, the adductors become paralysed and the vocal cord assumes the cadaveric position.'

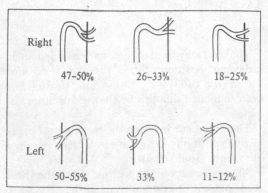

FIG. 30.1. Three chief relations between the right and left recurrent laryngeal nerves and the inferior thyroid artery. (Reproduced by permission from Hollinshead W. H. (1952) *S. Clin. North America* **32**, 1115.)

Differential innervation theory
Another theory of that era was based on the anatomic fact that the recurrent nerve branches outside the larynx with some branches presumably going to the adductors and others to the abductors. Injury to individual branches would thus cause paralysis of specific muscles.

Wagner and Grossmann theory
The most popular theory is that of Wagner [7] and Grossmann [8] which states that complete paralysis of the recurrent laryngeal nerve results in the cord being in the paramedian position because the intact cricothyroid muscle adducts the cord. If the superior laryngeal nerve is also paralysed then the cord will be in the cadaveric position because this adductive force will be lost.

This latter theory was confirmed experimentally by visual and electromyographic evaluation of thirty-three dog larynxes during section of the recurrent nerve, the superior laryngeal nerve and both nerves [9].

Further confirmation was obtained by the finding that the vocal cord was paralysed in the paramedian position with both gradual pressure and complete section of the recurrent laryngeal

nerve [10]. There is no evidence to prove that progressive pressure on the recurrent nerve causes first a paralysis of the posterior cricoarytenoid and then the adductors.

There are, however, many reported clinical inconsistencies in the Wagner–Grossman theory. According to this theory all intrathoracic lesions should produce a pure recurrent laryngeal nerve paralysis but many patients with lung cancer present with the cord in the cadaveric position. It has been suggested that retrograde atrophy of the vagus can occur up to the nucleus ambiguus and that stretching of the recurrent nerve by an enlarged heart or aortic aneurysm can pull the vagus down from the base of the skull thus injuring the superior laryngeal nerve.

A paralysed vocal cord can often be seen making attempts at adduction. It has been suggested that this is due to the bilateral innervation of the interarytenoid muscle as well as the intact cricothyroid muscle. That the latter muscle is predominant in carrying out this function is shown by bilateral paramedian positions in bilateral recurrent nerve paralysis with EMG-proven interarytenoid paralysis [9].

Changes in the cricoarytenoid joint and contracture of the paralysed muscle have been cited as determining the position of the cord [11]. While degeneration in the cricoarytenoid joint has been found [12], there is no evidence to show that a paralysed cord contracts. In unilateral paralysis the arytenoid body tilts forwards during inspiration but is level with the normal arytenoid in phonation. In the cadaveric position the vocal processes protrude medially and the body is displaced laterally so that the mobile arytenoid does not approximate tightly in phonation.

Paralysis of the superior laryngeal nerve is seldom diagnosed as a single clinical entity. It is claimed that the affected cord has an irregular, wrinkled or wavy edge and lies at a lower level than normal. The supraglottis and associated hypopharynx will also be anaesthetic. This injury must be as common if not more common than recurrent laryngeal nerve damage in thyroid and neck surgery. The nerve is certainly damaged in supraglottic laryngectomy but peculiar shapes of the cords have not been reported by surgeons who do this operation. The author has reviewed twelve of his own supraglottic laryngectomies and the cords looked quite normal in size, shape and position.

In practice it has been customary to wait for 6 months to see if any recovery occurs in a paralysed cord. This has been shown to occur experimentally [9]. The further away from the vocal cord that the recurrent nerve is crushed the longer it takes to recover. If it is crushed 8 cm from the thyroarytenoid in dogs recovery of function takes 45–85 days. Wallerian degeneration occurs followed by neuronal outgrowth with no significant axonal confusion.

Pathology

Vocal cord paralysis is a sign of disease and not a diagnosis. Because of its longer path the left recurrent laryngeal nerve is paralysed in 78% of cases, the right in 16% and both in 6%. Also since the commonest cause is malignant disease, the maximal age incidence is in the seventh decade. Men are affected eight to ten times as commonly as women.

A review of five large series of recurrent nerve paralysis [13–17] has shown the following percentage incidence of the various causes (rounded off to 0·5%):

	(%)
Malignant disease	24·5
Surgical trauma	20·5
Idiopathic	13·0
Inflammatory	13·0
Non-surgical trauma	11·0
Miscellaneous	11·0
Neurological	7·0
Total number 631	100·0

Malignant disease

One in four recurrent laryngeal nerve paralyses is due to cancer and of these, half are due to lung cancer, 20% to oesophageal cancer and 10% to thyroid cancer [18]. The remaining causes are nasopharyngeal tumours, chemodectomas of vagus, jugular and carotid bodies, metastatic cancer and lymphomas.

Because of the high incidence of malignant disease in the lung the cause of a vocal cord paralysis should not be regarded as unknown until at least 18 months after the first diagnosis.

Surgical trauma

Over the last 50 years surgery has developed for neurological, vascular and thoracic conditions which previously caused recurrent laryngeal paralysis as part of their natural history. However, this surgery has caused recurrent nerve paralysis in some of these cases. Examples are oesophageal and lung resection for carcinoma, carotid artery surgery, congenital heart surgery, surgical approaches to the cervical spine, mediastinoscopy, radical neck dissection, operation for pharyngeal pouch and partial laryngectomy.

Thyroid surgery has now reached such a level of technique that nerve damage should be very rare. Better pre-operative control of thyrotoxic glands and the earlier diagnosis of malignancy have made operative conditions much easier. Injury due to thyroid surgery is no longer the commonest cause of nerve damage.

Thyroidectomy without exposing the nerves causes a 5·4% paralysis rate of which 2·3% are irreversible [19]. If the nerve is routinely exposed, 8% of cords are paralysed but only 1·3% are irreversible [20].

Idiopathic causes

If the cause of a recurrent laryngeal nerve paralysis cannot be found the patient must be regarded as having a primary bronchial carcinoma until proved otherwise. Many paralyses due to viral infections have been described but actually proving the cause and effect relationship is difficult. Paralysis can occur in infectious mononucleosis [21] but the commonest cause is probably influenza. Many cases were described in the epidemic of A2/Hong Kong/1/68 virus in Europe in 1969–70. Only 20% of these recovered within 18 months [22].

Inflammatory causes

By far the commonest cause (95%) in this group is pulmonary tuberculosis either due to apical or mediastinal scarring or involvement with mediastinal glands.

Non-surgical trauma

Neck injuries due to automobile accidents are being recognized more frequently as a cause of nerve injury.

Stretching of the nerve by the enlarged left side of the heart in congestive failure, aneurysm of the aortic arch and a dilated pulmonary artery in mitral stenosis have been cited as causing paralysis. Unilateral and bilateral paralysis have been described in non-malignant thyroid disease [23] and as being due to a benign parathyroid adenoma [24].

Neurological causes

Central causes are cerebrovascular disease and brain stem ischaemia, epilepsy, Parkinson's disease, multiple sclerosis, syringomyelia, amyotrophic lateral sclerosis and head injury. Neuropathies can be due to alcohol or diabetes and this paralysis has also been described in the Guillain–Barré syndrome [25]. Neuritis due to vinblastine therapy can occur [26].

Miscellaneous causes

These include haemolytic anaemia, thrombosis of the subclavian vein, rheumatoid arthritis, syphilis and collagen disease.

Investigation

History

Consideration of the causes gives some idea of the possible associated symptoms in patients presenting with vocal cord paralysis. The type of voice (and therefore, presenting symptom) depends on the position of the vocal cords.

A whisper suggests an adductor paralysis whereas a fairly normal voice suggests an abductor paralysis. A voice which is normal in the morning and tires as the day goes on signifies a unilateral paralysis with a compensating normal cord.

Stridor, especially on exertion, occurs in bilateral abductor paralysis and aspiration in bilateral adductor paralysis, if it is organic as opposed to hysterical.

A reduced range and loss of singing voice is often associated with superior laryngeal paralysis but occurs with any vocal cord paralysis.

Examination

Again, consideration of the causes gives an indication of what to look for in general examination of the patient. Needless to say a full head and neck examination must always be done.

Of this latter examination, indirect laryngoscopy forms the most important part. It is very difficult to determine accurately whether the cords are in the paramedian or cadaveric position. Probably the best indication is the width of the membranous glottic chink in phonation. In the paramedian position it will be only about 1–2 mm since the normal cord does not need to compensate much. In the cadaveric position the gap will not only be greater but the tip of the vocal process will be directed medially as a definite prominence. A paralysed cord becomes bowed and atrophic and lies at a lower level than its fellow with anterior rotation of the arytenoid. In some patients, small rocking movements of the arytenoid may be seen due to bilateral innervation of the interarytenoid.

Radiology

If the cords are in the paramedian position the cause will almost certainly be below the larynx so that a chest radiograph including tomograms should be done. A barium swallow is also advisable and if a thyroid mass is palpable, a thyroid scan should be done.

If the cord is in the cadaveric position radiographs of the base of the skull, petrous bones and nasopharynx should be taken since the cause will probably be above the larynx.

Laryngograms have limited value but may show arytenoid rotation, change in level of the cord and atrophy, giving a sharper medial edge to the cord.

Laboratory studies

These have a very limited value. Every patient should have full blood indices measured: the differential white count, film and ESR may be of help in the lymphomas or tubercle. If mononucleosis is suspected, Paul–Bunnell and monospot tests are done; other viral studies can be started but since a change in titre is the finding of diagnostic significance, these take time. Neuropathy only occurs in well established previously diagnosed diabetes so that a glucose tolerance test is not needed. With the rise in venereal disease, a VDRL or WR should be done.

Endoscopy

Most patients require a panendoscopy comprising nasopharyngoscopy and biopsy of the fossa of Rosenmüller, oesophagoscopy, direct laryngoscopy with mobilization tests of the arytenoid to ascertain if the immobility of the cord is due to a muscle paralysis or a joint fixation, and bronchoscopy with a carinal biopsy if the bronchoscopy is normal. If a mediastinal cause is suspected mediastinoscopy should be done.

If definite clinical and radiological diagnosis has clearly been made then an endoscopy is done to confirm the diagnosis by biopsy. The more important group of patients is those in whom neither the history nor the radiographs are helpful – all of these patients should have panendoscopy.

Special tests

(1) *Respiratory function tests* may be done to find if the pulmonary reserve is affected by the inability to cough. If Teflon injection or cordopexy is planned these tests are the main measure of whether function has been helped or not.

(2) *Stroboscopy* shows an abnormal Bernouilli wave on the mucosa of the paralysed cord.

(3) *Laryngography* measures the quality, range, and pitch of the voice and air wastage.

(4) *Tape recordings* must be done to assess the effect of speech therapy or surgery.

Treatment

Unilateral abductor paralysis

The voice is almost normal and stridor and aspiration do not occur. Apart from speech therapy no treatment should be considered for at least 6 months. A few patients, usually professional voice users, demand further treatment. This should be by Teflon injection. Since the amount used is critical if the cord is in the paramedian position, a syringe which gives a measured quantity of Teflon paste, such as a Bruning syringe, should be used rather than a type which does not. The amount injected is critical, not only because of airway obstruction but also because too much Teflon alters the Bernouilli wave resulting in a high pitched diplophonia.

Unilateral adductor paralysis

Unless this is due to a carcinoma, the policy of 6 months watching and waiting accompanied by speech therapy should be followed. If the paralysis is due to a carcinoma, especially of the lung, then the distress of a weak voice and inefficient cough should be alleviated immediately with Teflon injection. This is done under local anaesthesia via an external approach with the cords inspected during injection by a fibre optic laryngoscope [27]. Injection in an adductor paralysis is not as successful as in abductor paralysis since it is difficult to close the posterior part of the glottic chink between the medial aspects of the vocal processes and arytenoids. There will thus always be some degree of air wastage.

If the paralysis is due to laryngeal trauma then injection of Teflon will not be successful due to the replacement of the thyro-arytenoid muscle with scar tissue. The best alternative is to attempt to add bulk laterally and hope to push the scarred glottis medially. This can be done by inserting sternohyoid muscle medial to the thyroid lamina [28] or by inserting a piece of thyroid cartilage between the thyroid lamina and its internal perichondrium [29].

Bilateral abductor paralysis

Since this is usually seen after a thyroidectomy, immediate re-exploration of the neck should be considered to see if the recurrent nerves can be resutured (which is not very successful) or to see if they have been caught in a ligature applied to the inferior thyroid artery.

The voice is good but there is stridor on exertion. A tracheostomy is required therefore and with a valved tracheostomy tube the patient can speak normally and carry on a normal life.

One question must be answered for every patient: 'Is a breathy voice better than a hole in the neck?'

If patients are given some months with a tracheostomy before being offered surgery it is the author's experience that most will opt to keep the speaking tracheostomy tube. It is advisable to wait at least 6 months to see if any recovery of function occurs and to see which side recovers most because an operation will then be done on the other cord.

A *cordectomy* has been advocated by some but is neither elegant nor satisfactory. Neither is the *operation described by Downie* of retracting the vocal process laterally with a wire. In the author's experience this is unsatisfactory in the long term because the scarring process pulls the cord back to the mid' position. About 6 months after the operation the patient develops stridor again and has to have the tracheostomy opened.

The most satisfactory method is *arytenoidectomy*, done externally as described by Woodman or internally via a thyrotomy.

The internal approach is easier since the access is good and the arytenoid can either be dissected out submucosally or arthrodesed to the cricoid with a screw. The disadvantage is the lack of control or judgement on how far apart the cords are at the end of the procedure.

Bilateral adductor paralysis

The commonest presentation of this is the commonly (but wrongly) named *hysterical aphonia*. Otolaryngologists of former days with a less enlightened view of psychiatry developed various 'cures' for this condition such as injections of sterile water, placing an overheated mirror on the soft palate in indirect laryngoscopy, and even standing on the patient's foot – all in an attempt to get the patient to shout, thereby persuading him that he could speak!

Many of these patients recover if given time to talk about their problems and perhaps this is the real use of speech therapy in the condition. A few patients who do not recover quickly need psychiatric help. Even with insight the same symptoms often recur when the patient finds himself again under stress.

Less commonly the cause is *organic*, usually a serious CNS disease such as a bulbar paralysis. These patients are not only aphonic but because they cannot produce a positive subglottic pressure the swallowing is inco-ordinated which, in the presence of abducted cords, causes constant aspiration of food and a consequent pneumonitis. Inability to close the cords also reduces the ability to cough so that in a very short time these patients are in grave danger. They nearly all need a tracheostomy for bronchial toilet and a nasogastric tube for feeding. Injection of Teflon into one vocal cord may help a little as may cricopharyngeal myotomy. If the neurological condition is not progressive a total laryngectomy should be seriously considered as the only way of protecting the lungs.

References

[1] BERLIN D. D. (1935) The recurrent laryngeal nerves in total ablation of the normal thyroid gland; an anatomical and surgical study. *Surgery, Gynecology and Obstetrics with International Abstracts of Surgery* **60**, 19.

[2] HOLLINSHEAD W. H. 1952) Anatomy of the endocrine glands. *Surgical Clinics of North America* **32**, 1115.

[3] KING B. T. & GREGG R. L. (1948) An anatomical reason for the various behaviour of paralysed vocal cords. *Annals of Otology, Rhinology and Laryngology* **57**, 925.

[4] DEDO H. H. & DUNKER E. (1967) Husson's theory, an experimental analysis of his research data and conclusions. *Archives of Otolaryngology* **85**, 303.

[5] ROSENBACH O. (1880) Zur Lehre von Doppelseitigen Totalen Lachmung des Nerv. Laryngeus Inferior (Recurrens). *Breslaver Aerztliche Zeitschrift* **2**, 14, 27.

[6] SEMON F. (1881) Clinical remarks on the proclivity of the abductor fibres of the recurrent laryngeal nerve to become affected sooner than the adductor fibres, or even exclusively, in cases of undoubted central or peripheral injury or disease of the roots or trunks of the pneumogastric, spinal accessory or recurrent nerves. *Archives of Laryngology* **2**, 197.

[7] WAGNER R. (1890) Die Medianstellung der Stimmbander bei der Rekurrenslahmung. *Archiv für pathologische Anatomie und Physiologie* **120**, 437; **124**, 127.

[8] GROSSMANN M. (1897) Experimentelle Beitrage zur Lehre von der 'Posticuslähmung'. *Archiv für Laryngologie und Rhinologie* **6**, 282.

[9] DEDO H. H. (1971) The paralysed larynx: an electromyographic study in dogs and humans. *Laryngoscope* **80**, 1455.

[10] ARNOLD G. E. (1961) Physiology and pathology of the cricothyroid muscle. *Laryngoscope* **71**, 687.

[11] ELLIS M. P. (Ed.) (1954) *Modern Trends in Diseases of the Ear, Nose and Throat*. London: Butterworth.

[12] KIRCHNER J. A. (1966) Atrophy of laryngeal muscles in vocal paralysis. *Laryngoscope* **76**, 1753.

[13] PARNELL F. W. & BRANDENBURG J. H. (1970) Vocal cord paralysis: A review of 100 cases. *Laryngoscope* **80**, 1036.

[14] STENBORG R. (1973) Cases of recurrent nerve paralysis in Gothenburg from 1968–71. *Acta Oto-laryngologica* **75**, 364.

[15] MAISEL R. H. & OGURA J. H. (1964) Evaluation and treatment of voice and paralysis. *Laryngoscope* **84**, 302.

[16] TITCHE L. L. (1976) Causes of recurrent laryngeal nerve paralysis. *Archives of Otolaryngology* **102**, 259.

[17] FRENCKNER P. (1936) The prognostic significance of paralysis of the recurrent laryngeal nerve. *Acta Oto-laryngologica* **23**, 85.

[18] DE GANDT J. B. (1970) Recurrent nerve compression. *Acta oto-rhino-laryngologica Belgica* **24**, 520.

[19] GLISSELSSON L. (1950) Laryngeal paralysis following thyroidectomy. *Acta chirurgica Scandinavica* **99**, 1950.

[20] WIDSTROM A. (1973) Vocal cord palsies following surgery for benign non toxic goitre. *Acta Oto-laryngologica* **75**, 370.

[21] KIFFER A. & DUFOUR P. (1971) Laryngeal and pharyngeal paralysis as a complication of infectious mononucleosis. *Revue d'oto-neuro-ophtalmologie* **43**, 157.

[22] FEX S. & ELMQUIST D. (1973) Endemic recurrent laryngeal nerve paresis. *Acta oto-laryngologica* **75**, 368.

[23] WORGAN D. *et al.* (1974) Recurrent laryngeal nerve paralysis and non malignant thyroid. *Journal of Laryngology and Otology* **98**, 375.

[24] ZORE J. M. *et al.* (1972) Parathyroid adenoma causing vocal cord paralysis. *Transactions of the American Academy of Ophthalmology and Otolaryngology* **76**, 1397.

[25] MATTUCI K. F. & CHODOSH P. L. (1970) Vocal cord paralysis in Guillain–Barré syndrome. *Eye, Ear, Nose and Throat Monthly* **49**, 318.

[26] BROOK J. & SCHREIBER W. (1971) Vocal cord paralysis. A tonic reaction to vinblastine therapy. *Cancer Chemotherapy Abstracts* **55**, 591.

[27] VERCOE G. S. & WILLIAMS G. T. (1976) Percutaneous teflon injection of vocal cord under fibre optic laryngoscopic control. *Clinical Otolaryngology* **1**, 183.

[28] BERNSTEIN L. & HOLT G. P. (1967) Correction of vocal cord abduction in unilateral recurrent laryngeal nerve paralysis by transposition of the sternohyoid muscle. An experimental study in dogs. *Laryngoscope* **77**, 876.

[29] KAMER F. M. & SOM M. L. (1972) Correction of the traumatically abducted vocal cord. *Archives of Otolaryngology* **95**, 6.

CHAPTER 31

Disorders of the Voice

Voice physiology

The larynx is a vital organ which protects the lungs and has important functions in respiration, coughing, deglutition and fixation but its most sophisticated function is the production of sound.

The necessary energy is produced during the expiratory phase. The air accumulating beneath the vocal cords sets them into passive vibration at different frequencies, according to the length and tension of the vocal cords.

The two best known theories of phonation are the myoelastic or aerodynamic theory and the neurochronaxic theory of Husson, but the latter is no longer tenable. The vocal cords are brought into vibration by the airstream which passes through the adducted vocal cords causing pressure dips (Bernouilli effect).

The voiced airstream is formed into words by the tongue, palate, teeth and lips, with added resonance from the pharynx, mouth and nose. The complicated centrally-controlled mechanism of speech develops during early childhood and language results through a tedious process of learning for which good auditory function is essential.

The normal human voice has a range of about four octaves, the average range for each person being about two octaves. The male voice ranges between 80 and 320 Hz for a bass and between 128 and 480 for a tenor; the female voice between 160 and 640 Hz for a contralto and between 256 and 1024 Hz for a soprano. Training of the voice will extend the range to three octaves and in exceptional cases to three and a half.

The range of the human voice is divided into registers according to the way the sound is produced. The vocal range includes three registers; the chest, middle and head register. The chest and the head register show a specific pattern of vibration and elevation of the larynx, while the middle register forms the transition between the two. In untrained voices the break between head and chest register can easily be heard as an abrupt change in timbre of the voice. In the chest tone, the vocal cords vibrate over their full length and thickness, while in head tone only the medial edge of the membranous part of the vocal cords are in vibration. The cricothyroid muscle is the main tensor of the vocal cords and together with the vocalis muscle it determines the pitch of the tone produced.

Investigation of dysphonia

History

The normal voice is clear, has adequate strength and can change according to the emotional state of the person. Loss of these qualities is a symptom of inadequate function and becomes evident in the most frequent presenting symptom of hoarseness. A more general term of inadequate vocal function is dysphonia, which indicates malfunctioning of the voice in a more general way. However, one should be aware that dysphonia is a symptom and not a disease.

Phoniatricians highly specialized in voice and speech diseases tend to favour the word dysphonia and maintain that malfunction is the primary cause of much laryngeal pathology, whereas laryngologists, who mostly deal with organic disorders, use the word hoarseness as a symptom of organic disease. While phoniatricians tend to accentuate the functional, psychological and habitual disorders as the primary cause, often leading to organic laryngeal disease, laryngologists dealing with gross pathology in the larynx tend to overlook important functional aspects.

When dealing with laryngeal pathology it often appears difficult to differentiate which aspect is the most important, the functional or the organic. Laryngeal carcinoma is not a functional disease, while singers' nodules are a typical example of a functional disorder leading to organic pathology. In between there is a broad spectrum of laryngeal and voice disorders in which both functional and organic factors are of aetiological importance.

Examination

Examination of the larynx is essential for the evaluation of voice disorders. In patients where it is impossible to perform indirect laryngoscopy it may be necessary to perform direct laryngoscopy. Usually this is done under general anaesthesia, which makes a functional evaluation impossible. Although helpful for diagnostic purposes, it is especially indicated for biopsies and for minor surgical procedures such as the removal of polyps or stripping of the vocal cords. The introduction of laryngoscopy using the operating microscope has allowed a more accurate examination and treatment of laryngeal disease.

The movements of the vocal cords can be studied more accurately by stroboscopy, which has proved to be an invaluable aid in the assessment of vocal cord movement. Laryngostroboscopy is performed with intermittent light pulses, the frequency of which should be close to the frequency of phonation, resulting in an optical illusion of slowly moving vocal cords, which allows the wave pattern of the vocal cords to be seen.

The modern electronic stroboscope couples the frequency of the vocal cord vibration accurately with the frequency of the light source. The vibration pattern of the vocal cord can be studied with ease allowing important conclusions to be drawn. Absent or reduced vibration of the vocal cord is often an early sign of organic disease within the vocal cord, even before lesions are visible by laryngoscopy.

When functional disorders are suspected the examination should be followed by a full assessment of the qualities of the voice including vocal range, medium speaking range, intensity and timbre.

Radiographs of the larynx are of limited value for the evaluation of the disorders of the voice. Glottography, electromyography and spectrographic analysis are as yet of limited value in daily practice, but remain important for research.

MUTATIONAL AND HORMONAL DYSPHONIA

During the hormonal changes of puberty the larynx undergoes accelerated growth. The concomitant change in vocal pitch and range is called mutation. The male voice drops about one octave, while the change of the female voice is restricted to half an octave. Both emotional and hormonal disturbances can affect this process and lead to disorders of the voice.

Mutational falsetto voice

This disorder is the persistence of falsetto voice in boys after puberty. It is generally agreed that it is primarily an emotional disorder although predisposing constitutional factors may be present. Psychological instability in boys during puberty may lead to habitual use of the falsetto register, which resembles the child's voice.

Examination of the larynx reveals normal development with normally functioning vocal cords. In some cases the behaviour is immature.

Pressure with the thumb on the thyroid cartilage (Gutzmann test) counteracts the contracted cricothyroid muscle with resultant slackening of the vocal cords and lowering of the voice. This test can also be used as a treatment to make the subject aware of the normal potential of the voice. The treatment also includes psychological and speech therapy.

Precocious vocal mutation

Endocrine disorders leading to precocious puberty also lead to precocious mutation and early development of the primary and secondary sex characteristics. The underlying cause is usually of gonadal, adrenal or pituitary origin.

These include hypertrophy and benign and malignant tumours of these glands.

Treatment should be directed towards the cause although the mutated voice will not regress. There also exists an idiopathic or genuine form of precocious puberty, which is usually of familial or inherited origin.

Incomplete vocal mutation

Incomplete mutation is classified by Arnold [1] into three clinical forms:

(1) Delayed mutation, which starts beyond the average age of puberty.

(2) Prolonged mutation, starting at the normal age.

(3) Incomplete mutation, in which the voice change is arrested.

Usually the sexual development is normal although minor signs of sexual immaturity may be present. Incomplete mutation is generally considered to be a constitutional disorder. Chronic upper respiratory infections can overstrain the larynx, which should be protected during a period of accelerated growth. The disorder sometimes occurs in boys who have strained their voice too much during puberty by frequent choir practices.

The main symptoms are hoarseness and instability of the voice. The vocal pitch is too high and sometimes the chest register is not used at all. The overstraining of the voice during this period can lead to serious phonasthenic complaints at a later age.

The treatment is varied according to the underlying cause. If hormonal deficiencies seem to be present a full endocrinological investigation is necessary.

Usually voice therapy, including respiratory exercises, will suffice although the disease can be very stubborn to treat. Attention should be paid to emotional instability either primary or secondary.

Eunuchoidism

Normal gonadal function is necessary for the development of the secondary sex characteristics.

Insufficiency of gonadal or pituitary function before puberty can lead to eunuchoidism in which the absence of secondary sex characteristics is most typical. The normal growth of the larynx in boys during puberty does not take place and the pitch remains at the level of the infant's voice. The range of the voice develops normally.

Treatment of hypogonadal and hypopituitary syndromes should be carried out by endocrinologists.

HABITUAL DYSPHONIA

The habitual dysphonias are primary functional disorders, which are caused by incorrect use of the voice and often by emotional disorders.

The dysphonias can cause secondary organic abnormalities such as vocal cord nodules or even chronic epithelial abnormalities.

Hypokinetic dysphonia

Hypokinetic dysphonia is characterized by hypotonia of the muscles of the vocal cord. In some cases this may be due to a congenital weakness or even hypoplasia of the larynx but it usually occurs in people who are emotionally unstable. Exceptionally, a hypokinetic dysphonia can arise from a hyperkinetic dysphonia.

The voice is weak and muffled and air escape can be heard.

The pitch of the voice is often higher than normal due to over-contraction of the cricothyroid muscle. The patient's posture is faulty with drooping shoulders, but during speech the neck is tense, and often accompanied by excess contraction of the accessory muscles of respiration.

Incomplete closure of the vocal cords is the most striking finding on laryngoscopy, and this may be assymetrical. This may be seen in the membranous part of the vocal cords resembling a paresis of the vocalis muscle, and also in the posterior part between the vocal processes.

When the patient speaks he barely opens his mouth; a hyperkinetic voice often occurs momentarily by way of compensation.

Treatment is difficult and is less successful than that of the hyperkinetic form. The most important facets of treatment are learning the correct pitch of the voice, control of respiration, and diminution of a compensatory hyperkinetic mechanism.

Hyperkinetic dysphonia

This term indicates excessive use of all the laryngeal muscles. In marked cases the voice sounds rough and heavy and the vocal attack is hard. The larynx is drawn upwards because of excess muscular contraction so that the resonating area is diminished. The respiratory muscles also show evidence of excess activity and the neck veins are frequently distended because of straining. This abnormality is often found in men who are short and squat, with a short muscular neck. Such patients are often men who talk and gesticulate a lot, and have an active social life.

Laryngeal examination is difficult because of oversensitive reflexes and excess muscular contraction of the pharynx; it is often necessary to use a local anaesthetic on these patients. The vocal cords are usually red and thickened and the false vocal cords are almost always closed tightly together.

Persistent friction of the true vocal cords eventually leads to epithelial alterations, similar to those found in chronic nodular laryngitis and chronic hyperplastic laryngitis.

As with hypokinetic dysphonia, treatment is often difficult and unrewarding. Secondary abnormalities are often irreversible and maintain the primary disorder.

Treatment is aimed at controlling the excessive activity of both the respiratory and the phonatory muscles. Behaviour therapy is also useful in understanding the underlying psychological problems.

Dysphonia ventricularis

The ventricular bands form one of the most important laryngeal sphincters for protection of the lower airway (the original and most important function of the larynx). The ventricular bands are most active during coughing, straining and swallowing, but normally play no part in phonation.

Dysphonia ventricularis arises when the ventricular bands play an active part in phonation.

The folds appose during speech and contribute to the formation of the voice. The ventricular bands were not designed for phonation, so that they produce a rough unmodulated sound with little carrying power.

This clinical picture is often seen in the worst cases of hyperkinetic dysphonia in which secondary organic abnormalities of the true vocal cords make good phonation impossible so that the voice is supplemented by use of the ventricular bands.

The larynx then contracts at two levels so that it may be difficult to see the true vocal cords during laryngoscopy. The ventricular bands often close first, and in long standing cases may be hypertrophic.

Treatment is primarily focused on the underlying cause, which is usually functional, but which can also be emotional or even of neurogenic origin. Treatment therefore consists of speech therapy with supportive psychotherapy.

Phonasthenia and vocal fatigue

Phonasthenia is a general term which indicates unsatisfactory function of the voice in the presence of normal laryngoscopic appearances. Although neurological or muscular factors can cause this disease it is primarily a functional disturbance produced by excessive demands on the voice. Thus the disorder often begins after a period of prolonged speaking or singing, especially in patients who place great demands on their voice for professional reasons [1].

Phonasthenia arises primarily from a combination of overtaxing and incorrect use of the voice.

The pitch of the voice is often too high, and the patient has difficulty in singing a note clearly and holding it at the correct pitch. Respiration is often shallow and spasmodic. After intensive use the voice gradually becomes weaker and loses its clarity, and can even become hoarse or completely absent (aphonia).

The patient complains of discomfort in the throat and neck, including the symptoms of globus hystericus and of retention of mucus in the throat. These patients often have other bad habits such as clearing the throat and coughing which can be regarded as nervous mannerisms.

The complex functional, emotional and sometimes organic factors demand if possible a causal approach. Much attention must be paid to the technique of voice production, and adaptation of the use of the voice to its capabilities. This can have far reaching consequences especially for professional voice users who should pay great attention to these matters in the choice of a career.

The help of a psychologist is often indispensable during treatment.

PSYCHOGENIC VOICE DISORDERS

The best known form is *psychogenic aphonia* in which the normal voice suddenly disappears and is replaced by a whisper. The symptom occurs almost exclusively in women and the term hysteria is often incorrectly applied to it. Indirect laryngoscopy shows that there is little or no movement of the vocal cords and that the pharyngeal reflexes are diminished. In other cases the appearances can be those of a paralysis of the vocalis or transverse arytenoid muscles. Typically in psychogenic aphonia a voiced cough can be produced in response to a request to cough.

As in other psychogenic reactions an emotional conflict is the basic cause of this disturbance. The inability to cope with certain traumatic experiences or to attract the attention of the outside world to past injustices can cause a flight into psychogenic aphonia. Fears and inadequate feelings which express themselves in an absence of the ability to communicate are sometimes important. The diagnosis is not difficult in complete aphonia but may be if the symptoms are limited to dysphonia. Psychogenic aphonia can be regarded in some patients as one of the conversion symptoms of the hysterical personality.

Management by an ear, nose and throat surgeon is usually limited to local treatment. Suggestive therapy consisting of faradic stimulation of the laryngeal skeleton supplemented by manual manipulation can restore the voice in a short time in many cases. The patient is thus led to believe that the treatment is responsible for the cure. In the absence of causal treatment the chance of recurrence is great and a speech therapist, a psychiatrist or psychologist is then needed to solve the underlying problems.

VOCAL CORD NODULES AND POLYPS

Vocal cord nodules or singers' nodules are one of the commonest laryngeal disorders due to abuse of the voice. They can occur at any age and begin during periods of excessive voice strain. Children, usually boys, who scream and shout are often afflicted, but also adults who by profession or otherwise demand much of their voice can develop vocal cord nodules. There seem to be predisposing factors as nodules often occur in endomorphs in which hyperplastic tissue reactions are more common. In contrast to polyps, vocal cord nodules occur nearly exclusively in females. Precipitating factors include allergic tendencies, thyroid imbalance and emotional instability; cigarette smoking and alcohol abuse are aggravating factors [2].

The diagnosis is easily established by indirect laryngoscopy. Usually symmetric on both vocal cords, the nodules appear on the medial edge in the middle of the membranous part of the vocal cord, which corresponds with the junction between the anterior one-third and the posterior two-thirds of the glottis (Fig. 31.1). It is generally assumed that they develop at this point where the maximal excursion of the vocal cord occurs. Through forceful phonation localized epithelial reactions occur characterized by epithelial thickening and stromal reactions. Because of the marked epithelial thickening the nodules are whitish or pink in colour and vary in size from a pin point to 3–4 mm. In some cases the protruding nodule on one side may fit into a small excavation on the other vocal cord.

Microscopically there is marked hyperplasia of the squamous epithelium and hyperkeratosis; acanthosis and parakeratosis are often present. The epithelial stroma is invaded by blood vessels and loose connective tissue, while signs of an inflammatory reaction are often present.

Treatment is primarily directed towards relief of the cause. A period of absolute vocal rest often gives dramatic results; even pronounced nodules can disappear after 2–3 weeks of vocal rest. It is advisable to start with such a treatment. After a period of vocal rest intensive speech therapy is necessary to prevent recurrence and to achieve a normal voice.

Only in long-standing cases with relatively large nodules which do not respond to conservative management should surgery be considered. Laryngoscopy for removal of vocal cord nodules should be done under the operating microscope

be present on the superior or inferior surface of the vocal cord (Fig. 31.2). Polyps may be pedunculated or sessile. The macroscopic appearance shows a wide variety of pictures with colour ranging from pink to deep red stained by blood. Some appear more solid through fibrotic changes, others are glazy and oedematous and may simulate Reinke's oedema. In contrast to nodules, polyps are rarely found in children and are far more common in males.

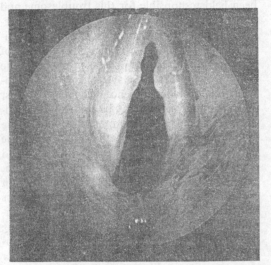

FIG. 31.1. Vocal nodules in the middle of the membranous vocal cords, a site which corresponds to the junction of the anterior third and posterior two-thirds of the glottis.

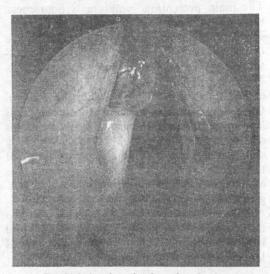

FIG. 31.2. A pedunculated vocal cord polyp.

with careful dissection [3]. Care should be taken not to damage the vocal ligament. Removal of vocal cord nodules is rarely indicated in children and should therefore not be done before puberty. After surgical intervention vocal rest is necessary for 10 days.

Generally *vocal cord polyps* are believed to be related to vocal cord nodules. Some authors believe that they are just another form of local reaction on the vocal cords due to vocal strain, but it is very doubtful if this is true.

The clinical picture is very different although mixed forms can be found. The vocal cord polyp is usually unilateral and appears anywhere on the vocal cord; as opposed to vocal nodules which always lie on the superomedial edge, polyps can

Although vocal strain can be a predisposing factor, this is usually more acute or episodic and the polyp often starts during an acute upper respiratory infection. In contrast to nodules, polyps do not disappear after a period of voice rest, and surgical intervention is indicated in most cases. Although a polyp is easily recognized by the trained laryngologist excision should be done to exclude possible malignancy. After meticulous removal the recurrence rate is very low.

ACUTE LARYNGITIS

Acute laryngitis is usually part of an upper respiratory tract infection like influenza or a common cold. However, it can also be a strictly localized infection limited to the vocal cords, usually of viral origin. Bacterial laryngitis used to be common before the days of vaccination against diphtheria and nowadays is only rarely seen as part of a streptococcal infection. Other non-infectious causes of acute laryngitis are toxic (smoke, irritating fumes) and mechanical (heavy voice strain).

Clinical features

The main presenting symptom is hoarseness, sometimes to such a degree that aphonia results. The throat feels rough and ticklish, leading to a dry cough. When an infection of the lower airways is present the cough becomes productive. The discomfort in the throat will turn into pain especially when irritation by coughing goes on. Only rarely will local swelling of the vocal cords lead to serious stridor, and a tracheostomy is seldom required in adults. This is not so in young children, however, because the narrow lumen of the larynx during an acute laryngobronchitis easily becomes obstructed necessitating emergency measures.

The diagnosis is made on the basis of the history and local examination. The laryngeal mucosa is red and swollen, and the vocal cords lose their normal light colour.

Treatment

Vocal rest is the most important measure to prevent further irritation of the laryngeal mucosa. Irritation by coughing should be dealt with either with antitussive agents or expectorants. Antibiotics are not of any help unless other signs of a purulent infection are obvious, such as sinusitis or bronchitis.

ACUTE EPIGLOTTITIS

A special form of acute laryngitis is epiglottitis, an acute localized swelling of the epiglottis accompanied by high fever and pain. Serious obstruction of the airway can result. Treatment is with bed rest, antibiotics and humidification and a close watch is kept for signs of respiratory obstruction.

CHRONIC LARYNGITIS

Pathology

The term chronic laryngitis indicates a chronic inflammation of the laryngeal mucosa. This may develop from an unresolved acute laryngitis, but more often is a disease of insidious onset. The voice complaints may be minor in the beginning, but the disease usually progresses and may lead to serious voice disability. Many causes have been held responsible for this troublesome and resistant condition and besides the external factors to be mentioned, there seems to be a constitutional factor. Chronic laryngitis may be part of a chronic inflammatory process prevalent in the upper and lower airway system, which is probably due to a failing defence mechanism against foreign invaders, or it may be a strictly independent process. The most important contributing factors are chronic suppurative infections of the upper respiratory tract such as chronic nose and sinus disease, chronic inflammation of the teeth, tobacco smoke, alcohol and the inhalation of irritating fumes. The exact role of voice abuse is not clearly understood but is certainly a contributing factor. The strain exerted in overcoming the slightest voice disability due to a minor inflammatory process is so great that further damage to the vocal cord results. The disease is, like most laryngeal diseases, commoner in men. Diabetes and malabsorption syndromes should be excluded although their causative significance is probably minor.

Clinical features

The diagnosis is made on the history and the clinical picture. Progressive hoarseness is the main symptom. The voice is usually worst in the morning because the mucus present in the larynx has dried during the night, but it becomes better after clearing the throat of this inspissated mucus. Gradually, as the day progresses, the voice deteriorates again. Compensatory mechanisms to maintain adequate sound production exert an unwanted strain on the tissues and muscles involved. Some degree of hyperkinetic dysphonia is therefore always present and when the true cords do not produce enough sound, ventricular fold voice may occur.

Examination of the larynx reveals a diffuse

redness of the laryngeal mucosa most pronounced on the true vocal cords. There is hardly any swelling or oedema and the mucosa is usually smooth.

In some cases the laryngeal mucosa reacts with visible tissue augmentation leading to the formation of polypoid growths. When this occurs the term *chronic polypoid laryngitis* is used. The swellings found on the vocal cords may be very extensive and simulate a tumour. These polypoid swellings therefore have also been named pseudo tumours. Although hyperplasia of the laryngeal mucosa can occur in all cases of chronic laryngitis, it is never the most prominent feature and therefore the term chronic hyperplastic laryngitis can be misleading.

Treatment

Treatment is often unrewarding, but can be effective especially in early cases with a short history. Elimination of any possible causative agent should be done as soon as possible. Vocal rest may also help, particularly in early cases. Antibiotics and corticosteroids may have a favourable effect when clear signs of inflammation are present but the value of inhalations and climatic treatment is difficult to estimate. There remains a group of cases resistant to all forms of prevention and therapy, probably because of the inferior nature of the respiratory mucosa. Some of these patients have a chronic resistant sinus disease and/or bronchitis and cannot be cured by any treatment presently available.

SPECIFIC LARYNGITIS

Tuberculosis of the larynx

Pathology

Since the advent of screening by chest X-ray and tuberculostatic drugs, tuberculosis has lost much of its sinister importance in the Western world. The detection of the disease in the lung at an early stage has markedly reduced the incidence of tuberculous laryngitis, since it is nearly always secondary to a focus in the lung. Parts of the world still exist where tuberculosis is common and secondary tuberculous laryngitis is found. It is generally believed that between 5 and 10% of patients with open pulmonary tuberculosis

develop tuberculosis of the larynx. The disease, caused by the human bacillus always has its primary focus in the lung and from there many other organs can be affected.

Other organs are usually involved by miliary spread but the laryngeal lesion is probably caused through direct contact with the tubercle bacillus. Dust, smoke, coughing and vocal abuse seem to be precipitating factors. When laryngeal manifestations are present, positive cultures of the sputum are nearly always found.

Clinical features

The disease presents as a local redness or inflammation, often of one vocal cord, and is therefore called a monocorditis; granulation tissue is also present in the vicinity of the arytenoid cartilage. Real ulceration does not occur at this stage of disease although loss of tissue can be apparent. Later, tuberculous nodules may develop in the submucosa of all regions of the larynx leading to caseation and ulceration.

Quite extensive destruction of the laryngeal mucosa and underlying tissues may be found, in extreme cases leading to perichronditis and necrosis of the cartilage. The picture may resemble tumour growth. The diagnosis should be suspected in any patient with pulmonary tuberculosis who develops hoarseness but also should be borne in mind when a monocorditis is found or the laryngeal picture otherwise suggests a granulomatous disease, in the absence of tuberculosis. Sometimes the diagnosis is made only after a biopsy has been taken and Langhans's giant cells are nearly always found in the granulation tissue.

Treatment

The treatment is primarily focused on the disease in the lung and consists of rest and tuberculostatic drugs. In most cases the laryngeal lesions heal leaving scars and sometimes cicatrical stenosis. The lesions may be very resistant to therapy in advanced cases and may even require life-long therapy.

Other specific laryngitis

Syphilis and *leprosy* occur rarely in the larynx in Europe and the USA. *Scleroma* is prevalent in Eastern Europe and is caused by bacillus rhinoscleromatis. *Wegener's granulomatosis* or mid-line granuloma is a tumour-like condition of unknown cause, usually starting in the nasal cavity or septum and leading to local destruction of the tissues. Both these latter conditions occasionally affect the larynx.

REINKE'S OEDEMA

Pathology
Reinke's oedema is characterized by an accumulation of fluid in the loose subepithelial space of the vocal cords (Reinke's space); the exact cause remains unknown. The condition may be the result of chronic inflammation of the upper respiratory tract especially of the paranasal sinuses, but a recent study [4] stresses the importance of the mechanical factor, i.e. misuse and over-use of the voice over a prolonged period. Contrary to chronic laryngitis, which is prevalent in men, Reinke's oedema also occurs quite frequently in women and children.

Clinical features
The diagnosis is readily established by laryngoscopic examination. The vocal cords show a thickened oedematous and sometimes flabby appearance and are covered by a thin translucent epithelium crossed by blood vessels (Fig. 31.3). Phonation is disturbed through interposition of the swollen mucosa.

Treatment
Treatment is by means of microlaryngoscopic methods. The mucosa is incised parallel to the vocal ligament, fluid or jelly-like substance is sucked out and the redundant mucosa is carefully removed. The mucosa of the anterior commissure should not be touched to prevent webbing. In some cases it is wise to treat each vocal cord at different operating sessions. The prognosis is good although the condition can recur.

EPITHELIAL HYPERPLASIA OF THE LARYNX

Normally two types of epithelium are present in the larynx, namely a non-keratinizing squamous epithelium present on the true vocal cords,

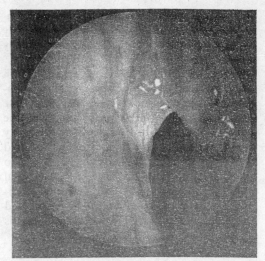

FIG. 31.3. Reinke's oedema. Vocal cords ballooned by oedema within Reinke's space giving the epithelium a thin translucent appearance.

between the arytenoids and on the edge of the epiglottis, and a ciliated respiratory epithelium covering the posterior surface of the epiglottis, the ventricular bands and folds, and the subglottis. The larynx forms the entrance of the lower respiratory airway and is an easy prey to irritation by inhalation, infection and mechanical trauma. Air pollution and smoking are considered highly irritating to the laryngeal mucosa and add considerably to the process of metaplasia of respiratory epithelium to squamous epithelium, a process which normally proceeds with ageing.

A large number of names have been used in the laryngological literature during the past 100 years to describe particular clinical entities which have in common some degree of epithelial hyperplasia with a varying degree of subepithelial inflammation. The names still currently found in the literature are hyperkeratosis, keratosis, pachydermia and leukoplakia.

Most authors, especially in the Anglo-Saxon literature, favour the word keratosis for laryngeal lesions of which epithelial hyperplasia and dysplasia are the most prominent features. The many confusing clinical names still in use today for the multi-causational lesions require at least a simple histological classification, which is gradually becoming widely accepted.

Aetiology

Although metaplasia of the respiratory epithelium of the larynx is part of the normal ageing process it is generally accepted that external factors influence this process. The vocal cords already covered by squamous epithelium are subject to frictional forces caused by voice production and coughing; in unfavourable circumstances the epithelium becomes hyperplastic. Chemical irritation, of which smoking is the most important and social one, has always been held the most serious factor leading to epithelial changes. The ill effects of smoking and air pollution on the laryngeal mucosa leading to metaplastic and hyperplastic changes have often been stressed [5]. This process may be partly reversible after many years when smoking is abandoned. However, the changes found in the larynx also appear to occur in non-smokers [6]. Other forms of chemical irritation include dusty atmospheres in mines, irritating fumes in factories and laboratories and inadequate climatic conditions.

Alcohol is also held to have an ill effect on the laryngeal mucosa, probably not by direct contact but through the ensuing hyperaemia.

The role of voice abuse and a faulty technique is generally considered to have an ill effect on the vocal cords, but the exact mechanism is not fully understood. The most common pathology caused by excessive voice strain is *vocal cord nodules* which are commoner in women and children who only rarely develop the same hyperplastic changes in the vocal mucosa as in men.

Many other factors have been suggested to contribute to the pathologic changes in the larynx of which chronic upper respiratory tract infection and vitamin-A deficiency are most often mentioned. Whatever the role of these contributing factors may be, in most cases a single factor is not found and an individual susceptibility must be present.

Clinical features

Hoarseness is the usual complaint for which the patient seeks advice. The onset of the symptoms is usually insidious; sometimes a preceding upper respiratory infection is held responsible by the patient. The speaking voice may be normal in the beginning and the hoarseness becomes apparent during singing as certain tones cannot be reached. Only minor discomfort or sensations in the throat are present, possibly accompanied by a spasmodic cough. Examination of the vocal cords with the laryngeal mirror not only reveals changes on the true vocal cords but also in other regions of the larynx. The lesions may be small and only slightly elevated from the adjacent tissue. The pink to whitish dusky appearance of the lesions is characteristic of the keratinization that is present and is in contrast with the shiny pink colour of the vocal cords. The degree of keratinization can be partly assessed by the degree of elevation of the lesion; excessive keratin can present as horns (cornu laryngeum). When extensive lesions are present the mobility of the vocal cord can be impaired.

Clinical types

The value of staging this pathological process on clinical grounds is debatable and, as previously stated, many names still in use correspond either with a certain clinical appearance (laryngoscopic image) or with a certain histologic picture. The clinical names used do not always correspond with the same histological picture.

Pachydermia, a term introduced by Virchow, is divided into two forms: diffuse and localized. The diffuse type is found typically on the posterior half of the vocal cords covering the vocal process of the arytenoids. The lesions have the appearance of a saucer-like swelling, with elevation at the edges and a central dip. They are usually present on both vocal cords. The current name is *contact pachydermia* and the picture resembles *contact ulcers* (Jackson) but it is not clear whether both conditions are exactly the same.

Sometimes the most pronounced epithelial changes occur on the posterior wall between the arytenoids, a region normally covered by squamous epithelium. The epithelium in this region can show reactive hyperplasia with quite pronounced swelling. Virchow called this *interarytenoid pachydermia* and more recently the term acid laryngitis has been used to indicate a possible relation with nocturnal gastro-oesophageal reflux [7]. Virchow's more localized form of pachydermia was named by him *pachydermia verucosa* because of the warty appearance of the lesions. In Virchow's time this condition was considered to be identical with squamous papilloma, a term nowadays reserved for excessively keratinizing lesions (Fig. 31.4). Their growth is usually slow with a definite tendency towards malignancy. The clinical behaviour is definitely different from juvenile papillomas.

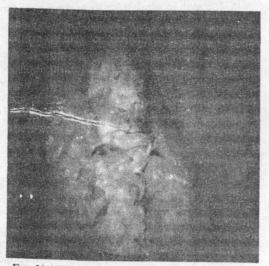

FIG. 31.4. Excessive laryngeal hyperkeratosis obstructing the laryngeal airway (squamous papilloma).

Keratosis laryngis and *leukoplakia* are more common and recent names in use today for epithelial lesions of the vocal cords. Although some authors adhere to definite characteristics of each name, there is little doubt that they, at least in part, cover the same disease of which hyperplasia and dysplasia of the epithelium are the most prominent features. The importance of staging this disease on histological criteria has been stressed by Kleinsasser [3].

Histological staging

The squamous epithelium of the larynx is of a non-keratinizing type. The epithelial layer is separated from the subcutaneous tissue by a thin basal membrane. The adjacent basal cell layer (stratum germinativum) consists of regularly arranged cylindrical cells with ovoid nuclei in which mitoses are common. More superficially the cell shape becomes polyhedral and the nuclei assume a spherical shape. Interconnecting bridges between the cells (desmosomes) become apparent. This layer is called the stratum spinosum. The most superficial layers of cells consist of flattened cells with small condensed nuclei. Keratin is normally not present.

The pathologic process described as epithelial hyperplasia is characterized by a thickening of the squamous epithelium with a varying degree of disturbance in the normal maturation process. The thickening can be caused by proliferation of any layer of cells. When the regular pattern of mitosis and maturation is retained simple hyperplasia is present.

This process can be accompanied by keratosis, the formation of keratohyalin in the cytoplasm of the most superficial cell layers. The superficial cells loose their nuclei and are shed off as keratin. If the nuclei persist in the keratinized cells the term parakeratosis is used.

Disturbance of the maturation process is generally called dysplasia, which may be light, moderate or severe. The cells and nuclei show aberrations such as irregular shapes, abnormal staining, atypical mitoses and individual cell keratinization to a varying extent. When the dysplasia is extensive the cells may be indistinguishable from squamous carcinoma cells, yet the infiltrative growth is lacking. Having been recognized as a definitely precarcinomatous stage the term carcinoma *in situ* (intraepithelial carcinoma) has come into use for the most serious degree of dysplasia.

The possible relation of epithelial hyperplasia and dysplasia with cancer, makes a histologic staging of the processes involved essential, but to date a simple and generally accepted classification is missing; it is, however, recognized that the degree of dysplasia should be the most important parameter to stage the disease. The classification of Kleinsasser has the advantage of being simple and corresponds with more descriptive classifications used by most pathologists:

Stage I. Simple epithelial hyperplasia; with or without keratosis.

Stage II. Slight to moderate dysplasia; with or without keratosis.

Stage III. Serious dysplasia; carcinoma *in situ*.

Relation to cancer

The relation of epithelial hyperplasia to cancer has proved difficult to assess. Although many laryngologists prefer to treat the most serious degrees of dysplasia and carcinoma *in situ* as cancer, it is far from certain that a substantial percentage of these cases progress to a real infiltrative carcinoma. Furthermore most cancers of the larynx develop without any previous history of disease of the vocal cords.

Several authors have attempted to assess the natural course of the disease and its relation to cancer [3, 6, 8, 9]. Although the degree of atypia is related to the chance of developing an infiltrative carcinoma the percentage of cases, over a prolonged period, developing cancer is very small. It is therefore doubtful whether any form of radical treatment is justified in these cases. Yet the presence of dysplasia in the laryngeal epithelium should arouse the suspicion of a carcinoma adjacent to the biopsied area or to the future evolution of a cancer.

Treatment

All degrees of epithelial hyperplasia should be treated by microlaryngoscopic removal, if possible of the entire lesion. Serial section of the excised tissue is necessary to assess the histological grade and to exclude the presence of an infiltrating carcinoma. Regular check-ups are necessary to follow the natural course of the disease. When the lesions are still limited a complete cure can be achieved, especially when the patients are prepared to give up smoking. In many cases however, the laryngeal picture will improve but never return to normal.

If definite lesions recur, the treatment should be repeated. When serious dysplasia is repeatedly found on histologic examination more aggressive treatment can be justified. A cordectomy by either microlaryngoscopy or laryngofissure is then the treatment of choice especially in the rapidly recurring squamous papilloma. A total laryngectomy or radiotherapy should be avoided.

References

[1] LUCHSINGER R. & ARNOLD G. E. (1965) *Voice, Speech and Language*. London: Wadworth.

[2] WITHERS B. T. (1961) Vocal nodules *EENT Monthly*, **40**, 35.

[3] KLEINSASSER O. (1976) *Mikrolaryngoskopie und endolaryngeale Mikrochirurgie*. Stuttgart: Schattauer Verlag.

[4] KOSOKOVIC F., CEPELJA I., VECERINA S. & KRAJINA Z. (1974) Experience with Reinke's oedema. *Acta Otolaryngologica* **78**, 150.

[5] RYAN R. G., McDONALD J. R. & DEVINE K. D. (1955) The pathologic effects of smoking on the laryngeal mucosa. *Archives of Pathology* **60**, 472.

[6] NORRIS C. M. & PEALE A. R. (1963) Keratosis of the larynx. *Journal of Laryngology and Otology* **77**, 635.

[7] DELAHUNTY J. E. (1973) Acid laryngitis. *Journal of Laryngology* **86**, 335.

[8] McGAVRAN M. H., BAUER W. C. & OGURA H. H. (1960) Isolated laryngeal keratosis. *Laryngoscope* **70**, 932.

[9] FECHNER R. (1974) Laryngeal keratosis and atypia. *Canadian Journal of Otolaryngology* **3**, 516.

CHAPTER 32

Tumours of the Nose and Sinuses

Most tumour registries keep no formal record of the incidence of benign tumours and the only indication of their frequency in the nose and paranasal sinuses is to be found in accounts of personal series. Not surprisingly, such reports concentrate on malignant epithelial and non-epithelial tumours which represent about 3% of all cancers involving the upper respiratory and alimentary tract and not more than 0·8% of all malignancies. Benign tumours are probably twice as common although this figure varies widely throughout the world.

Unfortunately, there is as yet no generally accepted classification for those tumours which arise within the nasal cavity and paranasal sinuses. Occasionally, they may be grouped together as 'nasal tumours' thus ignoring the essential differences in histopathology and natural history which separates tumours arising within the sinuses from those primarily developing within the nasal air passages. The close anatomical relationship of the paranasal sinuses to the nasal cavity does of course influence the spread of both benign and malignant tumours arising in both areas. However, variations in the incidence, histological types and behaviour of the multitudinous variety of tumours found in both the nasal cavity and sinuses require that these two areas be considered as separate entities.

TUMOURS OF THE NASAL CAVITY

Apart from those tumours which arise from mesenchymal structures, the majority of benign and malignant tumours develop from either:
(1) Pseudostratified columnar epithelium,
(2) Squamous epithelium,
(3) Melanocytes,
(4) Olfactory neuroepithelium [1].

For the purpose of both logic and clarity it is therefore sensible to divide nasal tumours, whether benign or malignant, into two groups based upon an epithelial or non-epithelial origin. Within such a division each anatomical site can then be considered individually.

Epithelial tumours

Adenomas

Although the pseudostratified columnar epithelium is the basic cellular pattern of the nasal epithelium benign adenomas are extremely rare. Ciliated and mucous cells are also seen in the papillary adenocarcinoma, most commonly found in the ethmoidal sinuses and specifically associated with the inhalation of irritant particles of wood dust, nickel or powdered tobacco. This condition will be discussed in detail when considering tumours of the paranasal sinuses.

Papilloma

Although squamous epithelium is not found at birth and in the infant nose, metaplastic foci can develop later in life secondary to chronic infection. Probably the commonest, and certainly the most controversial tumour arising from this squamous epithelium is the papilloma. In the vestibular region of the nose papillomas are similar to those found on squamous epithelium elsewhere in the body. However, within the nasal passages there is more confusion and since these lesions were first described by Bilroth in 1855 over fifty synonyms have been used for what are in general two quite distinct entities. Whether either are true neoplasms or merely a local response to trauma is open to doubt. Certainly, neither bears any direct relationship to allergy or chronic infection as was originally proposed by Ringertz. The exophytic lesion growing from a broad base attached to the nasal septum is a clearly recognized clinical entity. Epistaxis only occurs if there is superficial ulceration; removal with an area of surrounding septal mucosa prevents recurrence.

The controversial inverted papilloma, found almost exclusively on the lateral nasal wall or within the maxillary sinus, poses a greater clinical problem. In contradistinction to septal papilloma this lesion shows epithelial inversion into the underlying stroma on histological examination instead of proliferation outwards in the characteristic manner of other papillomas. These lesions also show microscopic mucous inclusion cysts not usually found in papilloma. Growth is considerable, and the firm, red to grey mass may extend from the anterior nares to nasopharynx. Obstruction is the main symptom though bone erosion from pressure may also be present.

Curiously enough these tumours are invariably unilateral; they have an incidence of around 2% of all nasal and sinus tumours. There is a male predominance of 5 to 1 with a median age of 40 years, though the condition has been seen in a 10 year old. Apart from some confusion over histopathological terminology, the term transitional cell papilloma now appears outmoded unless used to represent a transition between squamous and glandular epithelium. Inverted papilloma present a clinical challenge because it recurs locally. Although there are clear histological similarities between these lesions and papillomas arising in the remainder of the respiratory tract, there is a great difference in natural history possibly because the sinonasal epithelium (or Schneiderian membrane) is ectodermal in origin rather than entodermal as is the rest of the respiratory tract. Inadequate local removal will inevitably be accompanied by recurrence within a year; the maxillary sinus should always be inspected to ensure that it is not involved. Whether malignant change ever takes place is open to doubt although the development of an invasive squamous carcinoma within the same area as an inverted papilloma is well documented, particu-

larly in the elderly patient. The incidence of associated malignancy is usually quoted as around 10% and is a clear indication for histological examination of all papillomas removed from the nose, or indeed elsewhere. Even if the histologically benign papilloma is allowed to grow unrestricted secondary bone erosion may necessitate lateral rhinotomy to ensure adequate removal and also to minimize the risk of undetected associated malignancy. Radiotherapy no longer plays any part in the management of inverted papillomas since it is both ineffective and may induce malignancy. In most patients, intranasal or transantral ethmoidectomy is adequate as a primary procedure. Rapid regrowth, bone erosion or evidence of malignancy indicates a more thorough exploration, preferably by a lateral rhinotomy. It is a common misconception that the histopathologist can predict those papillomas which are likely to recur [2].

Squamous carcinoma

More than half of the primary tumours of the nose are malignant, the majority being squamous carcinoma, although a wide variety of histological types are recorded in the larger series. Nasal septal tumours are uncommon but are often not diagnosed until they are extensive. Since their behaviour is different from those arising in the nasal vestibule these two sites must be considered separately. Although malignant melanoma and basal cell carcinoma both occur in the nasal vestibule squamous carcinoma is the most frequent malignant tumour. This tumour occurs predominantly in men over the age of 60 years; extension into the columella, the floor of the nose or the upper lip indicates an aggressive local growth and is often associated with regional lymph node metastasis, usually to nodes around the facial artery or over the parotid gland. Except in small tumours primary treatment is usually by radiotherapy and almost any technique is successful. With more extensive tumours radiotherapy may still be used though residual disease or uncontrolled lymph node metastasis requires radical resection and possibly reconstruction. Absolute 5-year survival rates of 80% are quoted although the number of patients is small.

Primary carcinoma of the nasal septum

usually arises close to the mucocutaneous junction; the success of treatment is related to tumour size, degree of differentiation and the presence of regional metastases. Malignant lesions in this area are usually friable and bleed easily but can be confused with traumatic ulceration. Treatment may be by radical excision or radiotherapy but metastasis is common and the 5-year cure rate is less than 50%. There appears to be no place for prophylactic neck dissection.

Most squamous carcinomas seen within the nasal cavity arise from the associated paranasal sinuses. However, this tumour can arise from any part of the nasal epithelium although only associated with chronic infection in 10% of cases. Most are found on the lateral wall of the nose and will already have involved maxillary or ethmoidal sinuses on diagnosis.

Malignant melanoma

Until 1972, when melanocytes were demonstrated in the laryngeal mucosa and 2 years later dendritic cells containing melanin within the stroma of the nasal septum and nasal turbinals, there was doubt as to whether primary malignant melanoma occurred within the nasal cavity. This ignored the many authenticated cases of nasal malignant melanoma and the rarity with which metastatic melanoma is found within the nasal passages in patients dying from melanomatosis. Although junctional activity can occur within respiratory epithelium, nasal naevi are rare and it is likely that malignant melanomas in the nose arise directly from pre-existing melanocytes.

All published reports agree that malignant melanomas are rare in the upper respiratory tract. No valid figures are available but probably 2·5% of all melanomas occur in the mouth and respiratory tract, giving an approximate figure of 1% for the nasal passages. Most patients are over the age of 50 years on diagnosis but may be as young as 15 years; the sexes are equally affected. The commonest presenting symptom is unilateral nasal obstruction and epistaxis, for this is a vascular tumour. Not all tumours are pigmented and amelanotic lesions may be misdiagnosed unless intracytoplasmic pigment is sought; pigmentation does not appear to influence prognosis.

Tumours may arise from the nasal septum

(25%) lateral nasal wall or as polyps but bone erosion is uncommon as are regional and systemic metastases.

When planning treatment it is important to appreciate the near impossibility of carrying out a truely radical excision. It is possible that with this tumour, and adenoid cystic carcinoma, the

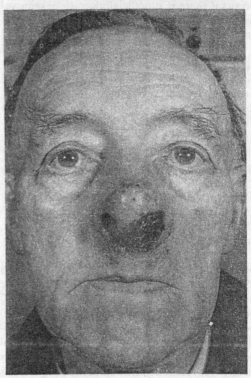

FIG. 32.1. Malignant melanoma involving nasal passages and body of nose. Treated by rhinectomy.

patient's own immunological resistance determines the eventual outcome. The surgeon's role is to remove as much tumour as possible. Radiotherapy appears to have little effect on most mucosal melanomas and merely wastes time. Isolated reports of dramatic resolution suggest either confusion with an anaplastic carcinoma or perhaps reflect the unpredictable nature of this disease.

Removal of the whole nasal mucosa by a lateral rhinotomy approach or total rhinectomy if the nose itself is involved (Fig. 32.1) reduces tumour bulk to a minimum. If regional metastases are present individual lymph nodes should be removed but radical neck dissection, whether prophylactic or curative, is not indicated.

Since it is our aim to stimulate the patient's immunological defences to destroy residual or undetected melanoma, systemic chemotherapy appears undesirable because of the risk of immunosuppression. However, intra-lesional BCG may prove effective in controlling local regrowth. Surgery may have three sequelae. The patient may die within a few weeks, from melanomatosis; no further melanomas may appear although follow up must continue for the remainder of the patient's life; or there may be local regrowth but without regional or systemic metastasis – a state of symbiosis. It is this group who may be helped by immunostimulation.

Recent reports indicate a 5-year survival rate of 30% although the 3-year figure is almost 50% [3]. These figures compare unfavourably with skin melanoma where a 5-year rate of 80% is reported in the absence of lymph node involvement.

Olfactory neuroblastoma

This is the term most widely accepted for malignant tumours arising from the olfactory sensory epithelium. The tumour was first recorded in 1924 and is uncommon, only 160 cases having been recorded since. It is now accepted that the tumour is neuroectodermal in origin and in most patients arises high in the roof of the nose on the lateral wall close to the ethmoidal labyrinth. There appears to be a slight preponderance of men but the age of diagnosis is spread evenly through all decades from 10–70.

The neoplasm is composed of nerve cells (neurocytes and neuroblasts), and although the histological pattern may vary there appears to be no rationale for subdividing the tumours into varying types since there is no evidence that this influences either management or prognosis.

The presenting symptoms are common to most intranasal neoplasms with obstruction, headaches and often severe epistaxis, for the tumour is extremely vascular. Grossly, the tumour is seen as a polypoidal mass, reddish-grey in colour and usually firm in consistency although this may be variable within the same tumour. Diagnosis is made on histological exam-

ination and additional confirmation obtained by assays of urinary and plasma catecholamines including dopamine, noradrenaline, adrenaline and 3-methoxy-4-hydroxy mandelic acid (VMA). All or some will be raised and catecholamines can be detected in biopsy material on electron microscopy.

At one time this neoplasm was considered as being only locally malignant but this is far from the truth for regional or systemic metastasis occur in over 25% of patients. However, a combination of radical surgery (at least a lateral rhinotomy) with radiotherapy can expect to produce a 5-year cure rate of 33% [4] and if patients surviving 5 years with disease still present are included, a survival rate of 50%.

The prime causes of death are systemic or regional metastasis and intracranial extension of residual tumour. It is possible that more effective surgical resection of the primary lesion combined with postoperative radiotherapy and possibly chemotherapy (mechlorethamine hydrochloride) may improve the long-term survival.

Non-epithelial tumours

It is perhaps surprising that malignant mesenchymal tumours comprise only about 10% of all malignant tumours arising in the nose and sinuses. Benign lesions are undoubtedly commoner if this definition is widened to include such conditions as juvenile angiofibroma. Despite the relative rarity of these tumours all mesenchymal tissues can be the origin of benign or malignant tumours; since many are exceedingly rare discussion will be limited to those seen most frequently or whose origin is primarily within the nasal cavity. Vascular tumours may develop anywhere in the lining of the nose and are probably the commonest benign tumours.

Haemangiomas

The 'bleeding polyp of the septum', a polypoidal or sessile nodular mass growing most frequently from the anterior end of the nasal septum, is probably a *capillary haemangioma*. The lesion is rare before puberty and produces both nasal obstruction and epistaxis – usually secondary to surface ulceration. Limited excision may lead to local recurrence unless a cuff of mucoperichondrium is removed around the base of the tumour.

Cavernous haemangiomas are more usually found on the lateral nasal wall, particularly the middle and inferior turbinals. When small they can be excised after preliminary cryosurgery but extensive tumours may require radiotherapy or even radical surgery.

Angiosarcoma

Angiosarcoma is the malignant counterpart of the benign haemangiomas and can be differentiated clinically by its tendency to invade. There is a greater likelihood of these tumours developing during childhood and although metastasis appears to be extremely uncommon, control of the local condition is frequently impossible with reported 10-year survival figures of less than 15%.

Although there is now ample evidence that juvenile angiofibroma arises from the posterior part of the nasal cavity, many people still think of this benign lesion as a primary tumour of the nasopharynx. This tumour and its management are described in Chapter 24.

Haemangiopericytomas

The haemangiopericytoma, which possesses a widespread distribution, is frequently found in the head and neck region (25%). This is a tumour of pericytic cells which are normally found surrounding capillaries; histologically it is both complex and variable causing difficulties in diagnosis and management. In the nasal cavity symptoms are related to the site and size of the tumour but obstruction and epistaxis are common. Growth is usually rapid but the clinical features, including vascularity, are too variable to predict with certainty. Diagnosis is only made after histological examination of biopsy material and initial treatment is usually radiotherapy unless the tumour is readily accessible to radical removal. An overall 5-year cure rate of 50% is quoted for all sites when treated by primary resection. Only a small number of patients with this tumour arising from the nasal cavity have been reported and combined surgery and radio-

therapy would appear to offer the best prospect of long-term palliation [5].

Cartilaginous tumours

Benign cartilaginous tumours arising from the nasal septum, cartilages or ethmoidal labyrinth grow slowly and project into the lumen of the nasal cavity or nasopharynx. They are uncommon and unpredictable regarding their rate of growth and risk of recurrence. Differentiation from *chondrosarcoma* may be obvious on clinical grounds but histologically *chondromas* demonstrate well differentiated hyaline cartilage, most cells showing single small nuclei. Despite this, wide surgical removal is necessary to avoid local recurrence since there is a suggestion that repeated recurrence may predispose to the development of chondrosarcoma. The latter is extremely uncommon in both the maxilla and the nasal cavity though it behaves like an osteogenic sarcoma. Histological assessment of malignancy in cartilagenous tumours depends on finding mitoses, double nuclei and pleomorphism. Both chondromas and chondrosarcoma occur in the second to fourth decades. In the established malignant tumour clinical differentiation presents little difficulty though even combinations of radical surgery and radiotherapy offer little prospect of long-term survival. High recurrence rates with aggressive local extension is frequently associated with pulmonary metastasis.

Peripheral nerve tumours

Benign tumours
Benign tumours originating from nerve sheaths are found throughout the body and occur occasionally within the nasal cavity. In general they are solitary and grow slowly being called *schwannomas* rather than neurofibromas [6]. Clinically they cannot be differentiated from other solid, non-vascular benign nasal tumours but should be removed completely either via an intranasal approach if small or a lateral rhinotomy if large (Fig. 32.2).

Malignant tumours
Malignant nerve tumours are rare and lethal. *Nasal gliomas* are not tumours at all but hetero-

topic brain tissue; their similarity to benign nasal tumours justifies their inclusion in this section.

The first description of a nasal glioma was in 1852 but only a 100 cases had been reported by 1966. Most appear shortly after birth, 60% being extranasal and 30% purely intranasal. The latter

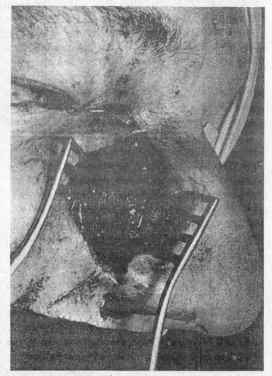

FIG. 32.2. Lateral rhinotomy approach to intranasal schwannomas.

are often mistaken for a nasal polyp and may displace the septum or nasal bones. Avulsion is accompanied by a flow of cerebrospinal fluid for the glioma has the same type of origin as an encephalocoele. From the third to the fifth embryonal week the posterior neuropore is open, being connected to the nasal cavity by an epithelial core. Herniation of the brain can occur along this track and if the meninges close behind the herniation an isolated mass of brain tissue is left in the nose. If the bony opening fails to close a small defect is left in the cribriform plate although this is rarely detected radiologically in reported cases with nasal gliomas.

It has been suggested that such gliomas are a

bridge between a purely anatomical defect and low-grade neoplasia. Recurrence after removal has been reported and growth may be unexpectedly rapid. Invasion or metastasis does not occur and histologically these masses are composed of brain tissue in which there is a significant gliosis, although the term glioma is really inappropriate.

It is rarely possible to differentiate gliomas in the nose from meningocoeles or encephalocoeles with a direct communication intracranially. These tumours grow slowly and, in the absence of spontaneous or induced cerebrospinal rhinorrhoea or gross external deformity, there is no great hurry to remove them. A diagnostic craniotomy is frequently indicated to determine the presence or absence of intracranial connections for failure to remove the mass completely may lead to regrowth. Intracranial extensions cannot be reached transnasally with safety. Most operations appear to be carried out when the child is between 5 and 10 years old [7].

Malignant lymphoma

Although malignant lymphomas localized to the nose or paranasal sinuses are uncommon, making up less than 10% of all malignant tumours seen at these sites, early diagnosis and treatment can result in a favourable long-term cure rate. Only 10% of those patients with generalized disease present with sinonasal lymphoma although no reliable information is at present available regarding the frequency of primary and secondary lymphomas in the head and neck [8].

Most malignant lymphomas seen in the sinonasal region are reticulum cell sarcomas (diffuse histocytic and stem cell types). When occurring in the maxillary or ethmoidal sinuses these tumours produce symptoms indistinguishable from the far commoner squamous carcinomas. When they occur in the nasal cavity alone, however, their granular appearance combined with local tissue invasion and destruction may lead to a diagnosis of midline granuloma or Wegener's granulomatosis. This is not entirely surprising since there is now ample evidence that the former lesion may well be a well controlled malignant lymphoma [9]. Wegener's granulomatosis is of course a completely different condition.

Surgery should be limited to obtaining a biopsy (which may be difficult) or providing temporary drainage in extensive sinus disease. A thorough clinical and haematological examination is essential and will probably include abdominal lymphangiography. In the absence of systemic disease or cervical lymph node metastasis, curative dosages of radiotherapy can expect to produce a 5-year survival rate of about 70% although there have been reports of delayed recurrence as late as 21 years after treatment. The effectiveness of multiple chemotherapy in systemic lymphomas may lead to its use even in the localized disease.

Plasmacytoma

Eighty per cent of extramedullary plasmacytomas occur in the head and neck. Once again symptoms of unilateral nasal obstruction, rhinorrhoea and epistaxis are caused by a bulky tumour mass. The more aggressive the tumour the softer and more friable it becomes, usually with evidence of underlying bone destruction. Occasionally, this tumour may be a manifestation of multiple myeloma but more frequently it is a primary plasmacytoma of soft tissue.

Ninety per cent of patients are over the age of 40 years with a male predominance of 2:1. Cervical lymph node involvement is uncommon and probably does not effect the prognosis. However, it has been suggested that some primary plasmocytomata are in fact undetected diffuse myelomatosis even though skeletal surveys and laboratory investigations, including bone marrow studies, are normal. Response to radiotherapy is variable but should be the initial form of treatment for both nasal and paranasal sinus tumours. Subsequent excision may be needed for residual or recurrent disease. A determinate 5-year survival rate of about 50% can be expected although published series are small and this tumour has an incidence of less than 5% of all sinonasal tumours [10].

Uncommon tumours

Many other uncommon tumours arise within the nasal cavity from mesenchymal elements such as muscle and fibrous tissue. Diagnosis is rarely made on clinical grounds and biopsy is essential. Differentiation between benign *fibromas* and the exceedingly malignant *fibrosarcoma* is obviously of great importance since the latter has a 5-year survival rate of less than 30%. In general most nasal tumours produce nasal obstruction, discharge and often epistaxis. Even benign lesions if allowed to grow will cause widening of the nasal framework from pressure alone. Malignant tumours invade surrounding structures such as the orbit and maxillary sinus. Examination under anaesthesia permits both assessment of tumour site and the taking of an adequate biopsy for both light and electron microscopy but interpretation of the latter may, however, require the aid of histopathologists particularly experienced in tumours of the head and neck.

TUMOURS OF THE PARANASAL SINUSES

Benign tumours arising within the nasal sinuses are uncommon, forming less that one-third of all tumours found in this region. A rigid definition of benign tumour and thus excluding odontogenic cysts, giant cell tumours and dermoids would reduce this figure to about 20%.

Benign epithelial tumours are extremely rare and are usually discovered accidentally. By far the commonest benign lesions found in the antroethmoidal and frontal sinuses arise from non-epithelial tissue. The lack of ready access to these sinuses and the dependence upon radiological assessment to determine site and extent, results in late diagnosis.

Osseous and fibro-osseous lesions

Osteoma
Although there is still considerable controversy and some confusion regarding fibro-osseous conditions affecting the cranio-facial region, osteomas are the commonest benign tumours found in the paranasal sinuses. Routine radiology of the frontal sinuses shows evidence of osteomas in at least 1% of all patients and this is certainly the commonest site of origin followed by ethmoidal, maxillary and rarely, the sphenoi-

dal sinus. Large tumours can produce an external deformity but smaller growths are associated with headaches, facial pain and occasionally chronic infection. Radiological examination shows the typically sharply defined radio-opaque calcified mass but not always the site of attachment (Fig. 32.3).

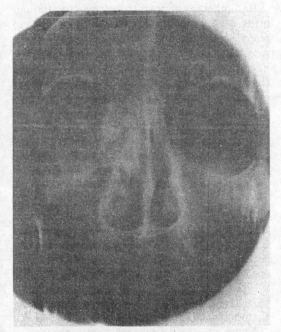

FIG. 32.3. Solitary osteoma involving left ethmoidal sinus.

Biopsy is not usually technically feasible but examination after removal shows these tumours to be either 'ivory', composed of hard, dense compact bone, or 'spongy' where a periphery of compact bone surrounds a cancellous lamellar centre and a mixture of the two types. Growth is always slow but growth rate and the incidence do appear to be greater in Arabs.

There are many theories of the aetiology of these tumours, the most popular being that of Fetissof who suggested that they arose from persistent embryonal periosteum, particular in areas where endochondral and membranous bones meet, i.e. at the junction of frontal and ethmoidal bones. Trauma or sepsis may stimulate such rests into activity and certainly most osteomas arise from a single pedicle which may fragment spon-

taneously allowing the tumour to sequestrate into nose or sinus cavity.

Treatment is only indicated if the patient has symptoms which can be attributed to the tumour but, of course, the smaller the osteoma the easier it is to remove. If the sinus cavity is completely filled with bone then the point of attachment may be difficult to find and fragmentation is necessary to avoid damage to the orbital floor or anterior cranial fossa. Regrowth may occur if the site of attachment is not completely removed; the site of attachment frequently proves to be in the immediate vicinity of centres of primary or secondary ossification.

It is important to bear in mind the association of cranio-facial osteomas, soft tissue tumours (sebaceous cysts and subcutaneous fibromas) and colonic polyposis found in *Gardner's syndrome*. This is an inherited systemic defect transmitted by an autosomal dominant gene; the mandible is the commonest site of the osteomas but all sinuses can be effected [11]. All the colonic polyps become malignant if untreated.

Fibrous dysplasia

Fibrous dysplasia is a term first used by Lichtenstein in 1938 to define a group of bony lesions previously called ossifying fibroma, fibrous osteoma; in fact over 35 synonyms had been used up to 1945. This condition constitutes 2·5% of all bony neoplasms and 7% of benign bony tumours but it is doubtful whether it is a developmental abnormality or simply a reaction to trauma. However, many bone pathologists use the term fibro-osseous lesions to cover a group of widely differing conditions ranging from a local monostotic focus found primarily in the maxilla to the diffuse polyostotic lesions of Albright's syndrome. Most patients with lesions confined to the maxilla do not have endocrine disorders or other bony lesions. Typically the disorder develops during the first two decades of life with painless facial swelling, deformity of the alveolar margin, perhaps with loosening of the teeth (Fig. 32.4) and occasionally nasal obstruction. Radiology is not conclusive but allows differentiation from osteogenic sarcomas. Histological examination of the often soft bone shows a mixture of fibrous and osseous tissue with the former predominating. Assuming that the biopsy is representative of the whole tumour the dysplasia may vary from an unusually active fibroma to virtually mature bone. More active forms are usually seen in the younger patient and with increasing age the connective matrix becomes more mature, with few mitoses and increasingly prominent bone component. The tumour stabilizes when the child stops growing.

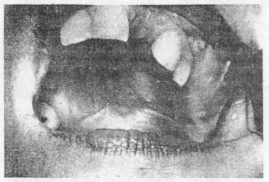

FIG. 32.4. Deformity of alveolar margin and palate from fibro-osseous dysplasia.

Unless these patients are irradiated there is no evidence that malignancy occurs and small localized areas should be left alone. If there is gross deformity the bone can be trimmed for cosmetic reasons, to enable dentures to be fitted or if the orbit is threatened. Major remodelling should be left until growth has ceased.

Osteogenic sarcoma

Although it is the commonest malignant tumour of bone, osteogenic sarcoma is a rare tumour and less than 7% are found in the jaws, the maxilla less often than the mandible. An incidence of less than 0·07 patients per 100 000 is quoted for the United States. The average age at diagnosis is about 30 years, which is older than when this tumour arises in the long bones. Apart from cases where the tumour is secondary to irradiation or associated with pre-existing Paget's disease, delay in diagnosis is only a few months since growth is rapid and often painful. Swelling of the face, loosened teeth, trismus and nasal obstruction are common symptoms but tomography invariably reveals extensive bony involvement though rarely pulmonary metastases. Radiological appearances are only characteristic of a pri-

mary bony tumour in 25% of patients and the so called 'sun-ray' appearance is rarely seen in the maxilla. Histological variants are common and appear to be unrelated to the prognosis [12]. The malignant supportive tissue is capable of producing osteoid and bone, the relative amounts vary within the same tumour, and may even produce cartilage.

Radiotherapy appears to be ineffective though often used to avoid the mutilation of radical resection. If the local disease can be effectively resected then the prognosis depends upon the likelihood of pulmonary metastases. Radical surgery is now followed by prophylactic courses of the cytotoxic agent Adriamycin which has proved useful as adjuvant therapy with long bone sarcoma. At present a 5-year survival rate of 25% is the best that can be expected but this may relate more to the extent of the primary disease than to the risk of pulmonary metastasis.

Ameloblastoma

The ameloblastoma is a locally invasive epithelial tumour with histological features bearing some resemblance to that of the enamel organ of the tooth germ. Although representing less than 0·1% of all tumours of the paranasal sinuses the mandible is affected five times more frequently than the maxilla and is easier to treat.

There are conflicting views as to the site of origin of the tumour; the histological appearances can be variable and may be confused with basal cell or adenoid cystic carcinoma. Growth is slow and, by extension into marrow spaces, produces resorption of bone at the growing edge. Consequently, the tumour is usually more extensive than appears on radiological assessment.

Symptoms are similar to those of other tumours affecting the maxilla although delay in diagnosis may be many months. This is a benign but locally invasive tumour and both radiotherapy and local resection are followed by regrowth of residual disease except in the unusually radiosensitive case. The early tumour should be resected widely with clear margins and this may eventually become necessary even in advanced tumours treated conservatively, for the natural history of this tumour is one of slow progressive local growth.

Myxomas

In 1971 Virchow used the term myxomas to describe a group of tumours that he thought histologically resembled the mucinous substance of the umbilical cord. Although this term was initially misused it is a clearly defined entity being a true neoplasm of mesenchymal origin which is locally invasive but does not metatasize. These tumours occur throughout the head and neck, particularly in the maxillary sinus, but are relatively rare. Macroscopically the myxoma is of variable consistency depending on the degree of fibrosis. The surface is slimy, mucoid and pale; growth is slow but locally invasive. By developing within the marrow of the maxilla the tumour produces a bony deformity like that of an ameloblastoma. Histological differentiation from more aggressive tumours is important, particularly from the sarcomas; local recurrence is only avoided by wide local excision with an adequate margin of normal bone for the tumour has a 'false capsule'.

Carcinoma of the paranasal sinuses

Pathology

Malignant tumours arising from the mucosal lining of the nasal sinuses make up less than 1% of all malignancies, only 3% of head and neck malignancies and approximately 15% of all neoplasms arising in the upper respiratory tract. Over 80% are squamous carcinomas with about 8% adenocarcinomas and a similar number of adenoid cystic tumours. Most occur within the antroethmoid complex where the close anatomical relationship between these two sinuses ensures rapid extension of tumours from one to the other. However, there is a definite variation in the natural history of all three tumours and considerable evidence associating ethmoidal adenocarcinomas with inhalation of irritant dust.

Adenocarcinoma

Whereas both squamous and adenoid cystic carcinomas most often occur in the maxillary antrum, adenocarcinoma invariably starts in the ethmoidal cells though eventually extending into the antrum. A high incidence of this tumour was reported from Oxford in 1965 where 49% of all paranasal sinus cancers were adenocarcinomas, almost all arising from the ethmoidal labyrint. This unusual incidence was directly related to a nearby woodworking industry and exposure to wood dust has now been confirmed as an aetiological factor in Belgium, Holland, Denmark, France and Australia. The main components of timber – cellulose, hemicellulose and lignin – are non-irritant and non-sensitizing. Minor components such as resins, terpenes and oils may cause contact dermatitis but wood irritants are mostly contained in the sap, and sensitizers in the heartwood. As yet the source of the carcinogen is unknown, but obviously there is a risk similar to that found in workers in the nickel industry. Squamous metaplasia has been found on the middle turbinate of workers exposed to nickel dust where an increased risk of respiratory tract neoplasia has been recognized for many years. However, the latent period for individuals exposed to wood dust and subsequently developing adenocarcinomas is around 30 years and working conditions must have been very different at that time.

Treatment with a combination of radiotherapy and radical surgery gives a 3-year cure rate of 50% compared with an expected 20% for squamous carcinoma. Certainly, adenocarcinomas carry a better prognosis than other sinus cancers although it has been suggested that death occurs at 7 years thereby giving an inflated 5-year figure. The finding of residual disease in the region of the cribriform plate is probably an indication for craniofacial resection in view of the relatively slow rate of growth of this tumour which presents early and in high risk industries should be detected and treated radically.

Adenoid cystic carcinoma

Adenoid cystic carcinoma (originally called cylindroma by Bilroth in 1859), however, arises from minor salivary glands and, although slow-growing, extends insidiously along the perineural sheaths. The maxillary antrum is the commonest site but management anywhere in the nasal cavity and paranasal sinuses is frustrated by an inability to resect the tumour effectively to include undetectable extensions. However, there appears to be some degree of immunological tolerance, for solitary pulmonary metastases may remain the same size for years and the primary tumour is usually extremely slow growing. Five-year survival rates are reported as between 5 and 10% which amply illustrates the seriousness of these tumours.

Squamous carcinoma

The majority of neoplasms arising within the maxillary and ethmoidal sinuses are squamous carcinomas: there may be some relationship between the development of neoplasia and chronic sinusitis. The long-term latent carcinogenic effect of residual thorium dioxide, a substance which was at one time used in diagnostic radiology, in the maxillary sinus has been recorded. However, it is doubtful if the relationship between the common sinus infections and the rare sinus neoplasms is any more significant than is the high incidence of middle ear disease in patients developing squamous carcinoma of the ear. Failure to cure more than 25% of sinus cancers is not due to any intrinsic mortality in this tumour but is related almost entirely to the advanced stage of the disease at diagnosis. Cure is almost directly related to the amount of extension into surrounding tissues; attempts have been made to document the latter for the purpose of classification and comparisons of treatment. Unfortunately, the ability to determine the exact extent of invasion of the tumour before operation is limited even with the aid of sophisticated radiological techniques. Retrospective classification after radical surgery frequently reveals unexpected extensions although pre-operative radiotherapy may confuse even this evaluation. Gross bony destruction of the orbit, pterygoid plates or bony walls, together with careful clinical examination, does enable many patients to be placed in the relatively broad classification suggested by Sisson *et al.* [13]. Few patients are diagnosed when the disease is confined to the maxillary antrum although the ethmoidal sinus neoplasm with its early symptoms of nasal obstruction and epistaxis may present relatively early. Extension outside the bony walls of the antrum is common but the actual extent is difficult to determine although it influences the final T grading and prognosis.

The use of hypothetical division lines to separate the maxillary and ethmoidal sinuses into supra, meso and infrastructure certainly reflects the seriousness of tumours involving the suprastructure but again suffers from an inherent difficulty in translating a three-dimensional disease into a two dimensional drawing. The histology of the tumour is not considered and is a defect in most staging systems. Fortunately, cervical lymph node metastases are uncommon even in advanced tumours when tissues with rich lymphatic supply, such as the facial skin, are involved.

Symptoms and signs

The symptoms of a carcinoma of the maxillary sinus may be orbital, nasal, facial or dental. Orbital symptoms are proptosis, diplopia and epiphora; nasal symptoms include blood-stained nasal discharge rather than frank epistaxis and obstruction due to the presence of a large polypoid mass; facial symptoms include swelling, numbness and pain and the dental symptoms are ulceration of the alveolus and loosening of the teeth if these are present, which is uncommon. The relative incidence of these symptoms is shown in Table 32.1 [14].

Examination

The following areas must always be examined – the nose, the nasopharynx, the mouth, the eye, the face and the neck. Depending on the main site of origin, examination of the nose often shows a friable mass filling the greater part of the nasal cavity; such a mass can also often be seen in the posterior choana when the nasopharynx is examined. Examination of the mouth shows ulceration of the alveolus or the superior buccoalveolar sulcus if the tumour arises in the lower part of the antrum; the latter area should always be palpated with a finger to assess if the tumour has broken through the anterior wall of the antrum. Whilst examining the mouth, the hard palate should be assessed for loss of sensation indicating involvement of the greater palatine nerve in the greater palatine canal. The face should be examined for swelling and for numbness indicating involvement of the infra-orbital nerve in its canal. The eye should be examined for diplopia in all positions of gaze and for prop-

Table 32.1. Incidence of presenting symptoms of a carcinoma of the maxillary sinus. Reproduced, with permission, from Lederman M. (1970) Tumours of the upper jaw: natural history and treatment. *Journal of Laryngology and Otology* **84**, 388.

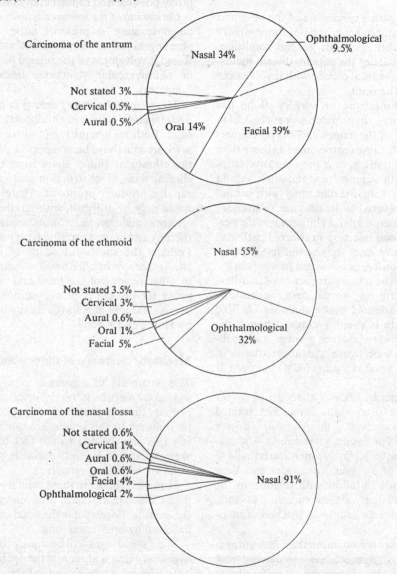

Carcinoma of the antrum

- Nasal 34%
- Ophthalmological 9.5%
- Facial 39%
- Oral 14%
- Aural 0.5%
- Cervical 0.5%
- Not stated 3%

Carcinoma of the ethmoid

- Nasal 55%
- Ophthalmological 32%
- Facial 5%
- Oral 1%
- Aural 0.6%
- Cervical 3%
- Not stated 3.5%

Carcinoma of the nasal fossa

- Nasal 91%
- Ophthalmological 2%
- Facial 4%
- Oral 0.6%
- Aural 0.6%
- Cervical 1%
- Not stated 0.6%

tosis; this examination should be carried out by an ophthalmologist to detect early degrees of involvement of the orbit. Finally the neck should be examined for enlarged lymph nodes.

Investigations

In addition to the routine investigations such as blood tests and chest radiographs, plain films, tomograms and possibly orthopantomograms should be taken of the sinuses. The patient should almost always be seen by an ophthalmologist (as outlined above) and by an oral surgeon who will take preliminary impressions from which a dental obturator will later be fashioned.

Treatment

Most patients with a carcinoma of the nose and sinuses are treatable but criteria of inoperability include advanced age, poor general condition, refusal on the part of the patient, distant metastases and massive local disease with involvement of the base of the skull.

Neither radiotherapy or surgery alone has proved to be more than moderately successful in treating cancer of the sinuses and it is now generally accepted, in those centres treating more than the occasional patient, that pre-operative curative dosage with supravoltage radiation should be followed by total maxillectomy with orbital clearance if required or in the case of primary ethmoidal cancer, a lateral rhinotomy with perhaps cranio-facial resection in selected patients.

Published cure rates vary somewhat depending upon the number of advanced tumours in the series and also the relative frequency of undifferentiated squamous carcinomas, adenocarcinomas and adenoid cystic tumours. A 30% 5-year cure rate is about average although the larger series tend to produce a lower, and probably more realistic figure. Adenocarcinoma of the ethmoid is good at 5 years (40%) but poor at 10 years (15%).

A recent paper by Sakai *et al.* reporting 3-year figures for maxillary sinus carcinoma treated with irradiation and 5-fluorouracil, surgery being reserved for failure, gives nearly 40% survivors for 80 patients [15]. No mention is made of the incidence of systemic metastases and their paper is difficult to follow with relation to the extent and histology of these tumours. It does, however, suggest an additional method of management.

Although uncommon, more than fifty authenticated cases of *frontal sinus carcinomas* have been recorded, many presenting primarily as mucocoeles [16]. Radiological evidence of bone destruction is present in over 60% of carcinomas at this site and is far in excess of that expected in mucocoeles. Sclerosis is also seen and may cause confusion with fibrous dysplasia, Paget's disease or chronic osteomyelitis. Extension into the sinus by tumours arising in the ethmoidal sinuses or the orbital lobe of the lacrimal gland is not uncommon but irrespective of whether it be primary or secondary invasion, radical resection is rarely possible and radiotherapy unsuccessful.

Carcinoma of the sphenoidal sinus is difficult to diagnose since it presents either as a nasopharyngeal or as a posterior nasal tumour. Rapid involvement of the related pituitary gland or neurovascular structures leads to severe symptoms.

Mesenchymal tumours arising in the maxillary and ethmoidal sinuses in childhood are invariably fatal. Both malignant lymphomas and rhabdomyosarcomas have been reported, particularly in the ethmoidal sinus; apart from the expected clinical signs of obstruction and epistaxis they rapidly produce proptosis. Histological diagnosis may be difficult without the aid of the electron microscope. Combinations of radiotherapy and limited excision have proved useless. Perhaps the successful usage of combination chemotherapy in childhood tumours occurring in other regions of the head and neck may improve the present hopeless outlook, and 5-year survival rates of 25% have recently been reported by Horch and Koch [17].

Metastatic carcinoma of the sino-nasal region

The possibility of a metastasis to the nose or paranasal sinuses is rarely considered because primary tumours are much more likely. Metastatic tumours to this region are rarely recognized but this may be due to the fact that complete skeletal surveys are not routine in patients with bone metastasizing cancers.

However, there are three primary sites of neoplasia which metastasize with some frequency to the maxilla. Foremost is the renal cell carcinoma followed by breast and lung.

The clinical signs will be similar to those found in primary sinus cancer and the age incidence will not differ markedly except in lung cancer which affects a somewhat younger age group. The marked vascularity of secondary renal carcinoma results in epistaxis being a frequent symptom and it is not uncommon for this metastasis to be detected before the primary tumour is suspected. Apart from renal carcinoma, the prognosis for patients with secondary neoplasia in the sinuses is the same as for carcinomatosis and diagnosis is made histologically rather than clinically. However, renal-cell carcinoma is unpredictable in behaviour and only 15% present with classical symptoms of haematuria, pain and a palpable mass. Treatment before metastasis gives a 5-year survival of over 60% but this drops to about a 2-year average survival once distant spread is discovered. Despite this, if the maxillary sinus is the only detectable metastasis then removal of primary and radical resection of the secondary has resulted in an occasional long-term survival [18].

NON-HEALING GRANULOMAS OF THE NOSE

It has long been recognized that a number of granulomatous destructive conditions occur within the nasal passages. Despite conspicuous differences in natural history and clinical behaviour these conditions have erroneously been grouped under the one heading 'non-healing granulomas'. Although attempts have been made to relate specific histopathological features to clinical entities considerable confusion and disagreement remains, largely due to the difficulties of obtaining representative biopsy material and the relative rarity of the condition.

In-depth studies of a large group of these patients by Harrison [19], and a unique histo-pathological study by Michaels and Gregory [20], have clearly established that there are most probably two different clinical conditions which may affect the nose. Their histopathology is quite different and so is the clinical management and possibly prognosis.

Malignant granuloma

Non-healing or malignant granuloma is a slowly progressing destructive ulceration of the tissues of the nose, sinuses, or occasionally pharynx. Soft tissues, bone and cartilage are eventually destroyed by a chronic inflammatory process leading to severe mutilation. If the condition remains uncontrolled, death from cachexia, hae-morrhage, or intercurrent infection occurs sooner or later (Fig. 32.5). McBride [21] is usually credited with the first description of this condition though this seems to have been based primarily on the failure of a pathologist to find evidence of either syphilis or tuberculosis in tissue removed at a subsequent necropsy.

The first clear account was published by Robert Woods [22] in 1921 when he aptly described the lesion as a 'wave of granulation tissue advancing irregularly into healthy parts, breaking down behind as it advanced in front, so that there was never any great depth of pathological growth present'. The term 'malignant granuloma' was suggested by his colleague Dr. O'Sullivan. In 1933 Stewart [23] published a detailed account of both clinical and histological features of the localized disease, but no better evaluation of the pathological features of granulomas can be found than that presented by Friedmann [24] in his Semon lecture of 1971. Nevertheless, persistent attempts to relate clinical manifestations to the histological appearances of often unrepresentative biopsy specimens have resulted in some degree of confusion ever since.

In essence the clinical behaviour is similar to that of a neoplasm, whose rate of growth has been accentuated to a varying degree by the individual's own immunological defences. Rate of destruction certainly varies considerably from patient to patient and there have been reports of patients dying with systemic metastases– usually malignant lymphomas. This proposition has now been confirmed by Michaels and Gregory who found common histological features in ten patients with a clinical diagnosis of 'midline granuloma' – widespread necrosis and atypical cells, collectively termed NACE (necrosis with atypical cellular exudate). The cytological features of these cells were such as to suggest malignancy and they believe that this neoplasm is a histiocytic lymphoma. Four of these patients had similar metastases in lymph nodes, although none had a classical lymphoma in the original nasal biopsy.

Because of the considerable necrosis and infection, there may be difficulty in obtaining adequate representative biopsy material. However, reports of non-specific inflammatory changes only are no longer acceptable, particularly if these changes are accompanied by considerable necrosis; further biopsies should be carried out.

Occasionally, local destruction is extremely

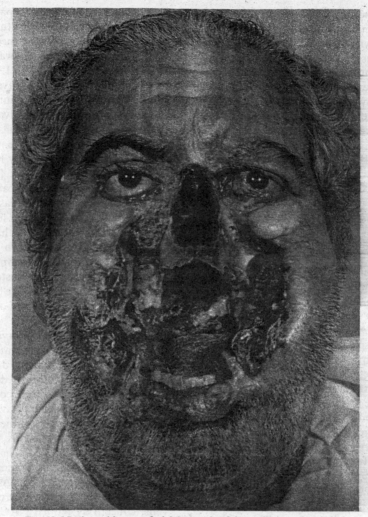

FIG. 32.5 Patient with severe facial destruction from malignant granuloma.

slow at first with any subsequent increase in rate being related to the appearance of a definite malignant lymphoma. Such patients may respond well to non-curative dosage of radiotherapy if treated at an early stage. In theory this condition, perhaps best called non-healing granuloma, should be treated with curative dosage of radiotherapy to both primary and regional lymph nodes on the assumption that this is in reality a histiocytic lymphoma. Many radiotherapists, however, may require a definitive histological report, which in many of the

more fortunate patients will not be available, before giving full tumouricidal dosage. It is usually sensible to follow radiotherapy, whatever the dosage, by local surgery to remove residual necrotic tissue (Fig. 32.6).

Dosage with steroids is not indicated and must be considered harmful in this condition for depressing the patient's immunological competence could accentuate tumour growth. The resulting deformity following disease control is best overcome with a purpose-built prosthesis rather than elaborate rehabilitative surgery.

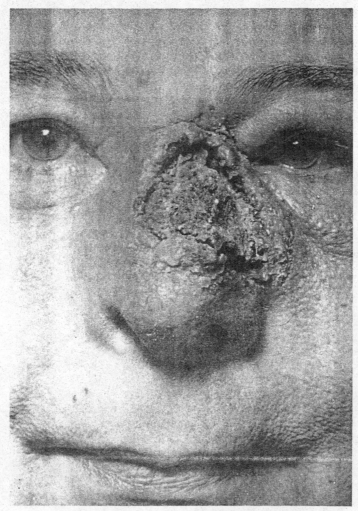

FIG. 32.6. Bone and skin necrosis following curative radiotherapy for a non-healing granuloma of left nose.

Wegener's granulomatosis

In 1939 Wegener [25] described three cases of another necrotizing granuloma which also affected the nose but which was associated with more lethal lesions in lung and kidneys. Good-man and Churg [26] 18 years later characterized the pathological features of this condition as: necrotizing granulomatous lesions in the upper and lower respiratory tract; generalized focal necrotizing vasculitis involving both arteries and veins, almost always in the lungs and more or less widely disseminated in other sites; glomerulitis characterized by necrosis and thrombosis of

loops of the capillary tufts, capsular adhesion, and development as a granulomatous lesion.

There are quite clear clinical and histological differences between this condition and the loca-lized non-healing granuloma. Onset of Wegener's granulomatosis is usually insidious with non-specific symptoms of infection in the respiratory tract. Constitutional upset is quite out of proportion to the severity of the local lesion, and the patient seeks advice initially because of malaise, fever or weakness [27]. Until recently the course of the disease was rapid, pro-gressing to death within 6 months from renal failure [28, 29]. Pathologically the disease is

left on this reduced dosage to test the significance of this finding for there is no guarantee that control will be possible on a second occasion.

The dangers inherent in long-term cytotoxic and corticosteroid therapy are well known and need no comment. Even the risk of sterility or genetic damage to children born of our younger patients cannot be ignored. Yet we can now increase the survival period of these patients from 6 months to many years, though with only their general condition and ESR to guide us in determining dosage. Even when it is possible to reduce therapy to minimal levels the risk of a sudden uncontrolled relapse remains and as yet this is a risk I am not prepared to take. It seems therefore that until satisfactory evidence of the action of these drugs is available and the means by which we can reliably monitor this action, each patient must be maintained on the dosage just sufficient to keep the ESR within normal limits and the clinical state as normal as possible. Awareness of the potential dangers of both the cytotoxic drug and corticosteroids used and the means to remedy any side effects are vital, and these patients need to be under the care of people experienced in the management of such problems.

Long-term follow-up of patients who have survived an initial 2 years following diagnosis reveal a number dying eventually from renal failure secondary to infection in their damaged kidneys which no longer possess reserves of function. The possibility of preventing this second phase tragedy by early renal transplantation may well offer selected patients with Wegener's granulomatosis the prospect of near normal expectation of life.

References

[1] MICHAELS L. & HYAMS V. J. (1975) Objectivity in the classification of tumours of the nasal epithelium. *Postgraduate Medical Journal* 51, 695.

[2] VRABEC D. P. (1975) The inverted Schneiderian papilloma: a clinical and pathological study. *Laryngoscope* 85, 186.

[3] HARRISON D. F. N. (1976) Malignant melanomata arising in the nasal mucous membrane. *Journal of Laryngology and Otology* 60, 993.

[4] BAILEY B. J. & BARTON S. (1975) Olfactory neuroblastoma. *Archives of Otolaryngology* 101, 1.

[5] FU YAO-SHI & PELZIN K. H. (1974) Non-epithelial tumours of the nasal cavity, paranasal sinuses and nasopharynx. A clinical study. *Cancer* 33, 1275.

[6] BATSAKIS J. G. (1974) *Tumours of the Head and Neck*, Chap. 16, p. 232. Baltimore: Williams & Wilkins.

[7] ENFORS B. & HERNGREN L. (1975) Nasal glioma. *Journal of Laryngology and Otology* 89, 863.

[8] SOFFERMAN R. A. & CUMMINGS C. W. (1975) Malignant lymphoma of the paranasal sinuses. *Archives of Otolaryngology* 101, 287.

[9] HARRISON D. F. N. (1974) Non-healing granulomata of the upper respiratory tract. *British Medical Journal* 4, 205.

[10] CASTRO EL. B., LEWIS J. S. & STRONG E. W. (1973) Plasmacytoma of paranasal sinuses and nasal cavity. *Archives of Otolaryngology* 97, 326.

[11] LEKAS M. D. (1975) Gardner's syndrome and nasal obstruction. *Rhode Island Medical Journal* 58, 471.

[12] GARRINGTON G. E., SCHOFIELD H. H., CORNYN J. & HOOKER S. P. (1967) Osteogenic sarcoma of the jaws. *Cancer* 20, 377.

[13] SISSON G. A., JOHNSON N. E. & AMIRI C. S. (1963) Cancer of the maxillary sinus. Clinical classification and management. *Annals of Otology, Rhinology and Laryngology* 72, 1050.

[14] LEDERMAN M. (1970) Tumours of the upper jaw: natural history and treatment. *Journal of Laryngology and Otology* 84, 388.

[15] SAKAI S., FUCHIHATA H. & HAMASAKI Y. (1976) Treatment policy for maxillary sinus carcinoma. *Acta Otolaryngologica* 82, 172.

[16] ROBINSON J. M. (1975) Frontal sinus cancer manifested as a frontal mucocoele. *Archives of Otolaryngology* 101, 718.

[17] HORCH H. H. & KOCH H. (1976) Malignant tumours in infancy and childhood in the maxillo-facial region. *Journal of Maxillo-Facial Surgery* 4, 157.

[18] BERNSTEIN J. M., MONTGOMERY W. W. & BALOUGH K. (1966) Metastatic tumours to the maxilla, nose and paranasal sinuses. *Laryngoscope* 76, 621.

[19] HARRISON D. F. N. (1974) Non-healing granulomata of the upper respiratory tract. *British Medical Journal* 4, 205.

[20] MICHAELS L. & GREGORY M.M. (1977) Pathology of 'non-healing (midline) granuloma'. *Journal of Clinical Pathology* 30, 317.

[21] McBRIDE P. (1897) Case of rapid destruction of the nose and face. *Journal of Laryngology* 12, 64.

[22] WOODS R. (1921) Observations on malignant granuloma of nose. *British Medical Journal* 2, 65.

[23] STEWART J. P. (1933) Progressive lethal granulomatous ulceration of the nose. *Journal of Laryngology* 48, 657.

[24] FRIEDMANN I. (1971) The changing pattern of granulomas of the upper respiratory tract. *Journal of Laryngology & Otology* 85, 631.

[25] WEGENER F. (1939) Uber eine eigenartigue rhinogene granulomatose des besonderer beiteiligung des arteriensystems und der nieren. *Beitrage zur Pathologischen Anatomie und zur Allgemeinen Pathologie* **102**, 36.

[26] GOODMAN G. C. & CHURG J. (1954) Wegener's granulomatosis, pathology and review of literature. *Archives of Otolaryngology* **58**, 533.

[27] MILLS C. P. (1967) Wegener's granulomatosis. *Hospital Medicine* **2**, 183.

[28] WALTON E. W. (1958) Giant cell granuloma of the respiratory tract (Wegener's granulomatosis). *British Medical Journal* **2**, 265.

[29] SINGH M. M., STOKES J. F., DRURY R. A. B. & WALSHE J. M. (1958) The natural history of malignant granuloma of the nose. *Lancet* **i**, 401.

[30] SHILLITOE E. J., LEHNER T., LESSOF M. H. & HARRISON D. F. N. (1974) Immunological features of Wegener's granulomatosis. *Lancet* **i**, 281.

CHAPTER 33

Diseases of the Salivary Glands

Salivary gland disease deserves a special place in medicine for at least two reasons. First, there are diseases that affect salivary glands and no other tissue in the body, and secondly, the close relationship of the major and minor salivary glands to nervous, bony and vascular structures necessary for the cosmetic and functional integrity of the individual makes surgical treatment of disease states in these glands especially vexing.

INVESTIGATIONS

History and examination

As with the rest of medicine, most diagnostic impressions are formed after completion of the history and physical examination. During these portions of the evaluation, several questions posed in the physician's mind can help to clarify that diagnostic impression:

(1) Is the disease localized to one gland or are multiple glands involved?

(2) Is the entire gland diffusely involved or is the disease localized to a discrete portion of a gland?

(3) Is the entire process located outside the salivary gland?

(4) To what structures outside the salivary gland has the process extended?

(5) Is this a local manifestation of a constitutional disease?

(6) Is the disorder metabolic or endocrine, traumatic, developmental, inflammatory, or neoplastic?

(7) Is the disorder obstructive or nonobstructive?

Historically, the chronicity of the disease is of great importance. The exacerbation, remission, or progression of pain or a lump over the preceding months or years is helpful in clarifying the diagnosis.

An often overlooked part of the evaluation is examination of the saliva. A diseased gland should not be palpated until its duct orifice is viewed to observe the character of the secretion (or its absence). A mucus plug, a bit of grit from a stone, or clear saliva may only be expressed by the first palpation of the gland; subsequently, there may be no discharge (and no diagnostic information). Microscopic and bacteriologic examination of the secretions may also be helpful.

Bimanual palpation of the major glands intra- and extraorally is a cornerstone of the physical exam. It is by this means that diffuse processes affecting the entire gland are distinguished from localized tumours. In the former, the gland is palpably enlarged in its entire extent and is not lobulated or localized. Tumours usually have edges which lie within the boundaries of the gland without palpably enlarged glandular tissue outside their limits; they are discrete, not diffuse.

Probing of the major salivary gland ducts often will provide an unequivocal diagnosis of stone. Palpation of the calculus by a lacrimal probe yields a diagnostic, gritty sensation. The use of graduated probes can dilate tight duct stenoses and allow trapped secretions to drain and be examined.

Radiology

Sialography
Sialography has established itself as a useful, clinical tool employed today in most hospitals. It is particularly helpful in the diagnosis of radiolucent calculi and duct strictures, and can provide valuable information in the assessment of

chronic inflammatory conditions. In the evaluation of masses, it is helpful in differentiating extra- from intrasalivary gland disease, diffuse conditions from localized tumours, and malignant from benign tumours. The technique is contra-indicated in acute inflammatory states and when the patient is allergic to iodinated compounds.

Radioisotopic scanning
Radioisotopic salivary gland scanning with technetium pertechnetate has been used primarily in the assessment of tumours. As is so often the case, initial optimism has been tempered with time. Demonstration of intraglandular tumours depends upon a difference in ^{99}Tc concentrating ability between the tumour and the surrounding glandular tissue. When the tumour concentrates less than the surrounding gland, it is described as 'cold' or radionegative and when the tumour concentrates more, it is 'warm' or 'hot', or radiopositive. When the two are of nearly the same concentrating ability, no tumour can be identified. Even with good contrast, the resolution of the technique usually precludes identification of tumours smaller than 1–1·5 cm and makes assessment of the tumour borders difficult. It was hoped that a particular scan pattern would have strong diagnostic or therapeutic implications, but recent reports have documented exceptions to the early guidelines: radiopositive epidermoid carcinoma, benign mixed tumours, and oncocytomas have all been reported [1]. It is not justifiable to make clinical judgements solely on the basis of radioisotope scans.

The technique may be useful in diseases other than tumours and possibly in determining if lateral neck masses represent metastases from salivary gland primaries.

Ultrasonic echography
The most recent addition to the diagnostic armamentarium is ultrasonic echography, where pulsed ultrasound waves are introduced into the tissues overlying salivary gland tumours, and the characteristics of the reflected sound waves are examined with an oscilloscope and photographed. An enormous advantage of the technique is that it is non-invasive, harmless, painless, and requires no anaesthesia and little subject cooperation. Its principle uses will probably be to distinguish unilocular cysts from solid tumours and encapsulated from non-encapsulated tumours [2]. Further use is needed to allow its reliability, validity and disadvantages to be determined.

Biopsy
Diagnostic incisional biopsy may be performed occasionally to clarify the diagnosis in diffuse glandular disease, to identify the cell type in suspected malignancy, or to obtain tissue for culture and examination when specific infection, e.g. tuberculosis, is suspected. In these situations needle biopsy is not recommended; exposure of the surface of the gland with direct incisional biopsy to obtain adequate tissue (avoiding the facial nerve in the parotid) is preferred. As the general rule, however, wide, local excision of tumours, with a generous cuff of normal surrounding glandular tissue and with facial nerve identification, dissection and preservation, avoiding wound contamination by tumour cells, is the procedure of choice when benign tumours or low grade malignancies are suspected.

TUMOURS
There are some special considerations distinguishing salivary gland oncology from that discipline in general. Some tumours which exist in salivary gland tissue are seen nowhere else in the body; the location of many minor salivary gland tumours as well as the presence of the facial nerve within the structure of the parotid gland makes traditional *en bloc* resection impractical. It is common to disregard the general oncologic principle of establishing the histologic diagnosis before definitive surgery by incisional biopsy because the pleomorphic adenoma, which comprises well over half of all salivary gland tumours, frequently recurs after incisional biopsy.

Nowhere is a close understanding between the surgeon and pathologist more important. The extirpative procedures for malignant tumours are sometimes functionally or cosmetically devastating to the patient or family; before these are undertaken there must be clear communication and agreement between the pathologist and surgeon regarding the diagnosis and its biologic significance.

Salivary gland neoplasms will be discussed from the viewpoint of the clinical-pathological correlations of individual tumour types followed by short sections on minor salivary gland tumours and tumours in children. That there have been so many classifications of salivary gland neoplasms suggests that none is ideal. The present one is utilitarian and includes the vascular malformations as well as the common epithelial tumours. Less common lesions are left to specialized texts.

BENIGN TUMOURS

Pleomorphic adenoma

By far the most common tumour of the salivary glands, the pleomorphic adenoma, or benign mixed cell tumour, occurs most commonly in the parotid gland where it comprises approximately two-thirds of all tumours. In the submandibular, or minor salivary glands, it constitutes less than half of all tumours, but remains by far the most common benign tumour. It occurs more commonly in women, and the peak incidence is in the fifth decade. Rarely there is more than a single tumour present. Rarely, also, does the tumour cause symptoms, the commonest presentation being a slowly enlarging, painless mass which has been present for months or years. On examination these tumours are smooth, rounded, firm or hard, non-tender, and not attached to skin, deep structures, or mucous membrane (the lack of normal mobility of the mucosa of the hard palate causes a tumour at that site to seem fixed). Benign mixed tumours rarely ulcerate or cause facial nerve paralysis.

The tumour is surrounded by a capsule of variable density and thickness, width and extent. Most apparently separate foci of tumour occurring outside the tumour capsule prove on serial sectioning to be outgrowths of the main mass; growth of these extracapsular extensions is the most plausible explanation of the recurrences after enucleation [3]. The histological appearances vary but both epithelial and mesenchymal elements are present. Epithelial and myoepithe-lial cells are arranged in variable patterns surrounded by variable amounts of a mucoid, chondroid, fibroid, or vascular stroma (Fig. 33.1).

Treatment is standard: complete excision with a margin of normal surrounding tissue with preservation of adjacent nerves, but in the palate full thickness resection of the palate to obtain a margin of normal tissue is not warranted.

Recurrence for pleomorphic adenomas is caused by incomplete excision of the tumour and may become manifest within months, but usually takes up to 5 years to do so. Recurrences are nodular and multicentric, and are usually fixed to the skin or facial nerve (in the parotid), or to deep structures. Once this tumour has recurred, it often recurs at different sites requiring several operations over many years. Occasionally adhesion to, and erosion of, the base of the skull further complicate management. The importance of the appropriate initial surgery is evident.

Warthin's tumour (papillary cystadenoma lymphomatosum)

The second most common benign salivary gland tumour, Warthin's tumour, occurs almost exclusively in the parotid glands, usually in the tail. It occurs bilaterally more commonly than any other tumour and is seen five times more commonly in men than women. While it has been reported in a $2\frac{1}{2}$ year old, it is decidedly a tumour of older people, the average age being over 55 years.

In many respects this tumour resembles the pleomorphic adenoma. It rarely causes symptoms, and usually the patient presents with a slow growing, painless mass which has been present for many months or years. It does not alter facial nerve function. Physical examination usually is helpful in the distinction (as is the patient's age and sex) with Warthin's tumours feeling soft and fluctuant, unless they are deeply placed, when they may feel firm.

The tumour is encapsulated and cystic or soft depending upon the number and size of the cystic spaces. The histological appearances reveal lymphatic tissue including follicles, and a double layer of oxyphilic staining cells in papillary projections in the cystic spaces (Fig. 32.2).

The treatment is excision. The tumour is

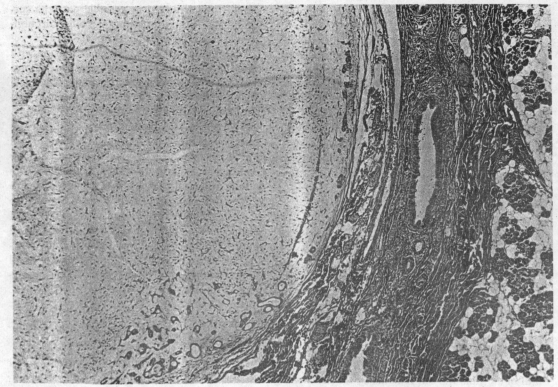

FIG. 33.1. Pleomorphic adenoma with thick capsule and predominant mesodermal derived elements in this section.

encapsulated and, if the clinical diagnosis is obvious, may be safely shelled out without fear of recurrence. If the diagnosis is at all in question, superficial lobectomy with facial nerve dissection is the preferred treatment. No treatment is indicated in a poor-risk patient if the clinical diagnosis seems certain. The prognosis with appropriate treatment is excellent.

Haemangioma

Most salivary gland haemangiomas occur in the parotid gland, manifest themselves before the age of 1 year, and occur in girls. The overlying skin is not usually involved, but, in over one-third of the patients, a concomitant cutaneous haemangioma is evident elsewhere. While they may be classified as capillary, cavernous, mixed, or hypertrophic, this is of little clinical help as all exhibit replacement of glandular parenchyma by

endothelial proliferation and vascular differentiation. The normal glandular lobulation is mantained, but the vasoformative elements surround the remaining acini and ducts.

The prognosis is excellent. Spontaneous regression occasionally occurs [4] so no surgery should be undertaken unless the tumour is definitely enlarging in proportion to the host. Recurrences after excision with preservation of the facial nerve are unusual unless surgery is undertaken in the first few months of life.

Lymphangioma

Like haemangioma, tumours of lymphatic origin usually are present at birth or detected in the first 2 years of life; female preponderance is again noted. While the most common site is the parotid, these tumours arise elsewhere much more commonly than haemangiomas and may be

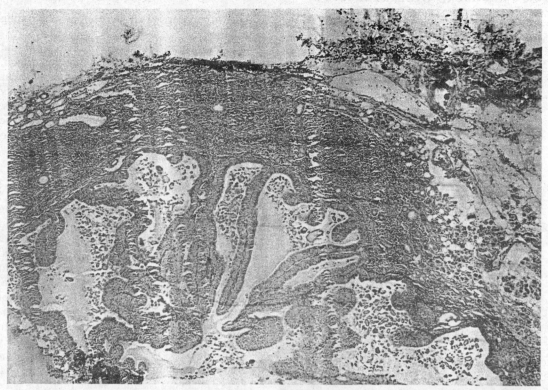

FIG. 33.2. Warthin's tumour with lymphoid and papillary elements and cystic areas well demonstrated.

classified as lymphangioma simplex, cavernous lymphangioma, and cystic hygroma with its variable size cystic spaces. In contrast to haemangioma, there is no replacement of glandular parenchyma, but rather, thin-walled lymph containing spaces occur in the interstices [3]. The same surgical guidelines are applicable as for haemangioma. There is probably no place for radiation therapy with these vascular tumours.

MALIGNANT TUMOURS

Adenoid cystic carcinoma

This relentless neoplasm occurs equally in the two sexes and over a wide age distribution. In any large series, numerous cases will be found in all decades from the third to the seventh and a few in other decades. While the tumour comprises only a small proportion of parotid tumours, it is the most common malignant tumour of the submandibular gland and the minor salivary glands, and comprises one-third or more of all malignant tumours of salivary tissue.

Although the tumour grows slowly, it commonly evokes clinical suspicion of malignancy because it tends to become fixed to skin or deep structures, to cause ulceration in the oral cavity, or to produce motor nerve paralysis (Fig. 33.3). Pain out of proportion to tumour size or growth rate is a prominent symptom. The tumour is firm but poorly demarcated and may present as an area of tender induration rather than a discrete tumour.

The tumour is invasive and exhibits a remarkable predilection to invade perineural sheaths and has a similar propensity for local recurrence. The character and amount of the stroma of the neoplasm varies; the interspersed cellular elements are uniform basaloid cells in clumps, masses, or cords.

The first treatment should be wide *en bloc*

resection with apparently normal tissue. In the parotid gland total radical parotidectomy, including the mastoid tip, with immediate facial nerve grafting is probably the minimum acceptable operation [4]. Resection at other sites must

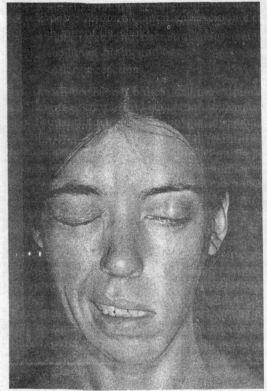

FIG. 33.3. Twenty-nine year old with left ear pain for 6 months and facial paralysis for 4 months. Hard, 3 × 3 cm, poorly defined, adenoid cystic carcinoma of left parotid. Exhibited extension to base of skull and haematogenous metastases despite radical parotidectomy with facial nerve graft and post-operative radiotherapy.

vary according to the patient's general health bearing in mind that the first operation is likely to be the only one with a chance of cure. The tumours are radiosensitive (but not radiocurable), and may disappear or regress and remain inactive for 2 or more years. Whether radiotherapy should be used after a resection where all tumour is felt to have been removed, or whether it should be reserved for recurrent unresectable tumours, is not clear. One should not give post-operative radiotherapy to compensate for inade-

quate surgery carried out in the hope of avoiding mutilation.

The short-term prognosis is fair to good and the long-term prognosis is poor to dismal. Tumours originating in the submandibular glands, the nose and sinuses, external auditory meatus and trachea have the worst prognosis. These tumours exhibit both regional lymphatic metastases, and haematogenous metastases to the lungs, brain, and bone.

Adenocarcinoma

This heterogenous group of neoplasms has long been surrounded by uncertainty of incidence and terminology. Often there are features suggestive of adenoid cystic carcinoma, mucoepidermoid carcinoma, acinic cell carcinoma, malignant oncocytoma, or malignant pleomorphic adenoma; in various series (especially older ones) some of of these tumours are grouped with adenocarcinoma making incidence figures difficult to assess. They appear to comprise approximately 3% of parotid neoplasms and 10% of neoplasms of the submandibular and minor salivary glands. The sex incidence is equal. While there is a wide age span, few occur before the age of 30 years. The tumours may present as an asymptomatic mass or cause symptoms typical of the malignant lesions discussed above. The tumours are usually firm or hard and are often attached to skin or underlying structures. They may be mucus-secreting or non-mucus secreting, papillary or non-papillary. Metastases occur both to regional lymphatics and via the blood-stream to distant organs. In the parotid the majority of these tumours occupy the isthmus, the deep lobe, or extend beyond the gland when first seen. Treatment must therefore be by radical excision. The place of postoperative irradiation and elective neck dissection is uncertain. In Blanck's series [5] the worst prognostic factors were the presence of regional or distant metastases and the local recurrence of the tumour. The determinate survival after 10 years is less than 50% [5, 6].

Squamous carcinoma

It is uncommon for this tumour to originate in the salivary glands and it almost never occurs in the minor salivary glands. Two-thirds of the patients are men, and the average age is older than that of patients with most other tumours; in Conley's series [6], thirteen of twenty-one patients were over the age of 60.

The tumour grows rapidly; pain, facial weakness, fixation, and ulceration occur as commonly, or more·so, than with any other malignant parotid tumour. Infiltration is aggressive and there is no encapsulation. While this is one of the most lethal of all salivary gland tumours aggressive surgery, often necessitating the use of a regional flap, followed by irradiation, may succeed.

Malignant pleomorphic adenoma

The considerable confusion and controversy surrounding this group of tumours is slowly being clarified. Two to five per cent of all pleomorphic adenomas are malignant. The average age of these patients is 10 years more than that for the benign counterpart and the tumour is commoner in women. Commonly, patients who have had a slow growing, painless mass for 10 or more years experience pain, rapid growth, and often progressive weakness of the facial muscles.

In most instances, the malignant tumour has developed within the pleomorphic adenoma invading and replacing the benign·mesenchymal elements. Metastases (which occur early and most commonly in regional lymphatics or lungs) represent only the. epithelial cell line and may resemble squamous cell carcinoma, undifferentiated carcinoma, or adenocarcinoma [6]. The biological behaviour is aggressive and usually reflects the behaviour of the malignant epithelial component. This tumour also has been reported to arise, *ab initio,* with histologically malignant epithelial and mesenchymal elements both in the primary tumour and metastases [3].

Aggressive surgical treatment comparable to that recommended for squamous cell carcinoma with facial nerve grafting and postoperative irradiation is recommended. The prognosis is poor but not as dismal as with squamous cell carcinoma.

Lymphoma

According to Conley [6], there are twenty to thirty lymph follicles and lymph nodes within the parotid gland as well as paraglandular nodes in the pre- and supratragal regions of the lateral, posterior, and inferior aspects of the gland. It is not surprising then that lymphomas occasionally arise in these locations. Lymphoreticular disorders are considered in detail elsewhere in this text but will be mentioned briefly here as they appertain to the salivary glands. The separation of malignant lymphomas into lymphocytic type, reticulum cell sarcoma, and Hodgkin's disease has long endured; their classification into diffuse or nodular patterns has also gained wide acceptance [3].

The overwhelming majority of malignant lymphomas in these areas represent disease arising in lymph nodes rather than primary extranodal salivary gland lymphoma. When the tumours do arise within the major salivary glands, they are usually lymphocytic type or reticulum cell sarcoma. The scarcity of Hodgkin's disease has been noted in all head and neck extranodal lymphomas [3].

The appropriate treatment for these neoplasms is radiotherapy (usually megavoltage) and/or chemotherapy, undertaken only after exacting clinical staging. The place of surgery in lymphomas of the salivary glands is essentially limited to obtaining material for histologic diagnosis. The tissue need be handled gently and expeditiously to avoid trauma and drying artifacts which make histologic diagnosis more difficult.

TUMOURS OF VARIABLE MALIGNANCY

While it is usual for the pathologist to be able to predict whether the tumour is benign or malignant by histological examination, this is by no means universal. Particular problems are encountered in Hurthle cell thyroid tumours, islet cell pancreatic tumours, and certain salivary gland neoplasms, notably mucoepidermoid tumours and acinic cell tumours and oncocytomas [3]. By strict histological or cytological criteria, it is not possible to predict reliably which tumours will behave aggressively and which will act as though they are benign. This presents an enormous dilemma to the surgeon. Biologically benign tumours (the overwhelming majority) need only limited resection, as for pleomorphic adenomas, but those which will behave in a malignant fashion (the minority) require radical resection. The surgeon must either treat all potentially malignant tumours of each group with radical resections, or judge each case individually, reserving radical surgery for those cases with some additional microscopic or clinical evidence of malignant behaviour. The three salivary gland tumours are considered separately, after which suggestions for management are given.

Mucoepidermoid tumour

Controversy surrounding this group of neoplasms has centred on whether they can be divided into benign and malignant subgroups which should be respectively termed mucoepidermoid tumours and mucoepidermoid carcinomas, or whether they are all malignant tumours with high- and low-grade forms. These tumours occur in all the salivary glands and they comprise between 5 and 10% of all salivary gland tumours. Both sexes are equally susceptible, and the tumours may occur at any age but the peak is in the fourth and fifth decades. While most tumours mimic the asymptomatic presentation of the mixed cell tumour, facial nerve involvement, skin fixation and ulceration, and regional and distant metastases are occasionally seen.

Grossly, the tumour is either poorly encapsulated or not at all, and may feel solid or cystic. Microscopically, several cell types are identifiable – maternal, intermediate, epidermoid, columnar, clear, and mucus. On the basis of histological criteria, many pathologists divide the tumours into low-grade (well differentiated) and high-grade (poorly differentiated) neoplasms, and some include an intermediate group.

In general, high-grade undifferentiated tumours comprise less than 10% of the total group and occur in older patients than the low-grade tumours. They also tend to be more solid unencapsulated tumours and have a much higher incidence of facial paralysis (when they occur in the parotid), skin fixation and ulceration, regional or distant metastases, and likelihood of causing death. Recurrences, metastases, and death are rapid, and there is little difference between 5- and 10-year survival figures. Two-thirds to three-quarters of patients with high-grade tumours die within that time [4, 7].

While the pathologist's diagnosis of a high-grade mucoepidermoid carcinoma provides significant (poor) prognostic information, it is the more common diagnosis of a low-grade tumour which presents a problem to the surgeon. A small percentage of the well-differentiated group will present clinical signs of malignancy or will behave in such a fashion. Of sixty low-grade parotid mucoepidermoid tumours in Conley's series [4] four had pre-operative facial paralysis and one had skin ulceration; six developed metastases. In Eneroth's series [5] of mucoepidermoid tumours, twenty-three were judged malignant because they metastasized or were the cause of death (twenty-two out of twenty-three). Of this group, seven tumours histologically were low- or intermediate-grade malignancies. It is evident that a small proportion (less than 10%) of low-grade tumours will behave aggressively and ultimately cause death, though the overwhelming majority will exhibit clinical behaviour and resemble the pleomorphic adenoma.

Acinic cell tumour

These tumours occur almost exclusively in the parotid gland where they comprise approximately 5% of all tumours. In most series, the ratio of female to male is 2:1 with the peak incidence in the fifth and sixth decades. Most patients present with an asymptomatic mass, but pain is common, and rapid growth, fixation, and facial nerve paralysis are also occasionally seen. Pathologically, the tumour is usually a well-defined but poorly encapsulated lobular mass which may have cystic spaces. Microscopically, the stroma is sparse and, occasionally, variable amounts of lymphoid tissue are seen. The neoplastic tissue resembles normal acinar tissue. Usually, the cells appear benign and have abundant granular cytoplasm; occasionally, the cytoplasm is clear.

An unusual feature is the propensity for late recurrence, even 30 or more years after excision; recurrences are often multilocular. The short-term prognosis is very favourable, and 20-year determinate survival figures are over 50% [8].

Oncocytoma

Oncocytes, derived from intralobular ducts or acini, for unknown reasons appear to undergo peculiar cytoplasmic changes eventuating in large cells with abundant oxyphilic cytoplasm. They may be seen singly or in small groups as an accompaniment of the ageing process, in association with other salivary gland tumours (adenoid cystic carcinoma, adenocarcinoma, Warthin's tumour), or as hyperplasias or as neoplasms. A diffuse multinodular hyperplasia is termed oncocytosis, and a solitary solid tumour is an oncocytoma. Oncocytomas usually present as painless, slow growing masses in elderly men. They are usually solid, encapsulated, and lobulated and are seldom seen outside the parotid gland. Mitoses are uncommon even in those very rare tumours which pursue a malignant course with local invasion and metastases [3].

Treatment policy

With these groups of tumours, the surgeon is not always able to make a rational therapeutic decision solely on the basis of the pathologist's frozen or paraffin section reports. With all three tumour groups, it is recommended that the extent of the resection be determined by the clinical presentation. Obviously, aggressive lesions with regional metastases demand vigorous excision. If facial nerve paralysis exists with these tumours, radical parotidectomy with grafting is indicated regardless of histologic appearance. Recurrences need aggressive surgery. Radiation therapy has only a palliative role for mucoepidermoid carcinoma but may have some adjuvant value in acinic cell carcinoma.

Minor salivary gland tumours

Approximately 15% of all salivary gland tumours arise from the minor glands of the upper respiratory or digestive tracts, and over half of these originate in the palate. Over 50% of palatal salivary gland tumours are pleomorphic adenomas, and nearly 40% are either adenoid cystic or mucoepidermoid carcinoma. Two-thirds are restricted to the hard palate, whereas less than 40% of palatal epidermoid carcinomas are limited to that region. Of the malignant tumours (including all mucoepidermoid tumours), slightly less than 30% are ulcerated when first seen and three-quarters of the palatal epidermoid carcinomas are ulcerated [9]. Excision without sacrificing underlying bone is usually adequate treatment, but if adenoid cystic carcinoma is present, a radical local excision is indicated. Pre-operative incisional biopsy is indicated if the tumour is ulcerated. The prognosis for palatal malignant salivary gland tumours is better for each tumour type than for the same tumour at any other site [9].

When these tumours arise in the nasal cavity or paranasal sinuses, they are usually either adenoid cystic carcinomas or adenocarcinomas; many arise high in the nose or in the ethmoid sinuses. They are aggressive and the prognosis is grim.

In contrast, salivary gland tumours arising in the lips have an excellent prognosis, because the overwhelming majority are pleomorphic adenomas which arise in the upper lip and which can be excised easily.

In the tongue, few of these tumours are benign and most originate in the posterior one-third. Adenoid cystic carcinoma again predominates, and the prognosis also is poor in the long term. Lesions of the retromolar trigone are almost exclusively pleomorphic adenomas or mucoepidermoid tumours.

Salivary gland tumours in children

The incidence of these tumours in children depends on whether the vasoformative lesions are included or not. If they are excluded and only solid tumours are compiled, under 5% of salivary gland tumours occur before the age of 16. In a recent review [10], the addition of several collected series revealed 169 vasoformative tumours (including 111 haemangiomas), 149 malignant tumours (including seventy-three mucoepidermoid tumours), and 110 benign tumours (including ninety-four pleomorphic adenomas). The vascular lesions are nearly all evident by the age of 2 years and can be distinguished clinically from solid tumours by their soft or fluctuant feel.

The pleomorphic adenomas tend to occur in older children. As in adults, they present in a single gland, usually the parotid, as an asymptomatic mass, and should be treated by excision with a cuff of normal surrounding gland.

After excluding the vascular lesions, nearly 60% of solid tumours in children are malignant, more than twice the adult incidence. Comparing Schuller's figures with Eneroth's data on 477 malignant parotid, submandibular, and palatal tumours [11] (which presumably include some childhood tumours), interesting differences occur. In children, mucoepidermoid tumours comprise 50% of all malignant tumours; in adults, they are less than 25%. They tend to occur in older children and both high-grade and low-grade varieties are seen. The second most common malignant tumour in children is the acinic cell tumour which makes up 10% of the total. This roughly equals the incidence in Eneroth's series. Other childhood malignancies in decreasing frequency are: undifferentiated carcinoma, adenocarcinoma, undifferentiated sarcoma, and malignant pleomorphic adenoma. Adenoid cystic carcinoma is rarely seen in children, while it composes more than 20% of adult malignant tumours.

Despite the intense emotional impact associated with oncology in infants and children, the basic surgical principles of adult salivary gland neoplasia are applicable to children as well.

NON-NEOPLASTIC DISEASES

Acute suppurative sialadenitis

As a rule, an acute bacterial infection involves a single gland, usually the parotid. The incidence is markedly decreased from the pre-antibiotic era, not because of antibiotics, but because of the improvements in the general and local care of all hospitalized patients. The debilitated, dehydrated, post-operative, surgical patient who developed an acute painful swelling in a parotid gland from retrograde infection with *Staphylococci* is now rare. Radiation therapy for head and neck malignancy with its subsequent sialostatic effects is now a more common predisposing event. Anything leading to decrease in salivary flow or

duct obstruction can also give rise to this problem. Purulent material for Gram stain, culture, and sensitivity can usually be expressed from the duct of the involved gland. Treatment is medical, with hydration and appropriate antibiotics, unless abscess formation supervenes *(vide infra)*.

Parotid abscess

There are certain clinical features of parotid abscess which distinguish it from uncomplicated sialadenitis and from abscess in most other parts of the body. Fluctuation is rarely appreciable despite some sizeable abscess cavities since the abscesses are usually multilocular rather than unilocular. Localized cutaneous 'pointing' of the abscess is uncommon and occurs late; rather, there occurs a wide zone of erythema, induration, and swelling. Finally, the oedema overlying the abscess frequently exhibits 'pitting' after pressure (Fig. 33.4). This is also seen with other deep neck space abscesses but rarely occurs elsewhere. Treatment requires drainage via a standard parotid incision and flap elevation. A haemostat is used to pierce the substance of the gland in multiple places and to spread it in the direction of the branches of the facial nerve minimizing the chances of nerve injury. The upper portion of the incision is closed and a rubber drain is brought out of the lower portion which is left open.

Recurrent suppurative sialadenitis

Occasionally, repeated suppurative episodes occur in one gland (rarely multiple glands). As in other areas of the body, there is often some local underlying abnormality decreasing the local tissue resistance to infection. Most commonly, in the parotid gland, there is glandular stasis with or without partial duct obstruction; the commonest clinical entities are congenital or acquired sialectasis, calculus disease, and duct stricture. Sialography is of the greatest diagnostic help in these patients and is essential for planning rational therapy [11].

Sialolithiasis

Over 80% of all salivary calculi occur in the

submandibular glands, and nearly all of the remainder are in the parotids. Usually only one gland is involved, and three patients out of four have only a single calculus. Sialolithiasis is a disease of middle age and men are more commonly affected. Calcium phosphate in the form

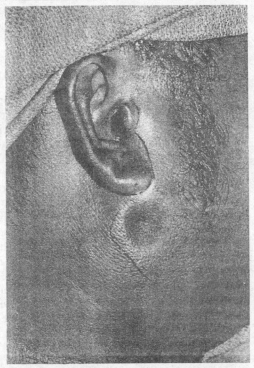

FIG. 33.4. Abscess demonstrating pitting after pressure in a 38-year-old man.

of hydroxyapatite forms the bulk of the inorganic content of the calculi.

Several facts suggest that the aetiology is related to local conditions that exist in the involved salivary gland. The calculi are usually unilateral and are rarely associated with calculus disease elsewhere in the body. Nearly two-thirds of the patients with chronic sialadenitis will have calculi in the involved gland. Finally, there has been ultrastructural support for the concept of initial organic nidus formation followed by deposition of inorganic material [12].

The symptoms, pain and sudden swelling of the affected gland, occur especially at meal times. Diagnosis is established by bidigital palpation of the calculus, by duct probing, or by radiography. For submandibular calculi, occlusal radiographs are the most accurate method of plain film detection and can demonstrate nearly 90% of calculi. Sialography will demonstrate the remainder. Since recurrent sialadenitis is the rule, the treatment is calculus excision if the stone can be palpated intraorally, or gland excision if it is at the hilum of the gland.

Allergic reactions

An occasional patient will have dramatic swelling of the parotid glands and sometimes the submandibular glands following ingestion of foods, drugs, or heavy metals; iodine is probably the most common offending agent. The glands are usually moderately tender, but the swelling and pain begin to subside within a few hours. Hydration is of some benefit.

Viral parotitis

Mumps, or endemic parotitis, is the most common cause of parotid swelling, but can be diagnosed clinically only during epidemics. Otherwise, the diagnosis is made by measuring serum antibodies to the S and V antigens, a titre greater than 1:192 indicating recent infection. The disease primarily affects children between the ages of 4 and 10; the incubation period is 14–21 days. During epidemics, the total clinical picture in patients with serologic evidence of infection may include parotitis, orchitis, pancreatitis, encephalitis, aseptic meningitis, and cochleitis. Asymptomatic subclinical cases may exhibit none of the above, while clinical cases may have any combination. The patients with parotitis have painful glandular enlargement with malaise and trismus. The attack usually lasts 7–10 days and complications are uncommon. Treatment is supportive. While parotid enlargement alone is the rule, the parotid and submandibular glands may be affected in any combination.

The virus of *lymphocytic choriomeningitis, ECHO virus, Coxsackie A virus,* and *parainfluenza viruses 1 and 3* have also been shown to cause parotitis with a similar clinical picture. These account for some of the serologic negatives in 'mumps' [3].

Benign lymphoepithelial lesions

The references review Mikulicz's case description, Schaffer & Jacobsen's separation of Mikulicz's disease and syndrome, Godwin's introduction of the term 'benign lymphoepithelial lesion', and Morgan & Castleman's contention that Mikulicz's disease is identical with localized Sjögren's syndrome [3, 13–16]. However, despite persistent confusion, patients continue to present to otolaryngologists with enlarged salivary glands and complaints referable to xerostomia. The glandular enlargement commonly affects both parotids diffusely and symmetrically, and occurs episodically, but with progressive enlargement between episodes. Considerable variation in the glands affected (lacrimal, submandibular, minor salivary) and the pattern of involvement is seen [14]. The complaints referable to the xerostomia may be simply a dry mouth, but sometimes difficulty in swallowing, trouble with dentures, or decreased taste are noted. The mouth may have fissures at the commissures, loss of filiform tongue papilli with a resultant shiny appearance, as well as a lack of saliva [15].

Usually there are additional features – keratoconjunctivitis sicca secondary to lacrimal gland involvement, and associated connective tissue diseases, most commonly rheumatoid arthritis, but occasionally systemic lupus erythematosis, scleroderma, haemorrhagic purpura, Raynaud's phenomenon and a host of others. When a diagnosis of Sjögren's syndrome is evident, the patients are usually menopausal women [16]. These patients have a higher risk for developing a 'pseudolymphoma' characterized by lymphadenopathy, nonthrombocytopenic purpura, and lymphocytic infiltration of the liver, spleen, lungs, or kidneys. These 'pseudolymphomas' and their symptoms respond well to corticosteroids or immunosuppressives, but rarely the patients develop reticulum cell sarcoma or Waldenstrom's macroglobulinemia to which they succumb [16].

It is evident that the management of patients with xerostomia and salivary gland enlargement dictates a thorough search for evidence of autoimmune disease. Serologic tests, ophthalmologic and medical consultations are advisable. There is no specific treatment for the xerostomia these patients experience since it results from a loss of secretion of both major and minor salivary glands. The duct wall changes and lymphocytic infiltration responsible for the loss of secretion have been well documented over the years. Management of the gland enlargement centres around recognition and prompt treatment of any suppurative episodes, and symptomatic treatment of the glands in between. Rarely is major gland excision necessary.

Manifestations of systemic disease

A host of diverse clinical diseases can be accompanied by non-inflammatory, non-neoplastic enlargement of the salivary glands. The precise cause is not known, but the process usually affects the parotid glands bilaterally, and the preauricular portion more than the tail. It is commoner in middle age and women are more often affected than men. There is usually a slow, painless enlargement unaccompanied by inflammation. Duct structure is usually normal. Histologically, there is acinar cell hypertrophy with interstitial oedema; variable degrees of fatty infiltration and glandular atrophy are also seen.

A host of ovarian, pituitary, thyroid, and pancreatic abnormalities have been associated with these findings as have malnutrition, hepatic cirrhosis, and drugs (e.g. phenylbutazone) [13].

References

[1] McGuirt W. F. & McCabe B. F. (1976) Limitation of parotid scans. *Annals of Otology, Rhinology, and Laryngology*, in press.

[2] Baker S. R. & Ossoinig K. C. (1977) Ultrasonic evaluation of salivary glands. *Transactions of the American Academy of Otolaryngology*, in press.

[3] Batsakis J. G. (1974) *Tumors of the Head and Neck: Clinical and Pathological Considerations*. Baltimore: The Williams and Wilkins Company.

[4] Conley John (1975) *Salivary Glands and the Facial Nerve*. New York: Grune & Stratton; Stuttgart: Georg Thieme.

[5] Blanck, C., Eneroth C.-M. & Jakobsson P. A. (1971) Mucus-producing adenopapillary carcinoma of the parotid gland. *Cancer* 28, 676.

[6] Evans, R. W. & Cruickshank, A. H. (1970). *Epithelial Tumours of the Salivary Glands*, ed. Bennington J. L., Vol. 1. Philadelphia: W. B. Saunders Company.

[7] ENEROTH C.-M., HJERTMAN L., MOBERGER G. & SODER-
BERG G. (1972) Muco-epidermoid carcinomas of the
salivary glands. *Acta Otolaryngologica* **73**, 68.

[8] ENEROTH, C.-M., HAMBERGER C. A. & JAKOBSSON P. A.
(1966) Malignancy of acinic cell carcinoma. *Annals of
Otology, Rhinology, and Laryngology* **75**, 780.

[9] HJERTMAN L. & ENEROTH C.-M. (1970) Tumours of the
palate. *Acta Otolaryngologica* **263**, 179.

[10] SCHULLER D. E. & MCCABE B. F. (1977) Salivary gland
neoplasms in children. *Otolaryngologic Clinics of North
America*, in press.

[11] ENEROTH C.-M. (1970) Incidence and prognosis of salivary gland tumours at different sites. *Acta Otolaryngologica* **263**, 174.

[12] WORK, W. P. & MCCABE B. F. (1964) *Otolaryngology*,
ed. Maloney W. H., Chap. 9, Section 1, p. 5a. Hager-
stown, Maryland: Harper & Row.

[13] MASON D. K. & CHISHOLM D. M. (1975) *Salivary Glands
in Health and Disease*. London: W. B. Saunders Company, Ltd.

[14] BLOCH K. J., BUCHANAN W. W., WOHL J. J. & BUNIM J.
J. (1965) Sjögren's syndrome. *Medicine* **44**, 187.

[15] MEDICAL STAFF CONFERENCE (1975) Recent clinical and
experimental developments in Sjögren's syndrome. University of California, San Francisco. *Western Journal of
Medicine* **122**, 50.

[16] SHEARN, M. (1971) Sjögren's syndrome. In *Major Problems in Internal Medicine*, ed. Smith Lloyd H., Vol. II.
Philadelphia: W. B. Saunders Company.

CHAPTER 34

Tumours of the Thyroid Gland

Malignant tumours of the thyroid are rare and the incidence of thyroid cancer as a cause of death remains fairly constant at 8 per million in the British Isles and 5 per million in the United States. The pathology of thyroid tumours has been thoroughly and frequently reviewed in recent years including the World Health Organization monograph [1]. The importance of an accurate pathological diagnosis of any thyroid tumour cannot be overstressed since the management will depend entirely on the pattern of the disease being treated.

PATHOLOGY

It is useful when considering thyroid malignancy to differentiate between the two different types of cell which are to be found in the thyroid gland. The great majority of thyroid cells develop from a downgrowth from the floor of the pharynx which later descends to lie as two lobes on each side of the upper part of the trachea, with an isthmus joining the two lobes and usually crossing the second, third and fourth tracheal rings. In addition there is a much smaller component of C cells otherwise known as parafollicular cells which arise from the neural crest and migrate forwards to be incorporated in many of the neck tissues. They are difficult to demonstrate in man.

The thyroid cells have the capacity of concentrating iodine from the blood-stream and manufacturing two hormones, thyroxin (T4) and triiodothyronin (T3); these cells give rise to fairly distinct groups of malignant tumours. On the one hand there are the differentiated tumours whose pattern is classified as papillary or follicular and it is usual to see a mixture of both elements in most tumours. However, those tumours which are not encapsulated and which show

papillary formation behave biologically in a quite different way from those which are purely follicular and encapsulated. Follicular tumours are frequently subdivided into those which show invasion of the capsule and blood vessels and which are well differentiated and completely enclosed within a capsule; the former group have a much poorer prognosis than the latter.

The other group of tumours which arise from thyroid cells are the undifferentiated ones which occur in an older age group and are usually referred to as anaplastic. In the past many other tumours have been included in this group and most of the so-called small cell anaplastic tumours were probably lymphomas, while others which resembled fibrosarcomas were probably arising from C cells.

The tumours which arise from the parafollicular or C cells have been called medullary since the original description as a clinicopathological entity [2]. Medullary tumours are relatively uncommon and do not usually constitute more than 8% of all the malignant tumours seen in the thyroid gland. Although many are sporadic there is also a very well-defined familial group; in these families a pattern of endocrine malignancy which includes phaeochromocytomas and neuromas constitutes what has been named the MEA 2 syndrome (multiple-endocrine adenomatosis 2). A simple diagrammatic representation of these various tumours and their origins is shown in Fig. 34.1.

CLINICAL FEATURES

The building blocks of the thyroid gland are the follicles which are made up of spheres of cells of single layer thickness with a collection of colloid in the lumen. These are the cells which concen-

1.

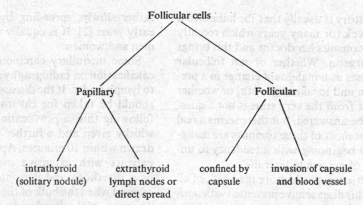

2. Undifferentiated – anaplastic carcinoma.

3. C-cells (parafollicular) – medullary carcinoma. This may be one aspect of MEA 2 (multiple endocrine adenomatosis syndrome type 2).

4. Lymphoid cells – lymphoma.

FIG. 34.1. Cell origins of thyroid tumours.

trate iodine and manufacture thyroid hormones which are then stored in the colloid. These follicles are grouped together in lobules of 40 or 60 which function on an end artery; the common nodule seen in endemic areas is the result of hyperplasia and hypertrophy of one of these groups of follicles.

Solitary nodule

When a solitary nodule is palpated in the thyroid gland the possibility of malignancy is always considered, but such clinically solitary nodules are accompanied by other smaller impalpable nodules in the thyroid gland in about 50% of the patients seen. It is useful to consider the clinically solitary thyroid nodule as an entity in its own right and the incidence of thyroid cancer in such nodules varies between 11 and 13% in different parts of the world. Usually the tumour is of papillary or sometimes follicular pattern, and malignant disease is commoner in areas of endemic goitre as shown by some of the statistics from Colombia. In such endemic areas follicular carcinoma is the type most commonly seen. The sporadic carcinoma encountered in areas where iodine intake is sufficient or in excess of normal requirements tends to be papillary in type. Most patients with solitary nodules are between 30 and 40 years, whereas the number of nodules which

are malignant is fairly constant throughout life, only being overshadowed in the middle decades by the great number of benign nodules which then occur.

Papillary carcinomas

Papillary carcinomas, which are the commonest, are spread by lymphatics and are frequently seen in young patients in whom the prognosis is good if removal is complete. The lymphatic drainage of the thyroid gland has been mapped both with dyes injected into the gland and with radio-opaque oil such as lipiodol which can be X-rayed as it spreads to the regional lymph nodes. These are found around the isthmus of the gland and in the groove between the trachea and oesphagus. They spread laterally especially in relation to the inferior thyroid artery reaching the jugular chain where they may be found extending from the clavicle below to the base of the skull above. Later they may spread to the mediastinum, usually in relation to the thymus, and also laterally to the areas above the two clavicles.

Follicular tumours

Follicular carcinoma tends to occur in a slightly older age group than the papillary tumours and its prominent feature is that it is encapsulated.

The patient's story is usually that she has noted a lump in the neck for many years which recently enlarged; she consults her doctor and this brings her to the surgeon. Whether or not follicular carcinoma arises as a malignant change in a previously benign and localized growth, or whether it is malignant from the very start is not a question that can be answered, but there seems a real possibility that most of these tumours are malignant from the beginning with a tendency to undergo a spurt of growth in later life.

In our experience a little more than 50% of all patients with this disease have presented with signs or symptoms due to metastatic spread of the disease. This spread is by the blood to lungs or to the flat bones, especially the ribs, pelvic girdle, skull, vertebrae and distal ends of the femora. Pulmonary metastases cause haemoptysis and later dyspnoea. Occasionally in a young patient the metastases are so vascular that a machinery murmur may be heard all over the chest. The metastases have been mistaken on radiography for sarcoidosis and miliary tuberculosis.

Some follicular tumours tend to spread to lung and others to bone, but only in the later stages of the disease are examples of both likely to be seen at the same time.

Anaplastic carcinoma

Typically anaplastic carcinoma occurs in patients over 60 years of age and is considerably commoner in women than men. The usual story is that the woman has noticed enlargement of the thyroid gland for many years and then it starts to enlarge rapidly causing hoarseness and pain, radiating to the ears.

The differential diagnosis of anaplastic carcinoma is in the first place lymphoma, then medullary carcinoma, and thirdly a florid form of Hashimoto's thyroiditis. For these reasons antibodies, especially thyroid auto-antibodies, should be looked for in the serum.

Medullary carcinoma

In 1959 Hazard, Hawk & Crile described this distinct clinico-pathological entity which is characterized by deposits of amyloid in the stroma of the tumour, occurs at any age, and usually grows rather slowly, spreading by lymphatics in the early years [2]. It is equally distributed between men and women.

Some medullary carcinomas show extensive calcification on radiography as do the metastases to lymph nodes. If the disease is suspected, blood should be taken for calcitonin estimation and following this, a provocation dose of 50 ml of whisky given and a further blood sample withdrawn within 10 minutes. Approximately 15% of patients with extensive medullary carcinoma have diarrhoea and it is interesting that this is relieved when the bulk of the tumour is removed. The cause of the diarrhoea is not clear but may be due to prostaglandins or kinins and it has been shown in some patients to be relieved by taking large doses of nutmeg daily.

A distinct variant of this tumour occurs in the form of the syndrome known as Multiple Endocrine Adenomatosis 2 in which there are phaeochromocytomas in the adrenal glands, which are often bilaterally involved, and parathyroid lesions. In a variant of this, MEA 2b, there are multiple neuromas of the tongue, eyelids and other mucous membranes. The patients may have an interesting bodily habitus resembling Marfan's syndrome, often complicated by club foot. The presence of phaeochromocytoma is suspected when there are attacks of paroxysmal hypertension and by the existence of a high urinary level of VMA (vanillyl mandelic acid).

INVESTIGATIONS

The most important single investigation is a very careful clinical history which should go into questions of geography in the first place, since in some areas of the world goitre is common and malignant change relatively more common than elsewhere. In addition, questions should be directed at the dietary habits of the patient since some never eat fish or other iodine-containing food. A history of radiation to the neck during fetal life or in childhood is extremely important, since ionizing radiation is carcinogenic in the developing thyroid gland. A family history of thyroid disease is also significant since other members of the same family often have simple, toxic and malignant involvement of the thyroid gland. Finally the typical physical habitus of the patient suffering from MEA 2 should be remembered, with the Marfan-like physique, neuromas of the tongue, eyelids and lips and the possibility of phaeochromocytomas and the hypertensive changes which accompany them.

Thyroid function tests are not of much value in aiding the diagnosis of thyroid cancer. It is an extreme rarity for thyroid cancer to produce thyrotoxicosis and although malignant disease is occasionally seen in a patient suffering from thyrotoxicosis as an incidental finding, it is rare. Scanning the thyroid gland with a radioactive isotope is by far the most useful test that can be done. The ideal isotope is technetium which has a very short half-life and is not a hazard from the radiation point of view. About 1 millicurie is injected intravenously and the gland is then scanned within the next half hour if possible; an extremely good pattern of uptake is shown where the thyroid tissue is functioning. Malignant tissue tends to take up very little or none of the isotope, in the presence of the normal thyroid gland, and thus appears as a 'cold' area. Radioactive iodine, ^{131}I can also be used, but the scan has to be done the following day and if the isotope is used in large amounts or frequently, it offers a radiation risk.

Plain radiographs of the neck and chest are valuable and show soft tissue shadows. A slightly underpenetrated lateral view and a more penetrating postero–anterior view provides the most information of the tissue outlines of the thyroid gland and any extensions it may have. A barium swallow should be done at the same time since the position of the oesophagus is helpful in outlining the gland.

Any patient who is to undergo a thyroid operation should have the vocal cords inspected by indirect laryngoscopy before operation since impairment or lack of movement of one cord is almost pathognomonic of a paralysed recurrent laryngeal nerve and this is likely therefore to be involved in the malignant process. In addition, if one vocal cord is paralysed it is imperative that great care should be taken to preserve the function of the opposite cord for, if this cannot be done, tracheostomy will almost certainly be necessary. When medullary carcinoma is suspected, as in members of a family where such a

tumour has been discovered, then calcitonin should be assayed in the peripheral blood. It is usual to repeat this test after giving something to provoke further secretion of calcitonin; the most useful way of doing this in our clinic has been to give 50 ml of whisky by mouth which stimulates a large rise and does not necessitate the injection of pentagastrin or an infusion of calcium. This use of calcitonin as a diagnostic aid in medullary carcinoma of the thyroid gland is also valuable in follow-up since it acts as a marker of residual or recurrent disease.

In addition it is wise to ask patients with medullary carcinoma if they have diarrhoea, since about 20% suffer from this and it is usually relieved when the tumour and its metastases are excised. It is surprising how rarely patients offer the information that they have diarrhoea probably because it has been present for so many years that they come to accept the frequent bowel actions as normal.

Finally, mention should be made of a non-specific test for malignant disease of the thyroid, the radio-immunoassay of colloid, which has been developed for this purpose and may be useful in the follow-up of patients.

MANAGEMENT

Papillary carcinoma

This is the commonest of all the thyroid carcinomas, and is a disease of young adults and, rarely, children. Typically it is slow growing and usually spreads by the lymphatics. As discussed already most papillary tumours show areas of follicular pattern and vice versa. Whenever a papillary pattern is detected in the thyroid tumour, however, it tends to behave in a particular clinical pattern and for this reason all tumours with any papillary processes in them, no matter how follicular they are, are usually included in the papillary category. The three factors which affect prognosis are the size of the tumour, which if less than 2·5 cm in diameter carries a very good prognosis. Secondly, spread of the tumour outside the thyroid capsule, when the prognosis is much worse, and finally the age of the patient when the diagnosis is made, for in those under 40 years of age the tumour progresses much less rapidly. A personal observation is that if the involved lymph nodes in the neck are found to be cystic in pattern the prognosis is excellent, for this means that the tumour is differentiated enough to manufacture colloid, which is seen as dark jelly-like deposits in the lymph nodes.

No operation for thyroid carcinoma is complete without a careful inspection of the lymphatic drainage of the gland. This has already been described and therefore it only remains to be said that a careful search should be made around the isthmus, in the groove between the trachea and oesophagus, and along the jugular chain. The surgeon should always dissect down towards the thymus gland, and with gentle traction withdraw it and have a good look into the mediastinum. If nodes are involved above the clavicle they should already have been felt clinically before operation. All apparently involved lymph nodes should be removed, but it is not necessary to remove the fascial planes and muscles with which they are related since the nodes tend to be so well encapsulated that they can be removed individually and with minimal dissection. The prognosis with this conservative removal is just as good as when more radical excision is carried out. In addition, as so many of these patients are young and female, a mutilated and scarred neck is something to be avoided if at all possible (Fig. 34.2).

Rarely a deposit of well-differentiated thyroid tissue is discovered in lymph nodes in the lateral triangles of the neck when nothing abnormal can be palpated in the thyroid gland. This is because the primary tumour is so tiny as to be 'occult', but it is still desirable to remove the thyroid gland with its focus of carcinoma in addition to the involved nodes.

What should be done at operation if a single nodule is palpated in the thyroid gland? The lobe in which it occurs should be excised in its entirety leaving the parathyroid glands and recurrent nerve intact. So long as no lymph nodes are involved, this operation, together with giving thyroxin by mouth afterwards for the rest of the patient's life, provides as good a result as more radical treatment. Indeed in the younger age groups the prognosis is the same as if the patient did not have a carcinoma at all (Fig. 34.3).

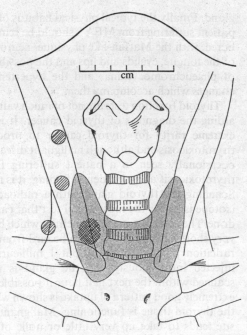

FIG. 34.2. Papillary carcinoma with lymph node involvement. Operation: total thyroidectomy and excision of individual nodes.

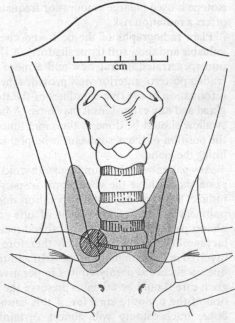

FIG. 34.3. A solitary thyroid nodule. Operation: lobectomy and removal of isthmus.

drainage system. Heavily contaminated clothing or bedding should be stored similarly. The maximum effect of the isotope is not usually seen for up to 3 months but meanwhile the patient is put on full replacement therapy with thyroxin so that any remaining thyroid tissue or metastases are not stimulated by the patient's own TSH. In those patients in whom the metastases are so well differentiated that the isotope is concentrated, excellent destruction of malignant tissue is seen and the bones usually recalcify more densely than the rest of the skeleton. There are reports of patients surviving for as long as 18 years after this form of therapy.

The occurrence of metastatic follicular thyroid carcinoma in children requires very different treatment. In these patients the metastases are almost invariably well differentiated and are hormone dependent, therefore the patients are given full doses of thyroxin replacement by mouth; the growth of the secondaries is inhibited and in some cases they disappear entirely. Dunhill [3] who first recorded this phenomenon was able to report three patients who survived until adult life and had normal pregnancies despite widespread disease when first seen.

Anaplastic carcinoma

Anaplastic carcinoma of the thyroid is a most unsatisfactory disease to treat since it grows with great rapidity and with very rare exceptions kills the patient in less than 1 year.

The clinical diagnosis is rarely in doubt and is best confirmed by doing a drill biopsy which should be followed as soon as possible by radiotherapy delivered through a variety of fields to the neck and upper mediastinum. There is no value in using radioiodine since the tumours are undifferentiated and do not take it up. Surgical ablation has hardly ever been attended by good results. There is a temptation to perform tracheostomy early in this disease but this is to be avoided since the patient often dies more peacefully from pulmonary causes so long as the tracheal obstruction is not severe.

Medullary carcinoma

The treatment of medullary carcinoma is surgical

excision of the whole thyroid gland and any lymph nodes which may be involved. Total thyroidectomy should always be performed if at all possible since it is known that C cells are scattered throughout the gland and it is quite usual for the disease to be multicentric. The parathyroid glands should be preserved and may be

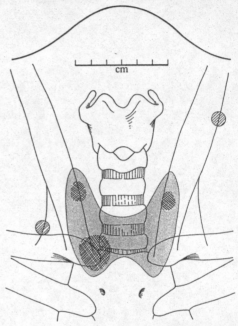

FIG. 34.5. Medullary carcinoma with involved nodes. Note lesions in both lobes. Operation: total thyroidectomy and excision of nodes.

seen to be enlarged and on occasion involved by adenoma formation. Lymph nodes should be removed completely if possible and this may entail sternal splitting and removal of lymph nodes and tumour tissue from the mediastinum and even pericardium (Fig. 34.5). Since this condition was not described until 1959 many patients who survived such major excisions have had the diagnosis made retrospectively.

Radiotherapy appears to arrest growth of the tumour in our series and two patients have been successfully irradiated after neck removal was incomplete. Finally, these tumours, although they grow slowly for many years, may suddenly enter a period of rapid growth in later life and metastases can then be widespread, even involving the skin and distant parts of the body super-ficially. The use of doxorubicin to control this tumour is now well documented and this should be tried when others means have failed.

Miscellaneous tumours

Malignant lymphoma is the commonest malignant tumour of the thyroid apart from those mentioned above and it occurs most commonly in the fifth and sixth decades. Its growth and presentation resemble anaplastic carcinoma. The presence of thyroid antibodies can be a key since some of these patients have Hashimoto's disease preceding the lymphoma. The diagnosis can be made by needle or drill biopsy. If an open biopsy is done the isthmus is removed since this has the added advantage of freeing the trachea. External radiotherapy usually causes local regression of the tumour but most of these patients have died between 1 and 3 years after the diagnosis has been made. Probably in the past these patients were diagnosed as small-celled anaplastic carcinoma.

Malignant teratoma is the rarest of all thyroid

tumours **and** is invariably fatal, the progress being extremely swift. The diagnosis is made histologically and the reported cases have so far all been in young adults.

Metastatic tumours. The thyroid gland is a common site for metastatic disease. Secondary deposits of melanoma, colonic carcinoma and hypernephroma of the kidney have all been recorded.

References

[1] HEDINGER C. E. & SABIN L. (1974) *World Health Organization International Histological Classification of Thyroid Tumours.* Geneva: WHO.

[2] HAZARD J. B., HAWK W. A. & CRILE G. JR. (1959) Medullary (solid) carcinoma of the thyroid: a clinicopathologic entity. *Journal of Clinical Endocrinology and Metabolism* 19, 152.

[3] DUNHILL T. (1937) Surgery of the thyroid gland. *British Medical Journal* 1, 460.

[4] MALT R. A. (ED.) (1977) Thyroidectomy. *Surgical Techniques Illustrated,* Vol. 2. No. 1, Boston: Little, Brown.

[5] HEDINGER E. (ED.) (1969) *Thyroid Cancer.* UICC Monograph 12. London: Heinemann.

CHAPTER 35

Tumours of the Ear

CARCINOMA

Cancer of the ear is an uncommon disease and, except in the auricle, is seldom diagnosed early. The incidence is estimated at between 1/5000 and 1/15 000 of all otologic pathological conditions. It can affect the auricle, the external canal and the middle ear and mastoid; the disease can involve more than one site and tumours of adjacent areas such as the parotid, the skin or the nasopharynx can invade any part of the ear.

Confusion often arises when determining the precise site of origin of a tumour affecting more than one area.

Malignant tumours of the inner ear are practically unknown although this site can be involved from tumours of contiguous areas.

Carcinoma of the auricle

Pathology

Most of these patients are referred primarily to a dermatology or general surgical out-patient department; tumours of the ear form 4–8% of all skin cancers [1]. The auricle is the commonest site to be involved in carcinoma of the ear, representing between 60 and 70% of all ear tumours. Between 80 and 90% occur in males and the peak age incidence is in the seventh decade [2]. Less than 2% occur in the first two decades. The male ear is not as effectively protected by hair or hats as the female ear and so is more exposed to the elements. While exposure to extremes of sun and frost are noted there is less evidence of the effect of lupus, psoriasis, eczema, old burns or wounds. Squamous cell carcinoma of the pinna is almost exclusively a disease of Caucasians; it is unknown in Negroes [3].

Over 70% occur on the helix and postauricular areas and less than 5% occur on the lobule and anti-tragus.

In a major UK series [2], 62% were squamous carcinomas and 21% were basal cell carcinomas, while in a major USA series [3] only 17% were squamous cell and 36% were of the basal cell variety. This no doubt reflects the different climatic conditions of the two countries. Other tumour types to occur at this site are basisquamous carcinoma and melanoma.

The incidence of lymph node metastases is from 7 to 18% [2, 5] and this is almost invariably unilateral.

Clinical features

Both squamous and basal cell carcinomas present with an ulcerating bleeding lesion which may be painful. Although the basal cell carcinoma classically shows rolled, elevated edges and a central area of depression, about one-third of squamous cell carcinomas present in this manner. A facial nerve paralysis, which occurs in less than 5%, indicates either extensive intratemporal spread or metastases.

In both tumour types about one-third of the patients will develop another primary malignancy in the head and neck regions, usually in the skin of the face, the nose or opposite ear. Ten per cent involve areas adjacent to the ear, usually facial skin, a fact which alters the treatment policy.

The majority of melanomas are asymptomatic and 10% are non-pigmented, suggesting a papilloma, haemangioma or cyst. The pigmented ones can show malignant change such as bleeding, pruritis or pain in a pre-existing mole (25%) or can appear as primary malignant growths. Exposure to sunlight in reported series does not appear to be a significant factor. About 10% will have a metastatic gland when first seen, and 30% will subsequently develop lymph node metastases.

With regard to squamous and basal cell carcinomas the only differential diagnosis is from keratoacanthoma, infective granulomas and discoid lupus erythematosus.

Although the diagnostic delay is generally of the order of a year, *in situ* changes are sometimes seen with marked epidermal dysplasia, usually with hyperplasia, hyperkeratosis and dyskeratosis.

Diagnosis is by biopsy but in the assessment of the patient special note must be taken of involvement of the external auditory canal, parotid gland and facial skin. The neck should always be palpated for lymph node metastases and it should be remembered that one-third of these patients will have another head and neck (usually skin) tumour. It is rare to find lymph node metastases, however, if the auricular tumour is less than 4 cm in diameter.

Treatment policy

Squamous carcinoma of the auricle has a worse prognosis than squamous cell carcinoma arising elsewhere in the skin of the head and neck [6]. The cartilage is invaded when the tumours are still macroscopically small because the elastic cartilage of the ear does not seem to form an effective barrier to the spread of cancer.

According to Lederman [2], the susceptibility of cartilage to radiation damage depends on:

(1) The precise character of the cartilage submitted to radiation. The yellow elastic fibrocartilage of the pinna, external nose and suprahyoid epiglottis is far more tolerant to irradiation than are the hyaline thyroid and arytenoid cartilages.

(2) Whilst normal cartilage tolerates therapeutic doses of radiation reasonably well, if these tissues are invaded by neoplasm or become infected then their tolerance to radiation is seriously diminished.

Although most North American surgeons advocate surgery, Lederman suggests pre-operative radiotherapy because healing is often obtained in spite of cartilage destruction and the need for disfiguring surgery can often be avoided. The sites where radiation is least successful are the concha and outer meatus. Involvement of the cartilage of the tragus, the free margin of the helix and the posterior surface of the auricle does not act so unfavourably against radiotherapy.

His indications for radiotherapy are as follows:

(1) Small superficial lesions situated anywhere on the pinna;

(2) Advanced inoperable lesions; and

(3) Extensive lesions affecting the anterior or posterior aspects of the projecting part of the auricle, the tragus or concha, even when there is extensive destruction of cartilage.

He suggests surgery when:

(1) The cartilage is invaded in the part of the concha surrounding the opening of the external auditory canal or on the mastoid boundary of the retroauricular sulcus or the squamous temporal bone;

(2) The tumour has recurred after previous radiotherapy or surgery; and

(3) Lymph nodes are palpable.

Using this policy he reports a 54% survival rate for squamous cell carcinoma and 62% for basal cell carcinoma.

A primary surgical approach gives 73% survival for squamous cell and 64% for basal cell carcinoma [4]. No patient survived when the cancer extended beyond the auricle into the ear, the temporal bone or parotid gland. The same series reports a 35% survival rate for melanoma treated by surgery. Tumours of the helix are excised in a V to facilitate repair. Conchal excisions can be repaired with a post-aural flap. Prosthetic rehabilitation after total auriculectomy is facilitated if a piece of auricle can be left. Local rotation flaps are preferable to split thickness skin if skin cover is required.

Survival data are difficult to evaluate because of the advanced age of patients at presentation.

Carcinoma of the external auditory canal

Pathology

This section is restricted to tumours obviously arising in the canal without affecting the middle ear. This is the second commonest site involved in tumours of the ear; approximately one in four tumours occur here. The sex incidence is equal and the peak age incidence is in the sixth decade.

When both the middle ear and canal are involved, the tumour probably arose in the middle ear. The behaviour of an external canal tumour depends on whether it arises from the bony or cartilaginous portions of the canal.

There is little to stop the spread of tumours arising in the cartilaginous portion either in an anterior direction into the parotid gland or posteriorly into the retroauricular sulcus. Invasion of the parotid gland may be accompanied by pre-auricular lymph node metastases or facial nerve paralysis. Lateral spread to the concha can also occur.

Tumours arising in the bony canal are prevented from spreading outwith the canal at an early stage and so they spread through the tympanic membrane to the middle ear.

By far the commonest tumour is the squamous carcinoma but adenoid cystic carcinoma and ceruminoma can also occur.

Very few factors can be incriminated in a search for the aetiology of this tumour. Analogies are often drawn between carcinoma in an ear affected by chronic otitis externa and carcinoma of the skin around a chronic osteomyelitis sinus (Marjolin's ulcer) but the implied role of chronic inflammation remains hypothetical. Although the sex incidence of carcinoma of the external auditory canal is said to be equal [7] the series from Michigan shows squamous carcinoma to be a disease of women (16/17 cases) [3]. This latter series also shows that over 90% were poorly differentiated.

Ceruminoma is a term applied to tumours arising from the apocrine (ceruminous) glands of the external canal. It is a common tumour in dogs and cats but rare in man. These tumours may be classified histologically into adenoma and mixed cell types [8]. Their innocuous histological appearance often belies aggressive biological behaviour. A small number of these tumours closely resemble adenoid cystic carcinomas.

This latter tumour is very rare as a primary tumour and often spreads into the canal from the parotid [9]. Its aggressiveness and ultimate inevitably fatal outcome are no different in this site than in any other.

Clinical features

A significant number of pateints give a past history of a previously benign lesion such as a papilloma or a polyp of the canal.

The usual symptoms are pain and discharge with an intact tympanic membrane. This latter feature often leads to an erroneous early diagnosis of otitis externa. It is only when this defies treatment for some time that one thinks of doing a biopsy. Bleeding, deafness and facial paralysis are much rarer than in carcinoma of the middle ear.

Ceruminoma usually presents as a polyp and so with the inevitable earlier biopsy the diagnosis is made more quickly.

Neck metastases are rare but assessment must be made of extension outside the canal. Examine the parotid, pre-auricular nodes, retroauricular sulcus and temperomandibular (TM) joint movement. Radiographs of the mastoid and TM joint are essential and simple hearing tests may obviate the use of audiometry to assess middle ear spread.

Treatment policy

According to Lederman [2], the treatment policy should be as follows:

(1) If the tumour involves both pinna and external canal, then the best treatment is pre-operative radiotherapy followed by surgery as and if necessary.

(2) If the tumour if localized in the external canal but does not involve the pinna or the tympanic membrane then radiotherapy should be used alone.

(3) If the tumour involves both the external canal and the middle ear it should be treated as a primary middle ear tumour.

Using this policy he reports a 25% 5-year survival.

Ceruminomas should be treated by a combination of wide excision and radiotherapy [10, 11]. There have been no reported cases of metastases from this tumour provided adenoid cystic carcinoma has been ruled out.

Using a policy of primary surgery, Conley & Schuller report a 28% 5-year survival [4]. Excision of an external canal tumour involves some form of modified temporal bone removal.

Carcinoma of the middle ear and mastoid

Pathology

These are the least common tumours of the ear, their incidence varying from 9 to 12% in different series. The sex incidence is roughly equal and the peak age incidence is the sixth decade. A much higher proportion of these tumours occur in patients under the age of 20 than in the other two sites and this is due to a higher incidence of mesodermal tumours in the young.

Fifty per cent of the patients give a history of chronic ear infections and 20% have a history of intermittent ear infection. It is well known that carcinomas may develop in relation to chronic bone sinuses and the relation between middle ear cancer and infection may be similar. It has been found that one patient in 208 with active chronic suppurative otitis media has a carcinoma [12]; the authors of the latter report suggested that every patient with chronic middle ear suppuration of more than 20 years' duration should be under regular otological supervision and routinely investigated by Papanicolaou smears. Eight cases of cancer of the mastoid process have been described in radium dial painters [13].

Over 90% of these tumours are squamous cell carcinomas but the following have also been recorded – rhabdomyosarcoma, adenocarcinoma, chondrosarcoma, lymphosarcoma, basal cell carcinomas, melanomas and secondary deposits.

Lederman classifies these tumours into two types, petromastoid tumours and tubotympanic tumours [2].

Petromastoid tumours include:

(1) Tumours limited to the tympanic cavity;

(2) Tumours limited to the mastoid antrum;

(3) Tumours involving the tympanic cavity and mastoid antrum; and

(4) Tumours involving the tympanic cavity and external auditory canal.

Tubotympanic tumours are uncommon and while they are basically petromastoid they produce some of the neuro-ophthalmological syndromes associated more usually with nasopharyngeal cancer. Spread, via the Eustachian tube, of a nasopharyngeal tumour to the middle ear is as rare as spread of a middle ear tumour to the nasopharynx via this route. It is considered that rather than passing up or down the cartila-

ginous tube the tumour passes into the fascial spaces around it, thus involving the trigeminal nerve and also the occulomotor nerves as it spreads to the cavernous sinus. Paralysis of the last four cranial nerves in middle ear cancer is due either to direct spread to the jugular foramen or to metastasis to the node of Rouvière which lies over the transverse process of the atlas in the lateral part of the parapharyngeal space.

Clinical features

The commonest presenting features of this condition are otorrhoea, deep ear pain, bleeding and deafness. About 10% of patients are asymptomatic and are diagnosed from altered appearances in a radical mastoid cavity or an ear with chronic ear disease. About 15% present with facial nerve paralysis and another 10% have spread to the temperomandibular joint or parotid when first seen.

On examination, there will be either granulations or a polyp in the ear or mastoid cavity. The diagnosis depends on a high index of clinical suspicion and biopsy must be performed. Very often the diagnosis is first suspected at the time of surgery and in this case frozen section should be requested. In a small proportion of cases the tumour may exist behind an intact tympanic membrane and one of the authors has in fact dealt with such a patient, who presented with a metastatic neck gland from an apparently unknown primary site; shortly after the neck dissection had been performed, the patient became deaf and the tympanic membrane was thereafter replaced by tumour tissue. Facial nerve function should be assessed not only clinically but also by electroneuronography.

Radiological examination is by means of plain films, and tomography is always necessary to gauge the extent of spread within and without the temporal bone and this will indicate the chances of successful treatment. Destruction is seen on plain films of the petrous bones and mastoids almost invariably, but tomography is required to assess the extent of destruction. A jugular venogram is occasionally helpful to see whether the tumour has invaded the jugular vein outside the skull or not. Angiography may show tumour circulation within the temporal bone but its real importance is in assessing cross circulation in case one internal carotid artery needs to be sacrificed at operation. Although very few of these patients have obvious metastases when first seen a chest radiograph must always be performed.

If there is any question that the tumour has spread outside the bony confines of the temporal bone then a brain scan should be done as well as computerized axial tomography (CAT).

Lederman [2] has pointed out the importance of the spine of the sphenoid in the submentovertical view. Invasion of the petrosphenoidal region medial to the spine of the sphenoid indicates a tubotympanic rather than a petromastoid tumour. This is of prognostic significance because destruction of bone in this region suggests that cure by any form of treatment is unlikely. On the submentovertical view one may also see destruction of the arch of the atlas especially if Rouvière's node and the last four cranial nerves are involved.

If, however, the tumour has arisen in an old radical mastoid cavity then radiography is of little value in assessing tumour extension.

Treatment policy

The choice of treatment lies among the following:

(1) Radiotherapy;
(2) Temporal bone resection;
(3) Combined radiotherapy and temporal bone resection;
(4) Radical mastoidectomy followed by radiotherapy;
(5) Radiotherapy followed by radical mastoidectomy; and
(6) Palliation.

In deciding the appropriate treatment the following facts should be borne in mind:

(1) Death from cancer of the middle ear and mastoid is slow and very painful;
(2) Before the introduction of en bloc temporal bone resection in 1951 [14, 15], the cure rate for this tumour at the Memorial Hospital, New York, with combinations of radiotherapy and radical mastoidectomy, was 6%; and
(3) Radiotherapy alone to middle ear cancers was not effective. Lederman reports no survivors at either 3 or 5 years [2].

It is therefore obvious that even the most reluctant surgeon will have to arrange some form of treatment for this most rare and painful of tumours. If the cancer is confined within the temporal bone and has not invaded the carotid canal then the choice of treatment is an en bloc temporal bone resection. Conversely, if cancer lies outside the bony box then to remove that box is illogical. Between this black and this white lies the inevitable grey area where dural invasion is noted during a temporal bone excision; in this case the en bloc policy is abandoned and the involved dura is excised and grafted as a separate exercise. Involvement of the petrous tip medial to the carotid artery is an area of a darker shade of grey; to remove this the carotid artery must also be removed and this carries dire risks of death and almost certain morbidity. Lewis [7] states that the en bloc resection must be abandoned because of tumour extension in 15% of operations.

Because of the absence of controlled studies and the rarity of the disease, the role of radiotherapy is in doubt, apart from the fact that if given on its own there are unlikely to be any survivors. Among the basic tenets of radiotherapy are the facts that if bone or cartilage is involved by tumour then its tolerance to radiation is much diminished, that if sepsis is present then radiotherapy is unlikely to be curative and that if there is extensive bone or cartilage invasion then surgery should be used also. Although radiotherapy is probably best administered before any operation because of the lack of scar tissue and good blood supply, some factors in petromastoid cancer suggest that it is used after operation. First, the temporal bone is a dense bone and there is almost always sepsis present if bone is involved. Secondly, a preliminary surgical exploration removing tumour bulk and dead bone will give some guide as to the full extent of spread of the tumour. And, thirdly, the patient is more comfortable when tumour bulk is removed and also a cavity is created for inspection and drainage.

An added advantage of radiotherapy used in conjunction with surgery is to deal with any possible spread to the spaces around the Eustachian tube.

The classical temporal bone resection includes

not only the temporal bone lateral to the internal carotid artery but also the TM joint and the ascending ramus of the mandible.

With temporal bone excision after pre-operative radiotherapy Lewis reports a 25% survival rate [7]. With various forms of surgery (radical mastoidectomy, modified temporal bone excision, *en bloc* temporal bone excision) followed by post-operative radiotherapy Lederman [2] reports a 34% 5-year survival.

It is rare for these patients to have concurrent neck gland metastases. If a neck dissection is required it should be performed after the temporal bone resection because if it is done first and the internal jugular vein divided, the pressure in the lateral sinus rises six to seven times, making operating conditions very difficult for the temporal bone resection. Thus, whilst in theory it is better to do these in two stages, the fact that survival with metastatic neck glands is a rarity makes it perhaps more sensible not to operate on the patient.

Complications of temporal bone dissection include:

(1) *Haemorrhage;* the temporal bone is surrounded by a lake of blood created by the sigmoid sinus, the superior petrosal sinus, the inferior petrosal sinus, the cavernous sinus, the jugular bulb, the internal carotid artery, the middle meningeal artery, the temporal artery and the maxillary artery. The main method of control of haemorrhage is tamponade of the sigmoid sinus, hypotensive anaesthesia and care around the internal carotid artery.

(2) *Hemiplegia* will occur in half of the patients who survive internal carotid artery ligation.

(3) *C.S.F. leak* arises from dural tears. Any tear or excised area should be repaired with temporal fascia.

(4) *Infection* is more liable to occur in the wound and the cavity if pre-operative radiotherapy has been given.

(5) *Facial nerve paralysis* can be dealt with either immediately by a facio-hypoglossal anastomosis, which is not usually favoured by surgeons who do many temporal bone resections, or later by fascial slings or face lift.

(6) *Mandibular shift and dental problems* are inevitable if part of the ascending process of the mandible is removed but generally they do not cause much distress.

GLOMUS JUGULARE TUMOURS

Chemoreceptor tissue lying in the dome of the bulb of the internal jugular vein was identified by Guild in 1941 [16]. He named this structure the glomus jugulare. The first tumour of this tissue was described by Rosenwasser in 1945 [17]. Since then it has been apparent that vascular aural polyps previously regarded as either haemangiomas or endotheliomas are in fact derived from chemodectomas growing in the middle ear or the jugular foramen.

Pathology

The maximum age incidence of glomus jugulare tumours is in the fourth decade with an age range from 15 to 80. Approximately three-quarters of all reported cases are women. Familial cases and multicentric chemodectomas have also been described.

The jugular foramen is formed by the jugular notch on the occipital bone and the adjacent temporal bone. It is subdivided into two parts.

(1) Posterolateral transmitting the internal jugular vein.

(2) Anteromedial transmitting the ninth, tenth and eleventh cranial nerves.

The glossopharyngeal nerve is anteromedial to the other two nerves and is separated from them by a fibrous septum. These cranial nerves are affected by direct spread from the adjacent tumour which also invades and encircles the vein. Only a thin plate of bone separates the bulb of the internal jugular vein from the tympanic cavity. Those tumours which arise in the jugular bulb rapidly destroy this plate of bone and then fill the tympanic cavity. A significant number also arise in and remain restricted to the ear [18]. They arise from similar chemoreceptor tissue lying under the mucosa on the medial wall of the middle ear or along the course of the tympanic nerve. Once the petrous bone has been invaded the facial nerve may be damaged. Access to the posterior cranial fossa is gained either through the petrous bone or through the jugular foramen itself. Spread into the pterygoid fossa and neck are well documented. These tumours characteristically grow very slowly. Metastases to lungs and lymph nodes have occasionally been recorded.

Microscopically all chemodectomas, whether from the carotid body or the jugular foramen, are identical. Characteristically one sees small tightly packed polygonal cells in small nests separated by venous channels varying in size from capillaries to large thin-walled sinuses. The degree of malignancy cannot be gauged from the histological features of the tumour.

Catecholamines have been detected in some and they may release potent monoamines into the general circulation [19].

Clinical features

Three main symptom complexes are recognized but there is considerable overlap in many patients.

(1) Aural.
(2) Cranial nerve.
(3) Intracranial.

Aural symptoms and signs

Evidence of middle ear disease is present in probably 95% of patients. Deafness, blood-stained otorrhoea, pain in the ear and tinnitus are the presenting symptoms. Auroscopy usually reveals a polyp in the external auditory meatus or visible through the tympanic membrane. A bruit is often heard on auscultation of the mastoid process. The deafness may be conductive or sensorineural depending on the extent of the tumour.

Cranial nerve symptoms and signs

Cranial nerve palsies do not in themselves indicate that the tumour has formed an intracranial mass. The tumour may invade or compress these nerves at various points in their extradural course. The ninth to the twelfth nerves are

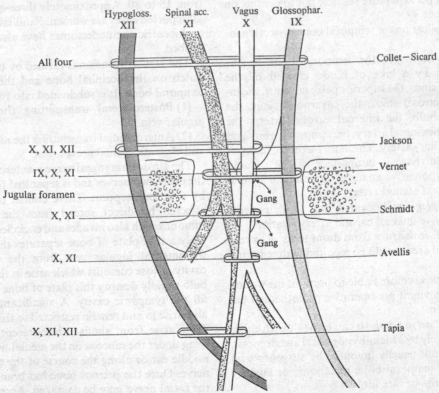

FIG. 35.1. The jugular foramen syndromes (from Gejrot T. (1968) *Disorders of the Skull Base Region*, eds Hamberger C. A. & Wersëll J. London: Wiley).

damaged by the tumour growing directly out of the jugular foramen. These latter nerves are most commonly affected at this stage of the disease. The fifth and sixth are much less commonly damaged but some patients may present initially with diplopia [20]. The symptoms resulting from glossopharyngeal damage include sensory impairment in the posterior third of the tongue, tonsils and the pharynx. Taste in the affected part of the tongue is also altered and a change in salivary secretion may be noted. Damage to the ninth nerve is diagnosed by testing taste and the pharyngeal reflex. A unilateral lesion of the vagus nerve may not necessarily give rise to symptoms. Changes in intonation, vocal cord and pharyngeal paralysis are however found on examination. Involvement of the accessory nerve results in paralysis of the sternocleidomastoid and trapezius muscles, the outline of the former muscle being abnormal with drooping of the shoulder. Weakness of the affected muscles is assessed by simple clinical tests. Involvement of

the hypoglossal nerve may also not create marked symptoms in the early stages, wasting, deviation and fasciculations being obvious only in the well-established lesion. These four cranial nerves are closely related both intracranially and at the base of the skull and a lesion affecting one is most likely to involve one or more of the others. A number of eponymous syndromes with differing combinations of nerve involvement have been described (Fig. 35.1). The differential diagnosis of these syndromes includes skull fractures, bullet and other penetrating injuries, osteomyelitis of the skull base, sinus thrombosis and other tumours of the skull base, e.g. chordomas and metastases.

Intracranial symptoms and signs
Symptoms of intracranial hypertension with suboccipital headache and vomiting, unsteadiness and limb weakness indicate a probable extension into the posterior cranial fossa. Papilloedema, nystagmus, ataxia and hemiparesis are

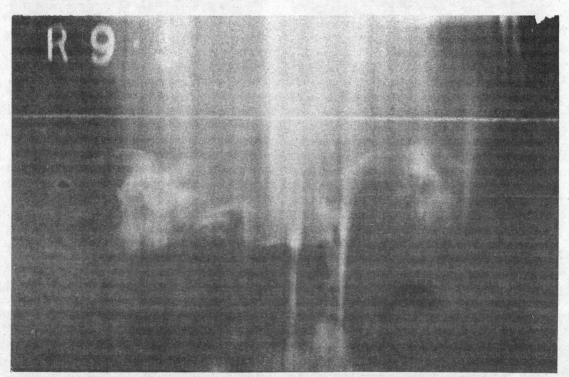

FIG. 35.2. Petrous bone tomogram showing extensive destruction of apex of petrous bone and jugular foramen (courtesy of Mr J. Block).

the cardinal features. Raised intracranial pressure is most often due to obstruction of the fourth ventricle and subsequent hydrocephalus; these features are rare as an initial presentation.

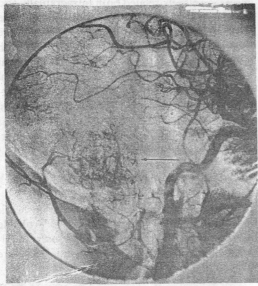

FIG. 35.3. Subtraction, magnification carotid arteriogram. Arrow indicates extensive fine tumour circulation.

Special investigations

A biopsy of an aural polyp may provide a pathological diagnosis if an adequate amount of tissue is obtained but this may be dangerous because of severe haemorrhage. The differential diagnoses in the early stages of the disease are considerable unless an aural polyp is present. To establish the diagnosis in these patients and to ascertain the size and extent of a definite tumour the following sequence of radiological investigations is recommended:

(1) Routine skull radiographs with special views of the jugular foramen. Petrous bone tomography is of considerable value. Sclerosis of the foramen, ill-defined margins, enlargement and destruction of the intrajugular process of the temporal bone, are the characteristic findings in the well established case (Fig. 35.2). Tumours arising in the middle ear do not show these radiological abnormalities. In about 50% of cases plain radiographs of the jugular foramen are positive and diagnostic.

(2) Common carotid arteriography with selective cannulation of the internal and external carotid arteries is essential. The subtraction technique is of inestimable value. The ascending pharyngeal branch of the external carotid artery is claimed to be the major blood supply to the

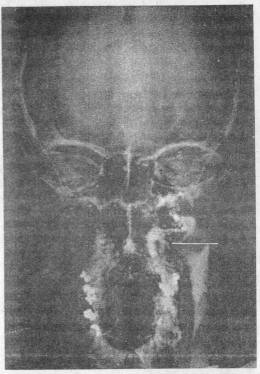

FIG. 35.4. Jugular venogram with filling defect indicated.

tumour [21], but fine tumour circulation and arteriovenous shunting may be obscured by the overlying bone and missed unless special temporal views are taken (Fig. 35.3).

(3) Internal jugular phlebography is very useful in differentiating other basal skull lesions [22]. The most characteristic finding is an intravascular filling defect with a convex distal contour and expansion of the vein, and sometimes external compression of the jugular vein and defects resembling intramural thrombosis (Fig. 35.4) [23].

(4) Vertebral angiography should also be performed to define the complete extent of the blood supply to the tumour. The vertebral arterial contributions are twofold – the anterior meningeal arteries and directly from the intracranial artery.

As with carotid arteriograms, rapid serial films with subtraction and magnification techniques are far more helpful than routine methods (Fig. 35.5).

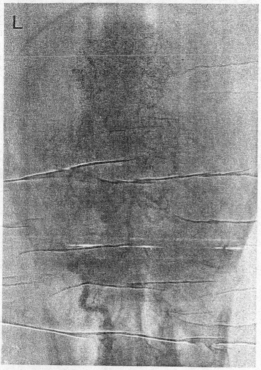

FIG. 35.5. Left vertebral angiogram with subtraction, showing extensive tumour circulation with a-v shunt (courtesy of Mr J. Block).

(5) The value of radioisotope scanning and computorized transverse axial tomography have not thus far been established. Probably only in the large intracranial extensions would these techniques be helpful but not diagnostic.

Treatment policy

Small glomus tumours arising from the promontory can be removed safely by tympanotomy. If the tumour is larger but confined to the middle ear a radical mastoidectomy and removal of the lesion is the treatment of choice. Opinion on the need for post-operative irradiation varies. The value of radiotherapy in slowing the growth of a glomus tumour has been doubted [24], but the extent and vascularity of the larger tumour makes surgical removal too hazardous in a number of instances. In these cases the only alternative is radiotherapy. Long periods of remission with considerable symptomatic improvement have been reported [25]. Recurrences do, however, occur [26] and a careful monthly review with an appropriate radiological reassessment is necessary in the follow-up of these patients. Surgical excision has been more often advocated recently [21, 24, 27]. Those authors recommending surgery argue that the tumours are radio-resistant and their very slow growth creates an illusion that they have indeed responded to irradiation. It may be possible to lessen the surgical problems by pre-operative irradiation or by intravascular sclerosis of the tumour with Silastic [28]. Despite recent resurgence of surgical enthusiasm in the treatment of these conditions, reports do not give mortality and morbidity figures [24] and long-term follow-up is of course not available.

References

[1] LEROUX-ROBERT J. & ENNUYER A. (1957) *Rapport Soc. franc. O.R.L.*, 64, part 1, Arnette.

[2] LEDERMAN M. (1965) Malignant tumour of the ear. *Journal of Laryngology and Otology* 79, 85.

[3] BATSAKIS J. G. (1974) *Tumours of the Head and Neck*, p. 325. Baltimore: Williams & Wilkins.

[4] CONLEY J. & SCHULLER D. E. (1976) Malignancies of the ear. *Laryngoscope* 86, 1147.

[5] SCHEWE E. J. & PAPPALARDO C. (1962) Cancer of the external ear. *American Journal of Surgery* 104, 753.

[6] HURIEZ C. *et al.* (1962) Etude de 126 tumeurs auriculaires malignes observées an 9 ans a la clinique dermatologique universitaire de Lille. *Bulletin de la Société française de dermatologie et de syphiligraphie* 69, 886.

[7] LEWIS J. S. (1973) Carcinoma of the ear. *Archives of Otolaryngology* 97, 41.

[8] WETLI C. V., PARDO V., MILLARD M. & GERSTON K. (1972) Tumours of ceruminous glands. *Cancer* 29, 1169.

[9] PULEC J. L. *et al.* (1963) Adenoid cystic carcinoma (cylindroma) of the external auditory canal. *Transactions of the American Academy of Ophthalmology and Otolaryngology* 67, 673.

[10] JOHNSTONE J. M., LENNOX B. & WATSON A. J. (1957) Five cases of hidradenoma of the external auditory meatus: so-called ceruminoma. *Journal of Pathology and Bacteriology* 73, 421.

[11] CANKAR V. & CROWLEY H. (1964) Tumours of ceruminous glands; a clinico-pathological study of seven cases. *Cancer* 17, 67.

[12] BRADLEY W. H. & MAXWELL J. H. (1954) Neoplasms of the middle ear and mastoid. *Laryngoscope* **64**, 553.

[13] LEWIS J. S. (1967) Cancer of the ear. In *Cancer of the Head and Neck*, ed. Conley J. Washington: Butterworths.

[14] CAMPBELL E., VOLK B. M. & BURKLUND C. W. (1951) Total resection of temporal bone for malignancy of the middle ear. *Annals of Surgery* **134**, 397.

[15] PARSONS H. & LEWIS J. S. (1954) Subtotal resection of the temporal bone for cancer of the ear. *Cancer* **7**, 995.

[16] GUILD S. R. (1941) A hitherto unrecognised structure the glomus jugulare in man. *Anat. Rec.*, Suppl. 2, **79**, 28.

[17] ROSSENWASSER H. (1945) Carotid body tumours of the middle ear and mastoid. *Arch. Otolaryngol.* **41**, 64.

[18] BICKERSTAFF E. L. & HOWELL J. S. (1953) The neurological importance of tumours of the glomus jugulare. *Brain* **76**, 576.

[19] HAMBERGER B. (1968) Cetecholamines in glomus tumours. In *Disorders of the Skull Base Region*, eds. Hamberger C. A. & Wersëll J., p. 269. London: Wiley.

[20] ALFORD B. R. & GUILDFORD F. R. (1962) A comprehensive study of tumours of the glomus jugulare. *Laryngoscope* **72**, 765.

[21] KEMPE L. G. (1970) *Operative Neurosurgery*. Vol. 2, p. 72. Berlin: Springer.

[22] QUENCER, R. M., TENNER M. S., ROTHMAN L. M. & LASTER D. W. (1976) Jugular venography for the evaluation of abnormalities of the skull base. *J. Neurosurg.* **44**, 485.

[23] GEJROT T. & LAUREN T. (1964) Retrograde venography of the internal jugular veins and transverse sinuses. *Acta Otolaryng. (Stockholm)* **57**, 556.

[24] KEMP L. G., VANDERARK G. D. & SMITH D. R. (1971) The neurosurgical treatment of glomus jugulare tumours. *J. Neurosurg.* **35**, 59.

[25] GLOVER G. W. & BLOCK J. (1972) Glomus jugulare tumours – radiotherapy or surgery. *Brit. J. Surg.* **59**, 947.

[26] FARRELL V. J. & HAWKINS T. D. (1967) Glomus jugulare tumours with special reference to their radiological features. *Brit. J. Surg.* **54**, 789.

[27] DENEKE H. J. (1969) Surgery of extensive glomus jugulare tumours of the ear. *Rev. Laryngol.* **90**, 265.

[28] HILAL S. K. & MICHELSEN S. W. (1975) Therapeutic percutaneous embolisation for extra-axial vascular lesions of the head, neck and spine. *Journal of Neurosurgery* **43**, 275.

CHAPTER 36

Tonsils and Adenoids

TONSILS

Pathogenesis of infection

Immunology of tonsils

A complete circle of lymphoid tissue, Waldeyer's ring, surrounds the beginning of the alimentary and respiratory tracts. It appears in the fifth month of gestation in relation to the first, second and third pharyngeal pouches and arches to form the palatine (faucial), lingual and pharyngeal adenoid tonsils. At birth, or in certain immuno-deficiency diseases, the tonsils are devoid of germinal centres. These germinal centres are strategically located immediately beneath the cryptal epithelium, forming a caplike aggregation of lymphocytes pointing toward the overlying epithelium. The germinal centres tend to be poorly vascularized, while the perifollicular areas contain a dense network of capillaries and post-capillary venules. The tonsils are a unique lymphoepithelial organ in that they have no afferent, but only an efferent, lymphatic circulation. Also, they possess both T and B lymphocyte subpopulations but the latter tend to be present in greater concentrations than the former, which is the reverse of the situation in the peripheral blood. The B lymphocytes are produced *de novo* by active lymphopoiesis while the T lymphocytes probably originate from the peripheral circulation since the numbers are similar in the tonsils and paired peripheral blood samples. Hence both cell-mediated and humoral immune effector mechanisms are demonstrable in human tonsils.

Three approaches have been used in the study of the physiological function of the tonsils: a phylogenetic, an ontogenetic and a direct ex-perimental approach. All three contribute to a unified assessment of these, as yet enigmatic, lymphoepithelial organs.

The phylogenetic approach, i.e. the development of the species from lower to higher verte-brates, indicates that the tonsils first appear in higher clasmobranchii (sharks, guitarfish, skates and rays) as aggregates of small and medium-sized lymphocytes lacking a distinct lympho-epithelial structure. The tonsils are well-developed lymphoepithelial organs in the amphibia where they present as primitive lymphoid nodules in the sublingual area. In the reptilia the tonsils appear as distinct lymphoepithelial organs at the same time as the species is adjusting to terrestrial life. All species developing later than this point of evolution possess tonsils. The tonsils and lymph nodes make their appearance after the thymus; thus, it is assumed that the thymus has a controlling influence over the maturation of these organs. Since the tonsils were retained during the evolutionary process they most probably have some phylogenetic advantage.

Ontogenetically, the human tonsils appear to be an integral functional part of the gut-asso-ciated lymphoid tissue (GALT) and humoral immunity as shown by an analysis of three immunodeficiency syndromes. There is a direct relationship between either atrophy or absence of the tonsils and related deficiencies in GALT. Hence, the immunological role of tonsils with respect to B lymphocyte immunoglobulin pro-duction is substantiated ontogenetically.

The experimental approach has provided the strongest evidence for the physiological role of human tonsils in the total immunobiology pic-ture. Removal of the tonsils and adenoids has repeatedly failed to compromise the immunolo-gical competence of experimental animals. In man the only effect of T and A is a depression of local specific antipolio secretory IgA of questionable clinical significance, with no detrimental effects on systemic immunity. Recent information has demonstrated humoral and cell-mediated immunity in tonsil-derived lymphocyte populations.

The complete sequence of cellular differentiation of B lymphocytes in human hyperplastic tonsils has been demonstrated. Also, direct fluorescent antibody procedures and quantitation of immunoglobulin synthesis by human tonsil-derived lymphocytes indicates the presence of lymphocytes producing all classes of immunoglobulins, some of which is specific antibody. In the presence of specific antigen it appears that an IgM specific antibody is produced *in vitro* by tonsil-derived lymphocytes from previously immunized individuals. Furthermore, lymphocyte migration from the germinal centres toward the lymphocyte caps with concomitant transformation to antibody-producing plasma cells has been demonstrated. The presence of recirculated T lymphocytes (sensitized) and their appropriate effector function as discrete immunological organs in the GALT has also been noted.

The known facts can be summarized as follows:

(1) The tonsils produce *de novo* B lymphocytes capable of synthesizing all classes of immunoglobulins and specific antibody.

(2) Immunologically functional T lymphocytes are present as concentrations comparable to those in peripheral blood and probably enter the tonsils by recirculation from this source.

(3) The tonsils are an integral part of the GALT for which there is phylogenetic, ontogenetic and experimental evidence.

(4) The tonsils are a first line of defence against invading respiratory micro-organisms but may also harbour latent viruses such as EBV or be the site of carrier micro-organisms (i.e. Group A *Streptococci*).

(5) Immunological memory cells for both humoral (B cells) and cell-mediated (T cells) immunity are present but the former appear to be much more active.

(6) Extirpation of tonsils and/or adenoids may alter local but not systemic immunity.

(7) At best the tonsils are strategically located

lymph nodes capable of generating a continuous supply of antigen-sensitized B cells.

Microbiology of tonsils and adenoids

Numerous authors have reported discrepancies between the surface and internal pathogenic microflora of the tonsils. Surface cultures of the adenoid often yield more bacterial pathogens than the palatine tonsils.

Before the antibiotic era the prominent bacterial pathogen isolated from acute adenotonsillitis was *Streptococcus pyogenes* (Group A). After the antibiotic era it became apparent that numerous patients with *S. pyogenes* (Group A) tonsillitis and pharyngitis became refractory to repeated oral antibiotic therapy. Also the isolation of antibiotic resistant *Staphylococcus aureus* increased. A high incidence of *Haemophilus influenzae* was reported in the adenoids of children with recurrent exudative tonsillitis. We have confirmed and extended these observations and the subsequent effects of T and A on the ecology of the oropharyngeal microflora. A shift in the oropharyngeal microflora, following repeated oral antibiotic therapy, from predominantly Gram-positive cocci to Gram-negative rods and *Candida* sp. may also occur. The appearance of penicillin-resistant *Streptococcus mitis* group normal microflora may occur in patients on prophylactic penicillin therapy.

The enigma of the inability to eradicate *S. pyogenes* (Group A) from all patients with exudative tonsillitis and/or pharyngitis persists. Explanations of this failure include insufficient therapy, co-colonization with penicillinase-producing *Staphylococcus aureus* and inability to achieve bacteriocidal levels of penicillin inside the tonsils. A segment of such a population studied by our laboratory has also revealed a high incidence of underlying infection with Epstein–Barr virus and a return of the complex pathogenic microflora to normal after T and A.

Other micro-organisms must be considered in the aetiology of adenotonsillitis. L forms or bacterial variants do not appear to play a significant role. However, *Mycoplasma pneumonia* can cause primary atypical pneumoniae, myringitis, and other upper respiratory diseases. *Mycoplasma hominis* Type 1 has been shown to produce an exudative pharyngitis in 95% of experimentally infected volunteers, but this microorganism has only rarely been isolated from naturally infected patients. An unconfirmed report of the isolation of two strains of *Mycoplasma* sp. from tonsils of 2/38 patients with scarlatina may have been a chance observation. The fungi rarely are considered as primary pathogens in adenotonsillitis, although there is at least one report of their isolation from tonsils. Most of the fungi isolated are saprophytes that become lodged in the crypts of the tonsils and might provoke respiratory allergic phenomenon.

The viruses pose another interesting question. After the original report of adenoviruses in the human adenoids, several confirming investigations followed. Most children have neutralizing antibodies to adenoviruses by 5 years of age.

Two patients out of three with recurrent exudative tonsillitis have had either a primary or reactivated infection with EBV. All such patients harbour latent EBV genomes as shown by the Epstein–Barr Nuclear Antigens (EBNA) test. These data in combination with the complex pathogenic oropharyngeal microflora offer an ecosystem which might provide a source for synergistic bacterial-viral recurrent disease.

To summarize, adenotonsillitis appears to have a bacterial-viral cause; the bacterial flora appears to be different from normal. From a quantitative and qualitative analysis of the total spectrum of bacteria found in children with recurrent exudative tonsillitis, as well as children with persistent non-suppurative otitis media, an increase in the number and types of bacteria which are associated with disease processes of the head and neck are found. These bacteria do not always fulfil Koch's postulates, and include *Streptococcus pyogenes, Staphylococcus aureus, Haemophilus influenzae, Streptococcus pneumoniae* species, *Candida albicans* (a fungus) and the enteric aerobes and anaerobes. Conversely, there has been found a quantitative and qualitative decrease in the commensals, notably *Streptococcus mitis* group, *S. salivarius, Micrococcus* sp. and *Neisseria pharyngitidis*.

Adenotonsillitis appears to have certain virologic characteristics, namely the presence in the tonsil and adenoid tissue itself of latent viruses. These viruses are primarily the Epstein–Barr

virus, adenovirus and perhaps herpes simplex. These viruses, at least in the case of Epstein–Barr virus, remain in the tonsils and adenoids for what appears to be the life of the human host. Adenovirus remains latent also for long periods of time. These viruses may be subject to activation by other viral infections, or specific and non-specific factors shown in Table 36.1. Could the acquisition of a latent virus account for the change in

TABLE 36.1. Host factors

Anatomic
  Neoplasms
  Metaplasia
  Anatomical variations, e.g. septal deflections

Immunological

Embryonic
  Genetic: mongolism, gargoylism, cystic fibrosis
  Remnant: thyroglossal duct, lateral cervical fistulae
  Structural: Kartagener's syndrome

Host variability

Environmental
  Chemotherapeutic agents and drugs
  Humidity
  Temperature
  Trauma
  Pollution
  Environmental antigens (inhalant and food)
  Hormonal
  Dietary

Metabolic
  Hormonal
  Diabetes
  Hepatic
  Renal

bacterial flora? This is a question one could speculate upon but not as yet answer.

Immunologically, these children have not shown any immunological deficit, either before or after adenotonsillectomy. Rather there is a hypergammaglobulinaemia with adult or better than adult levels of IgG and statistically significant elevation of IgA. The evidence for this review of the immunology and bacteriology of tonsillar infection, together with a full list of references, is given elsewhere [1].

Clinical features

Tonsillitis is much more common in children with a maximum age incidence in the 5–7 age group [2].

It is usual to recognize two types:

(1) Acute parenchymatous in which the whole tonsil is infected, with a marked generalized swelling of the entire tonsil. The surface of the entire tonsil is reddened and often that of the surrounding pharynx, but the orifices of the crypts do not exude pus.

(2) Acute follicular (lacunar) tonsillitis. Here the tonsils are covered in yellow spots due to exudation of pus from the crypts. Occasionally, the spots coalesce so that the tonsil is then covered by a false membrane.

The symptoms of both these types are similar and, furthermore, the different appearances do not indicate the causative organism, which is indeed also true of the symptoms.

The symptoms are as follows:

Sore throat;

Pain on swallowing;

Pyrexia high in children (up to 104° F) but usually not so high in adults (up to 100°); and

Earache, which is relatively common. It is presumably referred from the tonsil itself, though why this should be is not clear since this structure has no sensory nerve supply.

The general symptoms and signs of a fever – malaise, headache, oliguria, etc. – are also present. A young child may not complain specifically of his throat, and the tonsils should be examined in every child who has a pyrexial illness.

Investigations

History
This is as outlined above.

Examination
Examination shows the typical appearances of uniform redness and swelling if the tonsillitis is the parenchymatous form, and the yellow spots in the crypts in the follicular form.

The jugulodigastric lymph glands are virtually always enlarged.

Laboratory studies
A throat swab, for culture and sensitivity, is probably only useful in retrospect and in research projects; by the time the result is available the child will be better.

Blood tests will reveal the usual leucocytosis, but this is of little practical interest. Abnormal mononuclear cells and a positive Paul–Bunnell test occur in infectious mononucleosis.

Complications

Local suppurative

Acute suppurative otitis media
Although acute otitis media may be associated with adenoidal disease (v.i.) the available evidence is that tonsillectomy does not decrease the incidence of acute otitis media, so that presumably tonsillar infection is not as a general rule a cause of otitis media.

Rhinitis and sinusitis
It is possible that these diseases are a sequel of acute tonsillitis, but the evidence available is obscured by the fact that vague terms such as 'catarrh' are used [3].

Peritonsillar abscess and quinsy
This is a spread of infection to the peritonsillar space, almost always occurring as a sequel to streptococcal tonsillitis. A few days after an attack of acute tonsillitis the patient becomes ill again, his temperature rises, and he complains of otalgia, dysphagia and trismus. Talking is painful and muffled and the mouth is often full of retained saliva which cannot be swallowed.

Examination shows the tonsil to be displaced downwards and medially, and the soft palate is oedematous. Examination is, however, often difficult because opening the mouth causes pain and because of the retained saliva in the mouth. The jugulodigastric glands are also enlarged.

The treatment is to incise and drain the abscess under local anaesthetic by inserting a knife into the space above the superior pole of the tonsil. Often pus is not obtained. This indicates either that the infection has not proceeded beyond the stage of cellulitis, or that the diagnosis is wrong.

A swab of the pus is taken for culture, and the patient is given a full course of penicillin. It is also customary to isolate the patient but this is almost certainly an unnecessary left-over from a generation or more ago. It is also said that once a patient has had a quinsy that it is likely to recur causing spreading infection of the spaces of the neck. Due to the extreme rarity of the latter this also appears to be an atavistic statement but it remains the custom to advise patients who have had a true quinsy to undergo tonsillectomy.

As an alternative the tonsils may be removed in the acute phase (abscess tonsillectomy).

The differential diagnosis of a quinsy is a tumour of the tonsil – particularly one of the reticuloses.

The complications of a quinsy are now rare – parapharyngeal abscess is discussed elsewhere (p. 297).

Remote non-suppurative complications

Rheumatic fever
Rheumatic fever follows an infection of the upper respiratory tract with a Group A streptococcus, but the mechanism is unknown. Several hypotheses have been put forward:

(1) It results from persistence of streptococci or their variants in the patient.

(2) It is caused by toxic components or products of streptococci.

(3) It is a hypersensitivity or auto-immune disorder set off by Group A streptococci.

Although the third theory is popular and has been the subject of much research there is no evidence that it is true [4].

Rheumatic fever was formerly one of the most dreaded complications of streptococcal tonsillitis. The dramatic decrease in its incidence may be due only in part to the use of penicillin and may also be due to a change in the epidemiology of the streptococcus.

There is no evidence that tonsillectomy significantly alters the attack rate of acute rheumatic fever as a sequel of streptococcal infections, nor does it significantly reduce the development of valvular heart disease in patients with acute rheumatic fever [3].

Acute glomerulonephritis
Acute post-streptococcal glomerulonephritis (AGN) is a form of acute glomerular injury which follows as a delayed sequel of infection with certain nephrogenic strains of Group A β-haemolytic streptococci. Positive throat cultures, elevated antistreptococcal antibody titres, antistreptolysin O, anti DNAase B and anti NAD are prerequisites for the diagnosis.

Urinalysis shows proteinuria, haematuria, and the presence of red cell casts. Hypertension, anaemia and oliguria are usually mild, and full recovery is the rule, but recurrence may follow a fresh infection.

It appears that the glomerular injury may be mediated by soluble immune complexes [4].

Cardio-respiratory complications
Since 1956, 21 cases of severe respiratory and/or cardiac failure due to upper airway obstruction from enlargement of tonsils and adenoids have been reported [3]. Fifteen of these cases had pulmonary hypertension, and cor pulmonale, and of the fifteen at least ten had cardiac failure. One of these children died after a thoracotomy in a fruitless search for a heart defect, but all the rest showed striking improvement following removal of the tonsils and/or adenoids. Of the remaining six cases, three were deaths in children due to asphyxia from hypertrophy of tonsils and adenoids, one was a girl of 15 who died of cardiac failure and septicaemia due to tonsillitis, and two were children who had to undergo tracheotomy during an attack of acute tonsillitis because of enormous enlargement of the tonsils (these two recovered).

The largest group, the fifteen cases in which chronic hypoxia had led to cor pulmonale etc., nearly all had certain features in common: noisy stertorous respiratory efforts, worse in recumbency, somnolence or even coma, with lethargy and mental dullness when awake. These symptoms, together with hypoxia and hypercapnia, and otherwise unexplained pulmonary hypertension and perhaps right cardiac failure (when pulmonary stenosis and left to right shunt can be excluded), should point to the tonsils and adenoids as the probable cause.

With the decline in mortality from operations on tonsils and adenoids in Great Britain these dangers must be firmly borne in mind, otherwise the possession of tonsils and adenoids may in a few cases become more hazardous than their removal. [3].

Differential diagnosis
The differential diagnosis is from:
(1) Glandular fever (infectious mononucleosis);
(2) Agranulocytosis;
(3) Vincent's angina;
(4) Diphtheria; and
(5) Scarlet fever.

Treatment

At least half the attacks of tonsillitis are not due to bacteria, so that antibiotics are not strictly speaking indicated. But the parents often demand that something be done and penicillin is then usually given – 125 mg four times a day of oral penicillin (for a child). It is said that it must be impressed on the mother that the antibiotics should be continued for a full five days, but this is probably based on the authoritarian attitude of doctors rather than fact – virtually all haemolytic streptococci are dead within 24 hours of exposure to a full dose of penicillin.

The usual general measures such as aspirin, bed rest, fluids, etc., should be given.

Tonsillectomy

This operation has been the subject of enormous controversy over the last generation, and its place is still undecided, although it remains one of the commonest operations carried out today. Its earlier popularity was due to the fact that the sequelae of streptococcal infection were common, crippling and often fatal. The sequelae have gone but the habit lingers on.

Repeated investigations have shown that tonsillectomy is more often carried out in white people than in Negroes [3], in prosperous areas of the UK than in other areas, and in the children of the well-to-do than in working class children [2]. The reasons for this must remain a matter for individual contemplation.

In the almost total absence of any objective evidence of the benefit of tonsillectomy the following indications are advised:
(1) Those few children with cor pulmonale and right-sided heart failure secondary to enlarged adenoids and tonsils.

(2) Those children with three or more genuine episodes of exudative tonsillitis in a year, five attacks in 2 years, persistent abnormal bacterial microflora of the oropharynx and nasopharynx and/or elevated levels of IgG and IgA.

(3) Those children with persistent non-suppurative otitis media with no systemic immunological or metabolic deficit and no allergic disorder, but who carry a persistent abnormal bacterial microflora of the oropharynx and nasopharynx.

Tonsillectomy is now almost certainly not indicated in children who have had rheumatic fever or glomerulonephritis unless there are local indications.

Tonsillectomy is now generally carried out by the dissection technique under general anaesthetic, and the use of the guillotine has been largely abandoned. The destruction of the tonsil by the cryoprobe has also been described, but is almost certainly only applicable in certain conditions such as haemophilia.

Complications following removal

Complications following tonsillectomy and adenoidectomy are not uncommon: 1·5% develop serious complications.

Early complications
(1) *Death*. This is estimated at 1 in 10 000 operations but a considerable proportion should have been prevented.
(2) *Blood loss*. Several series [5, 6] have shown that a child loses up to 10% of its blood volume during tonsillectomy. Obviously blood loss of this order places the child at risk of circulatory collapse in the event of a reactionary haemorrhage.

Post-operative blood loss may be *reactionary* or *secondary*.

Reactionary haemorrhage comes from a vessel that was not ligated during the operation. It should be looked for by nursing the child prone so that blood trickles out of his mouth and can be seen, and by keeping a post-operative chart of vital signs. It should be treated by the well-known principles for dealing with post-operative bleeding:

Replacement of blood lost; and

Ligature of the bleeding point.

Other methods such as sedating the child are dangerous. Blood should be replaced urgently before the child is returned to theatre, and the anaesthetic must be given by a competent anaesthetist.

(3) *Temporo-mandibular joint dysfunction* due to bruising of the joint cartilage at operation from over-extension of the jaw (particularly in adults).

Intermediate complications

(4) *Speech disability.* This is due to palatal scarring and removal of the adenoid buttress, and injury to the blood supply to the uvula. This is particularly liable to occur in patients with submucous or complete cleft of the palate.

(5) Compensatory *hypertrophy* of the remaining lymphoid tissue comprising mainly the lateral pharyngeal bands and lingual tonsils. These tissues do not undergo atrophy in the usual manner and are very liable to viral infection.

(6) Production of *granular pharyngitis* due to drying, from inadequate moistening by a tight scarred palate, and aggravated by mouth breathing. Patches of hypertrophied tissue develop around the openings of tiny glands in nature's attempt to protect the pharynx from drying.

(7) *Psychological effect* on the child, which at times is considerable.

Late complications

(8) *Drying of the pharynx.* This is the commonest and most distressing of the late complications and is due to a tight palate. A varying degree of palatal scarring following tonsillectomy is inevitable, and as the scar tissue does not grow and stretch adequately with the normal growth of the palate, a palate which may function satisfactorily in the small child may become progressively inefficient as the child grows older. As the mucus from the nose cannot pass easily onto the dry pharyngeal area, it tends to accumulate, dry, and thicken, thus giving rise to the common complaint of catarrh or post-nasal drip.

(9) *Recurrent low grade infection*, usually viral, of the hypertrophied lymphoid tissues. In particular, irritation of the hypertrophied lingual tonsil and epiglottis area may cause a 'strain-swallow' syndrome and vicious circle with clearing of the throat and lack of relaxation of the throat and laryngeal muscles, causing a feeling of tightness.

(10) *Impairment of immunity mechanism* as an increased tendency to malignancy has been reported [7].

ADENOIDS

Adenoid tissue is present in the nasopharynx of all normal children, the amount varying from one child to the next and also varying with age. In a particular child the adenoid reaches maximum size between the ages of 3 and 7 and then undergoes involution. The clinician must decide whether the adenoid tissue in a particular child is present in abnormal amounts or whether it is irreversibly diseased.

Pathology

Two pathological processes can occur in the lymphoid tissue of the adenoid. First, and most commonly, the tissue can undergo hyperplasia due to enlargement and multiplication of the lymphoid follicles. Secondly, and much less commonly, the adenoid can be the site of chronic inflammation with the formation of abscesses. Abscess formation is a very rare occurrence and by no means as common as a similar process in the palatine tonsil. Similar micro-organisms can be isolated from nasopharyngeal and palatine tonsils. Polvogt & Crowe [8] cultivated the tonsils and adenoids removed from 100 children and the results are shown in Table 36.2.

Pathogenic viruses have also been cultured from the adenoid.

The hypertrophic adenoid may obstruct the posterior choanae interfering with nasal respiration and causing stasis of secretions in the nasal cavity. This stasis of secretions together with chronic infection in the adenoid may predispose to chronic sinusitis. The adenoid may also obstruct the pharyngeal opening of the Eustachian tube either mechanically or by oedema due to a salpingitis caused by the infected adenoid. A coexistent chronic sinusitis may also contribute to an inflammatory oedema of the Eustachian tube.

Clinical features of enlarged adenoids

Nasal obstruction

Because of obstructed nasal respiration the child may breathe through his mouth and snore at night. In addition he may have a constant nasal

TABLE 36.2. Organisms cultivated from 100 children

Number of patients	Organisms cultured
81	β-haemolytic streptococcus
8	Staphylococcus pyogenes
10	Staphylococcus from the adenoid, Streptococcus from the tonsil
1	No growth

discharge. Examination will reveal a child who keeps his mouth open and whose nasal mucosa is hyperaemic and bathed in secretion. However, these signs and symptoms may also be reproduced by allergic rhinitis or by chronic sinusitis. The former may be suggested by specific points of the history and the latter by radiology. It is the author's belief that many children thought to be suffering from enlarged adenoids have a disturbance of the immune mechanism which results in engorgement of the nasal mucosa.

Adenoid facies

The classical facial appearance said to be due to enlarged adenoids consist of:

(1) An open mouth with prominent upper incisors and a short upper lip.

(2) A thin nose, a hypoplastic narrow maxilla and a high vaulted palate.

Rather than a causal relationship between enlarged adenoids and this facial appearance it may be that children with this type of maxillary development are more liable to nasal obstruction due to the adenoid because of the particular anatomical development. If nasal obstruction

was responsible for growth changes one would expect those patients with unilateral choanal atresia to have asymmetrical facial development.

Cor pulmonale as a result of enlarged adenoids

Well-documented cases exist in which enlargement of the adenoid has resulted in pulmonary emphysema with cor pulmonale and right-sided heart failure. These pulmonary and cardiovascular complications have been reversed by adenoidectomy. Such cases, however, are exceedingly rare.

Investigations

A detailed history and careful clinical examination are an important part of the investigation of a child suspected of enlarged adenoids. In addition, radiology is the most reliable method of assessing the size of the adenoid. At the same time as a lateral radiograph to demonstrate the adenoid, an occipito-mental view will give information on the state of the maxillary sinuses.

Treatment

Indications for adenoidectomy

Nasal obstruction
In children whose nasal obstruction and mouth breathing are thought to be due to enlarged adenoids, adenoidectomy is the treatment of choice.

Serous otitis media
Although the aetiology of serous otitis is still the subject of debate, most practising otologists believe that the adenoid is responsible for the condition in a significant proportion of cases. Thus, the surgical management of serous otitis media consists of adenoidectomy with myringotomy and aspiration of fluid. Some surgeons insert a grommet at the first operation, others prefer to wait and insert a grommet only if fluid recurs.

Otitis media
Children with recurrent attacks of acute otitis

media or with persistent chronic suppurative otitis media of the safe type may benefit from adenoidectomy.

Chronic sinusitis

Huggill & Ballantyne [9] showed that the results of treating chronic sinusitis in children could be improved by removing the adenoids at the same time as treating the sinuses.

Contra-indications to adenoidectomy

(1) The relation between adenoidectomy and rhinolalia aperta is discussed in the next section. Any child who has had a cleft palate repair or who has a submucous cleft of the palate should not have adenoidectomy to avoid producing rhinolalia aperta.

(2) Although opinion varies on the age at which operation should be performed there seems little justification for adenoidectomy before the age of 4. In young children with serous otitis media perhaps the simplest procedure is to insert a grommet and leave adenoidectomy until the child is older.

(3) A recent upper respiratory tract infection is an absolute contra-indication to adenoidectomy as primary and secondary haemorrhage and pulmonary complications of the anaesthetic are more likely.

(4) Any child suspected of a bleeding disorder should be fully investigated before surgery. If operation is necessary in a child with a haemorrhagic diathesis deficiency of the clotting factors should be corrected before surgery.

Complications of adenoidectomy

Early complications

(1) *Haemorrhage*. The bleeding which accompanies removal of the adenoid ceases spontaneously in most cases. Persistent haemorrhage may respond to removal of adenoid remnants or insertion of a pack. It is essential that all haemorrhage has ceased before the child recovers from the anaesthetic. Primary haemorrhage, i.e. occurring up to 24 hours after surgery, must be treated very seriously. Minor bleeding may cease with sedation but persistent haemorrhage is controlled by returning the child to theatre and inserting a post-nasal pack under anaesthetic. Blood loss must be replaced. Most of the deaths associated with adenoidectomy are due to delay in the treatment of primary haemorrhage.

(2) *Trauma*. Hurried, careless surgery can result in damage to the soft palate or the posterior pharyngeal wall. Dislocation of the cervical spine can occur as a result of surgery but usually this is the result of infection affecting the anterior ligaments and causing subluxation of the atlanto-occipital joint about 1 week after the operation.

Intermediate complications

(3) *Secondary haemorrhage*. This occurs after 24 hours and before 2 weeks, usually between 5 and 10 days. It is due to infection and is treated by antibiotics and blood transfusion. Occasionally a post-nasal pack will be necessary to control bleeding.

(4) *Pulmonary complications*. Pulmonary atelectasis can occur after operation due to inhalation of mucus, adenoid fragments or blood clot. It is more likely in the presence of an upper respiratory infection at the time of surgery.

(5) *Earache*. Referred otalgia can occur after adenoidectomy but not as commonly as after tonsillectomy. Acute otitis media can be a complication of both operations.

Late complications

(6) *Rhinolalia aperta*. Hypernasality has been estimated to occur once in every 1450 adenotonsillectomies. However, the actual incidence of this complication is probably much higher because transient or minor defects may pass unnoticed [10].

To avoid this complication any suspicion of hypernasality before operation should be viewed with considerable caution and the patient assessed by a speech therapist. The finding of a bifid uvula before operation should also alert the surgeon. Beeden [11] has suggested that bifid uvula occurs at a rate of 1 in 70 in the population. A proportion of children with a bifid uvula will have a submucous cleft, diagnosed by feeling a notch in the palate and, in these, adenoidectomy should be avoided. The treatment of established rhinolalia aperta as a complication of adenoidectomy is speech therapy. Very occasionally, a pharyngoplasty will be necessary in severe cases.

Psychological effects of surgery

Levy [12] has described the emotional sequelae of surgery on young children and has advocated the following steps to reduce these complications.

(1) Avoidance of surgery in the very young;

(2) A careful explanation to the child of what he is going to experience;

(3) Close contact of the child with his mother immediately before and after the operation; and

(4) Adequate premedication.

Formation of scar tissue

A certain amount of fibrosis is inevitable in the post-nasal space following adenoidectomy and normally this will cause no harm. Damage to the Eustachian tube during the operation, however, may well lead to fibrosis which interferes with Eustachian tube function. An occasional case has been described in which almost complete obliteration of the post-nasal space by fibrous tissue has followed adenoidectomy.

References

[1] SPRINKLE P. M. & VELTRI R. W. (1976) The tonsils and adenoids. Clinical Otolaryngology 2, 153.

[2] FRY J. (1961) The Catarrhal Child. London: Butterworths.

[3] RANSOME J. (1900) Tonsils and adenoids. In Recent Advances in Otolaryngology, Vol. 2, pp: 253–274. London: Churchill Livingstone.

[4] STIEHM E. & FULGINITI V. A. (1973) Immunologic Disorders in Infants and Children. pp. 424 and 439. Philadelphia: W. B. Saunders.

[5] HOLDEN H. B. & MAHER J. J. (1965) Some aspects of blood loss and fluid balance in paediatric adenotonsillectomy. British Medical Journal 2, 1349.

[6] SHALOM A. S. (1964) Blood loss in ear, nose and throat operations. Journal of Laryngology 78, 734.

[7] GRAY L. P. (1977) The T's & A's problem. Journal of Laryngology and Otology, 91, 11.

[8] POLVOGT L. M. & CROWE S. J. (1929) Predominating organisms found in cultures from tonsils and adenoids. Journal of the American Medical Association 92, 962.

[9] HUGGILL P. H. & BALLANTYNE J. C. (1952) An investigation into the relationship between adenoids and sinusitis in children. Journal of Laryngology and Otology 66, 84.

[10] GIBB A. G. (1958) Hypernasality (rhinolalia aperta) following tonsil and adenoid removal. Journal of Laryngology and Otology 72, 433.

[11] BEEDEN A. G. (1972) The bifid uvula. Journal of Laryngology and Otology 86, 815.

[12] LEVY D. M. (1945) Psychic trauma of operations in children. American Journal of Diseases of Children 69, 7.

CHAPTER 37

Sensorineural Deafness in Childhood

Deafness affects children differently from adults. It is easier to compensate for deafness when language is firmly established than for deafness which occurs before the ability to speak exists.

It is difficult to test children's hearing because they may not be able to cooperate with tests which are relatively easy to adults. Play methods must be applied which require special techniques and environment. In very young children changes of behaviour as a result of sound stimulation must be carefully observed.

Rehabilitation is also different from that of adults and education is the important aspect of child audiology, because deafness also affects the child's learning ability.

A disability in a child is bound to affect the whole family. Considerable care is necessary to prevent family life from breaking down when under stress. Parental guidance forms an essential part of the care of deaf children.

Because we are dealing with a disability in a growing and developing individual regular reassessment is essential.

PATHOLOGY

It is important to diagnose whether the deafness is congenital or acquired. Children who have acquired a hearing loss when they have already heard and developed language and speech are trained and educated differently to those who were born with severe deafness. Also deciding whether the deafness is congenital or acquired acts as a guide to the cause.

Congenital deafness

Genetic

Almost half of all congenital deafness is of genetic origin.

The high rate of deafness in consanguinous parents shows that genetic deafness must often be recessive in type (probably 90% of all cases). Sex linked genes, which may be either recessive or dominant, contribute no more than 2% to the total of childhood deafness in the population [1].

There are many rare recessive genes causing deafness. One in four of the normal population is a carrier for at least one of the recessive genes causing childhood deafness.

The mating of two recessive deaf persons either produces all hearing offspring or all deaf offspring, depending on whether the two parents are deaf from different or the same recessive genes. If one parent is deaf due to a heterozygous dominant gene, half of the offspring are expected to be deaf, while if both are deaf due to dominant heterozygous genes, three-quarters are expected to be deaf.

Fifteen per cent of the total are due to matings involving two parents who are deaf due to the same recessive genes and 60% are between parents deaf due to two different recessive genes. The matings of parents deaf due to dominant genes contribute about 25% of the total. Thus the predicted pattern of families resulting from marriage of two hereditary deaf is as follows: 60% will have all hearing children, 15% all deaf children and 25% both hearing and deaf children. When a hereditary deaf person marries a spouse who has acquired deafness or hears normally, 80% of the resulting families will hear normally and 20% will have both hearing and deaf children.

It is not always possible to decide whether the same or a different gene is operating in two families with apparently similar abnormalities. Most genes are sensitive to change in their genetic background, and the pitfalls of assuming the identity of two genes on the basis of similarities of their effects, or the lack of identity on the basis of differences, need not be emphasized.

Generally it is difficult to place the great variety of types and degrees of deafness in children into a logical classification incorporating all aspects, such as pathological, symptomatological or those based on clinical findings. There is not even a satisfactory way of arranging the large number of inherited diseases of the inner ear in man into categories. Conditions clinically homogeneous may be heterogeneous as judged by mode of inheritance.

Embryopathic

Virus infections (principally rubella) during the first trimester of pregnancy are often incriminated, but the possibility of drugs should be always borne in mind. The site of the lesion in rubella deafness is the organ of Corti.

Perinatal

Neonatal anoxia, principally one beginning before delivery, can cause a high frequency loss, due to damage in the cochlear nuclei. Neonatal jaundice (hyperbilirubinaemia) causes a specific type of high frequency loss also as a result of damage to the cochlear nuclei [2].

Those children whose deafness was caused by a perinatal disorder are incorporated in the congenital group because it is impossible to separate with certainty the causes which may have started before delivery from those which are connected with the birth, or the immediate postnatal period [3].

It is not always easy to determine whether deafness is congenital or appeared during early infancy or childhood. During assessment, if no definite congenital cause can be discovered, one must consider whether the deafness was acquired during the intervening period from birth to the time when the child was diagnosed as deaf. The later the deafness is detected, the greater the uncertainty will be. Absence of conditions known to cause deafness after birth, combined with the history of the child's vocal performance or development of communication by speech and the results of clinical examination, help in making a correct assessment. The earlier the deafness

is detected the greater the possibility of correct assessment.

Syndromes associated with deafness

Most patients with sensorineural deafness present at birth do not have syndromes (whether or not genetically determined) with detectable anomalies of other systems.

However, there is a group of children whose deafness is associated with abnormalities in other systems of the body forming recognizable clinical syndromes.

Deafness in association with *abnormalities of the eyes* is the syndrome of retinitis pigmentosa [4].

Abnormality of the thyroid in Pendred's syndrome, in which thyroxine synthesis is affected, is associated with deafness as an independent effect of the gene [5].

Deafness in association with *abnormalities of pigmentation* appear as the Waardenburg or 'White forelock' syndrome, a dominant inheritance. There are other forms of 'pigmentation–hearing' disorders, genetically different, in which the pigmentation disorder is hypopigmentation, often mistaken as 'albinism' [6].

Deafness associated with *various connective tissue disorders* may occur in osteogenesis imperfecta, Hurler's syndrome (gargoylism), and achondroplasia.

Skeletal defects in the Klippel Feil syndrome are associated with severe deafness and in Treacher–Collins syndrome the deafness is conductive as a result of malformation of external and middle ear structures [7].

Abnormalities of the heart, in the rare Jervell and Lange-Nielsen's syndrome, associated with deafness, produces syncope which may occasionally be fatal [8].

Congenital renal disorders can be associated with deafness in Alport's syndrome (chronic haemorrhagic nephritis) and in renal anomalies with a small under-developed kidney.

Various *ectodermal abnormalities* can be associated. A recessive hereditary syndrome occurs with nail dystrophy and ectodermal dysplasia.

Of the non-genetic syndromes associated with deafness the most important are the rubella syndrome and athetoid cerebral palsy (due to haemolytic disease of the newborn).

All those who are concerned with the care of deaf children should gain a detailed knowledge of these conditions. This is essential for early detection and because each of them presents specific difficulties to the diagnostician and those concerned with training and education.

The frequency of the various causes of congenital deafness

The relative proportions due to the various causes vary from country to country, even clinic to clinic, because of variations in terminology, in criteria for assessment and differences in standards of paedoaudiology. But there are also true variations caused by prevalence of different types of congenital deafness.

TABLE 37.1

Cause	No. of Cases	Percentage
Genetic	244	36·0
Rubella	40	5·9
Anoxia	91	13·4
HDNB	83	12·2
Unknown	207	30·5
Other	12	1·7

An investigation of more than 600 patients with congenital deafness showed the results as illustrated in Table 37.1. In a sample of congenitally deaf children born after a major rubella epidemic, 24% of all children were deaf from maternal rubella. As a result of rubella immunization this cause may almost disappear. Also the genetic composition of the population may change.

Few reliable data exist concerning the true prevalence of congenital deafness of all types because of the lack of major population studies and the difficulty in obtaining complete ascertainment in a well-defined community.

Generally the prevalence of profound congenital deafness is estimated as 1:1000 in the population. Some countries such as Peru, Honduras and Japan exceed this figure, while the European and North American average is below it. These estimates may not include all cases of congenital deafness. A study of fully investigated children with congenital deafness in an area with good paedoaudiology facilities showed the distribution of types of hearing loss as illustrated in Table 37.2.

TABLE 37.2

Total 274	Number	Percentage
Residual hearing only	56	20·43
Predominantly high-frequency loss	105	38·32
Flat loss, moderate to severe	52	18·97
Predominantly low-frequency loss	9	3·28
Middle frequencies mainly affected	8	2·91
Highest frequencies only	8	2·91
Irregular audiogram (not classifiable)	7	2·55
Total deafness	4	1·45
No audiogram available	25	9·12

Severe deafness, with residual hearing only, occurred in 20%. Less severe deafnesses, which are not so easy to detect early, may remain undiagnosed for a long time during childhood and are often unrecognized as being of congenital origin. If these are included, the true prevalence of congenital deafness is 1:200.

Acquired deafness

Meningitis can cause a severe sensorineural deafness and mumps, as a result of cochleitis, can result in an almost total unilateral and rarely bilateral deafness.

Middle ear disorders of any type may cause deafness which is often variable and can affect children much more seriously than is generally realized.

Progressive sensorineural deafnesses developing during early childhood emerge from time to time. In some children a deafness may have been present at birth which gradually increases with age. Experience from audiology centres shows that such children do exist, but because of difficulties in discovering moderate degrees of deafness during early infancy, the natural history of early progressive sensorineural deafness in children has not been studied in great detail as yet.

Fracture of the temporal bone is a relatively rare cause of sensorineural deafness in children.

Of the new hazards, it is important to stress ototoxic drugs and noise exposure. Ototoxic drugs, both systemic and local, may cause sensorineural deafness [3].

Epidemiology of deafness in children

The prevalence of deafness in children and the composition of the child population with deafness is gradually changing. Rubella vaccination will eliminate the rubella syndrome as a serious cause of deafness in children. The genetic composition of populations may change, partly as a result of immigration and partly because of social changes.

An important development in the last century has been the increasing economic integration of the deaf with a corresponding increase in their fertility. This has led to an increase in the number of patients with dominant and, to a lesser extent, sex-linked recessive deafness and probably to an increase in autosomal recessive forms also. The social position of the deaf in society is changing again particularly because of the success of oral education. This may influence the prevalence of genetic deafness because of the decrease of intermarriage between the deaf. Larger numbers of deaf now integrate into normal society.

CLINICAL FEATURES

Consequences of severe deafness

The raw material from which human language is built is sound, so that it is very difficult for a child born with severe deafness to learn language spontaneously, as normal children do, simply by hearing speach.

Deaf children may not be able to learn language at all (unless specially taught) or they may do so slowly, and their speech may remain defective. They are also deprived of stimulation by environmental sounds which are of great practical and emotional significance.

We are surrounded by continuous background sounds originating from everyday activities. These become not only essential components of our emotional life but also keep us in continuous contact with the environment. Sensory deprivation in this respect plays an important part in shaping the personality of a deaf person and affects also the child's learning ability. Normally children learn about the outside world by a combination of several sensory stimuli arriving simultaneously or in quick succession and they learn the significance of individual components of this stream of signals. When a child hears a sound he first tries to locate the direction, then he turns his head in order to confirm the source visually and learns its meaning. This combination of the two most important sensory receptors is of great importance. Without it the process of learning slows down. The effects of a severe deafness in children is therefore much more complex than one would expect.

Many children show the same results on hearing tests, but there is a wide variety of difficulties which cannot be forecast from looking at the results of even a whole battery of tests. Without considering the patient's social context, his personality, learning ability, powers of discrimination, other abnormalities or disabilities, we cannot determine how he will be affected. The child's environment, age when deafness was diagnosed and the quality of training also modify the effects of the handicap.

The effects of high frequency loss

High frequency losses occur relatively often in children in slight, moderate and severe degrees. This type of impairment is still detected far too late. We have no reliable screening tests to detect the more moderate degrees of high frequency loss at a very early age. Children with a high frequency loss may even start to speak or learn to communicate fairly well by speech, but in unfavourable circumstances they have serious difficulties leading to a breakdown of communication. These difficulties are often not recognized as being caused by deafness and other causes are blamed for the child's frustration. Because the symptoms mask the true nature of the condition, hearing is not assessed properly and the children are often diagnosed as aphasic, emotionally disturbed or 'psychotic'.

In many respects a high frequency loss, especially when detected late, can cause greater frustration and disturbance than profound deafness.

Symptoms of hearing loss in young children

In infants the following early symptoms, as observed by parents, are reported: no reaction to sound; not waking from sleep when approached or called; not paying attention generally to sound stimulation; a 'very quiet baby'; frightened by sudden or unexpected visual stimulation. Later, when a child should develop greater variety in vocal performance, it does not produce babbling sounds. Babbling means production of syllables, such as 'ba-ba', 'ma-ma'; a 9-month-old child should be able to produce a clear four-syllable babble.

Young children 'do not pay attention'; they consistently confuse what is said, especially children with a high frequency loss. They are 'inattentive' and appear 'not to listen' or 'do not want to listen'.

Often it is not recognized that the cause of these difficulties is deafness and the child is accused of being 'naughty', 'lazy', 'slow in development', etc.

Many symptoms of deafness are shared with other conditions such as mental retardation, emotional disturbance, environmental deprivation, developmental retardation, autism, psychotic conditions, cerebral palsy, neurological orders, physical impediments and special language learning difficulties.

At the first stage of investigation the diagnosis must be established by a full hearing assessment. Difficulty in speaking is still one of the commonest reasons why children are sent for a more detailed examination of their hearing. This is also a symptom common to several other disorders.

At the initial stages two important possibilities should be considered – deafness or low mental ability. Although the cause of the difficulty is entirely different in these two conditions, initially there are similarities, and early differential diagnosis between the two possible causes is most important. However, deafness and low mental ability can coexist, in different degrees, in the same individual. It is then important to estimate correctly the degree of each disability separately and combined.

While the effects of severe congenital deafness in children are pronounced and, eventually, readily noticeable, one should not underestimate the effects of the less severe or even very moderate degrees of impairment. For instance, a moderate high-frequency loss can be extremely frustrating to a child and may cause severe emotional disturbance seemingly out of proportion to the deafness. Similarly, types of variable conductive deafness, relatively frequent in children, can have far reaching consequences on educational progress.

ASSESSMENT

The importance of early detection

Many difficulties, apparent later in the deaf child, are probably due to auditory deprivation from the very first hours of the child's life. These effects are cumulative and increase in complexity as time passes. The later the deafness is detected the worse for the child since many effects of late detection are permanent and irreparable.

Difficulties during infancy are caused by the absence of an effective universal screening test which would enable us to detect all types of deafness.

Detection, both by screening and by symptoms, cannot be considered as a once-for-all exercise but should be a programme extending over several years of childhood. Screening all children may not be possible at present but at least one should try to introduce a system which should ensure that all children who are at high risk due to their medical history should be tested. All children with symptoms such as absence of babbling at 9 months, late or slow speech development or with an articulation defect, should be tested routinely without exception. Suspicion by the parents that a child cannot hear well should be treated as a symptom and investigated.

A significant number of children born deaf have one of the many syndromes associated with deafness. All children who show signs of any of these syndromes should be screened and followed-up regularly until a full test can be carried out, if at all possible, by pure tone audiometry.

Developmental stages and hearing tests

There are three stages in a child's development

which determine the appropriate type of test. The first stage extends from birth to the time when the child starts to sit unsupported. During this stage we rely on involuntary reactions, such as blink, change of facial expression, change of behaviour, and movement of various parts of the body, which may occur as a result of sound stimulation. These reactions are not as consistent as head turning and are often difficult to note and interpret.

By 6 months a baby should sit up and keep his head vertical. A reflex has now fully developed which compels the child to turn his head towards the source of a significant sudden change in the environment. A normal baby turns the head briskly towards the source of a test sound, provided the sound does not merge into the general background noise and the child is not disturbed by other changes in the environment. This is the second developmental stage from the testing point of view.

The third stage begins at about 2½ years. From this age a physically and mentally normal child can be taught to cooperate, that is to carry out a movement as a game when a sound is produced. The movement can be, for example, placing toy bricks from one box into another or placing them on top of each other when a sound is produced. When this is achieved and a consistent reliable response is obtained full threshold audiometry should soon be possible.

Conditions for testing

It is not certain that in a normally hearing subject a reaction to a sound stimulus will occur every time.

Environmental and internal influences modify the probability of a response [9]. Anxiety can inhibit a reaction in a child. Other internal factors are distractibility, arousal, habituation and behaviour patterns. The environmental influences include size and quality of the room, the examiner himself and the method of applying the test sound. It is important to be aware of these influences when one sets out to test the hearing of children.

A child reacts to a test stimulus only when he is ready to respond. Environmental and internal factors interact and create 'readiness to respond', a condition which varies according to these influences. The environment must be specially designed for testing, both in a free field and by audiometry. The size and appearance of the room can be critical.

The examiner must be well trained in the various play methods used and be able to gain the confidence of children and reduce their anxiety to the minimum.

Screening tests in the newborn

Many attempts have been made to devise screening procedures to detect deafness at this very early age [10]. In most of these the startle response to high intensity sounds is used as the signal that it was heard. But this is a very unreliable test. Auditory screening tests for newborns, using only gross observation, establish only whether an infant responds to sound, on the basis of which an examiner can say nothing whatever about the integrity of the eighth nerve or any other system. Implicit in any pass-or-fail procedure is the notion that those who pass the test are normal, though in fact they may not be.

Electrophysiological procedures (such as electric response audiometry by electroencephalography) are used in newborn infants but they are not suitable for practical mass screening.

Screening tests in infants

When testing the hearing of infants we rely on some change of behaviour when a test sound is produced. These tests have to be carried out in 'free field' and therefore we cannot test at threshold levels. The intensity levels of the test sounds are about 40–45 dB.

The sounds are usually produced by hand-held objects (a rattle, bell, the tinkle of a spoon in a cup, rustle of paper, etc.). They are mixed sounds and therefore although the test helps to detect severe deafness it is not good enough to detect less severe deafness especially when the hearing is impaired for certain frequencies only. Acoustic conditions can influence the results considerably.

Hearing tests in free field

It is difficult to carry out accurate measurements in free field tests based on behavioural observation. However, when these tests are properly carried out, in a specially designed and acoustically suitable environment, hearing ability can be reliably assessed within certain limits. There is no need to wait for a full audiometric test before taking the necessary measures to train the child.

In spite of certain limitations, tests based on careful clinical observations are still the best we have although they could be improved. Observation and recording of the reactions can be improved by distant monitoring and videotape recording. The test sounds can be recorded and played back via a calibrated system into loudspeakers which improves the accuracy and standardization of these tests considerably [11].

Even if we had a truly 'objective' type of (electrophysiological) test, we could not discard behavioural observation of the child in free field, because this provides us with much additional information essential for assessment.

Screening audiometry at school

It is most important to detect deafness of any degree, even minor, in all school children; school screening audiometry is most effective in achieving this. It can be carried out in large numbers in a relatively short time because it is not a threshold test. The sound level is fixed at 20 dB and the child is asked to indicate whether frequencies from 250 Hz to 8000 Hz are heard. In young children play audiometry methods should be used and 50–60 children can be screened in a single session.

Those who fail to pass the screen should be tested by full threshold audiometry in a properly established audiometric room.

Pure tone audiometry

All children suspected of being deaf should be tested by pure tone threshold audiometry as soon as possible.

In physically and mentally normal children, when play audiometry is used correctly by specially trained examiners, cooperation can be achieved from about 2½ years.

Before a full test is carried out it is essential to prepare the child in stages, in surroundings which allow us to reduce his anxiety, to gain his confidence and achieve cooperation in the form of play.

During the first stage the child is taught to carry out a movement (which is the signal that the test sound was heard) when a sound is produced by a percussion instrument, so that the child can see and hear the sources of the sound. When he has learnt the game and performed reliably, the second stage follows during which the child cannot see the source of the test sound. When a reliable response is obtained the third stage follows, that is practising responses to pure tones produced with a small free field pure tone audiometer.

When a reliable response is obtained the fourth stage follows of introducing the child to the earphone. First, a single earphone is used in conjunction with the free field audiometer during a preparatory stage. Once a child has accepted it and responded reliably, the fifth stage follows: transfer to the audiometry room for a full threshold test. The large earphones are presented gently.

With some children even at this stage an intermediate stage of 'practice audiometry' is interposed.

Even with the best conditions a few children are difficult to test, or it may take much longer to achieve a full result. The child with a physical difficulty, especially cerebral palsy; the child of low mental ability; children with a narrow span of attention or high degree of distractibility, the anxious or extremely shy child; the totally unresponsive child; the hyperkinetic restless child; the autistic child. All these children need special conditions, that is an environment designed for the purpose and experienced examiners [12].

Speech perception tests

All children who are suspected of being deaf should have their speech perception ability tested as soon as possible. One can test speech hearing at a very young age. A 2½-year-old child (often even younger ones) can be presented with a series of pictures representing everyday objects or appropriate models of everyday objects and asked to point to them or handle them.

Speech perception tests can be carried out with older children in a variety of ways. If a child does not want to say anything or is unable to speak clearly he can be presented with a series of pictures representing everyday objects and asked in a conversational voice to point to the pictures from various distances. Alternatively the voice can be pre-recorded and played back at definite intensities, or monitored via a calibrated amplification system.

Normally before such testing begins the child is required to name each picture (provided this is within the limits of the child's ability) as it is placed before him and then to identify each picture as asked to do so by the test voice.

If a child can cooperate and his speech is intelligible it is most useful to carry out a simple test of hearing for speech in free field as follows: The child is asked to face the speaker who from a distance of 15 feet pronounces phonetically balanced test words and sentences and the child repeats them. If he is not able to do so the distance is gradually shortened and the distance at which the child can repeat consistently what the examiner said is noted. The same procedure is then carried out without lip reading. Each ear is then tested separately by masking one ear.

The room must be non-reverberating. The examiner must keep his voice at the same level whatever the distance and he must use phonetically balanced words and sentences. Provided the test is carried out properly it is highly informative, simple and most economical.

When a child who is known to be deaf is tested for speech perception ability, mainly from the point of view of hearing aid perception, his speech and speech thresholds are tested when the speech material is delivered via an amplifier. During such testing the child points to a corresponding picture when each stimulus is presented acoustically. The child's responses are recorded and scored. This simple test can be carried out in most children of 5 regardless of their deafness.

Full speech audiometry as applied to adults cannot be carried out below the age of 9 because special word lists must be constructed for each age group according to the child's language ability. Testing for speech perception ability should be part of the audiological investigation of children suspected of being deaf.

Differential diagnosis between conductive and sensorineural impairment

Bone conduction tests in small children can be difficult because they may be unable to distinguish clearly between vibration and hearing. Masking sounds can also disturb the child. For these reasons bone conduction thresholds in small children should be viewed with scepticism.

Differential diagnosis between conductive and sensorineural deafness should not be difficult. *Impedance measurements* should be carried out and children with abnormal tympanograms should have further investigation for conductive deafness [13].

A normal tympanic membrane without a history of middle ear disease in a severely deaf child indicates that the deafness is probably not conductive. When the deafness is so severe that it prevents the child from learning language it is unlikely that it is a purely conductive deafness.

Many children with a sensorineural deafness also have a superimposed conductive element which may change the pattern of the audiogram. If the hearing varies, one should always investigate the possibility of a superimposed conductive deafness.

Electric response tests

Tests based on recording physiological reactions to sound recorded by electrophysiological procedures are limited in their scope and value compared to tests based on behavioural observation, threshold pure tone audiometry and speech perception ability tests. Their principles are outlined in Chapter 1.

Children presented for assessment of hearing should be carefully observed in a variety of situations, including observation of their behaviour and their reactions to sound stimulation in free field. In some children both electrophysiological procedure and behavioural and clinical observation are necessary and are complementary.

Unfortunately those children who are difficult to test by behavioural observation are those who are often also difficult to assess with electric-response tests.

Children with athetoid cerebral palsy and high frequency loss, when the damage is in the cochlear nuclei, show normal threshold responses with ECoG although some changes in action potentials have been observed. ERA tests on these children, as with many others with behavioural difficulties or brain damage, conducted under sedation, may be confusing and unreliable.

Children with high frequency loss due to predelivery anoxia also show normal responses with ECoG; these are also often children with difficult behaviour or hyperkinesia and ERA tests under sedation are again very unreliable.

Even when responses to ECoG are present at high frequencies this does not exclude the possibility of considerable loss in the middle and low range. The deafness is often asymmetrical and in these children both ears must be tested by ECoG.

ECoG may be of some value in the most difficult children to test, for example in the deaf and blind child with the rubella syndrome, but one must be aware of the limitations.

The economy of testing must be also considered. When many children must be tested it would be impracticable to subject all the children to electric response tests, which are more expensive and time consuming.

Overall assessment

The best treatment, training and education require answers to the following questions:

Has the child other disabilities associated with the deafness?

What is the child's learning ability and if it is impaired is it because of abnormal intelligence?

What is the child's developmental status?

What is the family, social and genetic background?

How has the child, so far, been affected by the deafness (especially when it was discovered late)?

In a properly established audiology centre such assessment should be part of the routine investigation. As experience accumulates, the team becomes more expert in assessing many aspects and providing an all-round assessment of most children.

Some children can be upset by being examined by different people at different places, but all deaf children must be properly assessed to obtain the essential information, without which the best training and education cannot be determined.

Psychological tests

A test of learning ability forms an important part of the assessment of deaf children. This is normally carried out by one of the standardized tests for IQ. It is most important in children suspected of being deaf not to rely on verbal tests; rather the performance section of this test must be used. There are several standardized performance tests; those who carry out an all-round assessment of these children must fully understand the nature of these tests and be able to interpret them.

Learning ability in children can be impaired not only by low intelligence but also by emotional upset, sensory deprivation due to unfavourable environmental influences, cultural differences (for example, in immigrant populations) and additional disabilities.

Multiple handicaps and deafness

Search for additional handicaps must be part of the systemic assessment. We must distinguish between those abnormalities which are primarily part of the clinical picture and those which are secondary to the impairment (e.g. behavioural disorder or emotional disturbance). We must also recognize additional disabilities brought on by environmental influences, such as social conditions, parental inadequacy and unfavourable language background, for instance in immigrant populations, which modify the effects of the abnormality.

The combined effect of two or more handicaps is extremely severe and the care of the multiple-handicapped deaf child is probably one of the most difficult problems we face in child audiology.

MANAGEMENT

Objectives

Speaking and listening provide the most efficient method of transmitting language from brain to brain. The production of sounds and consequently oral language is a late phylogenetic development and it must have taken a long time for man to develop the fine neuromuscular coordination necessary for the voluntary movements which produce speech sounds for which hearing is the most important feedback control.

If a deaf child is to develop his intellectual abilities he must have language and should preferably be taught to communicate it by speech. Our aim should be to make him able to communicate in the normal hearing society without segregating him for ever. This oral and auditory training must begin as early as possible.

Home training

Early training means home training and depends entirely on the parents. Help and support for the parents of deaf children must be deliberately planned in all its aspects as part of the child's speech training.

Parents receive practical instructions on how to talk to the child (face to face at his own level), how to use amplified sound, how to speak clearly but without exaggerated mouth movements, and how to select their words.

Certain rules are essential; the understanding of speech must come first. If speech production is emphasized before there is understanding, the child soon notices the parents' anxiety and repeats whatever they say but cannot communicate; he then develops echolalia.

Informal (situational) speech training must be part of everyday life which goes on all day and in which all members of the family are involved.

When a deaf child approaches 3, placement in a nursery for normal children should be considered, to enhance social maturation which normally is slower in deaf children.

Parent guidance

It can be critical how the distressing news about the child's deafness is given to the parents. Parent guidance begins at this stage: they must be told in such a way that their anxiety is reduced to the minimum and they must be told that although it seems that the child is deaf, it can usually be helped. An optimistic outlook is fully justified because deafness is one of the disabilities in children which can be alleviated.

Detailed explanation of the cause of deafness, if known, is essential, or explanation why, if it is not known. Proper explanation about the type of

deafness and whether treatment is possible must be given. If the deafness is sensorineural we tell the parents firmly that no surgical or medical treatment is possible. We must give the parents some basic knowledge of the physiology and anatomy of the ear, about the causes of deafness and about the main difference between conductive and sensorineural deafness. In appropriate cases the parents should be referred for genetic counselling.

Amplification

When deafness is diagnosed the following questions should be answered:

Is amplification necessary?

Can amplification compensate for loss of sensitivity?

What kind of amplification and what kind of amplifiers should be used?

Deaf children must first be provided with the best wearable amplifier but this is not the only type of amplifier which may be needed. During language and speech training it may be desirable to use larger, non-portable amplifiers with good quality earphones, with separate adjustments for each ear, at home and at school.

We should never force a child to use a hearing aid and small children should use aids only under close supervision by an experienced teacher. If such supervision is not available it may be better not to use the aid at all. Parents must be instructed in detail about all types of amplification.

One should not use a hearing aid to make a diagnosis but one can legitimately carry out close observations of the reactions to amplified sound.

Undue amplification, mainly in partial deafness, especially of high frequency, must always be avoided. Incorrect amplification in high frequency deafness discourages children for a long time from using a hearing aid properly.

Compensation for the loss of sensitivity by amplification in high frequency deafness is difficult and remains unsolved. We probably need special types of amplifiers which should be 'consonant amplifiers'.

The most suitable hearing aid must be selected after careful consideration of the type and degree of deafness, additional disabilities, particular use (social; educational; specific occasions), cause of the deafness and the availability and degree of supervision and instruction. Close cooperation between the clinician, audiologist and teacher is essential.

Aided pure tone audiometric tests can be carried out with different hearing aids by using narrow band noise from a suitable audiometer. It is then possible to obtain amplified threshold audiograms. This gives valuable information in addition to the unaided pure tone threshold audiogram. In cooperative children this can be supplemented by a free field speech hearing test to compare the efficiency of various hearing aids in achieving the best possible intelligibility of speech.

Education

Deaf children, including those with profound deafness, should be educated as nearly as possible within the system for normally hearing children. Segregation of deaf children in special schools for the deaf is out of date and does not conform with the fundamental aims of integrating them into normal society.

Children with not only severe partial deafness, but also with profound deafness, are much better off with regard to social development and adjustment and ability to communicate by speech, when educated alongside normally speaking children [14].

Schools for the deaf will gradually disappear as larger segregated institutions and special classes or units within normal schools will develop as the system of choice for educating deaf children.

Organization of services

Audiology services for children should provide: early detection, diagnosis and assessment, parent guidance and programmes for training preschool children closely integrated with the diagnostic service.

Help should be provided for children in normal schools. Continuous reassessment of all deaf children is most important.

Facilities for systemic assessment must be so organized that the child is not examined by too many people at too many places. Continuity of care (within the child's community) must be ensured without fragmentation of the service into separate parts.

A comprehensive audiology service in which the medical, educational and social services closely cooperate, is essential but not easy to design. Adjustments must be made depending on the basic organization of health care delivery services in each country and according to the urban or rural character of each district.

Handicapped children cannot be cared for properly when the diagnostic services are divorced from training, rehabilitation and reassessment.

The focal point of this service should be an *audiology clinic* for children, staffed by an audiology team including an audiological physician, a teacher of the deaf, a psychologist, an audiology technician and a social worker. Help from an audiological scientist is often required.

The audiology centre should be responsible for diagnosis and assessment, for organizing, supervising and training of the pre-school child and deaf children who can attend normal schools. Recommendations for educational placement should be one of the important functions. Regular reassessment of children receiving special education should be carried out.

The following accommodation is essential: a general audiology examination room, an audiometric room, an observation room, a room for the teacher attached to the unit for auditory training and parent guidance, a psychologists' room, a room for taking impressions and issuing hearing aids, a room for electrophysiological testing and good storage facilities.

The environment in all rooms where children are tested should be so structured that the child's natural anxiety is reduced to the minimum.

References

[1] FRASER G. R. (1976) *The Causes of Profound Deafness in Childhood*. Baltimore: Johns Hopkins University Press.

[2] HALL J. G. (1964) *The Cochlea and the Cochlear Nuclei in Neonatal Anoxia*. Norwegian Monographs on Medical Science, Scandinavian University Books (Universitetsforlaget).

[3] FISCH L. (1969) Causes of congenital deafness. *Public Health. Journal of the Society of Medical Officers* 83, 68.

[4] SORSBY A. (1951) *Genetics in Ophthalmology*. London: Butterworths.

[5] FRASER G. R. (1964) Association of congenital deafness with goitre (Pendred's syndrome). *Annals of Human Genetics* 28, 201.

[6] FISCH L. (1959) Deafness as part of an hereditary syndrome. *Journal of Laryngology and Otology* 73, 355.

[7] WILDERVANCK L. S., HOEKSEMA P. E. & PENNING L. (1966) Radiological examination of the inner ear of deaf mutes presenting the cervico-oculo-acousticus syndrome. *Acta oto-laryngologica* 61, 445.

[8] FRASER G. R., FROGATT P. & JAMES T. M. (1964) Congenital deafness associated with electrocardiographic abnormalities, fainting attacks and sudden death. *Quarterly Journal of Medicine* 33, 361.

[9] FISCH L. (1971) The probability of response to test sounds in young children. *Sound* 5, 7.

[10] DOWNS M. P. (1976) Report of the University of Colorado Screening Project. In *Early Identification of Hearing Loss*. Nova Scotia Conference, Halifax, pp. 76–89. Basel: Karger.

[11] FISCH L. (1965) Recorded sounds for hearing tests in infants. *Journal of Laryngology and Otology* 79, 1077.

[12] FISCH L. (1975) Audiometry in children with difficult behaviour. *Bulletin d'Audiophonologie (Services technique de la Faculté de médecine et de pharmacie de Besançons)*, Vol. 5, 3, 67.

[13] FELDMAN A. S. & WILBER L. A. (1976) *Acoustic Impedance and Admittance: the Measurement of Middle Ear Function*. Baltimore: Williams & Wilkins.

[14] JOHN J. E. J. (1976) Some factors affecting the intelligibility of deaf children's speech. In *Disorders of Auditory Function II*, ed. Stephens S. D. S. London: Academic Press.

CHAPTER 38

Middle Ear Effusions

The classification of middle ear conditions connected with effusion varies a great deal and terms such as 'serous otitis media', 'catarrhal otitis media', 'secretory otitis media' and 'glue ear' are often used as synonyms. This confusion prevents accurate assessment of clinical and epidemiological studies and restricts the value of comparisons between the clinical and laboratory data.

It is appropriate to consider acute purulent otitis media as a different, well-defined entity whereas the other above conditions comprise middle ear effusions. For the sake of simplicity the subclassification into two groups on the basis of gross examination of the fluid is satisfactory. The first, serous otitis media, contains all ears with thin fluid and the second, secretory otitis media, all those with thick fluid. For a clinical otolaryngologist this division is not difficult to make; it divides middle ear effusions into two major groups, each with several different causes.

SEROUS OTITIS MEDIA

The fluid in these ears is watery, colourless or amber-coloured; clinical examination often shows a fluid line across the tympanic membrane. The mechanism of production of the fluid is reduced pressure in the middle ear with inward shift of the tympanic membrane. With the increase of negative pressure, slight damage occurs in the capillary walls allowing formation of a transudate type of fluid which lacks large molecular proteins. Generally the patients do not experience much pain but have a blocked feeling and deafness in the affected ear.

Serous fluid may be caused by several different conditions.

Adenoid hypertrophy

The commonest cause is a hypertrophic pad of adenoids blocking the Eustachian tube. Children thus affected may have an adenoid facies and be mouth breathers. The nasal secretion which is nearly always present also promotes the habit of frequent inward sniffing, the opposite of the Valsalva manoeuvre, causing further reduction in middle ear pressure and leading eventually to the formation of fluid.

Barotrauma

Patients with marginal Eustachian tube function and a swollen nasopharyngeal mucosa because of an acute or subacute infection cannot equilibrate decreased pressure in the middle ear by swallowing. This leads to typical barotrauma when flying. During the descent of an aeroplane the external pressure rises and exceeds the lowered middle ear pressure to a marked degree. This rather abrupt change causes pain and a transudate may form. In addition, more serious capillary damage may occur leading to a haemotympanum. An active and rather forceful Valsalva manoeuvre during descent should be made to prevent this condition. If the patient is known to have Eustachian problems he should apply vasoconstricting nasal drops in both nostrils an hour before the anticipated landing.

Nasopharyngeal tumours

Nasopharyngeal tumours such as carcinoma, sarcoma, malignant lymphoma or various types of leukaemia, can cause occlusion of the Eustachian tube either by direct invasion and tissue destruction or by submucosal infiltration with malignant cells. A painless serous effusion develops which may also extend to the pneumatic cell system.

Otitis media due to viruses

While the previous aetiological factors are not associated with ear infection, viral otitis, which causes slight symptoms, should be included in the serous effusions. Sometimes there is slight pain and the tympanic membrane may show some reddening. The disease may have started in connection with an upper respiratory infection, which would allow the clinician to place it under the heading of acute otitis media. Respiratory syncytial virus, adeno virus and para-influenza virus have been identified in cultures from these ears. The fluid is thin and nonpurulent and as such is indistinguishable from the effusion in serous otitis media [1].

SECRETORY OTITIS MEDIA

Clinical features

The fluid in these ears is thick, tenacious and gluelike in consistency and greyish or yellowish in colour. The tympanic membrane moves very sluggishly with the pneumatic speculum and the thick fluid does not usually form a fluid level. It lines the whole medial surface of the tympanic membrane which may be thickened but shows no signs of infection. The patients do not have pain but have some degree of deafness.

Pathology

The thick mucus in the middle ear is considered to result from the infective stimulus on the middle ear mucosa. Experimental infection of the middle ear of guinea-pigs produces such a secretion in less than 2 weeks [2], but in humans the timing of the onset of the disease has not been accurately defined. The neglect of paracentesis in acute otitis media and treatment with an inadequate antibiotic regime have been thought to be responsible for the world-wide increase of this disease. The onset may be very insidious and not precipitated by an acute inflammatory attack but the possibility always remains that the middle ear process may have started at some time during antibiotic treatment for an upper respiratory illness during the subclinical stage of acute otitis media.

In these ears the Eustachian tube is patent even if it is not capable of transporting the thick mucus out of the ear. The mucus itself is a mixture of fluids, partly derived from the capillaries in the form of exudate or transudate and partly derived from the newly-developed secretory elements of the middle ear mucosa. Indeed, the great increase in secretory epithelial cells and intra- and sub-epithelial glands is a feature characteristic of this type of effusion. Observations in human middle ears seem to indicate that this epithelial change takes place after an inflammatory stimulus of only a few days' duration.

Microbiology

The mucoid effusion, which was initially thought sterile, is now considered to contain bacteria. In one recent study [3], bacteria were cultured from 52% of the ears and seen in 77% of the aural smears. The most common bacteria were *Haemophilus influenzae* and *Staphylococcus epidermidis,* other bacteria occurring less frequently. Specimens taken from the ear canal showed virtually the same bacterial population as that in the middle ear. Mycoplasma seems to appear in about 5% of the thick effusions and evidence of viral infection is shown by raised serum titres in about 20%.

Immunochemistry

The secretory nature of the effusion has been conclusively demonstrated by immunochemical studies. Electrophoretic analysis with PAS and alcian blue staining has shown that the effusion contains at least one acid and one neutral glycoprotein which are not present in normal serum. Studies with anti-middle ear fluid sera, obtained from immunized rabbits, have revealed at least three middle ear specific protein fractions in the thick secretions [4,5].

In addition, the middle ear mucosa actively secretes various enzymes and immunoglobulins, including IgA, into the secretion. This is an important contribution to the serological defence mechanism. There has been no evidence of agammaglobulinaemia or even hypogammaglobulinaemia in the sera of patients with secretory otitis media.

The cellular pattern of the thick effusion consists predominantly of lymphocytes and polymorphonuclear leucocytes, with various types of mononuclear phagocytes occurring less commonly. Eosinophils and mast cells are so conspicuously absent from these secretions that a circulating IgE-dependent form of an allergic reaction is unlikely to play a role in the aetiology of secretory otitis media [6].

In recent years the middle ear mucosa has been shown to be a true mucosa from the immunological point of view. There is also a macro-molecular transport system by which the particles in the middle ear are carried to the retroauricular and junctional lymph nodes [7]. This may involve the participation of sensitized T-lymphocytes in a delayed type hypersensitivity reaction against various allergens, among them, possibly, food allergens. The limited data currently available suggest that the relative number of T- and B-lymphocytes in the effusion does not differ from their relative number in the blood.

DIAGNOSIS

In the diagnosis of middle ear effusions the otolaryngologist has to rely mostly upon the use of the Siegle's pneumatic speculum to determine the mobility of the tympanic membrane. In infants and small children a tympanogram which shows a typical flat curve during changes in pressure can be of great value. When in doubt, paracentesis and aspiration should be performed and the nature of the fluid determined by gross examination. A routine check should be made in paediatric wards of all infants with a respiratory infection with a cleft palate and all those having nasogastric tube feeding.

Audiometry or tympanometry may be used in screening programmes. Audiometry set at the 20 dB level allows many patients with effusion to be overlooked since hearing need not be severely affected especially in the early stages. Tympanometry, on the other hand, may result in false positives as ears with a high negative pressure need not always have effusion. Established cases of secretory otitis media will be diagnosed easily and the combination of both these methods produces the least number of false positives or negatives after screening. The percentage of pre-school children in need of specialist examination varies between 5 and 10%.

MANAGEMENT

The adenoid problem

Opinions on the effect of adenoidectomy in chronic secretory otitis vary; the work of Mawson et al. [8] is frequently cited to prove that adenoidectomy is of no help. However, this problem is not simple and the whole otitis media–adenoid problem needs to be reconsidered. Adenoid tissue is easily infected, it harbours bacteria and, when cultured for viruses, consistently reflects endemic infections for long periods. Furthermore, enlarged adenoids are an obstacle to good ventilation and also favour the development of rhinitis and maxillary sinusitis. The use of a postnasal mirror for evaluating upper respiratory infections in children should be routine since it may show an infected and inflamed adenoid mass associated with only minor changes in the palatine tonsil.

All parents of pre-school children should be advised that an adequate adenoidectomy should be done after one or two attacks of acute otitis media regardless of the size of the adenoids. The child should be intubated and the surgeon, after curettage of the main mass, should complete the operation using postnasal mirrors and angulated forceps. Adenoidectomy with the patient in a sitting position and quick removal by a curette should be condemned because tissue is always left in place high on the postnasal roof. On the other hand, surgical attack on the fossae of Rosenmüller themselves is not felt to be necessary or advisable. Early removal of the adenoids is effective in preventing a number of reinfections, and chronic secretory otitis media seldom develops. Once the condition is established, adenoidectomy can no longer be expected to give similar help; cure of the disease is prolonged and requires the help of tympanostomy tubes. Nevertheless, it is always our policy to do an adenoidectomy when grommets are inserted.

Ventilation tubes

The most effective current treatment is to use a grommet to provide ventilation from the ear canal. Once the mucus-producing elements in the middle ear mucosa have developed they can only be expected to disappear if there is free entry of air into the tympanic cavity. Even then, the average time for the mucosa to return to normal is 11 months in the ears showing a good tendency to heal. In more obstinate cases, the time before healing may well be doubled [9].

It is well established that infection alone rapidly leads to proliferation of the mucus-secreting elements. The role of allergic reactions, particularly in the form of a delayed type of hypersensitivity reaction, are poorly understood. It may well be that the adverse food reactions observed as immobilization, or disruption of the patient's leucocytes when brought into contact with food allergens, may play an important part in maintaining the chronic state. Milk, wheat and tomato sensitivity are quite frequent in children suffering from secretory otitis media.

Mastoidectomy

When the middle ear becomes infected and the patient is treated with antibiotics, a disease involving the mastoid system may remain silent but may still be the cause of chronic irritation of the middle ear mucosa. Mastoid radiographs should, therefore, not be omitted in the examination of these children. A complete cortical mastoidectomy should be done in all cases showing a cloudy mastoid air cell system; frequently the whole cell system is found to be full of glue. In these patients we occlude the aditus with a meatally based musculoperiosteal flap, as in chronic ear surgery. This prevents future spread of middle ear disease into the mastoid cavity.

Once the adenoid and mastoid parts have been found to be sufficiently healthy, grommets should be inserted through the lower quadrant of the drumhead and left in until they extrude spontaneously. Follow-up visits are done at 2-monthly intervals and if the disease is not

cured, after extrusion of the grommet in about 6 months, another one should be inserted. If the leucocyte cytotoxic test is available it should be used and a rotating diet arranged with all major irritants eliminated and the minor irritants allowed on a once-a-week basis.

Even untreated serous otitis media does not lead to middle ear adhesions but the mucoid secretion may be subject to tissue ingrowth and organization from small mucosal raw areas as a result of fibrocyte proliferation. The resulting adhesions lead to permanently damaged tubal function with very little chance of permanent improvement by any kind of subsequent surgery. If the condition becomes chronic, cholesteatoma may develop and the patient is then managed according to the principles used in chronic ear surgery.

References

[1] BERGLUND B., SALMIVALLI A. & TOIVANEN B. (1966) Isolation of respiratory syncytial virus from middle ear exudates of infants. *Acta Oto-Laryngologica (Stockholm)* 61, 475.

[2] FRIEDMANN I. (1963) The pathology of secretory otitis media. *Proceedings of the Royal Society of Medicine* 56, 695.

[3] LIU Y. S., LIM D. J., LANG R. W. & BIRCK H. G. (1975) Chronic middle ear effusions. *Archives of Otolaryngology* 101, 278.

[4] PALVA T., RAUNIO V. & NOUSIAINEN R. (1974) Secretory otitis media: protein and enzyme analyses. *Annals of Otology, Rhinology and Laryngology* 83, 35.

[5] PALVA T., RAUNIO V. & NOUSIAINEN R. (1975) Middle ear specific proteins in glue ears. *Acta Oto-Laryngologica (Stockholm)* 79, 160.

[6] PALVA T. & HOLOPAINEN E. (1976) Secretory otitis media: comparison of nasal and aural cytology. *Acta Oto-Laryngologica (Stockholm)* 81, 204.

[7] LIM D. J. & HUSSL B. (1975) Macromolecular transport by the middle ear and its lymphatic system. *Acta Oto-Laryngologica (Stockholm)* 80, 19.

[8] MAWSON S. R., ADLINGTON P. & EVANS M. (1967) A controlled study evaluation of adeno-tonsillectomy. *Journal of Laryngology and Otology* 81, 777.

[9] KOKKO E. (1974) Chronic secretory otitis media in children. (M.D. Thesis, University of Oulu.) *Acta Oto-Laryngologica (Stockholm)*, Supplement 327.

CHAPTER 39

Congenital Conductive Deafness

EMBRYOLOGY

There is no chronological uniformity in the development of the ear and ectoderm, mesoderm and endoderm all participate in its formation.

The inner ear

The first rudiment of the inner ear is the auditory plate which, induced by the notochord and the perichordal mesoderm, gives origin to the inner ear; it appears at about the tenth day. The auditory plate or placode becomes depressed and converted into the auditory pit; closure of its mouth soon forms the auditory vesicle or otocyst.

The first rough outline of the membranous endolymphatic labyrinth is present as early as the twenty-fifth day. From this vesicle various diverticulae appear, which later give rise to the entire endolymphatic duct system.

Surrounding the newly-formed labyrinth the mesodermal tissue is progressively converted into a cartilaginous capsule and forms the three layers of ossification of the otic capsule. It envelops the newly-formed perilymphatic system formed by a progressive vacuolization of the mesenchymatous tissue.

The middle ear

The middle ear cavity is developed from the first pharyngeal pouch which meets the ectoderm of the first pharyngeal groove to form the tympanic membrane. The first part of the tympanic cavity which appears is the inferior one, which joins the Eustachian tube. The antrum and the epitympanic recess appear progressively by resorption of mesenchymatous tissue and are invaded by the mucosal entodermal tympanic epithelium (Figs.

39.1 and 39.2). Aeration of these pneumatized cavities appears only at the end of fetal life. Its cavities are aerated before birth by homogeneous gas diffusion.

Between the tenth and the twelfth week the antrum and the aditus develop while individual ossicles with their ligamentous connections and the tendons appear. About the fifth month, the aditus ad antrum develops and, 1 month later, the antrum, followed by the progressive pneumatization of the mastoid.

The ossicles

The first outline of the *stapes* appears at the thirty-third day of fetal life. A patch of thickened mesenchymatous tissue on the dorsal end of the hyoid arch, supported by Reichert's cartilage, is, a few days later, crossed by the stapedial artery. The only remnant of its connection with the second arch is the stapedial muscle and its tendon.

This mesenchymatous tissue will form the superstructure of the stapes, which later will come into contact with the footplate, the latter originating from the cartilaginous otic capsule so that the stapes is formed from both origins; the stapes is formed around the forty-fifth day. The annular ligament, which gives these ossicles their motility, only appears later at the end of the third month. Ossification of the stapes appears from the fourth month on, so that 15 days before the end of fetal life the stapes has reached the adult stage [1].

The *incus* is derived from the first mandibular arch, supported by Meckel's cartilage. From the forty-fifth day on it grows progressively and by the fifty-fourth day the incudostapedial articulation is recognizable. Progressive ossification of the stapes starts during the fourth month.

The *malleus,* also derived from the first mandibular arch, maintains its continuity with Meckel's cartilage until the fifth month. The remnants of its connection with the proximal end of Meckel's cartilage become the anterior tympanomalleolar ligament, the latter being accompanied by the chorda tympani.

The tympanic ring is the second essential embryological element of this canal. The membranous ossification of this structure which forms the essential contribution to the formation of the bony external canal starts developing around the tenth week (Fig. 39.3). The embryological development of the tympanic ring has been particularly well described by Anson and Donaldson [2].

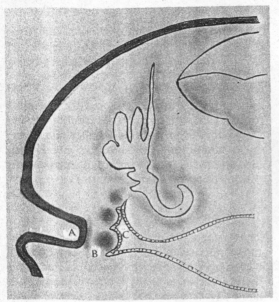

FIG. 39.1. A. First pharyngeal groove; B. Mesodermic layer; C. Mucosal entodermic layer of the first pharyngeal pouch.

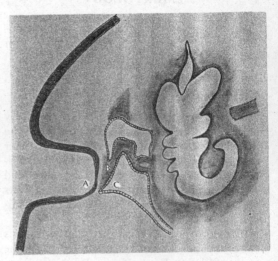

FIG. 39.2. As in Fig. 39.1.

The tympanic membrane

The external auditory canal develops from the first branchial groove, between the mandibular and hyoid arches. The primary meatus is formed by its extension inwards. An entodermal lining is acquired from the dorsal end of the first pharyngeal pouch and the mesoderm then extends between those two layers. The *tympanic membrane* is thus constituted in three layers.

The external auditory canal

The two arches which bound the depression of the first branchial groove form the external auditory canal. The cutaneous lining of the meatus originates from the ectoderm of this first groove and the underlying tissue from the mesoderm.

The pinna

The pinna is originated from a gradual differentiation of the tubercles around the margin of the first branchial groove. Those which appear around the forty-third day are called *colliculi* and there are three on each part of the groove.

There are two different theories concerning the development of the pinna from these tubercles [3].

First, that the three frontal tubercles are converted respectively into: (1) the tragus, (2) the crus helicis, (3) the helix, and the three dorsal ones into: (4) the crura anthelicis, (5) the anthelix (6) the antitragus and the lobe [4,5].

Secondly, that the entire pinna is developed from the second pharyngeal arch only and that the first pharyngeal arch is converted into the tragus only [6]. (Fig. 39.4).

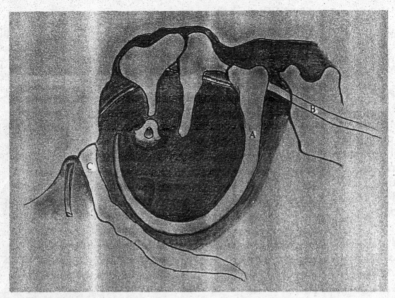

FIG. 39.3. A. Development of the tympanic ring at 15 weeks; B. Meckel's cartilage (Reitcher's cartilage).

Classification of malformations of the middle ear

Embryopathies can occur as an isolated lesion due to chromosomal, hereditary or teratogenous causes or secondary to an exogenous toxin or a viral infection. More frequently they are found in association with other malformations. The syndromes and their chronology are therefore better understood when their embryology is well known. These anomalies can be classified on an anatomopathological basis, in order to clarify the problems of surgical treatment.

The middle ear

Anomalies in the development of the middle ear are the most important ones, because their gravity determines the indication for and the prognosis of functional surgery.

(1) *Total absence of pneumatization of the middle ear cavity and of the mastoid,* which implies total absence of development of the Eustachian tube and lack of tubal function, is due to a maldevelopment of the first pharyngeal entodermal pouch. It is not amenable to any form of surgery.

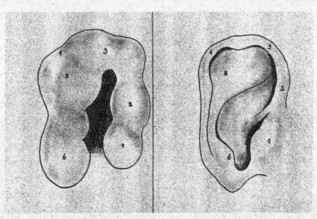

FIG. 39.4. Development of the pinna (see text).

A totally underdeveloped middle ear cavity and mastoid is classified as one of the most severe anomalies (Henner's Class III) [7].

(2) *Absence of mucosal lining in the middle ear.* The middle ear cavity remains full of embryonal mesenchymatous tissue. These anomalies are very often overlooked. In major atresia the disease is only discovered during operation but minor anomalies may be assumed to be a fibro-adhesive otitis. The prognosis for such patients is always bad because of poor function of the Eustachian tube.

(3) *Aplasia of the middle ear cavity* is generally associated with major atresia. It usually affects the hypotympanum, whereas the attic recess and the antrum are generally well developed

The ossicles

The stapes

(1) *Absence of the oval window* is generally associated with other anomalies. It is associated with fusion of the stapedial footplate to the embryonic otic capsule.

(2) *Absence of the stapedial annular ligament.* Both these anomalies are responsible for a congenital pure conductive deafness which can be confused with early otosclerosis. Surgical treatment is very successful if the ossicular chain, particularly the incus, functions properly. The surgical treatment is still controversial. Some [8], including the author, regard stapedectomy as the operation of choice. Others [9, 10] warn of the risk inherent in this approach. The fenestration operation is still advocated by some [11, 12].

(3) *Malformation of the crura.* The most common anomaly is lack of differentiation between the two crura and sometimes one crus is absent altogether, generally associated with a dehiscence of the facial nerve [13] (Fig. 39.5).

(4) *Congenital absence of the stapedial tendon* which may or may not be associated with the absence of the head of the stapes. These anoma-

lies are rare but do exist. The only symptom may be absence of the stapedial reflex associated with acoustic distortion. The only patient we have observed had a congenital defect of the incudostapedial joint.

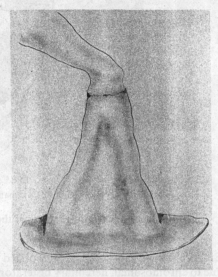

FIG. 39.5. Malformation of the stapes, lack of differentiation between the two crura.

(5) *Ossification of the stapedial tendon* which causes fusion between the posterior crus and the pyramidal process, by non-resorption of the end of Reichert's cartilage.

(6) *Persistent stapedial artery* (Fig. 39.6) due to non-resorption of this embryonic artery. This anomaly is often associated with an aberrant course of the internal carotid artery within the petrous bone. The stapedial artery is a continuation of the primitive hyoid branch of the internal carotid artery which terminates as the middle meningeal artery, but which normally regresses in the 24 mm embryo. Angiography of this anomaly is of great interest [14]. It can be part of an entire syndrome or an incidental finding.

(7) *Total absence of the stapedial superstructure* is generally associated with an absence of the oval window. Some cases have been described in association with a normal mobile footplate.

The incus

(1) *Absence of the lenticular process* or of the long process of the incus. Minor anomalies are usually incidental findings, but are also often associated with severe malformations.

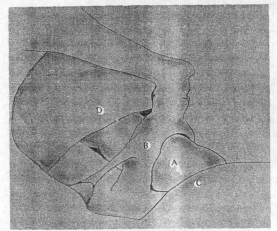

FIG. 39.6. A. Persistent stapedial artery; B. Stapedial arch; C. Promontory; D. Fallopian canal.

(2) *Agenesis of the body of the incus.* This very rare but functionally very important anomaly is generally part of the major atresia syndromes.

(3) *Fusion of the lenticular process with the bony facial canal* is the most frequent anomaly of the incus. Associated with a malformed stapes, also frequently fixed to the Fallopian canal, it is almost pathognomonic of the first arch syndrome (Fig. 39.7). Other types of fusion of the normally formed ossicles with the bony wall, e.g. of the short process of the incus to the fossa incudis, are generally associated with absence of tendon or ligament (Fig. 39.8).

The diagnosis between this anomaly and an acquired ectopic ossicular otosclerosis or from post-traumatic fusion origin, can only be made histologically [17].

The malleus

(1) *Absence of the malleus* or, more commonly, the presence of fused incudomalleolar remnants only, is a common malformation found in severe congenital atresia. The ligaments are generally

present, so that this disorganized ossicular chain remains mobile.

(2) *Fusion of the manubrium* to the tympanic ring is the most frequent malformation of the malleus. It plays a very important role in surgery because this bony fixation to the tympanic ring increases the risk of acoustic damage to the cochlea during surgery (Fig. 39.9).

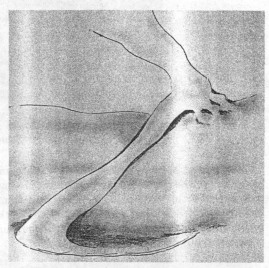

FIG. 39.7. Absence of the anterior crus of the stapes while the head of the stapes and the lenticular process of the incus are fixed to the bony wall of the Fallopian canal.

(3) *Fusion of the malleolar head* with the bony wall; the superior or anterior malleolar ligament may be ossified or absent. These present similar diagnostic problems to the one of incudal fixation.

(4) *Fusion of the incudo-malleolar joint* is the typical anomaly found in most than 3% of ear malformations, but seldom causes a functional disturbance.

The tympanic membrane

Malformations of the tympanic membrane cannot be considered separately from malformations of the external auditory meatus, and are always associated with anomalies of the tympanic ring. Nevertheless, in nearly all cases of

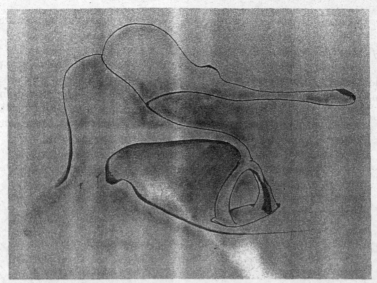

FIG. 39.8. Synostosis of the short process of the incus in the fossa incudis.

minor atresia of the external auditory canal some outlines of the tympanic membrane are present. Sometimes the tympanic membrane is completely formed of bone, which duplicates remarkably the shape and the landmarks of the normal membranous drum.

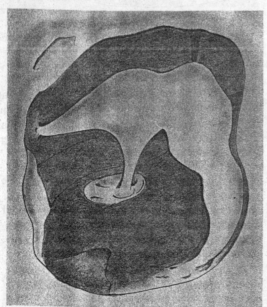

FIG. 39.9. Osteotic fixation of the malformed manubrium mallei.

The external auditory meatus

Abnormal direction and size of the external auditory meatus is a very common minor anomaly, which is found constantly in the first arch syndrome. The external auditory meatus loses its normal tortuosity to run straight anteroinferiorly.

Congenital exostosis of the external auditory meatus may present the appearance of a pseudo-atresia of the external auditory meatus which is compatible with a normal middle ear, external ear and pinna. This type of atresia can originate from the end of the body of the tympanic ring (spine of Henle) but usually seems to arise from the head of the tympanic ring. It corresponds with a maldevelopment of the squamotympanic suture or of the anterior tympanic spine.

Atresia of the external auditory meatus. Different types of this anomaly occur depending on the embryonic presence or absence of the external pharyngeal groove and, later, of the tympanic ring. Two types of true atresia are described (Fig. 39.10).

(1) When the external pharyngeal groove was embryologically active the atresia is the consequence of maldevelopment of the tympanic ring.

The facial nerve always follows its normal course, and anomalies of the ossicular chain are minimal. There is a fibrous or bony occlusion of the medial two-thirds of the external canal. In this type the characteristic space and the distance

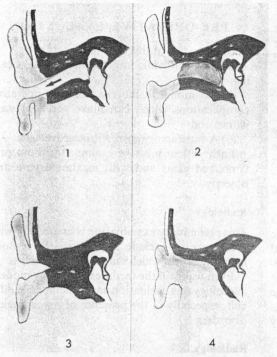

FIG. 39.10. External auditory canal malformations:

Type 1: narrow or abnormal direction of the external auditory canal.

Type 2: congenital exostosis of the external auditory canal.

Type 3: atresia of the external auditory canal with normal space between mastoid and glenoid cavity.

Type 4: congenital atresia of the external auditory canal without space between the mastoid and glenoid cavity.

between the posterior wall of the glenoid cavity and the anterior part of the mastoid are generally constant and normal.

(2) In severe atresia when the external pharyngeal groove was not active embryologically the maldevelopment is considerably worse. The space between the posterior wall of the glenoid cavity and the anterior part of the mastoid is characteristically absent and the latter is situated in the immediate neighbourhood of the temporo-

mandibular joint. The course of the facial nerve is always abnormal.

Everything works as if the space of the whole external canal was taken out as represented in Fig. 39.11.

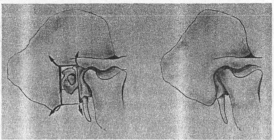

FIG. 39.11. Drawings showing the difference between type 3 and type 4.

ASSOCIATED ANOMALIES

One cannot study malformations of the middle ear without considering the associated problems often caused by the facial nerve, the malformations of the pinna, the often associated fistula and congenital cholesteatoma.

Facial nerve

The facial nerve, which is the branchial nerve of the second or hyoid branchial arch, is associated with a great number of malformations already described.

In the tympanic segment of the Fallopian canal the most frequent anomaly is *dehiscence of the bony covering*.

Duplication, reduplication and triplication of the nerve have been described.

Displacement has also been observed. The nerve or the duplicated neural fibres pass through the stapedial arch or may be situated inferior to this ossicle. In the mastoid segment a pronounced posterior dislocation has been reported; some cases also have been described with a facial nerve displaced, not only posteriorly but also laterally [16].

More severe anomalies such as *hypoplasia* or even *agenesis* of the facial nerve are unfortunately sometimes present in severe atresia.

In cases of type IV agenesis of the external

auditory canal modifications of the course of the nerves are well known [17]. In accordance with the embryological description of this anomaly, the nerve turns anteriorly at the level of the round window, instead of continuing inferiorly to the anteriorly situated stylomastoid foramen. This anomaly prohibits any drilling work inferiorly and anteriorly to enlarge the tympanic cavity. These anomalies of the facial nerve have been studied in particular by Miehlke [16] and Crabtree [18].

The pinna

Major malformations of the pinna are generally associated with middle ear anomalies and vice versa. A series of these malformations shows that the amount of development or maldevelopment has almost no relationship with the amount of deformity of the middle ear cleft [19].

A wide range of anomalies of the pinna has been described. They are all explained, from the minor architectural anomalies to the total absence of the pinna, by the embryological development pattern: microtia, dysmorphic auricles, accessory auricles, or the most common 'the question mark pinna'. In the majority of cases the outline of the tragus remains, which is very important from the cosmetic point of view.

The congenital aural fistula

The most frequent fistulae are located anterior to the pinna and are generally associated with minor ossicular anomalies. Cysts or fistulae originating from the first or the second branchial grooves are rare.

Those arising from the first branchial groove are situated between the lobe of the ear and the inferior part of the external auditory canal, and may pass through the parotid gland.

Those arising from the second branchial groove are more characteristic; the external orifice is situated anterior to the sternomastoid muscle, while the medial end lies in the middle ear cleft.

Cholesteatoma

The existence of congenital cholesteatoma has been proved by surgical findings. The disease is more frequent in teratological embryopathies, especially in severe congenital atresia, due to thalidomide which was responsible for the most severe ear malformation and fetal damage ever seen.

PRE-OPERATIVE EVALUATION

The main goals of this type of surgery are:

(1) A worth-while improvement of the hearing;

(2) To minimize the risks of post-operative complications which can make the final state worse; and

(3) A satisfactory cosmetic improvement.

Each patient must be examined without preconceived ideas and with maximum care and objectivity.

Audiology

This preliminary examination is carried out with great care to exclude any associated sensorineural deafness which makes surgery useless.

Even using all the facilities offered by modern audiology this evaluation can sometimes be difficult, especially in the presence of psychological disorders.

Radiology

Plain radiographs and tomograms are the most important parts of the pre-operative evaluation, and should never be omitted. The surgeon needs to know about the type of malformation before the operation, and if the lesion is too large or too extensive for surgical treatment.

The psycho-social evaluation

These considerations may also influence the decision to operate because some social situations or psychological disorders are incompatible with the required post-operative care or follow-up. The cooperation of a psychiatrist, paediatrician and psychologist are useful and sometimes indispensable.

The age of the patient

The average age compatible with this type of surgery is between 6 and 12 years of age. Most authors agree that surgery must never be carried out before 5 years of age. In our opinion, even in bilateral cases earlier operation is never indicated, because the audiophonetic effects of this conductive type of deafness can always be controlled by a hearing aid. An operation carried out too early rarely produces good functional results.

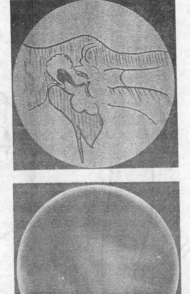

FIG. 39.12. Tomogram of a major congenital atresia showing a well-formed and probably functional middle-ear, ossicular chain and inner-ear structure (by courtesy of Dr E. Claus, Medisch Centrum, Antwerp).

Unilateral malformations

The dispute about surgery on unilateral severe malformations is still in progress. Most authors agree that surgery should never be proposed for unilateral disease. We believe that this attitude is conditioned by the present high rate of complications and the often poor functional long-term results. The use of homograft tympanic membrane and external auditory canal skin which give good anatomical and functional results has led us to change our policy; at present we advocate surgery for unilateral anomalies, provided

that the pre-operative evaluation suggests a good prognosis.

Cosmetic surgery

The new external auditory canal must be rebuilt in functional continuity with the middle ear cavity and ossicular chain. The canal must be

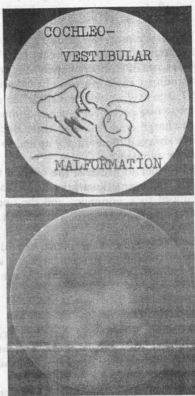

FIG. 39.13. Tomogram showing a margin congenital atresia associated with such inner-ear malformities incompatible with functional surgery (by courtesy of Dr E. Claus, Medisch Centrum, Antwerp).

reconstituted before any cosmetic surgery is carried out. Plastic surgery on the pinna is only acceptable if it is centred on the new meatus simultaneously or at a second stage and must never be done before the functional stage.

SURGICAL TREATMENT

General principles

Many complications can be avoided if certain main principles are kept in mind.

(1) The risk of acoustic trauma. If there is bony fixation of the ossicular chain, and more particularly of the handle of the malleus to the tympanic ring, drilling or the use of the cutting burr should be used as little as possible to avoid the risks of sensorineural deafness by acoustic trauma; the noise produced by such drilling is between 160 and 200 dB. Curettes should therefore be used in these areas.

(2) A full thickness skin graft is used preferably from the retroauricular area or the neck because of the absence of hair. Permanent hair growth in a new auditory canal is always troublesome.

(3) Large cavities which include the mastoid cells can cause persistent mucous or mucopurulent discharge from the ear; these discharging ears are always difficult to dry up and so cavities should be avoided.

(4) In order to preserve the surgical field for possible later cosmetic surgery the incisions must be reduced to a minimum and the underlying tissues must always be respected as much as possible.

Scar tissue around the pinna, caused by too extensive dissection or too large an incision, creates problems with later plastic surgery.

Surgical technique

Various surgical techniques have been proposed. Each of them has its advantages and disadvantages which cannot be discussed in detail in this work.

While for minor malformations, generally associated with a normal external auditory canal, classical middle ear surgical principles are applied, the severe malformations combined with deformities of the external canal and pinna require a more complex and well-defined surgical approach.

Different techniques have been described [11, 12, 17, 18, 20, 21] but our technique differs from these in the material used. A homograft is the only material which can provide long-term anatomical and functional results [22, 24].

The advantages of homograft material and the preservation method have already been described [23–25].

Because the entire fibrous auditory canal, including the annulus, the tympanic membrane

and possibly the ossicles, are now available as monobloc grafting material, congenital ear atresia has become one of the main indications for using a homograft.

Our technique has three advantages provided in one stage; valuable functional results, safe

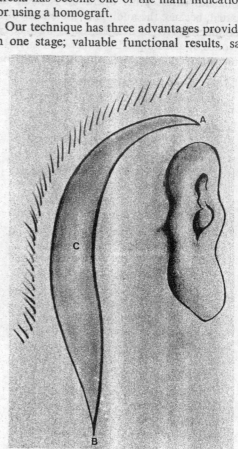

FIG. 39.14. Retro-auricular incisions of the skin (A–B); area for prelevation of a free skin graft (C).

anatomical restoration of the external auditory canal, and very acceptable aesthetic results.

The main points of this technique are:

(1) Incision: Starting at the level of the superior edge of the pinna the incision extends along the hair line inferiorly to the insertion of the sternomastoid muscle (Fig. 39.14).

(2) A large retroauricular area, with a possible extension to the neck, is thus provided as a donor site for a free full-thickness skin graft (Fig. 39.14C). This skin graft can, if necessary, be extended in length and width; a spear shape is particularly useful for the restoration of the external meatus (see Fig. 39.17).

(3) The skin is then elevated anteriorly; the posterior wall of the glenoid cavity is uncovered. A vertical incision traced posteriorly around the glenoid cavity is then made through the periosteum and dissected from the temporal bone; the periosteum is elevated backwards without any further incision to provide a good fixation point for the new external meatus (Fig 39.15).

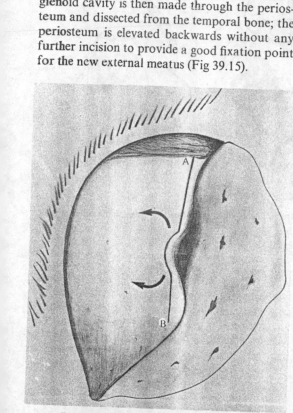

FIG. 39.15. Incision of the periosteum (A–B).

(4) As soon as the temporal and mastoid areas are exposed, the posterosuperior parts of the mastoid are drilled, the horizontal limit of the dura and the sigmoid sinus being used as landmarks. The posterior wall is reshaped by drilling the mastoid in order to create a triangular cavity as posteriorly as possible in the mastoid. This allows a check on the depth of the mastoid and the normal position of the posterior part of the atticus with the short process of the incus. As soon as this latter is spotted, the new external auditory canal is drilled out; this is made with maximum care especially in the deeper parts when the ossicular chain is reached. Excavation of the mastoid and of the middle ear cavity is similar to that obtained by the normal combined approach tympanoplasty (Fig. 39.16).

(5) The middle ear cavity is examined and the ossicular chain inspected. An ossiculoplasty is then done with great care in order to avoid acoustic trauma. Nevertheless, preference is always given to the use of the original ossicles which very often are functional. A bony annulus is then rebuilt by using the cutting burr.

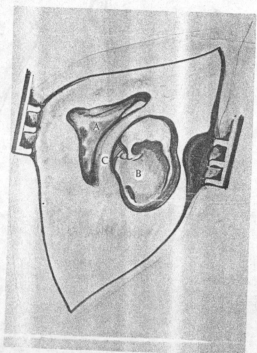

FIG. 39.16. A. Posterior superior exploration opening of the mastoid; B. New external auditory canal; C. Newly created posterior wall.

(6) The new external auditory canal and the bony annulus are reshaped until a tympanomeatal homograft can be placed in its normal position.

(7) The tympanomeatal homograft is put in place keeping in mind that the mobilized or rebuilt ossicular chain should be in perfect contact with the drum. Three or four holes are drilled in the lateral side of the wall of the new external auditory canal in order to pass 000 nylon threads which will closely fix the homograft and the skin autograft (Fig. 39.18).

(8) As shown in Fig. 39.17, a vertical incision is made behind the tragus in the distorted pinna. The posterior and superior part of the pinna is

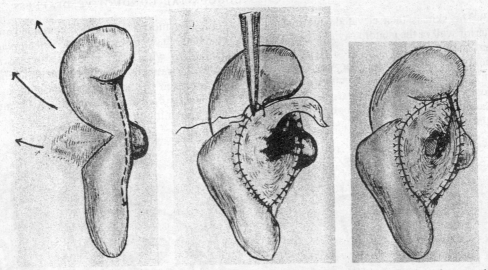

FIG. 39.17. Drawing showing the restoration, by means of a full free skin autograft, of the function between the external skin and the implanted meatal homograft skin.

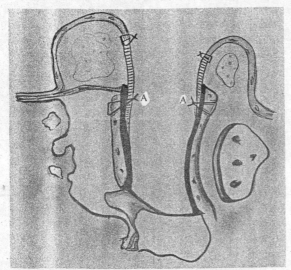

FIG. 39.18. Section showing the restored continuity between the external skin, the autografted skin and the homografted meatal skin.

then retracted upwards and backwards in order to obtain a normal curve. This curve will be facilitated by the repositioning of the retroauricular skin, and by the posterior retroauricular skin suture.

The skin autograft flap will then be sutured in

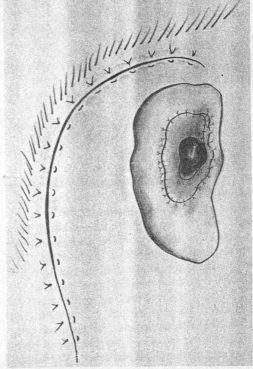

FIG. 39.19. Final stage showing the meatal and retro-auricular sutures.

a helicoidal way. The new meatus will be restored and the fusion between the skin of the pinna and the homograft will be obtained (Fig. 39.17b and c). The final results procure a perfect continuity between the original skin of the pinna anterior and posterior to the new external auditory canal and the homograft skin (Figs. 39.18 and 39.19).

The retraction of this retroauricular skin procures a new natural pinna with a satisfactory aesthetic effect.

(9) Packing is then done with artificial sponges inserted in the new external auditory canal. This packing will be held in place for 8 days.

This technique provides restoration of the external auditory canal, perfect overgrowth of the skin around this canal and the replacement of a natural physiological eardrum on top of the restored ossicular chain. So far rejection has not occurred.

References

[1] ANSON B. J. (1959) Development of the incus of the human ear. *Quarterly Bulletin of Northwestern University Medical School* **33**, 110.

[2] ANSON B. J. & DONALDSON (1973) *Surgical Anatomy of the Temporal Bone and Ear*, 2nd edn., pp. 32–49. London: Saunders.

[3] EYRIES CH. & PERLES B. (1962) Développement de l'oreille moyenne. *Encyclopédie Méd. Chirurg. Franc.* **20.0005 A**, 30.

[4] STREETER G. L. (1922) The development of the pinna in the human embryo. *Carnegie Contributions to Embryology* **14**, 111.

[5] GYOT R. (1934) Les fistules auriculaires. *Annales d'otolaryngologie* **12**, 1227.

[6] WOOD-JONES F. & WEN I-CHUAN (1934) The development of the pinna. *Journal of Anatomy* **68**, 525.

[7] HENNER R. & BUCKINGHAM R. A. (1956) Recognition and surgical treatment of congenital ossicular defects. *The Laryngoscope* **66**, 526.

[8] STEELE BURNS C. (1969) Congenital fixation of the stapes footplate. *Acta Oto-Laryngologica Supplement* **245**, 1.

[9] HOUSE H. P. (1958) Differential diagnosis between otosclerosis and congenital footplate fixation. *Annals of Oto-rhino-laryngology* **50**, 152.

[10] EDWARDS W. G. (1964) Congenital middle ear deafness with anomalies of the face. *Journal of Laryngology and Otology* **78**, 152.

[11] OMBRÉDANNE M. (1970) Malformation du conduit auditif externe et de l'oreille moyenne. *Encyclopédie méd. Chir. Or.* **20182 D**, 10.

[12] BELLUCI R. J. (1972) Congenital auricular malformations. *Annals of Oto-rhino-laryngology* **81**, 659.

[13] MARQUET J. F. (1965) Un curieux cas de surdité de transmission a début brusque. *Rev. de Laryngologie (Bordeaux)* **86**, 1126.

[14] GUINTO F. C. JR. GARRABRANT E. C. & RADCLIFFE W. B. (1972) Radiology of the persistent stapedial artery. *Radiology* **105/2**, 365.

[15] MARQUET J. F. (1971) Considérations sur le diagnostic des surdités de transmission par traumatisme de l'oreille. *Acta oto-rhino-laryngologica Belgica* **25**, 641.

[16] MIEHLKE A. (1973) *Surgery of the Facial Nerve*, 2nd edn. München: Urban & Schwarzenberg. Craltrec 9–21.

[17] BELLUCI R. J. (1960) The problem of congenital auricular malformation. *Transactions of the American Academy of Ophthalmology and Otolaryngology*, Nov.–Dec. 840.

[18] CRABTREE J. A. (1974) The facial nerve in congenital ear surgery. *Otolaryngologic Clinics of North America* **7**, 505.

[19] GILL N. W. (1969) Congenital atresia of the ear. *Journal of Laryngology and Otology* **83**, 551.

[20] GILL N. W. (1976) Surgery of meatal atresia. *Operative Surgery*, Vol. Ear 6-14. London: Butterworth.

[21] LIVINGSTONE G. H. (1966) Atresia–congenital and acquired. In *Clinical Surgery*, eds. Rob C. and Smith, R., pp. 18–29. London: Butterworth.

[22] COLMAN B. H. Congenital deformities of the ear. *Fifth International Otology Workshop. Chicago, February 1976.* (In press.)

[23] MARQUET J. F. (1969) Proceedings of the International Congress of Otolaryngology, Mexico. *Excerpta Medica, Amsterdam*, **206**, 151–159.

[24] MARQUET, J. F. (1977) Twelve years' experience with homograft tympanoplasty. *Otolaryngologic Clinics of North America*, **10**, 581–593.

[25] MARQUET J. F. (1971) Homogreffes typano-ossiculaires dans le traitement chirurgical de l'agenesie de l'oreille. *Acta oto-rhino-laryngologica Belgica*, 885.

[26] MARQUET J. F. (1976) Current status of tympanic membrane implants. *Fifth International Workshop on Middle Ear Microsurgery and Fluctuant Hearing Loss, Chicago, March 1976.* Huntsville, Alabama: Strode.

CHAPTER 40

Cleft Lip and Palate

The infant born with a congenital cleft is the catalyst within the family group for the production of an array of emotions which ultimately manifest themselves as questions to the professional undertaking the management of this patient. The typical questions from parents of an affected child (e.g. the chances of future offspring being involved, the number of surgical procedures needed, its effect on speech and dentition, etc.) make it obvious that these patients are handled most effectively by professionals representing a variety of disciplines. Surgical procedures on the lip and palate during a period of active facial growth, with the subsequent development of speech, dental, otologic, cosmetic and potential psychologic problems require long-term follow-up for as long as 21 years and possibly longer. The idea of a multidisciplinary team to deal with the patient in a comprehensive manner evolved to meet these needs.

There are certain specialities whose expertise is regularly needed during the routine periodic evaluations. Surgeons trained to deal with maxillofacial and otologic abnormalities, speech pathologists, orthodontists, and prosthodontists meet regularly to outline a plan of management for individual patients, following thorough evaluation by each specialist. In addition, there are certain specialties whose participation is occasionally found to be invaluable. A paediatrician with knowledge of genetic counselling, a social worker, and a child psychologist provide assistance when needed. The key to such a team approach is not just that the patient is evaluated by a variety of disciplines, but that the plan of management is designed in the milieu of multiple specialists jointly discussing the needs of individual patients.

PATHOLOGY

Incidence and genetics

Clefts of the lip and/or palate are one of the most frequent congenital deformities, being second in frequency only to talipes equinovarus (clubfoot). The frequency is higher in Caucasians (1·34 per 1000 births) than in Negroes (0·41 per 1000) [1]. There are certain American Indian tribes who also have a high frequency of clefts [2]. Therefore, variations in incidence reported from different States may be a reflection of differing racial proportions within the population of each. Most studies indicate a national incidence for the United States of 1:700 – 850 births.

Though such data may be useful in defining the proportion of a population which is involved, the recurrent risk rates are much more important in counselling families with a cleft child. These parents should be thoroughly informed about the risk of future siblings being similarly affected.

Patients with cleft lip, with or without cleft palate, are embryologically and genetically distinct from individuals with an isolated cleft palate [3] but the genetic factors for these two major cleft groups are similar and include:

(1) Mutant genes which undergo relatively simple Mendelian inheritance patterns which are manifest as a rare syndrome;

(2) Chromosomal aberrations (e.g. trisomies D and E); and

(3) Environmental teratogens (e.g. thalidomide); and multifactorial inheritance, encompassing the majority of cases [4].

Table 40.1 outlines the recurrent risk rates for clefts [5]; such information is very helpful to the parents of a child with a cleft. Genetic counselling for families is an obligation of the professionals involved with the total management of cleft patients.

Embryology

The embryonic face consists of one frontonasal, two maxillary, and two mandibular processes. Clefts were formerly felt to represent a failure in fusion of one or more of the adjacent embryonic processes of the face but it is now apparent that

TABLE 40.1. Recurrent risk rates

I. Cleft lip, with or without cleft palate Chances for child to have cleft:	
(1) One sibling has cleft No parent cleft	6%
(2) One sibling has cleft One parent cleft	14%
(3) No sibling has cleft	2%
II. Cleft palate, without cleft lip Chances for child to have cleft:	
(1) One sibling has cleft No parent cleft	2%
(2) One sibling has cleft One parent cleft	17%
(3) No sibling has cleft One parent cleft	7%

the isolated cleft palate is embryologically derived in a different fashion than that of a cleft lip, with or without cleft palate. Embryologic sequences which are involved in the normal closure of a palate include an initial intrinsic force which enables the palatal shelves to change from a vertical to a horizontal orientation, along with the anteroinferior migration of the tongue away from the shelves, to allow mesial growth of the shelves and midline fusion. Specific configuration of the base of the skull, size and migration aberrations of the tongue and/or mandible, and innumerable other factors not yet identified may be responsible for interrupting normal development and result in an isolated cleft of the palate [6].

Cleft lip, rather than representing a failure of fusion, results from a failure to maintain an epithelial bridge in an area with decreased meso-

dermal penetration in both the maxillary and nasal processes with subsequent breakdown of the epithelium. The probability of a cleft palate developing in association with cleft lip increases because of the existence of the cleft lip at an earlier stage of development. The lip discontinuity subsequently allows for obstruction of tongue migration by the median process of the primary palate. The tongue, not being permitted normal migration, then prevents horizontal alignment and ultimately prevents fusion of the palatal shelves with a resultant cleft palate [6]. Therefore, the cleft palate associated with cleft lip is a result of the earlier occurring embryologic insult to the lip. Once again, multiple mechanisms can cause the final anatomic defect.

CLASSIFICATION

A universally accepted system of terminology and classification for the variety of maxillofacial clefts does not yet exist. The obvious advantages of such a system in terms of communication and comparing results among medical centres have prompted numerous systems to be proposed. Kernahan & Stark [7] and the American Cleft Palate Association (ACPA) [8] classification systems are both based on embryological patterns (i.e. clefts of the primary palate and clefts of the secondary palate) and are commonly used at present. Whereas the Kernahan & Stark system leads to ambiguities as a result of its simplification of the multitude of cleft variations, the ACPA is somewhat cumbersome because of its specificity.

MANAGEMENT

Preoperative assessment

The top priority after the birth of a child with a congenital cleft is to reassure the parents about feeding the child. Even with wide clefts of the lip and/or palate, most newborn infants are capable of producing sufficient suction to feed from a nipple. The use of a large nipple such as a lamb's nipple or simply a premature infant nipple with an enlarged opening facilitates feeding. Because the infant tends to swallow a great deal of air while feeding, it should be carried out slowly and with periods for burping. With a basic understanding of the physical problems involved, most parents are capable of devising a system which works well for their particular child.

Because of the increased incidence of other congenital anomalies in these children, it is incumbent upon the physician to evaluate thoroughly all organ systems in the perinatal period. Such an evaluation should be completed well before any anticipated operation.

The pre-operative time is also important for parental counselling. The parents need and deserve an explanation of the deformity and all of its potential medical and psychological ramifications. They should be made to understand that feelings of guilt and other emotional stresses between spouses are a natural reaction. The family should also be counselled regarding those agencies which are available to help with the financial requirements of extensive long-term management. This pre-operative period is also a crucial time for the members of the team to establish good rapport with the parents, and thus establish a firm foundation for effective communication through the years.

Surgery

Detailed descriptions of the many operations used for correcting primary and secondary deformities associated with clefts of the lip and palate are not discussed here. However, certain techniques will be described to illustrate general principles of surgical management.

Surgery and facial growth

A primary consideration with any operation for a cleft, apart from cosmesis and function, is its effect on facial growth with all of the subsequent dental and speech ramifications. An understanding of the dynamics of facial and dental development in the presence of a congenital cleft is essential in planning surgical management.

Although there is considerable evidence that palate surgery is responsible for inhibition of facial growth [9–11] there has been a paucity of investigative work evaluating the role of the lip

closure. But a long-term study of pressures on rabbits with clefts of the lip, alveolus, and palate following closure of the cleft lip demonstrated increases in lip pressures following the surgical repairs (Fig. 40.1) and subsequent maxillofacial deformities [12].

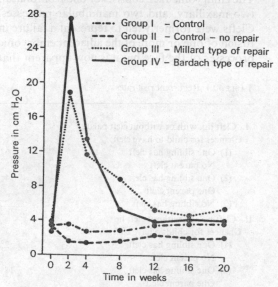

FIG. 40.1: Lip pressures in rabbits with clefts of the lip, alveolus, and palate following repair of the cleft lip only.

The optimal timing of palate surgery is the subject of considerable debate. Early repair with establishment of velopharyngeal competency may benefit speech development. For this reason some surgeons advocate closure of the palate when the child is 12–18 months of age. However, surgery before the appearance of the posterior molar teeth (18–30 months of age) is believed by many orthodontists to result in a high incidence of maxillary segment collapse. Bernstein's [13] evaluation of 325 patients with surgically corrected maxillofacial clefts revealed alteration of mid-third facial growth when palatoplasties were performed before the deciduous molars were in proper occlusion. He, therefore, recommended waiting for the establishment of this dental occlusion before palatal closure.

Primary lip repairs are usually performed when the child has met the requirements of the 'rule of 10s' (i.e. 10 weeks of age, 10 pounds in weight, and at least 10 grams of haemoglobin).

Surgery follows a careful search for other congenital anomalies.

Primary unilateral cheiloplasty

Though surgical repair of the unilateral cleft lip (cheiloplasty) may be performed in the neonatal period, most surgeons today prefer the child to be 10–12 weeks of age (see above). The unilateral cleft lip deformity consists of three basic components:

(1) A discontinuity of labial skin and muscle;

(2) An inadequate vertical dimension of the prolabial (medial) segment; and

(3) A deformity of the nose.

Surgical techniques are directed toward each of these components.

Figure 40.2 illustrates the rotation-advancement technique as described by Millard [14]. This technique incorporates a downward rotation of the prolabial segment with a medial advancement of the lateral segment. In so doing the nasal floor and sill may be closed, the medial lip segment is elongated, and the labial muscle and skin may be sutured (Fig. 40.3a and b). The resultant surgical scar should be nearly symmetrical with the opposite philtril column.

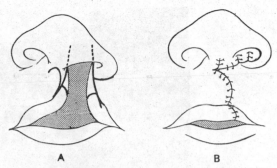

A   B

FIG. 40.2. The rotation-advancement technique of primary cleft lip repair as described by Millard.

Primary bilateral cheiloplasty

Though both sides of the cleft lip may be repaired simultaneously, many surgeons prefer to repair one side at 10–12 weeks of age, and the second side 4 weeks later. Though the basic components of the bilateral cleft deformity are similar to those of unilateral clefts, the severity of the deformity is frequently considerably greater.

The principles of surgical correction are similar to those for unilateral cleft lip, though modification may be necessary when the two sides are

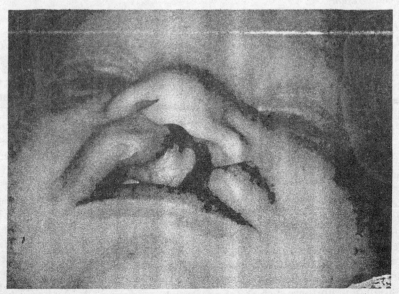

FIG. 40.3a. Pre-operative photo of an infant with a complete cleft of the lip, alveolus, and palate, demonstrating the typical lip and nasal deformities.

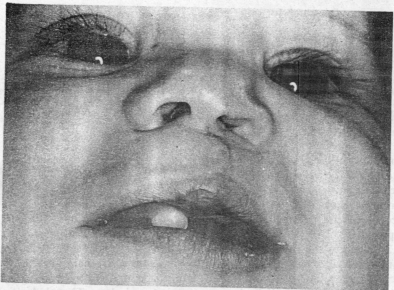

FIG. 40.3b. Post-operative photo demonstrating results following cleft lip repair using the rotation-advancement technique, but also with closure of the floor of the nose and reconstitution of the nasal sill.

closed simultaneously. The secondary deformities associated with bilateral cleft lip are generally greater and considerably more difficult to correct than those with unilateral clefts.

Primary cleft palate repair

The importance of timing in cleft palate surgery has been discussed previously. The goals of such surgery are an intact palate with sufficient length and movement to achieve closure of the velopharyngeal aperture during speech; i.e. the soft palate contacts the posterior pharyngeal wall to prevent the escape of air through the nose during speech. In addition, this should be accomplished without retarding maxillofacial growth and development.

Figure 40.4a–d illustrates the push-back palatoplasty as described by Wardill [15] and Kilner [16]. Most palatoplasty techniques combine the medial advancement of mucoperiosteal flaps to close the cleft with elongation techniques to lengthen the palate (Fig. 40.5).

Approximately 80% of cleft palate children may be expected to achieve acceptable speech following palatoplasty. The remainder will require implantation of a substance such as Teflon [17] into the posterior nasopharyngeal wall to give additional bulk, or a pharyngeal flap. The latter consists of a flap of constrictor muscle and mucosa from the posterior pharyngeal wall which is sutured to the soft palate, leaving only small lateral ports to be closed during speech.

Dental management

Long-term dental care is mandatory in achieving satisfactory results for the patient with a cleft. Orthodontic and prosthodontic treatment is intimately related to the timing of surgical procedures and the quality of results obtained. A simplified review of this dental management will serve to illustrate what type of long-term involvement is required.

Primary dental care is important not only in assessing the condition of teeth, but also in establishing good rapport with a patient who will need to be treated for many years to come. In children with cleft palate, supernumerary teeth (21%), dystrophied teeth (26·9%), and congenitally missing teeth (49·6%) are all more common than in a normal population [18]. Thus, the need for dental consultation arises early. In addition, because excellent oral hygiene is essential during

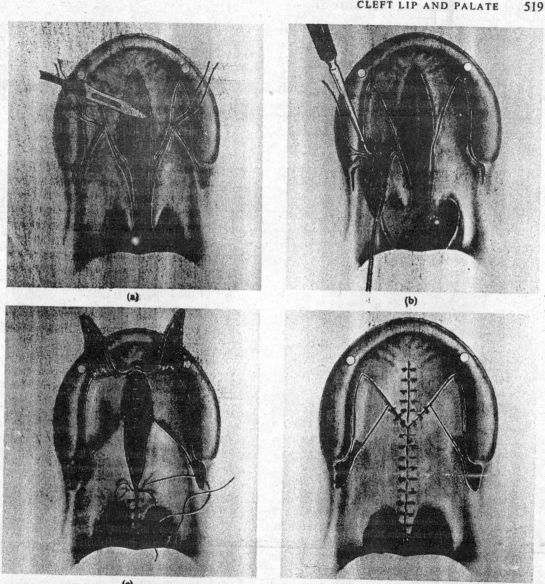

FIG. 40.4a–d. V–Y retropositioning of the palate as described by Wardill & Kilner.

the course of any orthodontic treatment, it is particularly important for these children to develop sound dental habits at an early age.

The orthodontic treatment may be complex and requires skilled personnel familiar with related abnormalities of the dentoalveolar segments. The goals of such treatment are to attain functional occlusion and to improve facial appearance. Long-term management can be divided into three phases [19]. Phase one involves

expansion of the maxillary segments when the child is 3 or 4 years of age. Spiit lingual expanders are effective means of widening the maxillary arch. Phase two involves treatment of mixed abnormalities of dentition. Extraction of certain deciduous teeth may be required during this period. The third and final phase does not begin until permanent dentition has erupted. Full band appliances are used to move teeth into proper occlusal relationships.

Prosthodontic devices provide an alternative to the surgical management of velopharyngeal incompetence and are especially valuable when there are medical contra-indications to surgery. Though prosthodontic obturators vary slightly in design, they generally consist of a palatal obturator which attaches to the teeth anteriorly and extends posteriorly as a bulb which touches the pharyngeal wall during speech.

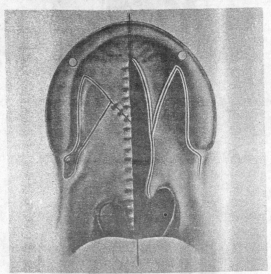

FIG. 40.5. Illustration of the palatal elongation achieved following an effective palatoplasty.

Speech therapy

Early guidance by a speech pathologist is important not only for the future success of the child's speech training, but also to alleviate the psychologic stresses which society imposes upon the individual with obvious 'cleft palate speech'. Any intervention which may improve the speech patterns therefore is beneficial. The efficacy of speech therapy in improving the speech of preschool children with cleft palate was established by Phillips and coworkers[20]. VanDemark [21] has similarly demonstrated the good results of speech therapy on articulation. However, the speech pathologist's responsibilities do not end with therapy, but include the gathering of valuable diagnostic information.

The speech clinician's diagnostic armamentarium includes speech assessments, oral manometric pressure readings, lateral soft tissue radiographs during phonation, and cineradiography. Not only does this data provide the opportunity to make conclusions about the effectiveness of velopharyngeal closure, but it aids in identifying those abnormal speech patterns due to causes other than velopharyngeal incompetence.

Otologic management

The Eustachian tube appears to be the anatomic origin of subsequent otologic problems in the cleft palate population, both before and after operation. The incidence of middle ear effusions in infants with cleft palate is high. The preoperative cause of these effusions may be a local inflammatory reaction about the nasopharyngeal orifice of the Eustachian tube as a result of the ease of food reflux through the palatal cleft [22]. This inflammation would then prevent proper tubal function. After operation the cause is alteration of the function of the tensor veli palatini, which opens the nasopharyngeal orifice of the tube, to a levator action by slipping the tendon off the hamulus during palatal closure.

Some investigators [23–25] have noted less hearing loss in children who had relatively early palatoplasties and concluded that the palatal closure restores proper Eustachian tubal function and therefore results in this decrease of auditory pathology. There are studies which challenge that hypothesis: advancing age may be the critical factor and not the palatoplasty [26].

Nevertheless, middle ear effusions in the young cleft palate patient are common and require continued otologic and audiologic assessments. The treatment of these effusions with multiple ventilating tubes also takes its toll. Therefore, these patients need continued follow-up to monitor the status of the often scarred and atrophic tympanic membrane.

References

[1] CHUNG C. S. & MYRIANTHOPOULOS N. C. (1968) Racial and prenatal factors in major congenital malformations. *American Journal of Human Genetics* **20**(1), 44.

[2] MILLER V. R. (1972) The use of registries and vital

statistics in the study of congenital malformations. New York: *Proceedings of 2nd International Conference on Congenital Malformations*, p. 963, pp. 334–340.

[3] FOGH-ANDERSON P. (1972) *Inheritance of Harelip and Cleft Palate.* Copenhagen: Nyt Nordisk Forlag-Arnold Busck.

[4] FRASER F. C. (1971) Etiology of cleft lip and palate. In *Cleft Lip and Palate*, eds. Grabb W. C. *et al.*, pp. 58–63. Boston: Little, Brown and Company.

[5] FOGH-ANDERSON P. (1972) *Inheritance of Harelip and Cleft Palate*, pp. 210–214. Copenhagen: Nyt Nordisk Forlag-Arnold Busck.

[6] FISHER J. C. & KOCHHAR D. M. (1974) Cleft lip and palate: a discussion of cause. In *Symposium on Management of Cleft Lip and Palate and Associated Deformities*, eds. Georgiade N. G. & Hagerty W. L., pp. 3–9. St. Louis: C. V. Mosby Company.

[7] KERNAHAN D. A. & STARK R. B. (1958) A new classification for cleft lip and cleft palate. *Plastic and Reconstructive Surgery and the Transplantation Bulletin* 22, 435.

[8] HARKINS C. S. BERLIN A., HARDING R., LONGACRE V. V. & SNODGRASSE R. (1962) A classification of cleft lip and cleft palate. *Plastic and Reconstructive Surgery and the Transplantation Bulletin* 29, 37.

[9] GRABER T. (1949) Cranial facial morphology in cleft palate and cleft lip deformities. *Surgery, Gynecology and Obstetrics with International Abstracts of Surgery* 88, 359.

[10] HERFERT O. (1958) Zur Chirurgie der Lippen-Keefer-Gaumenspalten Fortschr. *Kiefer-Geo-Chir.* XV.

[11] KREMENAK C. R. & SEARLS J. C. (1971) Experimental manipulation of mid-facial growth; a synthesis of five years of research at the Iowa Maxillofacial Growth Laboratory. *Journal of Dental Research* 50, 1488.

[12] BARDACH J. & EISBACH K. (1976) The influence of primary unilateral cleft lip repair on facial growth. Part I – lip pressure. *Cleft Palate Journal* 14, 88–97.

[13] BERNSTEIN L. (1968) The effect of timing of cleft palate operations on subsequent growth of the maxilla. *Laryngoscope* 78, 1510.

[14] MILLARD D. R. (1971) Rotation-advancement in the repair of unilateral cleft lip. In *Cleft Lip and Palate*, eds.

Grabb W. C. *et al.*, pp. 195–203. Boston: Little, Brown and Company.

[15] WARDILL W. E. M. (1937) The technique of operation for cleft palate. *British Journal of Surgery* 25, 117.

[16] KITNER T. P. (1937) Cleft lip and palate repair technique. *St. Thomas's Hospital Reports.* 2, 127.

[17] SMITH J. K. & McCABE B. F. (1976) Teflon injection in the nasopharynx to improve velopharyngeal closure. *Annals O.R.L.*

[18] MACKLEY R. (1958) Incidence of congenital anomalies in cleft palate patients. U.S.P.H. Undergraduate Research Fellowship Study, Northwestern University. Unpublished data.

[19] OLIN W. H. (1971) Orthodontics. In *Cleft Lip and Palate*, eds. Grabb W. C. *et al.*, pp. 599–615. Boston: Little, Brown and Company.

[20] PHILIPS B. J. (1971) Stimulating language and speech development in cleft palate infants. In *Communicative Disorders Related to Cleft Lip and Palate*, ed. Bzoch K. R. Boston: Little, Brown and Company.

[21] VANDEMARK D. R. (1974) Some results of speech therapy for children with cleft palate. *Cleft Palate Journal* 11, 41.

[22] LITTON W. B., SEVEREID L. R. & THARP R. (1971) Cleft palate and otitis media. In *National Conference on Otitis Media. Proceedings*, eds. Glorig A. & Gerwin K. Springfield, Ill.: Charles C. Thomas.

[23] YULES R. B. (1970) Hearing in cleft palate patients. *Archives of Otolaryngology* 91, 319.

[24] MASTERS F. W., BINGHAM H. G. & ROBINSON D. W. (1960) The prevention and treatment of hearing loss in the cleft palate child. *Plastic and Reconstructive Surgery and the Transplantation Bulletin* 25, 503.

[25] ASCHAN G. (1966) Hearing and nasal function correlated to postoperative speech in cleft palate patients with velopharyngoplasty. *Acta Otolaryngology* 61, 371.

[26] SEVEREID L. P. (1972) A longitudinal study of the efficacy of adenoidectomy in children with cleft palate and secretory otitis media. *Transactions of the American Academy of Ophthalmology and Otolaryngology* 76, 1319.

CHAPTER 41

Speech Disorders

In Britain approximately 14% of children between the ages of 5 and 10 have articulatory or language problems [1] and the incidence is similar in the United States [2–6].

The classification of speech disorders in childhood is fraught with difficulties. Phoneticians and linguists have made major advances in studies of normal speech development in children but have not yet applied their skills on any large scale to children with defective speech. In these circumstances it is necessary to classify speech disorders on the basis of disturbance of the primary elements of speech, voice, rhythm or articulation, and by associated clinical findings. The classification is shown in Table 41.1.

It will be seen that the present classification is essentially clinical; it is designed to encourage the doctor helping a speech therapist to classify appropriately.

DYSPHONIA

Between 3 and 4% of children referred to the speech clinic in the Royal Hospital for Sick Children, Edinburgh, suffer from hoarseness. This is most frequently the result of a combination of factors: intermittent upper respiratory tract infection, often acquired in poor social conditions, and excessive shouting. Laryngoscopy often shows nodules or thickened cords and, rarely, papillomas.

The treatment of dysphonia in young children is very difficult. The principles are that the voice should be rested and any infection treated.

DYSRHYTHMIAS

Speech dysrhythmia is the name commonly given dination between the activity of the respiratory and articulatory musculature. The common manifestations are hesitation, stammer (or stutter), blocking and the prolongation of syllables.

People not suspected of having any speech defect may produce as many 'non-fluencies' as patients who stammer. The difference between them and the stammerer is that the stammerer has become aware and anxious about what he considers is his speech disorder. Non-fluencies

TABLE 41.1. Classification of speech disorders

Dysphonia: usually due to laryngeal disease

Dysrhythmia: failure of synchronization between respiration and articulation

Dysarthria: structural or neurological abnormality of articulatory organs
    Structural causes: cleft palate; lingual disproportion; dental malocclusion; adenoid enlargement; palatopharyngeal disproportion
    Neurological causes: paresis or incoordination of lips, tongue, palate

Secondary speech disorders: retardation of speech development with no demonstrable abnormality of articulatory organs associated with:
    Mental defect
    Deafness
    True dysphasia
    Severe psychiatric disorders
    Social deprivation

The specific developmental speech disorder syndrome
    Articulatory defect with normal language development and comprehension
    Articulatory defect with retardation of language; normal comprehension
    Severe defects of articulation and spoken language. Defective comprehension
    Very severe defects of spoken language and comprehension; central deafness

are particularly frequent in children aged between 2 and 5 years [7]. It is possible that the efforts of anxious parents trying to correct the normal non-fluencies of their child at this age could result in true speech dysrhythmia at a later age. Parents belonging to families in which there was a history of stammering are particularly prone to notice any dysrhythmia in their children and pay undue attention to it.

Stammering may possibly be inherited as a Mendelian dominant characteristic in a proportion of patients, though the expression of the inheritance varies from patient to patient according to environmental circumstances and the way the child has been brought up [8].

Dysrhythmia may occur at any time but children are referred most frequently to speech clinics at the age of 2 or 3 years with 'cluttering', by which is understood a 'normal' tendency to repeat syllables, slur speech sounds and sometimes even repeat whole phrases. A second crisis point for the potential stammerer seems to be when he enters school at the age of 5 years. The stress is too much for him and he begins to have difficulty in spoken communication – he stammers. Another common time for the onset of stammer is between the ages of 7 and 8 years. The first onset of stammering at a later age is unusual (Table 41.2).

The treatment of stammering patients is difficult and requires a multi-disciplinary approach in which psychiatrists, psychologists, paediatricians, neurophysiologists and speech therapists may all require to be involved in order to make a useful diagnosis and plan further treatment.

There is no doubt that the introduction of training in so-called 'syllable timed speech' has brought symptomatic relief to many stammering children and adults in a very practical way. This treatment consists of teaching the child to put even stress on each articulated syllable in a rather deliberate manner. Even when patients fail to adjust their everyday speech to syllable timing, the technique is still useful when they are placed in conditions of stress, for they can resort to syllable-timed speech and know that they will not stammer. This is particularly important for adolescent stammerers and for school-leavers facing oral examinations and later interviews for jobs [8].

DYSARTHRIA

Structural causes

Cleft palate

Isolated cleft lip rarely gives rise to significant disorders of articulation even if it is not repaired. In unrepaired cleft palate there is frequently a

TABLE 41.2. The three patterns in the development of stammering.

Transient developmental stammering

'A transient period of difficulty in the smooth articulation of speech between the ages of 2 and 4 years' at the time when children are developing speech. This appears to be the same as cluttering as defined earlier and 'development stuttering' as described by Metraux [9] and Ingram [10].

Remitting stutterers

Those children who show speech dysrhythmia for a period of between 6 months and 6 years and then show remission. In these patients symptoms first appear between the ages of 3 and 11, the mean age being $7\frac{1}{2}$. It was found by Andrews & Harris [8] that males in this group tend to stammer for longer than females.

Persistent stutterers

This group comprises about 1% of the population. Commonly speech dysrhythmia appears between the ages of 2 and 8, persisting until the age of at least 15 and quite frequently into adult life. In this group male patients outnumber female patients. They form the large body of 'chronic speech dysrhythmics' or 'chronic stutterers' who require most clinical help if real distress in adult life is to be avoided.

---

history of nasal ejection of feeds during infancy and later difficulty in dealing with semi-solid foodstuffs. Even when the palate is repaired it may be found to be deficient in size or defective in movement so that nasal escape of air during speech occurs and there is hyperrhinophonia. A curious finding which has been demonstrated repeatedly in studies of children suffering from cleft lip and palate which have been repaired is that those who have an isolated cleft palate, without a cleft lip, score less well on tests of articulation than do those with clefts of both lip and palate [11]. Recent improvements in the surgical techniques of repair have greatly reduced the incidence of severe speech disorders attributable to cleft palate and its complications.

Hypoplasia of the palate results in hyperrhinophonia which is very similar to that found in cleft palate patients. The condition is often missed during infancy when the child may have regurgitated feeds nasally. Most children who suffer from short palate only come to paediatricians when it is noted that their speech at the age of 2½ or 3 years is abnormal and 'nasal'. As in cleft palate patients whose repairs have been unsuccessful, pharyngoplasty (an operation in which a partial obstruction of the nasopharyngeal orifice is made using tissue from the posterior pharyngeal wall and the soft palate) may be very helpful in diminishing the degree of nasal escape and dysarthria.

Lingual disproportion

Hypoplasia of the tongue is a very rare condition which does not seem to interfere significantly with infants feeding from the breast or bottle and has much less effect on speech development than one would expect. Commonly the tongue is found to be tethered by strands of fascia to the floor of the mouth (tongue-tie) and after release considerable mobility may be obtained [12].

Dental malocclusion

Appropriate occlusion of the jaws is influenced by many factors. Whenever malocclusion is found it is important to consider the interaction of the muscles which might have caused it. Far too often malocclusion is treated as 'a disease' whereas in fact it is the effect of facial weakness, excessive tongue thrust or prolonged mouth breathing. Even thumb-sucking, if it continues after the permanent incisors have erupted, may distort the occlusion of the jaws.

Adenoid enlargement

Enlargement of the adenoids is liable to cause hyponasality. Extreme enlargement of the adenoids restricts the movement of the soft palate required for clear articulation. Associated tonsillitis and peritonsillar inflammation, so often found in association with adenoiditis, further restricts palatal movement.

Palatopharyngeal disproportion

This syndrome consists of a disproportion between the size of the nasopharyngeal orifice and the size of the soft palate. It may be due to hypoplasia of the palate but is more commonly the result of relative hyperplasia of the maxilla.

The condition is often familial and the large cheekbones of parents, uncles and aunts leads to a striking similarity in facial appearance to many patients. The soft palate may appear to be normal in size, structure and function but is inadequate to close off the nasopharynx because the nasopharyngeal aperture is so very large. There is often a history of feeding difficulty with nasal regurgitation of milk feeds during infancy, and when speech appears it tends to be hypernasal. Later the hypernasality can easily be demonstrated by asking the child to produce an 'i' or 'e' sound and placing a finger below the nostrils. Normally there should be no nasal escape of air on production of these sounds but in the palatal disproportion syndrome nasal escape occurs. The 'cleft palate type speech' is commented on by many parents and is readily identifiable by speech therapists.

The effects of palatal disproportion may be masked to some extent if the adenoids are enlarged for the soft palate can then close off against them and the speech may even sound hyponasal rather than hypernasal. It is therefore important that if children require adenoidectomy on account of recurrent or chronic upper respiratory tract infections the surgeon should ensure that the palate will be adequate to close off the nasopharyngeal aperture after operation. X-ray palatography can be of great assistance in helping him to assess this type of hidden palatal disproportion and decide on what action he will take.

Neurological causes

Almost every disease of the central nervous system may cause a speech disorder in childhood.

Cerebral palsy

In cerebral palsy the paresis found in the limbs of

children suffering from bilateral hemiplegia or diplegic cerebral palsy may also involve the bulbar musculature. The slowness of voluntary movement, weakness and incoordination typical of ataxic cerebral palsy may be found in the movements of the lips, tongue and palate. The same type of unwanted involuntary movement that affects the limbs in dyskinetic cerebral palsy and interferes especially with fine voluntary movements may be observed in the movements of the lips, tongue and palate.

Approximately 60% of children who suffer from cerebral palsy have speech defects.

Peripheral nerve lesions

Peripheral nerve damage affecting the functions of the lips, tongue and palate are uncommon. Traumatic injury to the palatal nerve may occur in the course of tonsillectomy but is uncommon today.

Each year one or two children are brought to the speech clinic with a history of 'deteriorating speech', or 'cleft-palate-like speech', who are found to suffer from *facio-scapular-humeral dystrophy*. It is important to recognize that this condition may present as 'speech defect', and also realize that therapy is more likely to be frustrating to the patient, than to be helpful.

Acquired dysarthria

Acquired dysarthria occurs occasionally. It may result from damage to the cerebral hemispheres, as a result of meningitis, encephalitis, or head injury. Encephalitis, usually of viral origin, may cause severe impairment of the voluntary movements of the lips, tongue and palate as may traumatic damage to the brain stem: a condition which may be masked to some extent by associated dysphasic difficulties due to injury to the cerebral hemispheres. Damage to the lips, tongue and palate themselves resulting in permanent dysarthria is rare; partial amputation of a soft palate has been observed following tonsillectomy, and severe lacerations of the palate, usually as a result of a child falling onto a sharp object held in the mouth, are found occasionally. Quite severe dysarthria may be caused by the ingestion of caustic or acid substances. Frequently in such patients there is associated dysphonia secondary to laryngeal scarring.

SECONDARY SPEECH DISORDERS

The term secondary speech disorders was evolved in order to group together a somewhat diverse collection of speech problems in which the lips, tongue and palate and related structures were healthy but speech was defective because of other disease or adverse environmental factors.

Mental retardation

It would be out of place in this chapter to enter into a detailed discussion of the diagnosis of mental retardation in childhood, especially in view of the many recent advances in the recognition of diseases due to chromosomal abnormalities and metabolic disorders [13,14]. It is important, however, to emphasize the frequency with which mental retardation is responsible for delayed speech development, and that when a child is brought to the family doctor or specialist on account of slow speech development mental retardation should always be suspected. The diagnosis of a child with slow speech development is incomplete until the patient has been examined and fully investigated for the multiplicity of diseases which are associated with mental handicap.

He requires a carefully planned programme of stimulation and therapy worked out in conjunction with therapists and the parents which can often result in quite dramatic improvements in the child's use of spoken language, and consequently his ability to communicate.

A high proportion of these children have associated defects. These include hydrocephalus, with or without associated ataxic cerebral palsy; hemiplegic, diplegic or ataxic cerebral palsy; hearing loss; and associated developmental anomalies. Suspected mental retardation in a child coming to a speech therapy clinic should serve to encourage further investigation, not discourage it [15].

Deafness

The causes of hearing loss in infants and young

children have been discussed in Chapters 37 and 38. In spite of the improved methods of identifying hearing loss in the childhood population at a young age, a considerable number of children appear at speech clinics at the age of 3 or 4 years who are virtually speechless – and on investigation are found to be significantly hard of hearing.

Acquired childhood dysphasia

Children above the age of about 7 usually manifest the same syndromes of dysphasia as adults. Younger children, especially those under the age of about 3 years, who are subjected to brain injury as a result of disease or trauma, present a rather different picture [1]. Immediately after their cerebral injury children whose speech centres have been affected are remarkably mute. They may appear to understand what is said to them but are unable to respond using expressive language for a matter of weeks. When they do begin to speak their sentences are short and lack 'syntactical items'. They tend to 'talk in telegrams'. The majority learn to communicate using rather crude speech and gesture, but their speech is rarely fluent and the amount of speech they produce is small. Their major difficulties occur when they go to school for their difficulties with the written word tend to be considerably greater than those with the spoken word which they have experienced previously.

Psychiatric disorders

A high proportion of the children referred from child psychiatrists to speech clinics are found to be anxious because of their intrinsic speech defects. Their anxiety is often much relieved if their speech improves, with the help of speech therapy, and a certain gain in confidence and a feeling of improvement.

'Autism' is a shorthand description of behavioural abnormalities which requires neurological and psychiatric assessment. It is not a diagnosis. Nevertheless it must be admitted that there are a small number of children in the community who are withdrawn, idiosyncratic, completely self-absorbed, and 'live in a world of their own'. The speech of these children may be bizarre and in spite of their sometimes quite formatively large vocabulary, they have difficulty with pronouns, prepositions and sometimes articles. A few have difficulty in naming objects towards which they have any feeling, either positive or negative [16].

Elective mutism is a rare condition and is a term applied to children who speak only in limited circumstances, commonly only in the family. They are likely to remain mute at school and out of doors and behave strangely. Elective mutism tended to be regarded as a disease entity at one time but it has become increasingly apparent in recent years that there are at least two groups of children who suffer from the condition. The largest group consists of children who are very shy, withdrawn, uncertain and neurotic. With adequate psychiatric treatment and environmental control (rather than speech therapy) the prognosis for these children is good.

A small proportion of children who suffer from elective mutism are psychotic, and many of them possibly schizophrenic.

Social deprivation

The effects of the environment upon children suffering from speech disorders in general and specifically secondary speech disorders is not fully discussed here. Nevertheless it is often of great value to obtain a firsthand account from an experienced social worker of the conditions in which a child is living whose speech development is retarded, who shows other abnormalities of behaviour and whose development appears to have been deviant.

THE SPECIFIC DEVELOPMENTAL SPEECH DISORDER SYNDROME

This elaborate term was invented to describe a large group of children in the community who appear to be healthy in other respects but suffer from retarded speech development. The condition is often hereditary and affects boys much more severely and somewhat more frequently than girls. A family history of retarded speech development and/or stammering, and/or difficulties in learning to use the written word, are found in about 70% of patients. There is also an

TABLE 41.3 Classification of the developmental speech disorder syndrome

Severity	Description	Other terms
Mild	Retardation of acquisition of word sounds, language normal	Dyslalia
Moderate	More severe retardation of word sound acquisition and retarded spoken language development, comprehension normal	Developmental expressive dysphasia
Severe	Still more severe retardation of word sound acquisition and spoken language development, impaired comprehension of speech	Developmental receptive dysphasia, word deafness, auditory imperception
Very severe	Gross failure of speech development, impaired comprehension of language and significance of other sounds, often apparent deafness	Auditory imperception, central deafness

increased prevalence of weak laterality of handedness amongst relatives, and many are described as ambidextrous or weakly left-handed. It is not uncommon to obtain a history from parents that their own parents or their brothers and sisters played most games in a left-handed manner but wrote with their right hands.

An odd feature in the family history which is also found in children who suffer from so-called 'dyslexia' is that there is an excess of twins in the immediate family of patients suffering from specific retardation of speech development.

From the clinical point of view it is useful to classify the developmental speech disorder syndrome by degrees of severity [17] (Table 41.3).

The management of children suffering from the syndrome of specific retardation of speech development has been revolutionized in recent years since speech therapists began to use standardized tests of the ability to comprehend and produce spoken language and studied articulation by standardized tests. Many children suffering from this disorder progress, speech-wise, at their own rate and eventually produce acceptable speech patterns. Others fail to achieve this level of competence but speech therapists are now in a position using these specialized tests to identify the likely candidates who require speech therapy at a relatively early stage. That so many children who suffer from this syndrome later show difficulties in learning to read and spell should be much more widely known than it is. Unfor-

tunately there is often lack of communication between paediatricians and educational psychologists and teachers, and community medical officers and teachers when the problem of speech retardation is assessed. The probabilities of later difficulties in school are not adequately appreciated [18, 19].

References

[1] ALAJOUANINE TH. & L'HERMITTE F. (1965) Acquired aphasia in children. *Brain* **88**, 653.

[2] BLANTON S. (1916) A survey of speech defects. *Journal of Educational Psychology* **7**, 581.

[3] MILLS A. & STREET H. (1942) Report of a speech survey, Holyoke, Massachusetts. *Journal of Speech Disorders* **7**, 161.

[4] JOHNSON W. (1942) *The Iowa Remedial Education Program: Summary Report*. Iowa City.

[5] HAWK E. A. (1945) A survey and critical analysis of speech needs in the elementary schools of Ohio City of 15,000 population. Summarized by Travis L. E. (1959) *Handbook of Speech Pathology*. London: Peter Owen.

[6] IRWIN R. B. (1948) Ohio looks ahead in speech and hearing therapy. *Journal of Speech and Hearing Disorders* **13**, 55.

[7] JOHNSON W. (1955) *Stuttering in Children and Adults*. Minneapolis: University of Minnesota Press.

[8] ANDREWS G. & HARRIS M. (1964) *The Syndrome of Stuttering. Club Clinics in Developmental Medicine and Child Neurology, No. 17.* London: The Spastics Society & Heinemann.

[9] METRAUX R. (1950) Speech profiles of the pre-school child 18–54 months. *Journal of Speech Disorders* **15**, 37.

[10] INGRAM T. T. S. (1959) A description and classification of common speech disorders. *Archives of Disease in Childhood* **34**, 444.

[11] DRILLIEN C. M., WILKINSON E. M. & INGRAM T. T. S. (1966) *The Causes and Natural History of Cleft Lip and Palate*. Edinburgh: E. & W. Livingstone.

[12] ARDRAN G. M., BECKETT J. M. & KEMP F. H. (1964) Aglossia congenita. *Archives of Disease in Childhood* **39**, 389.

[13] BROWN J. K., INGRAM T. T. S., SHANKS R. A., SHAW J. F. & STARK G. D. (1973) Disorders of the central nervous system. In *Textbook of Paediatrics*, eds. Forfar J. O. & Arneil G. C., Chapter 14, p. 667. Edinburgh: Churchill Livingstone.

[14] BUIST N. M. R., FORFAR J. O. & HOLZEL A. (1973) Metabolic disorders. In *Textbook of Paediatrics*, eds. Forfar J. O. & Arneil G. C., Chapter 19, p. 1150. Edinburgh: Churchill Livingstone.

[15] INGRAM T. T. S. (1969) The new approach to early diagnosis of handicaps in childhood. *Developmental Medicine and Child Neurology* **11**, 279.

[16] WOLFF S. & CHESS S. (1964) A behavioural study of schizophrenic children. *Acta Psychiatrica Scandinavica* **40**, 438.

[17] INGRAM T. T. S. (1972) The classification of speech and language disorders in the young child. In *The Child with Delayed Speech*, eds. Rutter M. & Martin J. A. M. *Clinics in Developmental Medicine and Child Neurology, No. 43*. London: The Spastics Society & Heinemann.

[18] EUSTIS R. S. (1947) The primary etiology of the specific language disabilities. *Journal of Pediatrics* **31**, 448.

[19] INGRAM T.T.S. (1964) Late and poor talkers. In *The Child Who Does Not Talk*, eds. Renfrew C. & Murphy K. *Clinics in Developmental Medicine and Child Neurology, No. 13*. London: Spastics Society & Heinemann.

CHAPTER 42

Laryngeal Disease in Childhood

Any account of disease in childhood requires emphasis on the essential difference between children and the adult. The child will *develop* into an adult, the adult being already mature can never develop, he can only degenerate. Thus the normal spectrum of child development must always be weighed when offering advice or prognosis, or suggestions for treatment. The neonate's larynx is relatively and absolutely smaller than the adult's. It lies tucked under the base of the tongue and higher in the neck than in the adult. It descends gradually over the first months of extra-uterine life. The period of most rapid growth of the larynx is the first 2 years of life. After this there is a steady increase until puberty when the male larynx shows another growth spurt. The sensory nerve supply to the neonatal larynx is very easily triggered off and this is why the baby can hold its breath and choke over its feeds. Gradually as the child becomes more experienced the violence of the reflex action to laryngeal stimulation diminishes. For this reason gentle instrumentation is all-important when looking at the larynx. It is necessary too to appreciate the basic principles of laryngotracheal physiology for the larynx and the trachea spend their life working together as a single unit designed to cope with the intake and output of air and with the output of mucus. The stimulus to vocal cord abduction comes from the expiratory air thrust impinging on the subglottic mucosa. Mucus and debris are wafted up the tracheal wall by the ciliated epithelial lining. However, this directional cilial beat is enhanced by the respiratory air tide. Cine-endoscopy shows that mucus is only wafted out of the glottis when there is an expiratory tide and furthermore it demonstrates that this mucus emerges around the periphery of the whole glottis and not just over the posterior commissure as has been often recorded in previous books and papers. The patency of the whole airway is preserved by the flexible arrangement of incomplete tracheal rings separated by connective tissue bands. Thus the head can be bent in all directions while the lumen of the trachea remains patent. Therefore nothing should be done which interferes either anatomically or physiologically with this arrangement because the child's airway may be so prejudiced as to endanger his life.

SYMPTOMS AND SIGNS

Stridor

This may be inspiratory, expiratory or both, the so-called two-way stridor. The noise may be louder when sleeping or waking and may be changed by changing the child's position. Be that as it may, stridor always indicates obstruction to the airway. Inspiratory stridor usually indicates disease at the glottis or above. Expiratory stridor usually indicates obstruction in the bronchi. Two-way stridor indicates obstruction between the glottis and the bronchi. However, although careful attention to exactly where in the respiratory cycle the stridor comes will be helpful, it merely directs the attention to that part of the respiratory tract which must be examined in more detail. Over the past 30 years there have been many advances in this field of medicine. One of the most important has been in the field of anaesthesia, which has allowed the laryngologist to insist that all children with stridor should undergo endoscopy. Only in this way can an absolute anatomical and pathological diagnosis be made. The endoscopic findings may have an important bearing on the future management of the child. Textbooks of paediatrics are frequently reassuring in that they state that stridor in infancy disappears at 2 years of age. It may, but in the author's experience, it is more likely to persist to 5–7 years of age. In a significant number the stridor will get worse.

Hoarseness

A child who is born with a hoarse voice, a weak cry or an abnormal cry must always be suspected of a laryngeal lesion. In the neonatal period a weak cry may be associated with laryngeal paralysis and an abnormal cry with the cri du chat syndrome. In the young child hoarseness may be associated with webs between the vocal cords, subglottic stenosis or papillomas or an impacted foreign body.

Dyspnoea

A small baby with partial airway obstruction exhibits difficulty in breathing. It should be looked for in the alae nasi, the neck and the intercostal spaces. In extreme cases the whole sternum may be sucked in towards the vertebral column. These signs indicate that airway relief of some sort will shortly be required.

Feeding difficulties

Nearly all children with airway obstruction from whatever cause have difficulty in feeding. Feeds are taken slowly and sometimes spill over into the tracheobronchial tree. The child fails to gain weight; airway obstruction therefore may be a cause for failure to thrive. In other cases the airway obstruction only becomes apparent when the child has fed too well in the early weeks of life and has gained weight too rapidly. It is often necessary and usually unpopular to insist that the baby should lose weight.

Recurrent chest infections

Many children with airway obstruction develop chest infections. A decrease in the frequency and severity of the infection may indicate that the problem causing the obstruction is resolving, and that the surgeon should temporize and resist the temptation to seek radical surgical solutions to the problem.

INVESTIGATIONS

The *history* should note the replies to the following questions:
   (1) When was the stridor first noticed?
   (2) At what time of day or night is it loudest?
   (3) Is the voice or cry abnormal or weak?
   (4) Is the child a slow feeder?
   (5) Does feeding cause coughing, cyanosis or apnoea?
   (6) Have there been chest infections?
   (7) What is the weight? What was the birth weight? Has the child been slow to gain weight?
   (8) Was pregnancy, labour and delivery normal?
   (9) Did the baby cry immediately?
   (10) Have any other abnormalities been detected?

The *examination* should record the sex, size, weight and colour. Stridor should be timed in the respiratory cycle. The cry should be described. Cough should be noted. If the stridor is of acute onset the pulse rate should be noted. The patient should then be postured in the prone, right lateral, supine and left lateral positions, and the effect upon the intensity of the signs noted. A great deal of valuable information can be obtained by listening to the larynx with a stethoscope. The findings should be recorded if there is time. However, if the breathing is seriously embarrassed, the pulse rate high and the patient's colour poor, airway relief is the first priority.

Other writers have drawn attention to the value of *radiography* of the larynx. In this writer's experience radiography has not proved to be of value in acute respiratory difficulty except to exclude a primary chest condition. However when the child is to be investigated in an ordinary and leisurely manner a plain chest radiograph and a contrast examination of the swallow are helpful to exclude such conditions as tracheo-oesophageal fistula and dysphagia lusoria.

If these examinations do not suggest a diagnosis the larynx must be *examined under general anaesthesia* usually followed by a bronchoscopy and, if necessary, by an oesophagoscopy.

The surgeon should have a close working relationship with his anaesthetist. Both the surgeon and the anaesthetist should be able to carry out laryngoscopy, bronchoscopy and intubation. This is essential if the safety of the airway is to be assured. The surgeon records his findings in respect of structure and function: curarizing agents therefore should not be used except in an emergency. The anaesthesia should be light and the inhalational agents reinforced by the use of topical anaesthesia to the larynx. This allows inspection of the vocal cords and a check to be made of cord movements. Once anaesthesia is induced the laryngeal airway should be measured with a standard set of Portex endotracheal tubes and the size recorded in the notes.

CLASSIFICATION OF CONGENITAL LARYNGEAL DISEASE

Structural

Supraglottic
Congenital laryngeal stridor (laryngomalacia):
  Omega-epiglottis and short aryepiglottic folds
  True laryngomalacia
  Small, long epiglottis with funnel-shaped supraglottis.
Abnormality of the epiglottis:
  Bifid
  Broad quadrate
  Large overhanging.
Cysts:
  Mucous cyst
  Lymphangioma
  Laryngocoele.

Glottic
Atresia
Webs
Short cords
Tumours
Clefts

Subglottic
Stenosis
Webs
Tumours

Functional
Vocal cord paralysis:
  Unilateral
  Bilateral.

Extrinsic
Tumours
Vascular anomalies.

Inflammatory laryngeal conditions

Acute laryngitis
Acute epiglottitis
Acute laryngo-tracheo-bronchitis.

Supraglottic obstruction

Congenital laryngeal stridor (laryngomalacia)

Laryngomalacia is a particular variety of congenital laryngeal stridor of which there are three clearly defined types:

(1) The classical case of congenital laryngeal stridor has an omega-shaped epiglottis and short aryepiglottic folds.

(2) A minute epiglottic tip with a very small visible opening to the glottis and a long inverted funnel shaped supraglottis.

(3) A generally floppy laryngeal superstructure.

The varieties have certain points in common. The glottis accepts a tube of the right size for a child of that age. The noise is produced by the supraglottis being sucked into the glottis on inspiration, and there may be marked incoordination between the two sides so that one side may abduct while the other adducts. The noise is usually loudest when the child is relaxed and asleep. Generally speaking the noise tends to disappear as the child grows but the early years may be characterized by feeding difficulties, recurrent chest infections and poor weight gain. The patient should therefore be followed up until the noise has disappeared. Acute upper respiratory tract inflammation may lead to a sudden increase in laryngeal obstruction and this must be treated seriously; such patients are better managed in a paediatric respiratory unit where help is available immediately. If the stridor does not improve as the child grows older a further laryngoscopy should be carried out to confirm the diagnosis.

Abnormalities of the epiglottis

Previous writers have devoted much time to epiglottic abnormality. Operations such as amputation have been described for such conditions as bifid epiglottis. In general, abnormalities of the epiglottis *per se* are very rare. More commonly they are associated with other structural abnormalities and on occasion with genetic abnormality such as the cri du chat syndrome. For this reason attempts to correct airway obstruction on the basis of a diagnosis of isolated epiglottic pathology should be resisted. If surgery is decided upon it should be carried out only after a thorough search for other accompanying abnormalities.

Bifid epiglottis

This is an extremely rare condition. In over 3000 direct laryngeal examinations for stridor due to varying causes the author has never seen a bifid epiglottis. From textbook descriptions it appears that one-half of the epiglottis becomes sucked into the glottis and obstructs the airway. It is on this basis that amputation is advised. Viewed academically a more logical treatment would appear to be freshening of the edges of the cleft and an attempt at repair. In order to do this it would be necessary to carry out preliminary tracheostomy.

Quadrate epiglottis

This, as its name implies, is an epiglottis which is square in shape and which is in general much larger than usual by comparison with the rest of the larynx. It is one of the characteristic features of the cri du chat syndrome [1] associated with an abnormal gene on the short arm of chromosome 5. The glottis in such cases is rhomboidal and the vocal cords are very difficult to see. The other abnormalities include facial changes and poor muscle tone. Such children are generally retarded. This should be borne in mind when examination of a case of stridor reveals a large square-shaped epiglottis, a rhomboidal glottis, an abnormal cry and vocal cords which are hard to find. In view of the prognosis an early correct genetic diagnosis may do much to help when it comes to parent counselling.

Large overhanging epiglottis

This is seen commonly in small children early in life. The larynx lies high in the neck, tucked away under the base of the tongue. It is therefore difficult to see the anterior glottis because of the tendency for the large epiglottis to drop back over the glottis. The importance of this condition lies simply in the need for the endoscopist to appreciate that in the very young it is not always possible to get a complete view at the first session. Since no diagnosis can be made without a complete view it is necessary to carry out further endoscopy until a satisfactory inspection is possible.

Cysts

These may be of three types.

(1) They may be isolated, in which case they are cysts of mucous glands.

(2) They may be part of a generalized lymphangiomatous condition, in which case the treatment of the lymphangioma as a whole will have to be taken into account.

(3) They may be associated with a laryngocoele. These are seen later in childhood and may be diagnosed accidentally.

Cysts usually give rise to acute airway obstruction and this obstruction is seen when the cyst suddenly increases in size. When this is part of a lymphangiomatous process it is probably wise to carry out a tracheostomy and to wait because many of these tumours do not grow as fast as the baby. In this case no definitive treatment for the lymphangioma will be required and in due course it should be possible to remove the tracheostomy cannula and to leave a normal voice and airway.

Simple cysts occurring in mucous glands or in cystic laryngocoeles should be removed. Where these are small they may be removed endoscopically using microdissection instruments. The dissection must be very gentle, incisions must be made as far as possible from the laryngeal lumen and bleeding must be controlled meticulously. Larger cysts are better treated by the lateral pharyngotomy approach.

Glottic obstruction

Atresia

Total laryngeal atresia is incompatible with life. Partial atresia is extremely rare. When it occurs it is diagnosed at birth. The breathing is immediately embarrassed and direct laryngoscopy in order to carry out intubation will reveal the diagnosis. Half of the larynx will be present and intubation may be extremely difficult. Usually only a very small tube may be passed (2 mm), and this is not satisfactory for respiratory exchange. Since no definitive solution will be proposed for some years it is necessary to make a semi-permanent tracheostomy. A valved tracheostomy tube should be used to promote normal laryngotracheal physiology. In time the child will learn to speak. However, the voice will in general be high pitched and poor in volume. Any operation which is proposed for the relief and reconstruction of the glottis should be delayed until the child's neck is long enough and the larynx large enough to make a worthwhile solution feasible.

Webs

Webbing between the anterior ends of the vocal cords is well recognized. It is variable in extent and may fuse as much as two-thirds of the glottic area. Webs are associated with stridor, a weak cry and later in life with a hoarseness of the voice. Sudden inflammatory changes in neighbouring mucosa can narrow the glottis seriously so the web should be treated early.

Before describing the treatment recommended it is necessary to describe the surgical anatomy of the web. Some webs are merely thin membranes of epithelium with smaller amounts of subepithelial connective tissue joining the anterior portions of both vocal cords. Others are triangular in sagittal section with the broad base of the triangle anteriorly. The former may be treated by the passage of a bronchoscope or a bougie. The latter require more precise excision. The web is divided along one vocal cord, the triangular wedge of submucosal tissue is dissected away under the operating microscope and the mucosa thus left free is stitched into the anterior commissure. The vocal cords are held apart for 2 weeks with a Silastic sheet. This operation can give good results where simple division has failed.

Cleft

A congenital structural lesion which may involve all three regions is the congenital posterior laryngeal cleft.

Posterior laryngeal cleft is a rare condition. The cleft passes down through the posterior plate of the cricoid and a variable distance down the posterior wall of the trachea. If the cleft is wide it is likely to be incompatible with life for the child's first attempts to feed will be associated with massive overspill into the lungs. Thus, treatable clefts tend to be narrow and very difficult to diagnose. The diagnosis must always be borne in mind in the case of a child with stridor for which there is no other obvious cause, especially if the child has repeated chest infections. The posterior commissure should be examined under the microscope with particular care and gentle attempts made to pass a laryngeal probe between the two sides of the cleft. In long-standing cases nature may attempt to offset the cleft by throwing out folds of redundant mucosa to plug the gap. Once the diagnosis can be established the cleft should be closed in layers by lateral pharyngotomy.

Tumours

Benign tumours are seen every now and then in the stridulous child. The two common tumours are haemangioma and papilloma, although fibroma and lipoma have both been described as obstructing the glottis in a young child.

Haemangioma is usually associated with other haemangiomas and/or lymphangiomas in the head and neck region. Once early childhood is passed, provided that the glottis can be induced to grow more rapidly than the tumour, it is remarkable how little trouble the patients experience. Many surgeons know of elderly patients who have had laryngeal haemangiomas which have never troubled them. It is difficult therefore to propose anything other than the most conservative treatment. When active treatment is indicated cryosurgery probably offers the best hope of controlling the disease. For this purpose special small laryngeal cryoprobes are required.

Papillomatosis of childhood is not very common but it is difficult to treat. Evidence is accumulating that papillomatosis is of viral origin. The papillomas tend to seed themselves on any traumatized area. Papillomas may multiply so fast that the glottis may become totally obstructed early in the disease, requiring early and urgent tracheostomy. However, since tracheostomy itself involves trauma to the tissues, papillomas tend to seed to the tracheostomy tract; this is more likely to occur if a dead space is allowed to develop between the vocal cords and the tracheostome. It is therefore essential to use a valved tracheostomy tube which promotes normal mucus transport upwards towards the glottis during the expiratory phase.

The individual papillomas must be destroyed with no damage to surrounding healthy tissue and no bleeding. This may be achieved medically by the use of anti-viral agents or surgically by a physical agent which will destroy or remove the papilloma without causing bleeding. Thus ultrasound, cryosurgery, laser and diathermy have all been used and all are effective. The agent is not important, what is important is a total destruction of the papilloma without bleeding and with preservation of the maximum amount of normal mucosa.

Subglottic obstruction

Subglottic stenosis

Subglottic stenosis has been recognized as a clinical entity for about 20 years. Considerable variation in glottic size may be encountered. One of the difficulties is to achieve a universally agreed method of comparing the size of one subglottis with another and this is probably most easily achieved by measuring and recording the largest endotracheal tube which can be passed through the subglottis in comfort: subglottic stenosis is defined as any subglottis which accepts a tube two sizes smaller than that which is normally accepted at that age.

Subglottic stenosis may be either congenital or acquired. Using the measuring technique outlined above Mustapha measured several thousand larynges of healthy children undergoing surgery for any reason other than purely laryngeal disease and he found that 1% of children accepted a tube one size smaller or larger than the norm for the age and one in a thousand accepted a tube two sizes below or above the norm. From this we can deduce that some degree of subglottic stenosis occurs once in a 1000 live births. On top of this must be added those patients who acquire subglottic stenosis as the result of damage to the subglottic area later in life. Clearly those children born with subglottic narrowing are more likely to develop conditions for which intubation may be required but it is prudent to remember, too, that children with an unusually large larynx may acquire subglottic stenosis as a result of the passage of an abnormally large endotracheal tube. Subglottic stenosis produces a characteristic unmusical barking type of stridor present in both phases of the respiratory cycle. Patients with subglottic stenosis experience respiratory difficulties aggravated by upper respiratory tract infections which often cause further narrowing due to mucosal swelling. Respiratory infections are common and these children are slow feeders and found to be underweight for their age.

Management

The subglottis enlarges as the child grows, particularly in the first 2 years, and the condition will right itself provided that adequate air is inspired. However, when there is a marked subglottic narrowing there may be insufficient inspired air to produce an adequate expiratory thrust. This expiratory thrust is probably instrumental in providing the stimulus for laryngeal growth. Thus, for the child with marked narrowing, repeated chest infections and failure to gain weight, a tracheostomy may prove to be the short-term management of choice. Since the expiratory thrust is translaryngeal only when an expiratory valve is fitted, a valved and fenestrated tube must be used. If the condition is diagnosed early enough and the tracheostomy established early sufficient stimulus will be provided to promote laryngeal growth and the subglottis will enlarge. This may mean a tracheostomy life of about 2 years; it is essential to maintain the child at the normal weight and height for his age. In those children who do not respond to such management surgery may have to be considered. Many attempts have been made to develop a satisfactory procedure to treat this condition. The fundamental problem is how to preserve the ciliated mucosa in the area of the narrowed cricoid cartilage. Very satisfactory results can be obtained by the use of Evans's laryngotracheoplasty [2].

Tumours

Haemangioma and *lymphangioma* may involve all the regions of the larynx.

There is, however, one benign tumour which has a predilection for the subglottic area. This is the rare *chondroma* which may present in childhood and tends to push in from the lateral side of the cricoid causing subglottic narrowing. Untreated chondroma has on occasion undergone malignant change and so the tumour should be excised even if it is not producing sufficient airway narrowing to give rise to respiratory embarrassment.

Functional disorders of the larynx

Paralysis

Paralyses of one or both vocal cords are widely recognized causes of stridor and dyspnoea in children. Unilateral paralysis may be associated with birth trauma. Bilateral paralysis may be due to birth trauma or to increased intercranial pressure such as is often seen in hydrocephalus when the rising CSF pressure may force the brain stem down through the foramen magnum producing stretching of the vagus.

Patients with laryngeal paralysis have inspiratory stridor which is usually inaudible when the child is asleep but which becomes very audible on crying, straining or feeding. Where one cord is paralysed there may be an asymmetrical action of the cricopharyngeus and milk or food may 'bounce' on the unrelaxed portion and be inhaled causing recurrent chest infection.

Idiopathic unilateral paralysis

This usually either resolves or the patient compensates for the condition. This may take up to 2–3 years. There may be problems with feeding in early life but these usually become less when weaning foods are introduced. Chest infections are more likely to occur because of the danger of inhaled food. When they do, treatment with physiotherapy and antibiotics is indicated. It is unusual to attribute symptoms to unilateral paralysis after 3 years of age.

Bilateral vocal cord paralysis

Bilateral vocal cord abductor weakness is seen periodically. It presents with stridor, dyspnoea, occasional cyanosis and feeding difficulty. The diagnosis is confirmed most easily by means of cine-photography in slow motion. Where the respiratory embarrassment is severe a tracheostomy with all its attendant disadvantages will have to be made. Arytenoidectomy should be deferred until the end of adolescence. Bilateral vocal cord weakness associated with internal hydrocephalus is of the gravest prognostic importance. Probably no useful purpose is served by surgical treatment. In six cases seen five had died within 6 weeks of the diagnosis being made.

Extrinsic causes of stridor

Dysphagia lusoria

Pressure on the larynx or trachea from without can cause signs of respiratory obstruction. In dysphagia lusoria the aortic arch may be duplicated or abnormal vessels may pass between the trachea or the oesophagus. In this case a pulsating narrowing of the trachea may be seen on bronchoscopy and indentation of the oesophagus and separation of the oesophagus from the trachea may be noted in the contrast radiogram of the swallow. Once the diagnosis is made the patient should be referred to the cardiothoracic surgeon for correction of the vascular anomaly.

Tumours

Tumours in the neck not directly arising from the larynx or trachea can cause pressure and therefore obstruction. A high percentage of head and neck tumours in childhood are of neural origin: *neurofibromatosis* and *embryonic neuroblastoma* may both cause extrinsic stridor. The treatment depends on the cause.

Inflammatory disease of the larynx

Childhood is above all a period of continuing respiratory infection and inflammation.

Acute croup

Acute inflammation of the larynx is common and can give rise to acute stridor. Formerly the most common and most fatal cause of croup was diphtheria; however, diphtheria immunization in the United Kingdom has made this a most uncommon disease, although sporadic cases still do occur. Greatly improved transport over the world must keep the physician on the alert for diphtheria arriving from countries which do not have an immunization programme. In the United Kingdom currently the two most important types of acute lower airway inflammation are acute epiglottitis and acute laryngotracheal bronchitis.

Acute epiglottitis

Acute epiglottitis is due to the *Haemophilus influenzae*. There appears to be evidence suggesting that the condition arises as part of a *Haemophilus influenzae* septicaemia. Some cases are associated with meningitis and some with toxic myocarditis. Onset of the symptoms may be very sudden and it is quite possible for the patient to progress from a state of mild irritation to gross respiratory obstruction in as little as half an hour. Unless urgent treatment is established the outcome will be fatal.

Acute laryngo-tracheo-bronchitis

This condition is characterized by an acute inflammatory reaction in the subglottis and trachea which may spread into the bronchi. *Haemophilus influenzae* and streptococci are frequently found on culture of the secretions. Pathological findings include cilial death and ulceration of the mucosa. The blood released as a result of the ulceration combines with the fibrinous exudate to produce tough dark brown crusts which obstruct the airway still further and which the child has great difficulty in coughing up. Death results from respiratory obstruction and from toxaemia.

Apart from these two clinical entities other forms of acute catarrhal laryngitis are found which are similar to those seen in the adult.

Management of acute inflammation in childhood

(1) Protect the airway.
(2) Humidify the air.
(3) Identify the causative organism, and treat it.
(4) Control the inflammatory reaction.

The first requirement of treatment in acute inflammation must always be to safeguard the airway. This means that there must be an accurate clinical appraisal of the cause and the pathological state reached. If the stridor is marked, cyanosis present and the pulse thready and rapid, a laryngoscopy should be carried out and an attempt made to pass an endotracheal tube. If this fails a tracheostomy must be made immediately. However, this is not always necessary if the condition is seen early enough. If there is a suspicion of deterioration supported by a rise in the pCO_2 mechanical relief of the airway must be considered. Many children will respond to being placed in high humidity and treated with a broad spectrum antibiotic, with or without the addition of anti-inflammatory agents such as hydrocortisone. Hydrocortisone is of considerable value in the *early* case but of much less value later in the disease, particularly when the respiratory obstruction has become severe. A high dose (100 mg) is administered and then the dose is rapidly reduced over the next 24–48 hours.

The key therapeutic measures are airway protection and humidification. Most patients can be managed by the intelligent use of these two lines of treatment, but it is absolutely necessary to identify the infecting organism. Secretions are always sent for culture and sensitivity testing and a blood culture will often reveal the causative organism. Other measures which may be required include the removal of crusts from the trachea and bronchi. This manoeuvre can be helped considerably by the instillation of 1 ml of sterile water immediately before the attempted removal of the crusts. After recovery the airway should always be checked for such possible predisposing causes as subglottic stenosis or an unsuspected sinus infection.

References

[1] LE JEUNE J. (1966) Cri du chat syndrome. *Journal of American Medical Association* 197, 40.
[2] EVANS J. N. & TODD G. B. (1974) Laryngo-tracheoplasty. *Journal of Laryngology and Otology* 88, 589.

CHAPTER 43

Congenital Nasal Conditions

SEPTAL DEFORMITIES

The fetal skull may receive severe pressures during pregnancy or parturition – particularly with oligoamnios. These pressures may cause two basic types of nasal deformity which may occur singly or in combination. They are caused by pressures acting in different ways [1, 2].

Anterior cartilage deformity

This is a bend localized to the anterior quadrilateral septal cartilage, with or without dislocation from the anterior nasal spine (Fig 43.1a). If the pressure is great enough to produce obvious external deformity still present 3 days after birth, then there is also distortion and depression of the nasal bones (Fig. 43.1b). The deformity is due to direct pressure on to or across the nose, particularly if the head is extended during internal rotation [2, 3]. Its incidence is shown in Table 43.1. This deformity can also be caused by trauma at any age.

Combined nasal deformity

The normal septum lies in the mid line, its growth being controlled by the opposing tissue pressure of the quadrilateral cartilage and the perpendicular plate of the ethmoid on the vomerine bone (Fig. 43.2).

The bimalar diameter is the widest part of the face so that bilateral pressure tends to compress the maxilla, and elevate and narrow the palate. The resultant force is directed up the septum, compressing it against the firm base of the skull (Fig. 43.3a). This causes an 'S'- or 'C'-shaped compression deformity which may be severe enough to widen the septum and cause subperichondral extravasation of blood (Fig. 43.3b).

This septal deformity does not increase with the growth of the nose.

If the pressure is predominantly unilateral, one side of the maxilla is compressed (Fig. 43.4a) with ipsilateral narrowing and elevation of the palate. The vomer is tilted towards the opposite side, causing a kinking of the vomer-cartilage junction (Fig. 43.4b). This deformity increases with growth and age. On the concave side of this kinking there always develops compensatory hypertrophy of the lateral wall of the nose and turbinates.

This deformity cannot be initiated after birth.

Assessment

Septal deformity can be detected by the degree of difficulty of passing struts sized 6 mm by 2 mm, along the floor of the nose hugging the septum. The incidence of deformity detected by routine testing is shown in Table 43.1. Only about 20% of adult skulls have straight septa [2].

The disabilities arising from these deformities may be immediate or delayed. The delayed troubles of nasal blockage, sinus disease, ear disease, headache and malocclusion are mentioned to emphasize the importance of this type of facial deformity. These disabilities only occur if a combination of septal deformity, allergy and infection are present.

The immediate problems are discussed below.

Nasal discharge and noisy breathing

The nose of every baby becomes infected to a varying degree after birth. This causes little trouble unless there is impairment of the airway by septal deformity which causes impaired drainage leading to increased infection and excess secretion. Treatment by simple sucking of

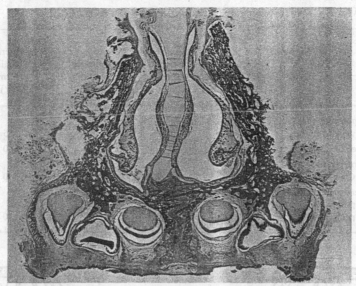

FIG. 43.1a. Section of anterior end of septum at birth demonstrating dislocation of septal cartilage and anterior end of vomer off the maxillary spine.

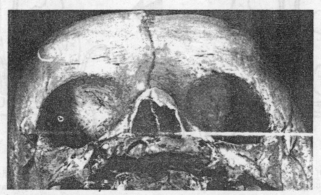

FIG. 43.1b. Skull of new-born baby demonstrating depressed fracture and distortion of nasal bones with septal deformity. Note also parietal bone moulding. (Reproduced by permission from Steinder A. (1959) *Maryland Medical Journal* 8, 557.)

the anterior nares with an open-ended catheter before feeds is often all that is required. The catheter should *not* be passed down the nose as this traumatizes the delicate nasal mucosa perpetuating the obstruction.

Feeding problems, slowness or irregular sucking, cyanotic attacks and minor vomiting

If the baby cannot breathe adequately and suck simultaneously he has to interrupt the sucking rhythm to gasp a breath causing undue swallowing of air. If the air is regurgitated in large amounts it may cause vomiting, but if the cricopharyngeal sphincter relaxes only a little, a small amount of fluid wells up posteriorly into the larynx, causing laryngeal spasm and a cyanotic attack. These problems have been found to be closely related to septal deformity and are greatly relieved by manipulation.

Eye problems

If a baby develops puffy eyelids from parturition pressure, the lacrimal secretion may overflow causing a type of moist intertrigo which usually

TABLE 43.1. Results of routine testing by nasal struts

Type	Straight septum (%)	Bilateral deformity (%)	Unilateral deformity (%)	Anterior cartilaginous deformity (%)
Spontaneous vaginal delivery	40	25	30	5
Elective Caesarean	50	25	25	0
Non-elective Caesarean	40	35	25	0
Persistent occipito-posterior presentation	20	35	35	10

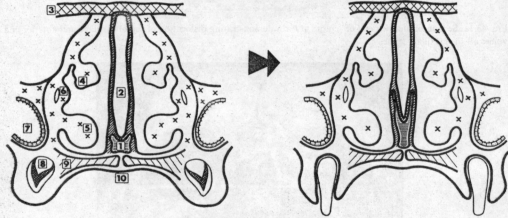

FIG. 43.2. Diagram of normal septal growth from birth: 1, vomer bone; 2, septal cartilage; 3, firm base of skull; 4 and 5, middle and inferior turbinates; 6, ethmoidal bulla; 7, antrum; 8, developing tooth; 9, bony palate; 10, roof of mouth and palate.

does not develop until 2–3 days after birth. This is best treated by regular simple eye bathing with saline. However, the moist skin area can become infected from the surrounding skin saprophytes, causing a sticky eye due to conjunctivitis. This is often associated with blockage of the nasolacrimal duct, from oedema or distortion from facial compression, which may require probing later. There is a close association of facial compression with sticky eyes, and a high incidence of septal deformity has been found in these patients. This syndrome is to be distinguished from the acute purulent conjunctivitis due to bacterial infection.

Treatment

If the anterior cartilage deformity is still obvious after 3 days it should be reduced [2].

The main indications for treatment of the combined septal deformity are nasal stuffiness, feeding problems, and severe sticky eyes. Manipulation can be done readily and efficiently without anaesthesia, particularly in the first 2–3 weeks, but it is worth attempting even up to 9 months of age.

In cases with unilateral obstruction there is minimal nasal reaction. The immediate results of

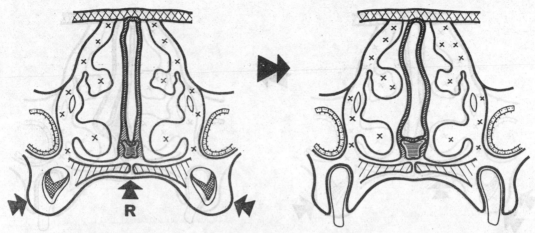

FIG. 43.3a. Diagram of effect of bilateral maxillary pressures producing compression of the septum and splaying out of vomer-cartilage junction.

manipulation are very good, with relief of symptoms with 75% achieving considerable permanent improvement in septal contour. In cases with bilateral obstruction there is usually an accompanying rhinitis, and routine anterior nasal suction before feeds may be required for 2–3 days, followed by the instillation of antibiotic-cortisone drops.

CONGENITAL ANOMALIES

Apart from cleft lip and palate and posterior choanal atresia, which occurs in about 1 in 5000 births, nasal malformations are quite rare.

Posterior choanal atresia

This may be unilateral or bilateral, complete or incomplete, or bony. The obstruction is at the posterior end of the nose, a few millimetres anterior to the bony edge of the hard palate. There is a higher incidence of unilateral atresia with preponderance of the right side, and it is commoner in females than males. Embryologically it is due to the persistence of the 'temporary' bucconasal membrane formed at the posterior end of each nasal sac, which should rupture at about 40 days of fetal life. Some association with maternal thyroid disease has been observed which could be due to autoantibody reacting with complemen-

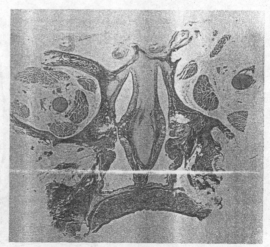

FIG. 43.3b. Section of middle third of septum at birth of a patient with bilateral obstruction. Note the splaying out and compression of the septum with vertical fracture line and subperichondral reaction.

tary deoxyribonucleoprotein, interfering with chromosomal separation at cell division [4]. Multiple abnormalities may be present (45% in unilateral and 60% in bilateral cases), particularly affecting the head and heart, and often the alimentary system. This is not unexpected for the bucconasal membrane is practically in the middle of the developing head and heart.

Unilateral atresia may cause very few symptoms

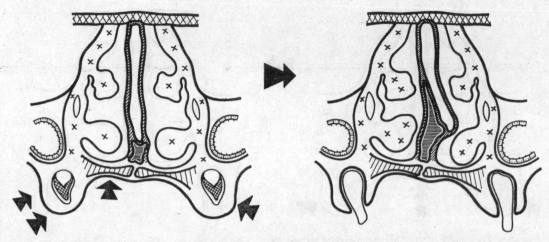

Fig. 43.4a. Diagram of effect of unequal maxillary pressures producing narrowing and elevation of the palate and tilting of vomer to opposite side. Note also with growth, unequal growth of the vomer, irregular hypertrophy of the lateral nasal wall and changed alignment of the teeth.

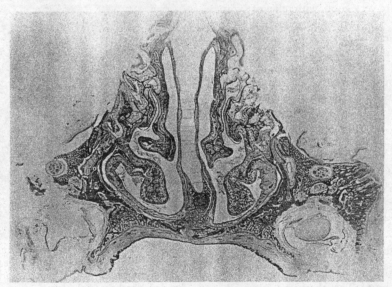

Fig. 43.4b. Section of middle third of septum at birth of a patient with obstruction to strut testing of the nose on the right side of the section. Note elevation of the palate on the left and kinking of the vomer-cartilage junction on the right with no perichondral reaction because it is a simple bend.

at birth and may not be diagnosed for years. It usually causes a continuous mucoid, at times purulent, rhinorrhoea. There is usually normal middle ear and Eustachian tube function and mastoid aeration. It is very successfully treated by the transpalatal approach after the age of 6 months.

Bilateral atresia causes obvious respiratory difficulty at birth with cyanosis, characteristically temporarily relieved by crying and aggravated by feeding. A few babies may quickly adapt to oral breathing but usually an oral airway must be inserted. Intranasal choanotomy is then performed as soon as possible. The diagnosis is

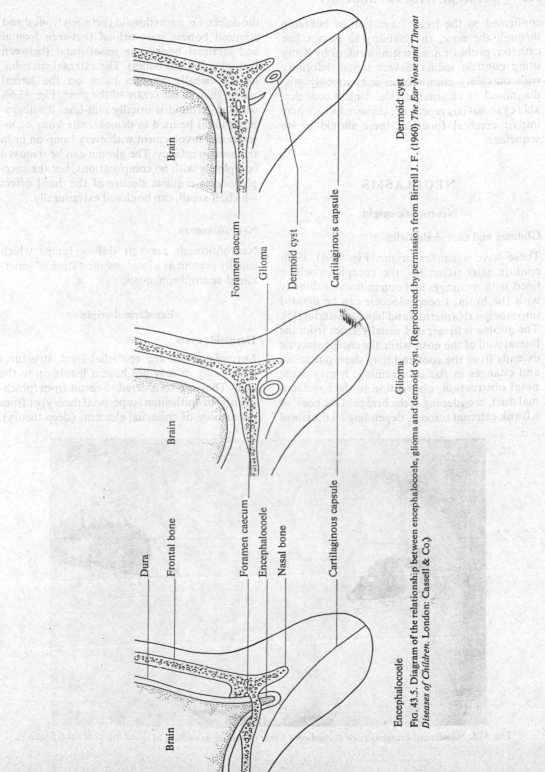

Encephalocoele

Glioma

Dermoid cyst

Dura

Frontal bone

Foramen caecum

Encephalocoele

Nasal bone

Cartilaginous capsule

Brain

Foramen caecum

Glioma

Cartilaginous capsule

Brain

Dermoid cyst

Cartilaginous capsule

Fig. 43.5. Diagram of the relationship between encephalocoele, glioma and dermoid cyst. (Reproduced by permission from Birrell J. F. (1960) *The Ear Nose and Throat Diseases of Children*. London: Cassell & Co.)

confirmed by the lack of aeration or bubbling through the nose, the inability to pass a fine catheter, probe or nasal testing strut, or by X-ray using contrast media. Severe septal deformity with maxillary compression is commonly mis-diagnosed as choanal atresia. Unless consider-able cyanosis has repeatedly occurred which may impair cerebral function, there should be no sequelae.

NEOPLASMS

Neurogenic origin

Gliomas and encephalocoeles

These have a similar origin (Fig. 43.5). Both contain glial tissue but the encephalocoele is lined with meninges and communicates directly with the brain. Encephalocoele can be divided into sincipital (anterior) and basal (posterior) [5]. The glioma is firmer and usually arises from the lateral wall of the nose, while the encephalocoele extends from the roof and may show pulsation, and changes in size on straining. It may cause nasal obstruction, obstruction to the nasolacri-mal duct, broadening of the bridge of the nose, or a frank external tumour, depending on the site of

the defect, i.e. nasoethmoid (between frontal and ethmoid bones), naso-orbital (between frontal and lacrimal bones), or nasofrontal (between frontal and nasal bones). The external encepha-locoele usually appears more on the lateral aspect than in the centre of the nose (Fig. 43.6), while a dermoid is usually mid-line. Radiogra-phy should be used to demonstrate bony or in-tracranial involvement with every lump on or in the nose in infancy. The glioma can be removed completely with no complications, but the ence-phalocoele requires closure of the dural defect which, if small, can be closed extradurally.

Neurofibromas

Neurofibromas are soft diffuse lumps which usually present as a local manifestation of gener-alized neurofibromatosis.

Ectodermal origin

Dermoid cysts

Dermoid cysts are epithelial-lined structures which may or may not have a fistula on to the skin. They are considered to result from 'pinch-ing off' of epithelium (superficial theory) or from persistency of epithelial elements (deep theory).

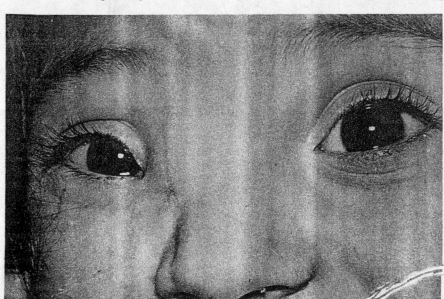

FIG. 43.6. Nasofrontal encephalocoele in child aged 1 year presenting as swelling of lateral aspect of nasal bones.

The deeper cyst may be central or lie along the lateral side of the nose. The superficial cyst is a mid-line mass, usually communicating with the skin by a fistula anywhere from the glabella to the subalar area. The track is rarely in the lateral line of the nose. The diagnosis is suggested by the presence of a central hair in the opening, or epithelial cells in the secretion. The track usually extends upwards, in front of or behind the nasal bones. Radiography, with or without contrast media, shows the extent of the track or erosion of bone. The cyst is removed via a lateral rhinotomy [6].

Haemangiomas

Haemangiomas are recognized by their colour, and may be inside or outside the nose. There are two main types:

(1) the *strawberry* or *capillary type* which is usually on the surface, and

(2) the *cavernous type* which is soft, collapsible, of bluish colour and deeper placed.

The strawberry type is best left alone and will atrophy. The cavernous type may require surgery, although injection of sclerosing agents may be used.

References

[1] GRAY L. P. (1972) Early treatment of septal deformity and associated abnormalities. In *Modern Trends in Diseases of the Ear, Nose and Throat*, ed. Ellis M., p. 19. London: Butterworths.

[2] GRAY L. P. (1974) Septal and associated cranial birth deformities, types, incidence and treatment. *Medical Journal of Australia* 1, 557.

[3] JEPPESEN F. & WINDFELD I. (1972) Dislocation of the nasal septal cartilage in the new-born. *Acta Obstetrica and Gynecology Scandinavia* 51, 5.

[4] SCOTT J. S. (1966) Immunological disease and pregnancy. *British Medical Journal* 1, 1559.

[5] DAVIS C. H. & ALEXANDER E. (1959) Congenital nasofrontal encephalomeningoceles and teratomas. *Journal of Neurosurgery* 16, 365.

[6] SKOLINIK E. M., MAJOR T. M., CAMPBELL M. C. & MEYERS R. M. (1971) Dermoid cysts of the nose. *Laryngoscope* 81, 1632.

CHAPTER 44

Foreign Bodies

FOREIGN BODIES IN THE EAR

Foreign bodies are inserted into the ears more commonly by school children than by toddlers, and it is usually a deliberate act. There seems to be no reason why a child should decide to insert an object into an external auditory meatus, but the child frequently confesses to the act, although some maintain a bland assertion of innocence of the event.

Clinical features

The objects may be organic or inorganic. *Organic foreign bodies* include paper, cotton-wool, india-rubber, seeds, orange pips, etc. Paper, cotton-wool and seeds are hygroscopic and swell from the absorption of water either during washing or during ear syringeing. The organic objects may give rise to otitis externa by local irritation of the epithelium of the meatal walls. This produces itching or even pain and there is a discharge of pus and debris. Cotton wool which has been put into the ear and forgotten is the most common cause of this. *Inorganic objects,* such as beads, ball-bearings, stones, crayons and even milk teeth do not, as a rule, cause otitis externa, and may be found accidentally. Apart from otitis externa there are few symptoms attributable to a foreign body in the external meatus, although deafness may occur if the lumen is occluded.

The object may be seen easily on inspection, but if it has lain in the meatus for some time it may become covered with wax. A piece of red crayon or a red bead may resemble a polypus or granulation tissue, but gentle palpation with a fine wool-tipped probe will demonstrate its hardness.

Treatment

In most cases it is unwise for those unskilled in handling children's ears to attempt a removal in the conscious child. Inorganic objects which do not occlude the meatus may be removed by syringeing, although this is uncomfortable and may prove painful. Organic objects may swell on contact with the solution and so resist removal. However tempting it may be to try to remove a foreign body in the conscious child with a pair of forceps this manoeuvre is fraught with danger. An object may be pursued too far along the external meatus and cause a rupture of the tympanic membrane. Most otologists will have had to deal with the results of this by making a post-aural incision, removing part of the posterior bony meatus, incising the soft tissues of the posterior meatal wall and extracting the object. The traumatic injury to the tympanic membrane may take some time to heal, but there are greater problems if the ossicles have suffered damage.

With the operating microscope and using fine wax curettes or hooks most foreign bodies may be removed safely and speedily under general anaesthesia. Once the object is out, the tympanic membrane is examined to ensure that it has not been damaged. If the object is organic and otitis externa has occurred, the meatal walls are cleaned and a length of ribbon gauze impregnated with a suitable medication, such as oxytetracycline and hydrocortisone (Terra-Cortril®), dexamethasone, framycetin and gramicidin (Sofradex®) or triamcinolone, neomycin and benzocaine (Audicort®) may be inserted, and this dressing is repeated until the meatal skin is healthy.

FOREIGN BODIES IN THE NOSE

In children a nasal foreign body will have been deliberately inserted. Young children learn about their natural orifices by palpation rather than by looking in a mirror, and there is a constant temptation for them to push something into an orifice which can be felt. Usually the insertion is done in privacy, while playing by themselves, when left in a bath, or when in bed. Nasal foreign bodies are most commonly found in children of the 2–3 year age group.

Clinical features

From the clinical standpoint one may divide foreign bodies into organic and inorganic. The inorganic foreign bodies, metal, plastic, stone, china, buttons, beads, etc. produce little in the way of symptoms and may be discovered accidentally during a routine examination for an unrelated complaint. There may be a unilateral nasal discharge, usually mucoid, and there might be a unilateral stuffiness if the object is large enough.

Organic foreign bodies, on the other hand, are irritant and the surrounding nasal mucosa eventually becomes involved in an inflammatory reaction. This group includes wood, paper, peas, nuts, and, most common of all, sponge rubber. The symptom is a unilateral nasal discharge, at first mucoid, then mucopurulent and finally of stinking mucopus tinged with blood. It is quite remarkable how long parents tolerate this, and how long the child is treated with a barrage of antibiotics before inspection with a good light source reveals the cause. A unilateral nasal discharge in children is due to a foreign body in 95% of cases.

Initially the object lies in the nasal vestibule or just inside the nasal cavity where it is easily seen and equally easily removed with a probe or forceps. Once it enters the nasal cavity it becomes coated with mucus, and is thus slippery and difficult to grasp with forceps. Constant sniffing draws the object posteriorly and it is usually held up in the region of the olfactory cleft. An organic object may swell because of absorption of water from nasal secretions. Once the nasal lining becomes infected from the presence of an organic object, there is production of mucopus and inflammatory oedema of the surrounding mucosa which arrests the posterior movement as the child sniffs. Finally a foul stench is noticeable to the parents and to the examiner at a distance of a few feet.

Treatment

Removal in the conscious child is only possible if the object lies anteriorly, either in or just beyond the nasal vestibule. This may be accomplished with forceps or a probe. A simple expedient is to allow the child to smell pepper and, as he sneezes, to occlude the healthy nostril so that the blast will expel the foreign body. Should the object lie more posteriorly in the nasal cavity and be covered in mucus it may be removed in the conscious child by an expert, but it is seldom easy for this to be done in the casualty department by untrained personnel. If the attempt fails the child will seldom allow a second try. It is much safer and more certain to admit the child as a day patient and to remove the foreign body under general anaesthesia.

At operation the mucus or mucopus is aspirated and the object removed. A blunt-pointed probe with the terminal 0·5 cm bent to a right angle copes with most objects. It is passed point downwards above the foreign body which is brought to the floor of the nose and raked anteriorly. Thin objects, such as buttons, or soft organic objects such as sponge rubber should be grasped with forceps with cup ends. Sometimes sponge rubber which has lain for weeks or months may adhere to the mucosa and there is bleeding on removal. The nasal cavity should be examined in case there is another foreign body more posteriorly, and the other side of the nose should also be examined. Occasionally an irregular metal object may defy attempts to withdraw it, and it may be necessary to push this into the nasopharynx, with a finger tip in the appropriate choana, and to remove it from there.

The possibility of a rhinolith developing around a longstanding foreign body in the nasal cavity must be borne in mind.

FOREIGN BODIES IN THE NASOPHARYNX

It is rare to find a foreign body being retained in the nasopharynx. Not infrequently food or fluid may enter the nasopharynx during choking, coughing or laughing while swallowing, and this causes pain behind the nose until the object descends into the pharynx and oesophagus.

Clinical features

The pain felt is similar to that experienced when a Eustachian catheter is passed unskilfully. A large object may be retained in the nasopharynx to cause pain or discomfort. Little may be seen on pharyngoscopy, but radiography of the post-nasal space will reveal an opaque foreign body. We have seen a marble and a small metal bell in this situation and reports in the literature mention seeds or grains of corn being removed from the nasopharynx. Occasionally a nasal foreign body may be pushed into the nasopharynx either to lodge there or to be removed from this situation.

One object which is difficult to locate in the heat of the moment is the blade of an adenoid curette, either the Popper or the St. Clair Thomson model, which may break during removal of adenoids. In the presence of blood the broken piece may be difficult to see or palpate, so it is wiser to X-ray the nasopharynx on the day after operation and, if the broken blade is still there, to remove it at a planned operation.

Treatment

All removals should be done under general anaesthesia. In order to remove a large object it is advisable to retract the soft palate anteriorly with two soft rubber catheters. Smaller objects may be palpated and removed by grasping them with suitably curved artery forceps which may be guided along the palpating finger.

FOREIGN BODIES IN THE PHARYNX

Foreign bodies are arrested in the pharynx of a child less frequently than in the pharynx of an adult.

Clinical features

The most common object is a fish bone which lodges in the tonsil and usually protrudes from its surface to give rise to a stabbing pain on swallowing. The probable causes for the relative rarity in childhood are that, in most homes, fish is examined for bones before being given to a child,

and that a fish bone is felt by the child in its mouth more easily than by an adult, especially if the adult wears dentures. A toothbrush bristle may be found embedded in lymphoid tissue in a child's pharynx, but again less commonly than in adults. If the bone or the bristle protrudes into the pharynx it is more easily seen on examination than if it lies along the surface of the tonsil. In children a foreign body in the lingual tonsil is rare, but it is common in adults. Occasionally a young child may swallow a large object which cannot enter the oesophagus but which may be held up in the hypopharynx, oropharynx or even the nasopharynx, and this gives rise to pain and retching.

Treatment

It is not always possible or desirable to remove a foreign body from the pharynx in the casualty department. A good source of light is essential, and reflected light from a bull's-eye lamp or a strong light from a mains-operated headlamp is necessary to see the object. In the older child who is not frightened it is often possible to extract a bone from the tonsil swiftly and painlessly, but if the manoeuvre does not succeed at the first attempt it may prove less easy to grasp it subsequently.

In young children, in second attempts in older children, and, especially, if the projecting point of the object is not readily seen, it is much safer to remove it under general anaesthesia. If the object is not seen easily on inspection the pharynx should be palpated with the ungloved finger in an effort to locate it.

If no object is palpated, then the symptoms of pain and salivation will have been produced by the probing of a parental finger causing scratching before the child is brought to hospital. When a foreign body is discovered it is removed with any suitable pair of forceps, from a pair of crocodile forceps in the conscious child to a pair of straight or curved artery forceps in the anaesthetized child.

Instant cure is the usual result, but some children who have choked on a large bolus of food, e.g. tough apple skin, hard crust, half-chewed meat or a plum stone, may suffer from a functional dysphagia for some weeks if presented with the same food. These symptoms occur more often if a finger has been thrust down the throat of a choking child. The epiglottis is often palpated on these occasions, and it may be traumatized by the finger nail.

FOREIGN BODIES IN THE TRACHEA AND BRONCHI

Most inhaled foreign bodies enter the right main bronchus, which is larger and more directly continuous with the trachea, than the left. A smaller proportion lodge in the left main bronchus and very few indeed find their way into an upper lobe bronchus. Foreign bodies too large for the bronchial lumen remain in the trachea.

Clinical features

In the conscious child a foreign body, before entering the tracheobronchial tree, must produce spasmodic choking and coughing, often with cyanosis, as it enters the larynx but if the child is asleep or unconscious this phase may pass unnoticed. Once the object enters the trachea there is a symptomless interval which may last for many hours, and it is usually at this stage that the child is seen by the practitioner or at the hospital emergency department. The child seems well; there is no stridor; clinical examination of the chest is unrewarding and radiography is negative unless the foreign body is radio-opaque. All too often the parents are reassured on this examination, but it cannot be too strongly emphasized that any history of choking and spluttering, especially if food is in the mouth, should be investigated endoscopically. Visual evidence is the only justification for reassurance, and if there is an inhaled foreign body present its removal is immeasurably easier within the first few hours.

About 80% of patients are under the age of 3 years and the majority have a history of more than a week between the choking spasm and being seen in the department. By this time the object may be firmly wedged into the lumen of the bronchus with inflammatory oedema of the mucosa.

The subsequent clinical pattern depends upon the size of the foreign body. The larger object which is retained in the trachea gives rise to some inspiratory and expiratory stridor but the characteristic sign is a palpable 'slap' on expiration as the object is blown against the inferior aspect of the vocal cords when the child is lying flat. Should the foreign body enter a bronchus and occlude the lumen the earliest sign is a prolongation of expiration over the affected lobe. Later there is wheezing on expiration, some degree of dyspnoea, and radiography shows an opacity of the distal lung segment. Stridor is not common but there may be intercostal indrawing. Clinical examination reveals adventitious sounds initially, while later there is dullness on percussion and absent breath sounds. If the object is organic it gives rise to surrounding mucosal oedema with inflammation while in the distal lobe there is mucopurulent stagnant secretion. The patient will be pyrexial and may develop a lung abscess. Every year many children still die from the consequences of inhaling an organic foreign body.

A small thin object, such as a piece of eggshell, may lodge in a bronchus without causing occlusion. Inspiration is unimpaired, but on expiration the foreign body may rotate so that in the narrowing bronchus not all the air is exhaled. The patient will have a slight cough, while on auscultation there is prolonged expiration possibly with a slight wheeze, and eventually radiography will show emphysema in the obstructed lobe.

Small metallic objects such as pins tend to migrate peripherally and cause slight spasmodic coughing as they move.

Instrumentation

At birth and in early childhood the subglottic diameter, which measures 5–7 mm, is 1 mm less than that of the trachea, and its lax mucosa is prone to oedema from the passage of a bronchoscope. This is a complication of bronchoscopy which may be avoided by using a suitably sized instrument which can pass through the subglottis without force. In selecting the instrument it is the outside diameter which is important, not that of the lumen. However, it is the lumen through which the bronchoscopist makes his diagnosis and manipulates his instruments, and it is obvious that, even with fibre lighting, it is extremely difficult to recognize details in the small baby unless the abnormalities are gross. A 3 mm lumen tracheoscope is used up to the age of 3 months, 4·1 mm from 3–24 months, 5·4 mm from 2–5 years, and 7 mm in school-children.

Apart from limitation of vision, limitation of proper oxygenation is a major difficulty in bronchoscopy in the young child. The standard bronchoscopes only have two fenestrations on each lateral wall. This means that when the bronchoscope is rotated to enter one main bronchus the opposite main bronchus is virtually occluded by the blank wall of the bronchoscope and hypoxia develops rapidly. For 25 years the author has used modified standard bronchoscopes with six smaller fenestrations on each of three walls, the only blank wall being that carrying the light source. This allows a much safer bronchoscopy for a much longer time.

Safety in bronchoscopy depends upon the skill of the anaesthetist and upon complete cooperation between him and the endoscopist. Some anaesthetists induce intravenously, spray the laryngeal entrance with xylocaine, and maintain oxygenation and anaesthesia through a nasopharyngeal tube, while others maintain oxygenation through a small-bore injector (19 swg for infants and 22 swg for children) within the lumen of the bronchoscope. Some induce by cyclopropane inhalation and maintain the level by halothane delivered hrough the in-built aspiration tube in the bronchoscope. There is little margin for error in any method and the skill of the anaesthetist is paramount in obtaining a good level of anaesthesia, maintaining oxygenation, and ensuring a fast return of the cough reflex. During bronchoscopy the anaesthetist monitors the pulse rate, blood pressure and respiratory exchange, and warns of the imminent hypoxia as shown by slowing of the pulse rate. In this event it will become necessary to discontinue bronchoscopy immediately to resuscitate the child, and so the endoscopist must be prepared to withdraw the instrument without hesitation.

Gentleness is paramount for successful bronchoscopy in children; the tissues must be handled with care, and patience should replace speed in manipulations. With limited vision through bronchoscopes, especially when aspiration tubes or forceps occupy so much of the lumen, the instinct for haste must give way to prudent care.

There are many forceps available for the removal of foreign bodies in the bronchus, and each surgeon has learned to rely on those which he can manipulate most easily. They must be kept in good condition because rust may result in a blade breaking off during use, and this may have to be removed also. Those who have to deal with this age group infrequently may find a long very fine pair of crocodile forceps the most useful instrument.

Treatment

Inorganic objects may be located accurately by X-ray and it is usually easy to get a firm grip on them with forceps. Some, such as molar teeth inhaled under anaesthesia, present problems not only in grasping the object but in withdrawing it through the triangular glottis, especially if the level of anaesthesia is too light and the vocal cords are moving. Pins which have migrated out of vision may be brought into a large bronchus by the use of a magnetized probe and then removed with forceps.

The most common organic foreign bodies are nuts, the peanut being the most frequent. Should the toddler be seen within 48 hours of inhalation the nut is generally sufficiently firm to be grasped without crumbling. It will be located in the mouth of a bronchus, either covered by its brown husk or seen as a smooth whitish mass, only the edge of which may be visible. It is tempting to grab at this edge, but it often crumbles and the rest of the nut is pushed deeper into the bronchus. If the nut is not firmly impacted it may be brought proximally by suction through a large aspiration tube, and it may then be gripped.

In cases in which the nut has lain for some time it becomes softer and will disintegrate with attempts to grasp it and it is in these cases that most patience is required. Vision, limited by the lumen of the bronchoscope, is reduced further when the aspiration tube or forceps are introduced. All secretions must be aspirated and the forceps gently coaxed between the mucosa and the nut. An image intensifier may be of help in preventing the mucosa being nipped between the blades of the forceps. The nut may have to be moved gently within the bronchus to obtain a firm hold. Once this is felt to have been achieved slow steady traction is used to disimpact it. It is unwise to try to bring the foreign body within the lumen of the bronchoscope because it may be too large to enter. The forceps and bronchoscope are withdrawn together, care being taken to see that the nut is not dislodged in the glottis. The bronchoscope should be reintroduced immediately to remove any secretion and crumbs or a second piece of nut. At this stage anaesthesia is lightened so that the cough reflex is restored rapidly, and occasionally further crumbs may be coughed out.

Those children in whom the inhaled nut has not been diagnosed for several weeks present the greatest problem. Bronchoscopy should be preceded by antibiotic therapy. The mucosa is inflamed and oedematous around the nut, and granulations may be seen. The mucosa bleeds readily and this obscures vision. The nut may have disintegrated and much of it may be aspirated through a wide-bored tube as it is often too soft to be removed by forceps. Antibiotics and physiotherapy may be continued and a further bronchoscopy carried out in a week.

Should bronchoscopy fail on one or two attempts the assistance of the thoracic surgeon should be sought with a view to bronchotomy. Some surgeons advocate bronchoscopy through a tracheostomy prior to this, because it allows the use of a wider bronchoscope and it removes the possibility of subglottic oedema from prolonged bronchoscopy. The occasional paediatric bronchoscopist may require an hour for a successful removal, but those with greater practice and facilities may accomplish this in less than half the time for an impacted nut and in a few minutes if the object is not impacted. Time is unimportant if there is an expert anaesthetist, and it is wise to postpone bronchoscopy until one is available. Gentleness of touch and patience are the keys to success.

FOREIGN BODIES IN THE OESOPHAGUS

Swallowed foreign bodies are common in children, over 75% occurring in the 1–3 age group. A foreign body may be arrested most commonly immediately below the cricopharyn-geus muscle, then at the lower end of the oesophagus, or thirdly at the point in the oesophagus where it is crossed by the left main bronchus. The act is normally confessed to, but if not, a foreign body may lie in the lumen for a considerable time before discovery.

Clinical features

The oesophagus is insensitive apart from stretching or scratching in which case there is pain on swallowing, and this may be acute if a sharp object has been swallowed. Dysphagia will infrequently be total. Radiography will show radio-opaque objects, but it is important that the film includes the mandible or objects held at the cricopharyngeus may be missed. A barium swallow should not be ordered if the object is not opaque because the barium will have to be aspirated before the foreign body can be seen at oesophagoscopy. In all cases of suspected swallowing of a foreign body oesophagoscopy should be performed.

Perforation of the oesophageal wall may be caused by a sharp foreign body, or the wall may be gradually eroded by a long-standing disc-shaped or irregular object.

Instrumentation

Measured from the upper incisor area the hiatus is found at 17 cm at birth, 21 cm at 3 years and 25 cm at the age of 10.

In childhood the standard oesophagoscope measures $23 \times 7 \times 10$ mm for younger children and $33 \times 8 \times 10$ mm for those over the age of 5. The infant's oesophagus will not accommodate the smaller of these, and so if an infant oesophagoscope is unavailable, a bronchoscope with a lumen of 5·4 mm may be employed. Gentleness is essential for safe oesophagoscopy in children because of the thinness of the walls of the oesophagus.

Treatment

Disc-shaped objects, such as coins, form the greatest proportion and when they are located they are grasped with crocodile forceps, making certain that no oesophageal mucosa is contained in the bite. The oesophagoscope is then pushed downwards to meet the coin and the forceps and oesophagoscope are removed together. The coin should never be pulled up to meet the oesophagoscope because this will nip a fold of mucosa with consequent tearing on removal.

Irregular objects which are not sharp may have to be rotated into a favourable position before removal.

Sharp foreign bodies, such as bones, must be disimpacted gently from the wall of the oesophagus and one end rotated into the lumen of the oesophagoscope before removal. Drawing pins or safety pins lying point uppermost should be grasped if possible by the point after disimpaction and the point brought into the lumen of the oesophagoscope before removal. If this proves impossible with a strong safety-pin, special wire-cutting forceps may be used and the object removed in two pieces. A safety-pin lying point down poses fewer problems because it may be caught at the ring and removed. The trailing point may scratch but will not perforate the oesophageal wall. Any damage to the wall of the oesophagus calls for intravenous feeding, hourly recording of vital signs and careful observation.

It is not uncommon for a child with a stenosis of the oesophagus, whether congenital or due to caustic burn or surgical anastomosis, to swallow a large bolus of food which cannot pass the stricture. This leads to vomiting and rapid dehydration requiring immediate oesophagoscopy and removal.

Index